Rheumatology Teaching

Yasser El Miedany

Rheumatology Teaching

The Art and Science of Medical Education

Springer

Yasser El Miedany
King's College London
Darent Valley Hospital
Dartford
Kent
UK

Rheumatology and Rehabilitation
Ain Shams University
Cairo
Egypt

ISBN 978-3-030-07467-8 ISBN 978-3-319-98213-7 (eBook)
https://doi.org/10.1007/978-3-319-98213-7

Softcover re-print of the Hardcover 1st edition 2019

This Springer imprint is published by the registered company Springer Nature Switzerland AG
The registered company address is: Gewerbestrasse 11, 6330 Cham, Switzerland

"I touch the future, I teach".
Christa McAuliffe (1948–1986)

To my teachers whose dedication made it possible for me to be where I am today.

To every teacher who loves to teach and feels the joy of teaching.

Foreword

The word "rheumatology" derives the Greek root "rheum", meaning "flow". Thus rheumatology is the study of "that which flows". This word was first ascribed to "rheumatism" and so-called rheumatic disease because of the nature of reported symptoms and observable signs in certain of the "rheumatic diseases" which seemed to spread, or flow, within a patient's body. And the word "flow" might also be applied to the evolution and revolution in thinking about this family of conditions that we have witnessed over the last two generations. It seems extraordinary in the contemporary era to think that only two or three generations ago, many of the conditions that we now regard as diseases, or even syndromes, defined by phenotype, were lumped together into a heterogeneous group of pathologies known as rheumatic diseases. And it seems equally extraordinary today to think that Sir William Osler, writing in *The Principles and Practice of Medicine* published in 1892, stated that "Arthritis deformans is an incurable disease …… Too often it invades successively all the articulations and in 10, 15 or 20 years the crippling becomes general and permanent", going on to recommend that "it is useless to saturate the patient with iodide of potassium, salicylates or quinine. Arsenic seems to do good as a general tonic….Hydrotherapy, with carefully performed massage, is best for the alleviation of the pain…..When good results, it is largely from change of scene and climate and careful regulation of diet…" How times have changed, as have the nature of unmet needs for rheumatology patients. And for many rheumatological conditions, enormous advances in understanding pathobiology together with concurrent advances, initially in protein engineering and more recently in chemical engineering, opened the gateway to an era of highly efficacious targeted therapies of which the armamentarium continues to expand at a rate. These advances are gradually encouraging us to reformulate the way in which we classify rheumatic diseases. A new immunotaxonomy is beginning to emerge, and the potential for precision medicine is paving the way towards the concept of "pathotype" rather than "phenotype".

Appreciation of the importance of early treatment intervention and a preventative approach to multimorbidity is also changing the contemporary landscape in rheumatology. The never ending quest for improved outcomes has seen increasing protocolization in the management of rheumatic diseases which in some cases, of which treat-to-target is a notable example, there is abundant evidence for reduced morbidity, mortality and improved quality of life at a cohort level. Arguably, however, some of these trends have come at the price of neglecting our heritage as rheumatologists for the art of compassionate care of those people living with chronic inflammatory disease. Osler himself wisely reminded us that "The good physician treats the disease but the great physician treats the patient who has the disease". And of course, as rheumatologists, it is our duty to apply the clinical and basic science discoveries that have been validated in patient cohorts and trials to the needs of the individual person with a rheumatic disease who attends our clinic.

Thus in routine clinical care, we all need to practise both the art and science of rheumatology and to keep up with the dizzying pace of change in practice and clinical advance. And all this needs to be attended to in an era of information overload.

Good education in its many guises is therefore crucial to ensuring the best achievable quality of life for any given patient at any point in time. At every stage of our training and subsequent careers as rheumatologists, we need to be nourished by education that should ideally be delivered in manner that both informs and delights! And as practising rheumatologists, we all have a role in educating our peers, patients and colleagues. We learn from one another. Contemporary advance in information technology has made the ease of access to data and learning materials available in a manner that could only be dreamed of three generations ago in Osler's age.

For all these reasons, I welcome this volume on *The Art of Teaching Rheumatology* by my friend Dr. Yasser El Miedany. It has been a pleasure to learn from his wisdom and experience about the art of science and learning in rheumatology and how to apply a bewildering range of new pedagogical methods to the next generation of rheumatologists. And in doing so, Dr. El Miedany will be passing on the best of the heritage of our past learnings and to integrate them with novel advances in understanding of disease. This volume will be of enormous value not only to those who educate and to the recipients of education. Importantly, the learnings will ultimately be to the great benefit of the many people who continue to live with a rheumatic disease as well as those in whom a rheumatic condition arises in future.

Peter C. Taylor, MA, PhD, FRCP, FRCPE
Botnar Research Centre
Nuffield Department of Orthopaedics
Rheumatology and Musculoskeletal Sciences
University of Oxford
Oxford, UK

Preface

Over the years, there have been requests for a book to be published that handles the art and science of medical teaching; this is the book. It serves two purposes, introducing new medical teachers to the exciting opportunities and challenges facing them, whether they are working in undergraduate, postgraduate or continuing medical education. It also assists more experienced educators to review and assess their own practice and gain a new perspective on what is new in medical education as well as an update about recent trends in teaching. In writing the book, the constraints on teachers' time have been considered; hence every effort has been made to make the chapters succinct and clear. Bearing in mind Albert Einstein's words, "Any intelligent fool can make things bigger and more complex", I have done my best to make this book unnecessarily complex and to the point.

There is no magic bullet to becoming a competent teacher, but this book can point teachers in the right direction. It has been written in the belief that teaching is both a craft and a science and that with better understanding of their work, poor teachers can become good teachers and good teachers can become excellent teachers. The information, algorithms and suggestions offered are based on my extensive experience in teaching medicine and rheumatology, curriculum planning and in the organization of courses in rheumatology education at both the basic and advanced levels. In writing the book, there have been three main aims in mind. The first was to provide hints and clues attained over years from my practical experience that will help teachers to create powerful learning opportunities for their students while retaining a practical focus. The second aim was to introduce clearly some key basic principles that underpin the practical advice given and help to enhance clinical practice education development. This has been based on the belief that effective teaching demands much more than the acquisition of technical skills, and that an understanding of teaching and learning is essential if the teacher is to be able to respond to the recent developments in the learning context as well as the demands over time for change. The third aim of the book was to discuss the basics of all the new and recent tools of education and how to implement them in the standard medical teaching process, recognizing that there is no single best method of teaching; the reader can choose the best model of teaching, which he/she feels comfortable with for his/her own teaching.

After an introduction about the education and whether it is art or science, Part II of the book introduces the reader to basic sciences in education and its impact on the teaching process. This provides a valuable lead-in to the following part regarding the art of teaching, with the principles explained in separate chapters handing the teaching of primary care, undergraduate students as well as postgraduate medical trainees, nursing and patient education. A separate part has been dedicated to the modern and innovative tools of teaching such as reflective learning, e-learning, simulated teaching, TED Talks, virtual reality as well as motivation. This is followed by two parts about mentoring as well as the art and science of facilitating. The final part highlights the essence of teaching, reclaiming the art and science of education.

Medical teaching has entered a new era, and there is a growing attention in the development of the educational process worldwide. Technology and modern teaching styles have given the teaching process a 3D dimension. What makes teaching exciting is that each situation is different and that through responding to the challenges, teachers will achieve more satisfaction and enjoyment in their work. Good teaching can bring its own joy. Perhaps the greatest reward is knowing that through teaching the teacher is helping to shape the next generation of doctors. Christa McAuliffe was to be the first teacher in space but died tragically when her spaceship disintegrated 70 s after take-off. Earlier when asked about her work, she replied "I touch the future, I teach". Personally, I have taken much pleasure in updating and developing my teaching skills as well as learning new techniques while reviewing the literature and writing this book. I hope you will find this book useful too, in your own educational practice.

Meopham, Kent, UK Yasser El Miedany

Contents

About the Author

Yasser El Miedany is Consultant Rheumatologist and Honorary Senior Clinical Lecturer, King's College, London. He is a clinical rheumatologist with research interests and expertise in the diagnosis and management of inflammatory rheumatic diseases including rheumatoid arthritis, lupus, psoriatic arthritis and ankylosing spondylitis. He is also a lead clinician for bone health and metabolic bone disease. He has a special interest in musculoskeletal ultrasonography, particularly its use for diagnosis and monitoring of arthritic patients.

Professor El Miedany attended medical school at Ain Shams University, Cairo, Egypt, and trained at the Royal Infirmary, Glasgow. He is a member of international committees and organizations like the American College of Rheumatology, the European League Against Rheumatism (EULAR) as well as the British Society for Rheumatology. He has developed strong local and international partnerships with clinical and academic colleagues, centred on his role as clinical lead and researcher in rheumatology.

Professor El Miedany has unique interest in medical education. Over the past years, he has actively contributed to educational leadership programmes and medical education courses at both undergraduate and postgraduate levels, delivering an excellent student experience through teaching, assessment and administration processes. He implemented new teaching approaches such as simulated teaching and flipped learning in standard teaching protocols. He has also undertaken high-quality research relating to educational leadership.

Part I
Introduction: Investing in Education

Chapter 1
Teaching: Art or Science?

Introduction

There is no teaching gene, as "great teachers" are made, not born. Teaching does not emerge as a package of innate abilities or temperament. Teaching skills are learned, absorbed, honed, revised and tweaked and occasionally dumped and retrofitted, multiple times in a long-term teaching career. However, while techniques can be taught and refined, good teachers cannot be produced on an assembly line. The talent to communicate must be nurtured, and teachers should be encouraged to use their individual gifts in the classroom. This what makes some teachers memorable. However, some of the memorable teachers may have been quite forgettable to others. It is a fact that good teaching is a highly subjective matter. As in all such fields, most artists may not be memorable, but they should be highly competent. To reach that goal, teachers with intelligence, positive personalities and a feeling for others should be kept, encouraged, got motivated and given the opportunity to mentor junior colleagues or trainers.

Every day there are more and more teachers entering the field of education. However, overall the big question is, what makes an effective teacher, and can we create more of them? Teaching can be stratified into two categories, teaching qualities and teaching quantities. In fact, there's a big difference between the two teaching styles and how the teaching process is delivered. Another question is how an effective teacher can be assessed, and whether scientific research can be used to measure how well teachers are doing.

A good teacher not only includes how effective he/she is or what qualities the teacher possesses but also how able the teacher is to lead and teach a group of students sitting in a classroom. "Teaching the teacher" preparation programmes are designed to prepare the teacher to be a confident educator and provide him/her with the knowledge and skills required to be an "effective teacher".

The overarching theme is that effective teaching begins with first identifying and then breaking down what can be quite formidable barriers to student learning, which

Y. El Miedany, *Rheumatology Teaching*,
https://doi.org/10.1007/978-3-319-98213-7_1

Table 1.1 Principles of teaching

	Teaching principle
Teaching principle 1	Effective teaching strikes a delicate balance between the self confidence that students must develop to become independent thinkers and the humility they must maintain to recognize how much more they have to learn
Teaching principle 2	Effective teaching entails transmitting the subject matter on a number of different "frequencies" to accommodate the heterogeneous nature of how students learn
Teaching principle 3	The effectiveness of the lecture is limited by the students' willingness to "buy" what the teacher is "selling"
Teaching principle 4	The effective teacher never confuses indoctrination with teaching because the objective is to develop thinkers, not "parrots"
Teaching principle 5	The use of the soft Socratic method is superior to the traditional Socratic method because teaching by facilitation is more effective than teaching by interrogation
Teaching principle 6	The effective teacher uses his research to enhance his teaching and his teaching to enhance his research while recognizing the importance of taking the long view
Teaching principle 7	The dissemination of knowledge is maximized when the teacher develops multiple communication pathways and encourages interdisciplinary thinking
Teaching principle 8	Effective teaching is less about providing students with the right answers and more about developing in them the ability to ask the right questions
Teaching principle 9	The effective teacher crafts his lectures to play to his strengths in communicating the material in the classroom, be it through humour, music, poetry, etc.
Teaching principle 10	The well-planned lecture like the general's battle plan should be sufficiently flexible in design to allow for real-time adjustments necessary to address unforeseen obstacles encountered in the course of the "struggle"
Teaching principle 11	We fail our students when we teach them the material without also instructing them on the most effective methods to communicate what they have learned
Teaching principle 12	The teachers' effectiveness is not measured by the numbers on the teaching evaluations at the end of the term but by what they have helped their students to achieve over the course of a lifetime

can be considered as "science". However, effective teaching should strike a delicate balance between the self-confidence that students must develop to become independent thinkers and the humility they must maintain to recognize how much more they require to know and how to learn from their failures. These are considered an "art", as it requires a special skill to deliver. In both scenarios, teaching principles remain the same for all the students. Table 1.1 summarizes the main teaching principles as reported by Weisman in 2012 [1].

The Effective Teacher

Every day there are more and more teachers entering the field of education who are unprepared or inexperienced and may create an unsuccessful environment for their students. Overall the big question is, what makes an effective teacher and can we create more of them?

In the last decade of the twentieth century, the picture of what constitutes an effective teaching became much clearer. Among elements such as a well-articulated curriculum and a safe and orderly environment, the one factor that surfaced as the single most influential component of an effective teaching is the individual teacher within the educational system.

Many studies have quantified the influence an effective teacher has on students' achievement which is relatively independent of anything else that occurs in the educational authority [2–4]. Of these studies, the one by Nye et al. [4] is the most compelling, as it involved random assignment of students to classes controlled for factors such as the previous students' achievements, class size, gender, socioeconomic status, ethnicity and the availability of an aid in the class. Among several outcomes, the study could answer the question of how much influence the individual teacher can have on his/her students' achievements. The study summarized the outcomes as follows:

> The findings would suggest that the difference in achievement gains between having a 25th percentile teacher (a not so effective teacher) and a 75th percentile teacher (an effective teacher) is over one-third of a standard deviation (0.35) in reading and almost half a standard deviation (0.48) in mathematics. Similarly, the difference in achievement gains between having a 50th percentile teacher (an average teacher) and a 90th percentile teacher (a very effective teacher) is about one-third of a standard deviation (0.33) in reading and somewhat smaller than half a standard deviation (0.46) in mathematics. These effects have certainly large enough effects to have policy significance.

Another group of researchers investigated whether it helps to have a teacher who has earned a teaching certification or a master's degree and found that neither makes a quantifiable difference in the classroom. Test scores, graduate degrees and certifications – as much as they appear related to teaching prowess – turn out to be about as useful in predicting success as having a quarterback throw footballs into a bunch of garbage cans [5].

Taking it a step further, the teacher should enable the student to "do it right" to demonstrate for the class's benefit. An effective teacher also develops the skill of reading for his/her students and measuring comprehension and then adjusts the lesson to accommodate the needs of the group [6].

In conclusion, the studies that comprised the science part of teaching revealed that the single most important factor affecting student learning is the teacher. Effective teachers appear to be effective with students of all achievement levels, regardless of the level of heterogeneity in their classrooms [7].

The Science of Teaching

Science is a systematic and precise body of knowledge in a specific field. It seeks to discover the general laws regulating the phenomena in that field through observation and experiments. As per this definition, education must be taken as a science since it is a systematic body of knowledge accumulated through ages by observation and experiments. It has its own theories and laws for educational activities arrangement as well as organization. In fact, the science part of effective teaching is founded on decades of research that has provided guidance for the general categories of behaviours, which in turn constitute effective teaching, as well as for the specific techniques that can be employed within those general categories. This has, over years, endorsed education as a science. Teachers have been considered like scientists, trying new teaching practices and changing them if it didn't work. Furthermore, science of teaching implies that good teaching will at some stage be attainable by closely following vigorous laws that yield high predictability and control. This paved the way for the science of teaching to be defined as the accumulation of information and the improvement of teaching practices based on the information gained [8].

The accumulation of information can be viewed on three levels (Fig. 1.1) [9]. The most basic set of information would be the acquiring of knowledge in one's subject area in order to be able to teach it. Without it, there would be nothing to teach. The next level can be labelled as "there is a scientific basis for the art of teaching", describing the set of information which can be acquired from the study of research performed by others. For teachers, this scientific base is found chiefly in the social sciences and in the research on learning generated by the disciplines of psychology, sociology and speech communication. Naturally, the "knowledge" produced by the social sciences, like that of the physical sciences, is growing and ever-changing, subject to correction and open to new findings. But a knowledge base exists and is there to be known and understood by teachers.

Lastly, there is the information gained by the teachers in their own classroom. To be an effective teacher, it is essential to be aware of what is known about how people learn [10]. This information provides a framework for how we can affect the learning of others. Most educational research is based on observation, and the effective teacher implements methods and strategies learned from studying other scientists' research then observes its impact in the classroom. In fact, teachers perform educational research every day in their classrooms, particularly new teachers. They try

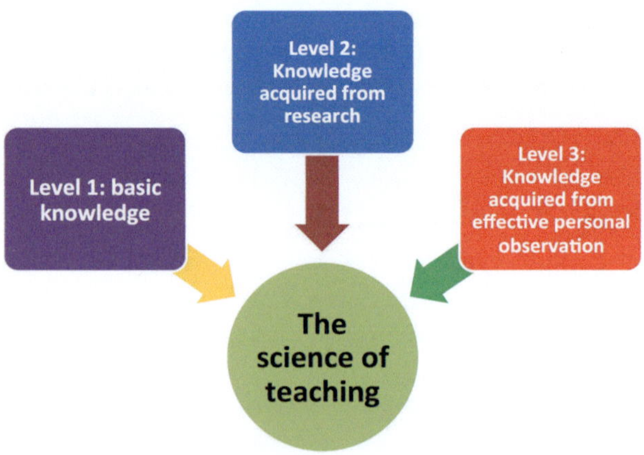

Fig. 1.1 Levels of information that form the pillars for the science of teaching

different theories and approaches, changing a variable here and a strategy there, and then observe its impact on the classroom environment. This continual building of a knowledge base throughout a teacher's career is essential to the science of learning and to be an effective teacher.

Therefore, it can be concluded that there are basic tenets of good practice and fundamentals that must be mastered for any art, whether it's painting, film, architecture or teaching. One must explore the science of the field before one can practice the art [11]. However, research will never be able to identify instructional strategies that work with every student in every class. What the best research can do is tell us which strategies have a high probability of working well with students. Individual classroom teachers must determine which strategies to employ with the right students at the right time [12]. It is the application of the science that constitutes the art.

The Art of Teaching

In its simplest form, effective teaching can be seen as the art of applying education research. Mere research cannot provide answers for every student in every situation; an example is that the same behaviours can be employed in a different order and fashion by two different teachers with equally beneficial results [13]. In fact, a teacher cannot be effective unless he/she is able to integrate both the science and the art of teaching. If the teachers are unable to communicate their knowledge effectively, they cannot impart that knowledge onto others. Conversely, one may be an excellent orator, able to mesmerize the audience, yet he/she needs to have a knowledge of the subject, learning theories and teaching strategies, as well as an understanding of the needs of his/her own students' in order to gain the trust that is essential to creating an effective learning environment.

The art of teaching involves not only knowing what to do and how to do it but also when to do it and in what situations not to do it. It is this kind of thinking process that takes teaching from a scientific base to an art form [8]. These kinds of decisions are not easily made. Effective teachers build these skills over time. As teachers gain experience, they learn to read and understand their student's abilities and needs. Through the application of information learned, they build a foundation of strategies and the knowledge of when and how to apply them. To get through to a student, a teacher must be creative. The creativity that is involved in changing the classroom environment based on study and observation is where the art shines through [14]. The art of teaching is presentational as well as improvisational. The lesson should be planned and scripted, but an effective teacher should be ready for the unexpected teachable moment [5].

While the science of teaching is essential (knowledge of subject matter, learning theories and instructional strategies that form the foundation of teaching), it is the mastery of the art of teaching that defines truly effective teachers. Perhaps, this is the reason why even the proponents of the scientific method in education did not consider teaching itself to be a science but a combination of art and science. In the article written by Makedon [13], it was stated that "If there were an opposition between science and art, I should be compelled to side with those that assert that education is an art".

With the recent technical developments and development of social media, the term "educational technology" was introduced consisting of all media, methods and materials being utilized for optimum development of education. That is, results of the art in combination with different sciences were being utilized in education for the growth and development of the individual as well as the society [15].

In conclusion, the debate of teaching art or science and which one outwits the other is an eternal one. If science is about fact, art is about performance. If science delves into the world and beyond, art is about searching within. To be an effective teacher, one must not only stay abreast of the latest research and findings in the field of education but must also continually practice the art of applying this information, assessing what works and refining their approach in order to create an effective learning environment.

References

1. Weisman D. An essay on the art and science of teaching. Am Econ. 2012;57(1):111–25.
2. Haycock K. Good teaching matters … a lot. How well qualified teachers can close the gap. Thinking. 1998;K-16, 3(2):1–14.
3. Marzano RJ. What works in schools: translating research into action. Alexandria: Association for Supervision and Curriculum Development; 2003.
4. Nye B, Konstantopoulos S, Hedges LV. How large are teacher effects? Educ Eval Policy Analyses. 2004;26(3):237–57.
5. Gladwell M. Most likely to succeed. 2008. http://www.newyorker.com/reporting/2008/12/15/081215fa_fact_gladwell?currentPage=all#ixzz0dSOzyI82.
6. Reynolds T. The art and science of teaching. 2006. http://www.associatedcontent.com/article/22648/the_art_and_science_of_teaching.html?cat=4.
7. Marzano RJ, Pickering DJ, Pollock JE. Classroom instruction that works; classroom instruction that works: research-based strategies for increasing student achievement. Alexandria: Association of Supervision and Curriculum Development; 2001.
8. Friendly Teacher. The art and science of teaching. 2005. http://www.associatedcontent.com/article/16569/the_art_and_science_of_teaching_pg4.html?cat=4.
9. Is teaching an art or a science? Online portfolio of Todd Philipp. https://toddphilipp.weebly.com/is-teaching-an-art-or-a-science.html.
10. Davis JR. Better teaching, more Learning. 1997. http://www.ntlf.com/html/lib/btml_xrpt.htm.
11. Qualters D. The art and science of teaching with a little help from my friends. 2002. http://www.stthomasu.ca/publications/teaching/spring2002/qualters.htm.
12. Marzano RJ. The art and science of teaching. 2007. http://www.ascd.org/publications/books/107001/chapters/Introduction@_A_Question_Answered.aspx.
13. Makedon A. Is teaching and art or a science? 1990. http://www.eric.ed.gov/ERICDocs/data/ericdocs2sql/content_storage_01/0000019b/80/22/de/39.pdf.
14. Cain C. Is teaching an art or a science? 2007. http://www.associatedcontent.com/article/111558/it_teaching_an_art_or_a_science.html?cat=4.
15. Nikiphorou E, Studenic P, Jani M on behalf of EMEUNET, et al. OP0313 the use and impact of social media in modern rheumatology practice based on a survey by the Emerging Eular Network (Emeunet). Ann Rheumatic Dis. 2015;74:191.

Part II
The Science of Teaching

Chapter 2
Rheumatology Teaching: The Need to Review

Introduction

There is no other time in the history of rheumatology when progress has been so fast. The numbers of treatment options, diagnostic guidelines and treatment approaches have exploded so greatly. This phenomenon could be unique to rheumatology, where a relatively short time interval has been recorded between the introduction of new therapies and an almost simultaneous entry in treatment guidelines. While this situation should engender great excitement and optimism, there are nevertheless reasons for concern. Several challenges have been noted over the past period in both the developed and developing world, and individual countries may face more specific local challenges. Limited understanding of the burden of musculoskeletal condition among public health professionals and policymakers means that these diseases are often not considered a public health priority [1]. This was paralleled by limited time and resources dedicated for rheumatology education. This might be the reason for both undergraduate students and postgraduate young doctors to opt out of choosing rheumatology speciality as a future career. The objective of this review is to address musculoskeletal challenges on both local and global scale and the need to review current rheumatology teaching approaches to encourage junior doctors choosing musculoskeletal medicine as a profession.

Reflection from Current Musculoskeletal Practice

According to the WHO, a key component of a well-functioning health system is to provide equitable access to people-centred care. Availability of healthcare workers, clinical services, affordability of care and cultural acceptability of treatment are all important factors [2, 3]. Any disparity or inadequacy in patient access to healthcare professionals, including primary care providers, rheumatologists, orthopaedic

Y. El Miedany, *Rheumatology Teaching*,
https://doi.org/10.1007/978-3-319-98213-7_2

surgeons, physical medicine and rehabilitation specialists, nurses, occupational therapists and physiotherapists, can significantly delay the diagnosis process as well as treatment initiation, both of which are key to minimizing disease progression and improving patient outcomes [4, 5].

Musculoskeletal conditions are common and place an enormous burden on health resources. In a study done by Day and Yeh in 2008 [6], they reported that MSK problems accounted for about 15–30% of all primary care encounters in the United States. In addition, MSK chronic conditions have been linked to significant healthcare expenditures and associated with high prevalence of population morbidity. Results of a survey of eight countries, including Denmark, France, Germany, Italy, Japan, Norway, the United States as well as Netherlands, revealed that arthritis had the highest negative impact on health-related quality of life [7]. Despite the high prevalence of MSK disorders and the fact that MSK symptoms might be the initial presentation of variable systemic disorders, patients with MSK complaints are often overlooked. Earlier studies [8–11] reported virtually full documentation of cardiovascular, respiratory and gastrointestinal systems examinations but almost a major neglect of MSK examination. A wide spectrum of medical specialists, including internists, orthopaedic surgeons, paediatricians and general practitioners, share the delivery of MSK care; however, they usually handle the patients' MSK case as part of the general medical or surgical concept rather than through a dedicated focussed MSK service. Such overlooking of MSK examination and delay of diagnosis mostly lead to serious complications both on the short- and long-term patient's care.

Furthermore, studies looking into competencies among medical trainees and physicians reported significant limitations of the essential MSK skills. A cross-sectional survey of 297 primary care physicians indicated that MSK complains make up 30–40% of daily practice. However about 80% of participants reported a low level of confidence in performing a musculoskeletal physical examination [12]. Another study indicated that 79% of respondents, including medical students, residents and staff physicians, failed the essential MSK cognitive examination [13]. The reality is that the current musculoskeletal practice as well as teaching is facing vital challenges at all levels.

At the undergraduate level, investigators reported that the principles of MSK examination were overlooked in residency education and undergraduate programmes [14–17]. These findings were supported by a survey carried out by Ramani et al. [18], which depicted that new medical graduates have lower competence in demonstrating physical examination especially for MSK and cardiovascular system. In another study done by Di Caprio and his colleagues [19], about 50% of the US medical schools had no obligatory MSK basic sciences course or clinical clerkships [19]. Harvard medical students considered MSK medicine as the third most important topic in a physician's career, yet they presented low levels of confidence in MSK examination [20]. Medical school curricula pay scant attention to MSK medicine: it is estimated that only 3% of most US undergraduate curricular is devoted to MSK medicine [21]. In UK undergraduate teaching, MSK education is included among "long-term conditions module" (King's college MBBS Curriculum

2020), which is usually covered over 8-week block Stage 3 Integrated Clinical Practice (years 4 and 5) [22].

The underrepresentation of MSK in medical curricula has been highlighted by the Association of American Medical College (AAMC). Recommendations regarding the essential competencies for medical graduates were stressed [23]. This concurred with the United States Bone and Joint Initiative (announced Project 100), which recommended that 100% of US medical schools should have a musculoskeletal course. Accordingly, medical schools developed their MSK curriculum. However, most of these initiatives did not meet the expected results of improving medical students' competencies in MSK medicine [24–26].

At the foundation level, in the United Kingdom (UK), Nammari et al. (2009) [27] highlighted that UK Foundation Programme currently provides inadequate training in MSK medicine. The MSK training exposure was limited; about 15% of the 112 respondents had any exposure to orthopaedics during the foundation programme, and only 13% felt they had adequate exposure to MSK medicine. This concurred with Nigerian study that revealed inadequate musculoskeletal competency of the pre-internship Nigerian medical-school graduate, evaluated by the Freedman and Bernstein test for musculoskeletal competency [28].

In the postgraduate programmes, the same limitations have been emphasized since the 1980s: directors of residency programmes indicated that rheumatology was not adequately covered as cardiology or gastroenterology in internal medicine residency programmes [29]. General dissatisfactions of MSK training were reported by internal medicine residents and family medicine practice. US residents expressed their dissatisfaction of their competence in performing MSK examinations at various parts of the body and attributed that to the inadequate or poor training [30]. Two hundred sixteen internal medicine residents, from 13 English language Canadian internal medicine programmes, reported poor self-confidence in rheumatology diagnoses (5.24/10): They achieved considerably lower scores than all three comparator subspecialties, including cardiology, respiratory medicine and gastroenterology [31]. Another study reported that orthopaedics residents' achieved s significantly low score in the multiple-choice decision-making MSK patient examinations [16]. Adding a year of training had no association with higher self-confidence for rheumatology [31] nor improved residents' competence in MSK patient's examinations [16]. Many studies highlighted the essential need to review the residency training programmes.

Educational Challenges in Musculoskeletal Medicine Teaching

The frequently identified gap between theory and practice has led practitioners in many professions to conclude that theory belongs in its ivory tower, neither useful nor relevant to those in practice. Education is no exception. However, as the processes that underpin educational practice are better understood, it is clear that theory has the potential both to inform practice and to be informed by it.

Unfortunately, medical education research is not as well understood or established as is basic science or clinical research. The reasons for this are many, but most importantly, there is insufficient funding for medical education research and paucity of skilled and dedicated medical education researchers. New regulatory requirements at all levels of physician training demand assurance that physicians are competent to practice in the current healthcare environment and provide optimal patient care. Documenting the relationship between education and patient outcomes represents one of the biggest challenges and greatest opportunities in medical education research. Unfortunately, there is no research infrastructure in place to support such outcomes studies, and the majority of medical education research that is currently being done is supported by volunteer faculty time and resources. Compared with medicine specialities in general, these challenges are augmented in rheumatology, where less funding resources as well as skilled investigators are available to carry out rheumatology education research. Building a critical analysis of rheumatology education and identifying the challenges facing it would be vital to address the issue and find ways forward towards improving the service. Medical education as we know it today spans three sectors: undergraduate, postgraduate and the continuing professional development of established clinicians. The challenges facing these three sectors will be discussed in the following section.

Challenges at the Medical School Level

Early exposure of medical students, residents and students of other relevant health professions to rheumatology "culture" is vital to improve awareness of the MSK disorders and increase the number of students and residents considering this field of study. To date, rheumatology education has not been a high priority in many medical school curricula and consequently does not allow sufficient exposure of students to the MSK diseases [32]. Several studies revealed that total average time spent in musculoskeletal physical examination teaching was just 4–7 h over 4 years of study and 58% of teaching was performed by non-MSK experts [22, 33, 34]. Furthermore, in the final years' OSCE exams, musculoskeletal cases are not one of the standard cases, in comparison to heart, chest and abdomen assessment, which form main and regular components of OSCE tests; hence, the student might get graduated without having a single musculoskeletal clinical assessment.

Challenges at the Primary Care Level

As expected, the insufficient exposure to musculoskeletal training as medical students has reflected on the primary care physician's (PCP) standard practice. In many countries, PCPs lack knowledge of the nuances of MSK disorders, leading to misconceptions about the most appropriate treatment options, delayed diagnoses and a limited awareness of conditions such as the spondylarthropathies. In part, this may be attributed to the limited number of rheumatologists and other health professionals trained educators and educational leaders, who can combine their expertise in both MSK and education to increase focus on rheumatic diseases across the education continuum.

A US survey of primary care physicians evaluated their experience in using disease-modifying drugs (DMARDs) for rheumatoid arthritis (RA) patients. Results revealed that only a minority initiated this therapy option and PCPs generally had a high level of discomfort prescribing DMARDs [35]. A similar US survey to assess the use of European and American gout treatment recommendations found that of 838 primary care physicians respondents, only half reported optimal treatment practices for the management of acute gout, and <20% for inter-critical or tophaceous gout, raising concerns regarding adequacy as well as quality of care [36]. Typically, PCPs services are extremely stretched, taking care of several other chronic diseases, such as obesity, hypertension and diabetes. This may explain their restricted time devoted to increased understanding of MSK disorders. In a survey of undergraduate nursing, occupational therapy and physiotherapy courses in the UK, educationalists reported only limited coverage of rheumatology [37, 38]. In a trial to help sorting out the problem, the American Association of Rheumatology Health Professionals (ARHP) started offering a programme called "Advanced Practice Rheumatology", with a modular online course and hands-on training for advanced practice nurses and physician's assistants. Other societies offered similar programmes such as the Rheumatology Nurses Society (RNS), committed to the education of nurses working in rheumatology. In the Latin American countries, a PANLAR-endorsed multinational rheumatology e-learning as well as a training diploma programme for nurses and health professionals includes a hands-on and theoretical MSK ulstrasonography course. Greater provision of online training courses in developing countries, at reduced costs, could further enhance training opportunities.

Challenges at the Physicians' Level

With the growing geriatric population, instances of rheumatic and musculoskeletal diseases are on the rise. This spurs the need for more rheumatology awareness and an increase in the global practice of rheumatology. Well-equipped rheumatology centres offering people-centric care are mandatory. However, availability of such centres, affordability of the care offered and clinical services are few of the many arising challenges in this field. Any disparity created only prevents the early diagnosis of MSK disorders and delays the whole process. In addition, there are still many clinically challenging issues including early diagnosis of inflammatory arthritic condition, the waiting time until a primary as well as secondary care appointment is given, formal barriers to the rapid use of biologicals as well as the local economically driven guidelines.

On another front, paediatric rheumatology represents another bigger challenge. Awareness of these conditions in childhood is lacking, and patients are often misdiagnosed as growing pains and hence are referred late which results in poor long-term outcomes. Therefore, paediatric rheumatology is a particular area in which primary care physicians as well as paediatricians require further education. A review of the barriers constraining access to appropriate paediatric rheumatology care found that, in general, paediatricians had little or no training in MSK health and had relatively poor physical examination and diagnosis skills [39]. Introduction of a mandatory musculoskeletal rotation for paediatric residencies could help to improve awareness and understanding of these cases. The American College of Rheumatology (ACR) currently funds visiting paediatric rheumatology professorships, to bring in-depth training to paediatric programmes and provide much needed support for paediatric care in developing countries.

Challenges in Specialist Training

Collaborations between rheumatology associations and universities could help strengthen existing teaching, provide core knowledge of the MSK disorders to all practitioners and encourage rheumatology as a specialty within that region. The ACR provides training and research grants for medical students, residents, fellows and clinicians in rheumatology and has convened an international task force to assess the need for, and distribution of, educational tools. Similarly, the EULAR Committee for Education and Training (ESCET) offers bursaries for students and rheumatologists worldwide to attend online and postgraduate courses on rheumatic diseases. The Emerging EULAR Network (EMEUNET) is a working group of young rheumatology clinicians across 77 countries that facilitates education in RMDs. EULAR also offers a subsidized online rheumatology course. Nevertheless, there is a general lack of training opportunities for those considering specialization as rheumatologists. For example, in Nigeria, there is only one rheumatology training centre in the country. In Thailand, there are only 15 rheumatology training positions available each year, but this could be improved by increasing the number of grants available from the Thai Ministry of Public Health [40]. Of the current rheumatologists practising in India and Pakistan, 20% and 50%, respectively, received their training elsewhere. In the United Arab Emirates, Bahrain and Oman, all rheumatology training takes place overseas, while in Kuwait, Qatar and Saudi Arabia, residents have hybrid programmes of local and international training. Although overseas accreditation can be beneficial, the majority who train in the West do not return to their native countries to practice rheumatology [41].

Continuous Medical Education

Developing and maintaining professional performance are mandatory for every doctor in recent medical climate. Physicians are asked to show they are competent in all aspects of their work, including management, research and teaching, must keep their professional knowledge and skills up to date and regularly take part in activities that maintain and develop your competence and performance. In addition, all physician should prove that they have taken steps to monitor and improve the quality of their work.

Fortunately, over the past years, regional and national rheumatology leagues have launched several courses, workshops and scientific meetings with clear curricular goals. The Chinese Rheumatology Association is working with medical schools to provide intensive training sessions, lectures and comprehensive curricula for the purpose of continuing medical education (CME) [42]. The ACR Rheumatology Research Foundation also has programmes for this, plus nascent programmes to attract college students to rheumatology and other rheumatology health professions. Reduced registration fees or sponsorship to attend international congresses presents an ideal opportunity to promote “rheumatology without borders” so that physicians worldwide can learn about the latest advances in the treatment of RMDs [43]. The impact of educational forums could be broadened via free post-congress web links that disseminate talks and workshops (using podcasts, videos, slide sets, handouts and translated materials) to target audiences that are unable to attend the congress due to lack of time or funding, travel requirements and language barriers. In addition, world rheumatology leaders could travel to developing regions to share their knowledge and expertise, e.g. the International Advanced Abu Dhabi Rheumatology Review Course (and numerous other meetings around the world). CME programmes are currently offered by ACR, EULAR, American Board of Medical Specialties (ABMS), Royal College of Physicians (RCP), Asia Pacific League of Associations for Rheumatology (APLAR), PANLAR and African League against Rheumatism (AFLAR). However, there is a general lack of programmes in Africa, Asia and the Middle East. The International League of Associations for Rheumatology (ILAR) Grants Program also provides opportunities to advance the education and clinical practice of rheumatology in developing countries but has limited resources, with grants totalling $150,000 in 2014. A successful ILAR-supported project running from 2012 to 2013 addressed a particular need in Zambia to enhance paediatric and adult rheumatology education and practice [44]. Similarly, the ILAR-funded UWEZO Musculoskeletal Health training project aims to provide medics in Kenya with appropriate training to diagnose and treat RMDs (UWEZO means “capability” in Swahili). Trained medics can then go on to train community health workers in their region. The Arthritis Alliance of Canada has developed a coordinated national framework for models of care for patients with inflammatory joint diseases. Similarly, the Canadian Rheumatology Association (CRA) is a strong and committed organization for RMDs, forming alliances with the Canadian Medical Association and the Royal College of Physicians and Surgeons and increasing relationships with other organizations including ACR and PANLAR.

Improving Musculoskeletal Education Is Necessary

Medical education’s ultimate aim is to supply society with a knowledgeable, skilled and up-to-date cadre of professionals who are able to provide a patient-centred care and maintain their expertise over the course of a lifelong career. Rheumatology has a privileged position in medicine as it is a primary presentation for several diseases; meanwhile, it can also impact on most of the body organs. In a complex and uncertain world, it is important to make the best decisions about MSK education, training and development. For this, it is vital to address the weaknesses in our education curricula and identify the appropriate scholarly medical educators and educational scholars. It would be considered negligent for a medical graduate to be incompetent at adequately assessing the heart or lungs, yet it is quite common for students to leave medical school without being able to make a general assessment of the musculoskeletal system [45, 46]. Furthermore, training in orthopaedics and rheumatology is rarely mandatory in systems with rotating internships or in family practice training programmes, despite the large number of patients treated by doctors in these programmes [47].

A number of different medical specialties are involved in treating patients with musculoskeletal complaints, usually working in teams with other health professionals, such as physiotherapists, but often without a multispecialty focus. In order to truly improve the outcome of treatment for musculoskeletal conditions, it is important that experts in the various specialities work more closely together and look for commonality of approach, as they often treat the same patients but from different angles.

For the future, it is essential that education at all levels pays proper attention to training in musculoskeletal conditions, in view of their prevalence in society and the need for doctors to be able to manage them appropriately.

In conclusion, in spite of being the fourth leading cause of disability worldwide, the importance of musculoskeletal conditions is under-recognized in undergraduate curricula of medical schools as well as general postgraduate training programmes in most countries. The reasons for this lack of recognition are not uniform but relate to lack of awareness of the magnitude of the MSK diseases impact, the variable disease panorama and genetics of individual countries or regions throughout the world and, most importantly, to the conventional false belief of both doctors and the public that there is a lack of treatment possibilities. Increased awareness of this imbalance between needs and educational priorities is the first step towards change and improving the situation. Agreeing upon recommendations for an educational curriculum in musculoskeletal conditions represents a major step forward.

References

1. Al Maini M, Adelowo F, Al Saleh J, Al Weshahi Y, Burmester G, Cutolo M, Flood J, March L, McDonald-Blumer H, Pile K, Pineda C, Thorne C, Kvien T. The global challenges and opportunities in the practice of rheumatology: white paper by the world forum on rheumatic and musculoskeletal diseases. Clin Rheumatol. 2015;34:819–29.
2. Key components of a well-functioning health system. World Health Organization, 2010. http://www.whoint/healthsystems/EN_HSSkeycomponentspdf?ua=1. Accessed 15 Dec 2017.
3. Putrik P, Ramiro S, Kvien TK, Sokka T, Pavlova M, Uhlig T, Boonen A, Tafaj A, Harutyunyan R, Radner H. Inequities in access to biologic and synthetic DMARDs across 46 European countries. Ann Rheum Dis. 2014;73(1):198–206.

4. Fiehn C, Hajjar Y, Mueller K, Waldherr R, Ho A, Andrassy K. Improved clinical outcome of lupus nephritis during the past decade: importance of early diagnosis and treatment. Ann Rheum Dis. 2003;62(5):435–9.
5. Nell V, Machold K, Eberl G, Stamm T, Uffmann M, Smolen J. Benefit of very early referral and very early therapy with disease modifying anti-rheumatic drugs in patients with early rheumatoid arthritis. Rheumatology. 2004;43(7):906–14.
6. Day CS, Yeh AC. Evidence of educational inadequacies in region-specific musculoskeletal medicine. Clin Orthop Relat Res. 2008;466:2542–7.
7. Alonso J, Ferrer M, Gandek B, Ware JE Jr, Aaronson NK, Mosconi P, Rasmussen NK, Bullinger M, Fukuhara S, Kaasa S, Leplege A. Health-related quality of life associated with chronic conditions in eight countries: results from the international quality of life assessment (IQOLA) project. Qual Life Res. 2004;13:283–98.
8. Almoallim H, Bukhari E, Amasaib W, Zaini R. How to avoid delay in SLE diagnosis and management. In: Almoallim H, editor. Systemic lupus erythematosus. Croatia: InTech; 2012. p. 219–42. https://doi.org/10.5772/26498.
9. Almoallim H, Khojah E, Allehebi R, Noorwali A. Delayed diagnosis of systemic lupus erythematosus due to lack of competency skills in musculoskeletal examination. Clin Rheumatol. 2007;26:131–3.
10. Beattie KA, Bobba R, Bayoumi I, Chan D, Schabort I, Boulos P, Kean W, Obeid J, Mccallum R, Ioannidis G, Papaioanno A, Cividino A. Validation of the GALS musculoskeletal screening exam for use in primary care: a pilot study. BMC Musculoskelet Disord. 2008;9:115.
11. Akesson K, Dreinhöfer KE, Woolf AD. Improved education in musculoskeletal conditions is necessary for all doctors. Bull World Health Organ. 2003;81:677–83.
12. Abou-Raya A, Abou-Raya S. The inadequacies of musculoskeletal education. Clin Rheumatol. 2010;29:1121–6.
13. Matzkin E, Smith MEL, Freccero CD, Richardson AB. Adequacy of education in musculoskeletal medicine. J Bone Joint Surg Am. 2005;87:310–4.
14. Freedman KB, Bernstein J. The adequacy of medical school education in musculoskeletal medicine. J Bone Jt Surg. 1998;80:1421–7.
15. Skelley NW, Tanaka MJ, Skelley LM, Laporte DM. Medical student musculoskeletal education: an institutional survey. J Bone Joint Surg Am. 2012;94:e146.
16. Beran MC, Awan H, Rowley D, Samora JB, Griesser MJ, Bishop JY. Assessment of musculoskeletal physical examination skills and attitudes of orthopaedic residents. J Bone Jt Surg. 2012;94:e36.
17. Comer GC, Liang E, Bishop JA. Lack of proficiency in musculoskeletal medicine among emergency medicine physicians. J Orthop Trauma. 2014;28:e85–7.
18. Ramani S, Ring BN, Lowe R, Hunter D. A pilot study assessing knowledge of clinical signs and physical examination skills in incoming medicine residents. J Grad Med Educ. 2010;2:232–5.
19. Di Caprio MR, Covey A, Bernstein J. Curricular requirements for musculoskeletal medicine. J Bone Joint Surg Am. 2003;85:565–7.
20. Day CS, Yeh AC, Franko O, Ramirez M, Krupat E. Musculoskeletal medicine: an assessment of the attitudes and knowledge of medical students at Harvard Medical School. Acad Med. 2007;82:452–7.
21. Craton N, Matheson GO. Training and clinical competency in musculoskeletal medicine. Identifying the Problem. Sports Med. 1993;15:328–37.
22. Curriculum 2020. King's College school of Medicine. (https://www.kcl.ac.uk/lsm/education/meded/mbbs/index.aspx).
23. AAMC. Report VII contemporary issues in medicine: musculoskeletal medicine education, medical school objectives project no. VII. Washington, DC: Association of American Medical Colleges; 2005.
24. Wise EM, Walker DJ, Coady DA. Musculoskeletal education in general practice: a questionnaire survey. Clin Rheumatol. 2014;33:989–94.
25. Queally JM, Kiely PD, O'Daly BJ, O'Byrne JM. Design and implementation of a system-based course in musculoskeletal medicine for medical students. J Bone Joint Surg Am. 2009;91:1276–7.

26. Bilderback K, Eggerstedt J, Sadasivan KK, Seelig L, Wolf R, Barton S, Mccall R, Chesson AL Jr, Marino AA. Design and implementation of a system-based course in musculoskeletal medicine for medical students. J Bone Joint Surg. 2008;90:2292–300.
27. Al-Nammari SS, James BK, Ramachandran M. The inadequacy of musculoskeletal knowledge after foundation training in the United Kingdom. Bone Joint J. 2009;19:1413–8.
28. Nottidge TE, Ekrikpo U, Ifesanya AO, Nnabuko RE, Dim EM, Udoinyang CI. Pre-internship Nigerian medical graduates lack basic musculoskeletal competency. Int Orthop. 2012;36:853–6.
29. Goldenberg DL, Dehoratius JK, Mason J, Meenan R, Perlman SG, Winfield JB. Rheumatology training at internal medicine and family practice residency programs. Arthritis Rheum. 1985;28:471–6.
30. Clawson DK, Jackson DW, Ostergaard DJ. It's past to reform the musculoskeletal curriculum. Acad Med. 2001;76:709–10.
31. Katz SJ, Oswald AE. How confident are internal medicine residents in rheumatology versus other common internal medicine clinical skills: an issue of training time or exposure? Clin Rheumatol. 2011;30:1081–93. Matzkin E, Smith MEL, Freccero CD, Richardson AB. (2005). Adequacy of education in musculoskeletal medicine. J Bone Joint Surg Am. 87:310–4.
32. Freedman KB, Bernstein J. Educational deficiencies in musculoskeletal medicine. J Bone Joint Surg. 2002;84(4):604–8.
33. Oswald AE, Bell MJ, Snell L, Wiseman J. The current state of musculoskeletal clinical skills teaching for preclerkship medical students. J Rheumatol. 2008;35(12):2419–26.
34. Thompson AE. Improving undergraduate musculoskeletal education: a continuing challenge. J Rheumatol. 2008;35(12):2298–9.
35. Garneau KL, Iversen MD, Tsao H, Solomon DH. Primary care physicians' perspectives towards managing rheumatoid arthritis: room for improvement. Arthritis Res Ther. 2011;13(6):R189.
36. Harrold LR, Mazor KM, Negron A, Ogarek J, Firneno C, Yood RA. Primary care providers' knowledge, beliefs and treatment practices for gout: results of a physician questionnaire. Rheumatology. 2013;52(9):1623–9.
37. Almeida C, Clarke B, O'Brien A, Hammond A, Ryan S, Kay L, Hewlett S. Current provision of rheumatology education for undergraduate nursing, occupational therapy and physiotherapy students in the UK. Rheumatology. 2006;45(7):868–73.
38. Hewlett S, Clarke B, O'Brien A, Hammond A, Ryan S, Kay L, Richards P, Almeida C. Rheumatology education for undergraduate nursing, physiotherapy and occupational therapy students in the UK: standards, challenges and solution s. Rheumatology. 2008;47(7):1025–30.
39. Henrickson M. Policy challenges for the pediatric rheumatology workforce: part I. Educ Econ Pediatr Rheumatol Online J. 2011;9:23. https://doi.org/10.1186/1546-0096-9-24.
40. Louthrenoo W. An insight into rheumatology in Thailand. Nat Rev Rheumatol. 2014. https://doi.org/10.1038/nrrheum2014142.
41. Gibson T. Rheumatology in India and Pakistan today. Rheumatology. 2014;keu306.
42. Li Z, Yang Y. Rheumatology in China: challenges and development. Rheumatology. 2012;51(10):1733–4.
43. Lau C, Feng P. Rheumatology without borders. Nat Clin Pract Rheumatol. 2007;3(6):305.
44. Chipeta J, Njobvu P, McGill PE, Bucala R. Progress made towards enhancement of rheumatology education and practice in Zambia: review of an ILAR-supported project. Clin Rheumatol. 2014:1–6.
45. Pinney SJ, Regan WD. Educating medical students about musculoskeletal problems. Are community needs reflected in the curricula of Canadian medical schools? J Bone Joint Surg Am. 2001;83:1317–20.
46. Williams JR. The teaching of trauma and orthopaedic surgery to the undergraduate in the United Kingdom. J Bone Joint Surg Br. 2000;82:627–8.
47. Rasker JJ. Rheumatology in general practice. Br J Rheumatol. 1995;34:494–7.

Chapter 3
Barriers to Learning Rheumatology

Introduction

As rheumatology practice becomes more complex, practitioners in the field are required to learn, develop and implement new skills as well as knowledge [1]. However, research concerning the use of scientific knowledge in clinical practice has shown that professionals experience difficulties in implementing the basics and outcomes of evidence-based knowledge into their standard clinical practice as well as keeping up to date within their professional fields, leading to questions concerning conditions for professional learning [2–4]. It would not be unreasonable to surmise that the difficulties in keeping up to date in the professional field of rheumatology would be similar to those experienced in other fields.

Rheumatology medical practice has undergone many changes in the last 20–30 years, with many new research findings in such areas as genetics, biological therapies and diagnostic as well as investigational radiology [5]. The first discovery was that of disease-modifying antirheumatic drugs (DMARDS) which have shown a very good impact on the disease activity as well as progression when administered early, rather than at later stages of the disease course. In primary care, early recognition of persistent symptoms has since been recommended, with rapid referral to specialist care [6].

A second significant development was the introduction, around the year 2000, of the biologic therapy. Although the costs of biologic drugs are much higher than for traditional DMARDS, the cost-effectiveness ratio was shown to be in favour of the biologics. The drugs have been shown to reduce disease activity and improve both functional ability and quality of life [7, 8]; hence, the use of these drugs has expanded significantly since their introduction to the day-to-day rheumatology practice. Used initially only for severe cases or refractory RA, the use of biologics has got widespread now targeting variable cytokines, covering wide spectrum of rheumatic conditions, with good results.

Y. El Miedany, *Rheumatology Teaching*,
https://doi.org/10.1007/978-3-319-98213-7_3

The advancements in diagnostic and therapeutic technology mandated the need for a parallel approach towards high-quality and enthusiastic rheumatology teaching. Unfortunately, there have been several barriers to delivering this teaching in an effective manner. Research concerning the use of scientific knowledge in clinical practice has shown that professionals experience difficulties in keeping up to date within their professional fields, leading to questions concerning conditions for professional learning [2].

This chapter will discuss barriers to rheumatology learning, educational need of the junior and training rheumatologists and ways to tackle these barriers.

Defining the Concepts: The Learning Process

Summarizing a wide range of theoretical approaches to learning, Illeris (2011) [9] proposed that learning is "any process that in living organisms leads to permanent capacity change and which is not solely due to biological maturation or ageing". Therefore, and in spite of the fact there is no generally accepted definition of learning, there is considerable consensus among learning theorists that the experiencing of changes is inherent in the concept of learning [10]; hence, it can be considered that the learning process has been successful and effective when the learner changes from his/her pre-learning state [11, 12].

In general, a barrier to learning is anything that stands in the way of a learner being able to learn effectively. Though, any learner may experience one or more barriers to learning throughout his or her education on the way to achieve the expected full academic/clinical potential; when identifying the barriers to learning, it is important to look at the candidate's holistic abilities as well as needs. Barriers to learning are not limited to intrinsic barriers (such as individual cognitive or learning skills) but also to educational environmental (learning experience and progress in clinical attainments, behaviours and actions) as well as academic environment (Fig. 3.1). This highlights the need not to solely focus on the learner, and what he or she can or cannot do, but to look at the clinical skill that is being taught, the expectations being placed on the learner and the learner's readiness for the task. This is crucial for successful learning. Success can usually be acquired if the learner achieves; therefore, it is important to ensure the task is achievable.

Barriers to Learning Rheumatology

The rheumatology learning process faces multiple barriers from both systems and personal domains, which may reflect negatively on the education process and expected teaching outcomes. The good news is that many of these barriers are modifiable and future efforts should focus on implementing strategies to overcome these barriers.

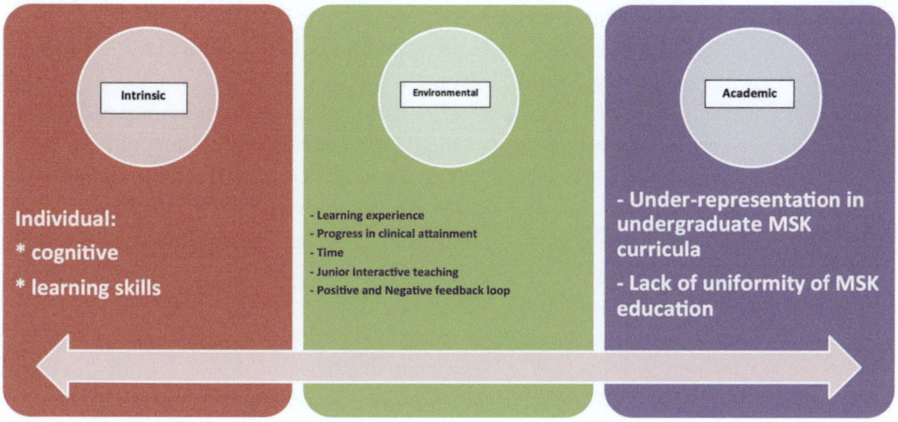

Fig. 3.1 Barriers to rheumatology learning

Intrinsic Barriers

Though the common concept is that teaching is about transmission only, i.e. the transferral of knowledge and standard processes into a students' brain without change or challenge, the reality is that what we are asking is for learners to change the way they practice. Intrinsic barriers or individual characters refer to those attributes and capabilities that are associated with an individual learner. Broadly speaking, this area fits into three categories: (1) personal environment and background, including work commitments, finances and resources available to the trainees and previous educational experiences (which can determine a learner's expectations and attitudes to learning in a new context); (2) commitment, beliefs and perception of self, which include motivation, aspiration, academic confidence, self-efficacy and individual perception of challenge; and (3) academic facilities which refers to amenities that help the trainees in their learning context. Relations with colleagues at work also play an important role in the education and training loop [13]. Positive and negative feedback loops appear to be important in the resident-fellow interaction, with positive interactions strengthening future ones and negative interactions creating additional barriers.

Educational and Academic Barriers

Educational environment is perhaps the most obvious area of academic influence as it encompasses several aspects. Perhaps the starting point would be the level of interest paid to musculoskeletal (MSK) diseases teaching. Unfortunately, in spite of the high frequency of MSK disease, the locomotor system is often overlooked and not given the same attention as other bodily systems [14]. Evidently, MSK examination is seen as a neglected skill by practising clinicians [15–17]. This is paralleled by a global inadequacy in MSK clinical skills teaching [18] and lack of confidence on the educators' front [19].

From the academic point of view, another major obstacle to the enhanced education of MSK examination has been its underrepresentation in undergraduate curricula [20]. There has been little agreement about what "core" standards are expected of students [21]. This is paralleled by the inter-professional way in which MSK clinical skills are often taught, in that learners often report inconsistency and confusion in the way that teaching is delivered. It is discernible that the focus of examination will be different when trainees are taught by different specialists, although there is consensus that MSK clinical teaching should be simplified and standardized.

On the postgraduate level, there have been barriers reported at both the basic level and the continuous progressive development aspect. A number of barriers for young rheumatologists to participate in postgraduate education were identified in an earlier published study [22]. The study revealed that the commonest barriers identified by the participants were lack of resources, time, English language skills, lack of support, mismatch between offerings and needs and having low expectations. Furthermore, even if postgraduate education for trainees in rheumatology is available, there was a lack of insight into the educational offerings. The ratings were found to vary among regions and countries, underlining the need for a tailored educational approach.

A major area of disagreement and deficiency in MSK teaching is related to the lack of a standardized approach not only in MSK teaching but also examination. Earlier published comparative cross-sectional survey which evaluated the current state of undergraduate teaching in rheumatology and orthopaedics, including preferred teaching methods, attitudes towards MSK examination and barriers to effective teaching [23], revealed that a large proportion of clinicians preferred to have their own teaching style rather than use the standard teaching methods, e.g. the Gait Arms Legs and Spine (GALS) method for examination [24, 25] (Table 3.1). This finding echoes the wide variation in examination styles seen in clinical practice across and within specialties, as clinicians adopt individualized ways to detect abnormalities. Unlike other body systems, there is no "one-size-fits-all" approach to the locomotor examination; therefore, it may come as no surprise that GALS method has largely been abandoned. Furthermore, although GALS has been validated for use in the undergraduate curriculum [26], its underrepresentation in day-to-day clinical teaching may reflect a change in attitude towards the screening tool across both specialties and is likely to explain why the uptake of GALS in the patient clerking has diminished [14, 16, 27, 28]. Given the fact that no orthopaedic educators were using GALS to assist in clinical diagnosis, it is unsurprising that only around 7% of respondents utilized this screening tool in their teaching practice. Interestingly, over 75% of rheumatologists declared that they teach using GALS despite only 21% using this in the day-to-day clinical setting. Most of the MSK examination focus on more thorough "regional examination" [15].

These disparities are compounded by the finding that educators are often not familiar with the undergraduate curricula, and consequently there is a desire to

Table 3.1 Gait Arms Legs and Spine (GALS) locomotor screen

Position/activity	Observation
Gait	Symmetry, smoothness of movement (legs, arm swing, pelvic tilting)
	Normal stride length
	Normal heel strike, stance, toe off, swing through
	Ability to turn quickly
Spine	
Inspection from behind	Straight spine (no scoliosis)
	Normal, symmetrical paraspinal muscles
	Normal shoulder and gluteal muscle bulk/symmetry
	Level iliac crests
	No popliteal swelling
	No hindfoot swelling/deformity
Inspection from the side	Normal cervical and lumbar lordosis
	Normal (mild) thoracic kyphosis
Inspection from in front	
Head on shoulders	Normal cervical lateral flexion
Touch toes	Normal lumbar spine (and hip) flexion
Palpation from behind	
Press over the midpoint of each supraspinatus	Note any tenderness
Arms	
Arms behind the head	Normal glenohumeral, sternoclavicular and acromioclavicular joint movement
Arms straight	Full elbow extension
Hands in front	No wrist/finger swelling or deformity
	Ability to fully extend fingers
Turn hands over	Normal supination/pronation (superior and inferior radioulnar joints)
	Normal palms (no swelling, muscle wasting, erythema)
Make a fist	Normal power grip
Fingers on thumb	Normal fine precision pinch/dexterity
Squeeze across second to fifth metacarpals	Note any tenderness
Legs	
Inspection	Normal quadriceps bulk/symmetry
	No knee swelling or deformity (varus/valgus)
	No forefoot/midfoot deformity
	Normal arches
Flex each hip and knee while holding the knee	Confirm full knee flexion with no crepitus
Passively internally rotate each hip in flexion	No pain or restriction

(continued)

Table 3.1 (continued)

Position/activity	Observation
Press on each patella	Note tenderness or effusion
Squeeze across the metatarsals	Note tenderness
Inspect the soles	Note any callosities, reflecting abnormal weight bearing

The development of the Gait Arms Legs and Spine (GALS) locomotor screen in the 1990s was a step forward towards standardized musculoskeletal examination. GALS comprises three screening questions: (1) Do you have any pain or stiffness in your muscles, joints or back? (2) Can you dress yourself completely without difficulty? (3) Can you walk up and down the stairs without difficulty? Followed by a more detailed assessment of the locomotor system (regional examination)

increase awareness of learning objectives and how best to teach these. Traditionally, clinical educators have a duty to align their teaching methods with the course objectives and intended outcomes, although this notion would appear aspirational when one considers that 16% of clinical teachers are unacquainted with the curriculum contents or examination style. If one is to refine the teaching of MSK clinical skills, it is imperative that clinical educators as well as medical school faculty are up to date with the desired competencies for learning.

Educational Needs for the Rheumatologist

In spite of the large interest in education among undergraduate students as well as postgraduate junior clinicians, with ample opportunities to implement and/or adjust existing offerings to better suit their needs, MSK clinical skills remain a challenge to most of the trainees in standard clinical practice. Identifying the educational needs for those interested in MSK medicine might be the first step towards crossing that hurdle (Fig. 3.2).

Perhaps the first requirement for MSK teaching is to agree a definition of what should be taught. Though this sounds to be a logic and simple requirement which was enforced by a number of recent recommendations about curriculum requirements for musculoskeletal education [28–30], it has not yet been achieved. Leading rheumatology teachers at UK medical schools have expressed a wish for national agreement about core requirements in musculoskeletal education [31]. The advantages of such an agreement would include the possibility of consistent teaching of MSK skills across disciplines as well as education centres. There were complaints reported by students as well as trainees that they are taught differently by rheumatologists and orthopaedic surgeons and differently again in general practice. An agreed "core list" of musculoskeletal regional examination skills was suggested to ensure fairer assessment, increased confidence in the use of these skills and, ultimately, better practice and consequently benefits for patients. Such a core list would need to be acceptable to rheumatologists, orthopaedic surgeons, general practitioners, medical students, trainees, MSK teachers as well as deans of medical schools.

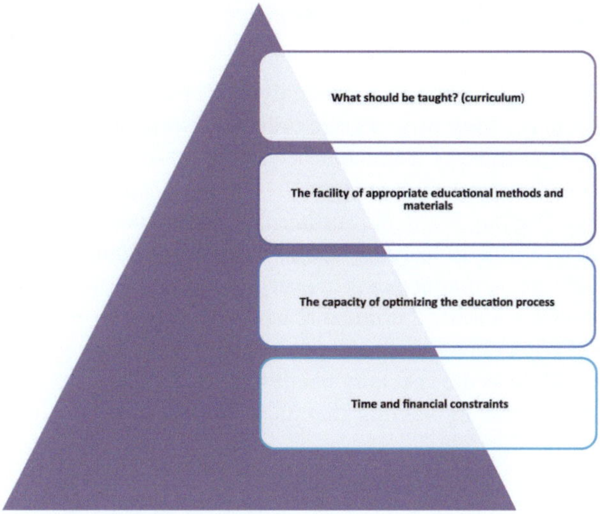

Fig. 3.2 Educational needs for the rheumatologist

The subsequent next requirement to "what should be taught" need to be addressed is the facility of appropriate educational methods and materials. Naturally assessments and examinations can be better defined if the required skills are agreed. Assessment and feedback are expected to drive learning, particularly among trainees and students. Use of the history taking and examination skills in clinical practice is likely to be encouraged by increased confidence in the usefulness of the taught tests and by the experience of successful identification of treatable abnormalities. Using standard models such as GALS or regional examination would prepare the trainee for practice and be a starting point for postgraduate training in their chosen specialty. The effect of rheumatology undergraduate training is retained in clinical practice many years later [32, 33] and is influential in later career choice [34], and so it is important that this task has got the right way.

A third requirement is the capacity of optimizing the education process. This core set suggested usually includes the "basic minimal requirement" and is a good starting point on which to build an MSK teaching programme. Further modification of this set of clinical skills might be required tailored to the learners needs. A study carried out by Vlieland and colleagues in 2016 [22] addressed gaps in the core set of topics identified in the MSK curriculum including non-pharmacological treatment, adolescent health and transitional care as well as connective tissue diseases [35]. The junior clinicians should have the opportunity to highlight such limitations in the key areas and have these topics addressed and taught [36].

Finally, in addition to the general need to better underscore the benefits of properly trained rheumatologists for the quality of care for people with MSK symptoms/ diseases, offering postgraduate education in such a way that time and financial constraints are minimized is another requirement that need tackling. Online courses/ education represents a potential solution as it appears to fulfil these requirements, giving the trainee the opportunity to study the topic in their own time at no/low cost.

How to Tackle the Barriers

Medical education has certainly made considerable strides in recent years. However, there is a long way to go in order to shift the focus of medical education from information delivery – which is becoming less critical, given the ready access to information that most learners have – to helping learners become effective critical thinkers and lifelong learners. Furthermore, in graduate medical education, it is difficult to devote time to learning due to patient care demands. Taking advantage of the teachable moment that exists in every consultation request is a tremendous opportunity to enhance learners' clinical reasoning skills and enhance workplace-based learning.

What changes would you make to rheumatology education going forward, particularly as the specialty needs to attract more residents? Figure 3.3 depicts the main approaches to tackling rheumatology learning barriers.

Enhance Exposure to Rheumatology

Though there are many attractive aspects to rheumatology, however, students and residents often have little exposure to rheumatology and may be dissuaded from considering the field by their relative lack of clinical skill and knowledge about the specialty in comparison with other subspecialties. Maximizing rheumatology teaching opportunities during medical school and residency is an important component of the effort to attract trainees to rheumatology. Studies have shown that subspecialty trainees have an impact on internal medicine resident career choice [37, 38]. Fellows/registrars have the most opportunity to interact with students and residents during inpatient consultation. Therefore, enhancing fellow/registrar teaching skills may make an impact on attracting residents to the rheumatology specialty.

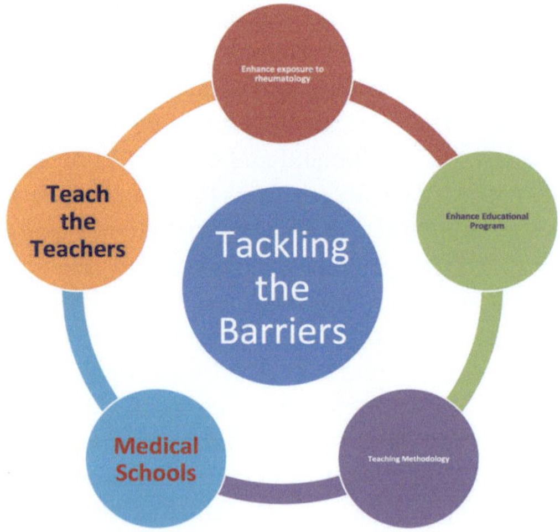

Fig. 3.3 Main approaches to tackling rheumatology learning barriers

Enhance Educational Programmes

- Education should ideally consist of a combination of courses addressing knowledge and skills as well as training on the spot. In the United Kingdom, the availability of a validated rheumatology-based course, combined with a structured programme of work-based supervision and training to ensure consistency of clinical competency and knowledge for all the physicians working in rheumatology, has been suggested [39]. In the United States, the "Fellow as Clinical Teacher" (FACT) curriculum was developed aiming at applicability in any fellowship programme [40]. The curriculum focuses on two major aspects of teaching during consultation: (1) overcoming barriers to teaching in the setting of inpatient consultation, such as time constraints, and hospital-based barriers such as communication, and (2) developing an effective technique for teaching during consultation, a setting that can make it challenging to assess the learners, their interests, strengths and knowledge gaps. Using video examples, the curriculum helps fellows overcome barriers to teaching and use the teaching opportunities they are able to create effectively and efficiently.

Integrating Specialities

Another example of tackling deficiencies in MSK teaching was reported by Tim Blake in 2014 [23], who highlighted notable opportunities such as an integrated "specials" block on musculoskeletal disease. This approach was reported to help bridging the gap between different specialties and deliver a more consistent teaching programme. This style has gained popularity in several UK medical schools and has been shown to be an effective vector for students' knowledge, confidence and satisfaction. Nevertheless, such a heuristic package of teaching requires the motivation and subsequent reward of multiple educators, many of whom are engaged in busy clinical duties. A key theme to emerge was that clinicians were more likely to respond to teaching requests when they had been primed with the course objectives and given adequate time and financial recompense.

Medical Schools

In the current climate, it is crucial that clinical teaching is contextual and reflects the ever-increasing burden of musculoskeletal disease. Competence in MSK examination is essential for all students prior to qualification, although how this is delineated is more complex. Clearly, medical schools should be the drivers for this change in medical education. In the first instance, it has been proposed that a core "list" of MSK regional examination skills should be agreed upon by curriculum planners

[41, 42]; however, this is likely to be influenced by the style of medical curriculum and local resources. Medical schools should embrace evidence-based instructional methods of learning and work more closely with clinicians to facilitate meaningful and consistent teaching practice. They should also ensure that the curriculum is reflected in the assessment.

Teaching Methodology

Though the traditional methodologies of teaching clinical skills have been the standard in most of the teaching session, modern teaching techniques started to gain some ground and popularity. It is expected that using innovative, interactive and contextual ways of teaching will equip medical learners with the necessary knowledge, skills, attitudes and behaviour to bring about improvements in clinical diagnosis of MSK disorders. It is likely that advances in medical science and education will further drive development of evidence-based and values-based practice.

It is important to note that the number of teaching hours does not always guarantee an improvement in learner's clinical skills; thus, in order for MSK specialists to optimize teaching opportunities and offer more efficient learning, they should embrace new teaching strategies and learning styles that are being driven by new medical curricula. More recent evidence-based strategies include use of small group interactive teaching sessions, patient educators and computer-assisted learning (CAL) programmes [37].

Regarding the mode of delivery, the interest in online provision of education has been high. This finding is in line with Hay's report [43] on undergraduate rheumatology education. In that work, innovative delivery methods were proposed, with collaboration between educationalists, clinicians and patients being strongly recommended. Apart from e-learning, the use of clinical videos and interactive games was among the suggestions. Moreover, education should ideally consist of a combination of courses addressing knowledge and skills and training on the spot.

Previously, at the national (UK) level, the availability of a validated rheumatology-based course, combined with a structured programme of work-based supervision and training to ensure consistency of clinical competency and knowledge for all HPs working in rheumatology, has been advised [44].

Teach the Teachers

Whatever the level of seniority or changes at local institutional level, one should take individual responsibility for their state of teaching and seek to improve skills accordingly. This may involve attending update courses on aspects of teaching or through regular appraisal. Educators of the MSK system need to be aware that their interpretation of research findings will be coloured by their experiences and values, which may influence decision-making. One solution to these conflicts may be to adopt a collaborative approach in education practice, akin to the healthcare environment, so that the personal and professional values of several healthcare workers are taken into account [45]. One such approach to bringing about change in organizations and communities is termed Appreciative Inquiry [46]. Another approach is learning from the trainees' feedback and reflection on the teaching content and approach. Including separate sections on the physician's/rheumatologist's appraisal for education reflection and teaching outcomes would help in enhancing the educators' responsibility towards their teaching role.

In conclusion, there are challenges to rheumatology teaching which has negative impact on the learning process. There is a need to overcome the identified barriers if musculoskeletal clinical teaching to medical students and junior rheumatologists is to be improved. The fact that the uniformity in the way that MSK clinical skills are taught is still missing can only add to the confusion and frustration of medical students and young healthcare professionals. There is a need to shift the focus of medical education from information delivery to helping learners become effective critical thinkers confident of their history taking and clinical examination skills. It is hoped that modern styles of teaching such as newer evidence-based strategies can be used for teaching and get embedded in the educational curricula.

References

1. Woolf AD. Healthcare services for those with musculoskeletal conditions: a rheumatology service. Recommendations of the European Union of Medical Specialists Section of Rheumatology/European Board of Rheumatology 2006. Ann Rheum Dis. 2007;66(3):293–301.
2. Forsman H, et al. Use of research by nurses during their first two years after graduating. J Adv Nurs. 2010;66(4):878–90.
3. Nutley SM, Walter I, Davies HTO. Using evidence: how research can inform public services. Bristol: The Policy Press; 2007.
4. Squires JE, Moralejo D, Lefort SM. Exploring the role of organizational policies and procedures in promoting research utilization in registered nurses. Implement Sci. 2007;2:17.
5. El Miedany Y. MABS: targeted therapy tailored to the patient's need. Br J Nurs. 2015;24(16 Suppl 1):S4–13.
6. Deighton C, et al. Management of rheumatoid arthritis: summary of NICE guidance. BMJ. 2009;338:b702.
7. Chen YF, et al. A systematic review of the effectiveness of adalimumab, etanercept and infliximab for the treatment of rheumatoid arthritis in adults and an economic evaluation of their cost-effectiveness. Health Technol Assess. 2006;10:1–229.
8. Nam JL, et al. Current evidence for the management of rheumatoid arthritis with biological disease-modifying anti-rheumatic drugs: a systematic literature review informing the EULAR recommendations for the management of RA. Ann Rheum Dis. 2010;69(6):976–86.
9. Illeris K. The fundamentals of workplace learning – understanding how people learn in working life. London: Routledge; 2011.
10. Merriam SB, Caffarella RS, Baumgartner LM. Learning in adulthood: a comprehensive guide. San Francisco: Jossey-Bass; 2007.
11. Argyris C, Schon D. Theory in practice: increasing professional effectiveness. San Francisco: Jossey Bass; 1974.

12. Ellström PE. Integrating learning and work: problems and prospects. Hum Resour Dev Q. 2001;12(4):421–35.
13. Miloslavsky E. The resident-fellow interaction: limiting barriers and maximizing learning. American College of Rheumatology conference 2013. Abstract number 2814. http://acrabstracts.org/abstract/the-resident-fellow-interaction-limiting-barriers-and-maximizing-learning/.
14. Doherty M, Abawi J, Pattrick M. Audit of medical inpatient examination – a cry from the joint. J R Coll Physicians Lond. 1990;24:115–8. Google Scholar.
15. Walker DJ, Kay LJ. Musculoskeletal examination for medical students: the need to agree what we teach. Rheumatology. 2002;41:1221–3. https://doi.org/10.1093/rheumatology/41.11.1221.
16. Marshall RW, Hull RG. For crying out loud: musculoskeletal assessment of inpatients referred to rheumatology. Rheumatology. 2004;43:1447.
17. Rigby JC, Oswald AG. An evaluation of the performing and recording of physical examinations by psychiatric trainees. Br J Psychiatry. 1987;150:533–5. https://doi.org/10.1192/bjp.150.4.533.
18. O'Dunn-Orto A, Hartling L, Campbell S, Oswald AE. Teaching musculoskeletal clinical skills to medical trainees and physicians: a best evidence in medical education systematic review of strategies and their effectiveness: BEME guide no. 18. Med Teach. 2012;34:93–102. https://doi.org/10.3109/0142159X.2011.613961.
19. Lanyon P, Pope D, Croft P. Rheumatology education and management skills in general practice – a national study of trainees. Ann Rheum Dis. 1995;54:735–9. https://doi.org/10.1136/ard.54.9.735.
20. Dequeker J, Esselens G, Westhovens R. Educational issues in rheumatology. The musculoskeletal examination: a neglected skill. Clin Rheumatol. 2007;26:5–7. https://doi.org/10.1007/s10067-006-0288-0.
21. Coady D, Walker D, Kay L. The attitudes and beliefs of clinicians involved in teaching undergraduate musculoskeletal clinical examination skills. Med Teach. 2003;25:617–20. https://doi.org/10.1080/0142159031000137454.
22. Vlieland T, van den Ende C, Alliot-Launois F, Beauvais C, et al. Educational needs of health professionals working in rheumatology in Europe. RMD Open. 2016;2(2):e000337. https://doi.org/10.1136/rmdopen-2016-000337.
23. Blake T. Teaching musculoskeletal examination skills to UK medical students: a comparative survey of rheumatology and orthopaedic education practice. BMC Med Educ. 2014;14(1):62.
24. Doherty M, Dacre J, Dieppe P, Snaith M. The GALS locomotor screen. Ann Rheum Dis. 1992;51:1165–9.
25. Plant MJ, Linton S, Dodd E, Jones PW, Dawes PT. The GALS locomotor screen and disability. Ann Rheum Dis. 1993;52:886–90. https://doi.org/10.1136/ard.52.12.886.
26. Fox RA, Dacre JE, Clark CLI, Scotland AD. Impact on medical students of incorporating GALS screen teaching into the medical school curriculum. Ann Rheum Dis. 2000;59:668–71.
27. Lillicrap MS, Byrne E, Speed CA. Musculoskeletal assessment of general medical in-patients – joints still crying out for attention. Rheumatology. 2003;42:951–4.
28. Jones A, Maddison P, Doherty M. Teaching rheumatology to medical students: current practice and future aims. J R Coll Physicians Lond. 1992;26:41–3.
29. British Orthopaedic Association. Guidelines for undergraduate teaching on the musculoskeletal system. London: British Orthopaedic Association; 2001.
30. Doherty M, Woolf AD. EULAR standing committee on education and training. Guidelines for rheumatology undergraduate core curriculum. Ann Rheum Dis. 1999;58:133–5.
31. Kay LJ, Deighton CM, Walker DJ, Hay E. Undergraduate rheumatology teaching in United Kingdom Medical Schools: a survey of current practice and changes since 1990. J Rheumatol. 2000;39:123–6.
32. Glazier RH, Dalby DM, Badley EM, Hawker GA, Bell MJ, Buchbinder R, et al. Management of common musculoskeletal problems: a survey of Ontario primary care physicians. Can Med Assoc J. 1998;158:1037–40.

33. Meenan RF, Goldenberg DL, Allaire SH, Anderson JJ. The rheumatology knowledge and skills of trainees in internal medicine and family practice. J Rheumatol. 1988;15:1693–700.
34. Lambert TW, Goldacre MJ, Parkhouse J, Edwards C. Career preferences of doctors who qualified in the United Kingdom in 1993 compared with those of doctors qualifying in 1974, 1977, 1980 and 1983. Br Med J. 1996;313:19–24.
35. McDonagh JE, Southwood TR, Shaw KL, on behalf of the British Paediatric Rheumatology Group. Unmet education and training needs of rheumatology health professionals in adolescent health and transitional care. Rheumatology (Oxford). 2004;43:737–43.
36. Hewlett S, Clarke B, O'Brien A, et al. Rheumatology education for undergraduate nursing, physiotherapy and occupational therapy students in the UK: standards, challenges and solutions. Rheumatology (Oxford). 2008;47:1025–30.
37. Hanly JG. Manpower in Canadian academic rheumatology units: current status and future trends. Canadian Council of Academic Rheumatologists. J Rheumatol. 2001;28(9):1944–51.
38. Horn L, Tzanetos K, Thorpe K, Straus S. Factors associated with the subspecialty choices of internal medicine residents in Canada. BMC Med Educ. 2008;8:37.
39. Miloslavsky EM, Criscione-Schreiber LG, Jonas BL, et al. Fellow as teacher curriculum: improving rheumatology fellows' teaching skills during in-patient consultation. Arthritis Care Res (Hoboken). 2016;68(6):877–81.
40. Saleh K, Messner R, Axtell S, Harris I, Mahowald ML. Development and evaluation of an integrated musculoskeletal disease course for medical students. J Bone Joint Surg Am. 2004;86-A:1653–8.
41. Woolf AD, Walsh NE, Akesson K. Global core recommendations for a musculoskeletal undergraduate curriculum. Ann Rheum Dis. 2004;63:517–24.
42. Hays RB. Practice-based teaching: a guide for general practitioners. Melbourne: Eruditions Publishing; 1999.
43. Fulford KWMB, Peile E, Carroll H. Essential values-based practice: clinical stories linking science with people. Cambridge: CUP; 2012.
44. Thistlethwaite JE. Values-based inter professional collaborative practice: working together in healthcare. Cambridge: CUP; 2012.
45. Carr A. Defining the extended role for allied health professionals in rheumatology. ARC Conference Proceedings No: 12. Chesterfield: Arthritis Research Campaign; 2001.
46. Cooperrider DL, Srivastva S. Appreciative inquiry in organizational life. Stamford: JAI Press; 1987.

Chapter 4
Evidence-Based Rheumatology

Introduction

Evidence-based medicine, whose philosophical origins extend back to the mid-nineteenth century, is based on integrating individual clinical expertise and the best external evidence. Recently, in the healthcare sector, there has been a drive towards implementing evidence-based medicine and evidence-based practice in standard day-to-day clinical setting. Evidence-based medicine integrates (Fig. 4.1) best research evidence with clinical expertise and patient values to facilitate the clinical decision-making process [1]. Individual clinical expertise means the proficiency and judgement that individual clinicians acquire through clinical experience and clinical practice. Best available external clinical evidence includes clinically relevant research, often from the basic sciences of medicine, particularly from patient-centred clinical research into the accuracy and precision of diagnostic tests (including the clinical examination), the power of prognostic markers and the efficacy and safety of therapeutic, rehabilitative and preventive regimens. However, while healthcare professionals do their best to adopt the best standard of care to their patients, healthcare academics and clinical educators do not apply the same concept of best practice strategies and pedagogical approaches in the teaching of their students [2, 3]. This might be attributed to several challenges, with pressures of improving student learning and satisfaction, while maintaining educational excellence. Challenges include growing number of diverse learners, fluctuating levels of tertiary education funding, variable curricula delivery, fast growth of information technology as well as ensuring the availability of enough number of efficient clinical educators [4].

Health professional education does not occur in isolation. In health profession, many educators are clinicians who practised for many years before adding academia into their activities and taking on an educator role. Therefore, these healthcare professionals/educators play a dual role: that of healthcare profession with specific knowledge and experience and an educator with general pedagogical knowledge.

Y. El Miedany, *Rheumatology Teaching*,
https://doi.org/10.1007/978-3-319-98213-7_4

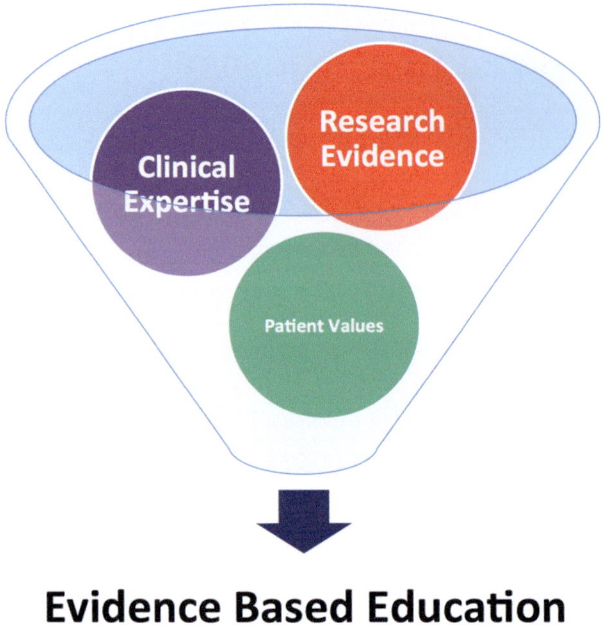

Fig. 4.1 Pillars of evidence-based education

When the healthcare professional educator blends these two components, it is referred to as "pedagogical content knowledge," a concept framed by Shulman [5]. This definition fits with the three key elements for evidence-based education: (1) scholarship of learning and teaching, (2) pedagogical content knowledge and (3) teacher–learner interaction. Ginsberg et al. [3] have defined evidence-based education as "an educational approach in which current, high quality scholarship or teaching and learning research evidence is integrated with pedagogical content knowledge; and teacher-learner interaction in making education decisions to maximise student learning outcomes". Evidence-based education is important for several reasons [4, 6–8]. First, it ensures a high level of contemporary education that is based on teaching and learning best practices supported by high-quality evidence. Second, it inspires academics to keep abreast and revise the teaching curricula. Refreshing, updating, benchmarking and internationalizing of the curriculum make it relevant to the higher education market needs, which in turn ensure receiving cost-effective education, particularly in publicly funded educational centres. It also promotes critical reflection about the implemented educational methodologies. Furthermore, evidence-based education can provide the underpinnings for optimal learning experiences for students. Therefore, evidence-based education is crucial for every educator, as it facilitates and enhances the ability to change and begin to consciously monitor what is happening within the classrooms, make decisions about how to meet the learning outcomes for their students and maximize information learning and retention [9].

Given these challenges, healthcare educators need to find the best evidence for teaching and learning. This chapter will provide an overview of key concepts relevant to rheumatology evidence-based practice as well as evidence-based education.

The Relationship Between Evidence-Based Practice and Evidence-Based Education

Evidence-based practice is an attitude and structured process that is scientifically based. The traditional mainstream teaching approaches, including the delivery of "sage on the stage" lectures and the apprenticeship clinical education model, may be based on personal views or may lack a scientific basis for what is being taught. Evidence-based practice does not call for an upside-down change in the education system, but it does provide a structured approach in which change can be justified based on the evidence, not personal beliefs, word of an authority or current fads. Evidence-based practice can be used to substantiate a current process and support the move to another new teaching approach based on a significant level of evidence. Alternatively, it may stop the transition to a different education process if it proves to have worse outcomes supported by the evidence.

Evidence-based education, like evidence-based healthcare, is a set of principles and practices which can alter the way people think about education and the way they go about education policies and the basis upon which they make professional judgement and deploy their expertise [10]. It is not enough to be an expert health professional and an excellent educator. Many such educators work hard to implement innovative strategies for their students. This also reflects on their practice. Health professional educators are increasingly applying evidence in their clinical practice to improve the health outcomes in their standard practice. A vital component to evidence-based education practice is the teachers' ability to appraise what is credible and useful to make determination about, apply or build upon the findings of others. The scholarship of learning and teaching (SOLT) reflects the quality improvement questions asked by educators every day. The scholarship of learning and teaching is based on "five As" which act as key concepts or a framework for evidence-based education (Fig. 4.2) [11]. These are Asking questions, Accessing, Appraising, Answering questions and Applying the SOLT evidence. Adopting a systematic approach to generating, applying or disseminating educational evidence assists the health professional educator in building a coherent basis for practice. When practice recommendations are applied, assessment as to whether the targeted aims were achieved is essential. Evaluating the outcomes serves to reveal consistent or conflicting findings while producing new evidence. Table 4.1 shows the advantages and disadvantages of evidence-based education.

Undertaking small studies with students can ascertain if what is being taught is meeting their learning expectations. Results of such study can then direct the

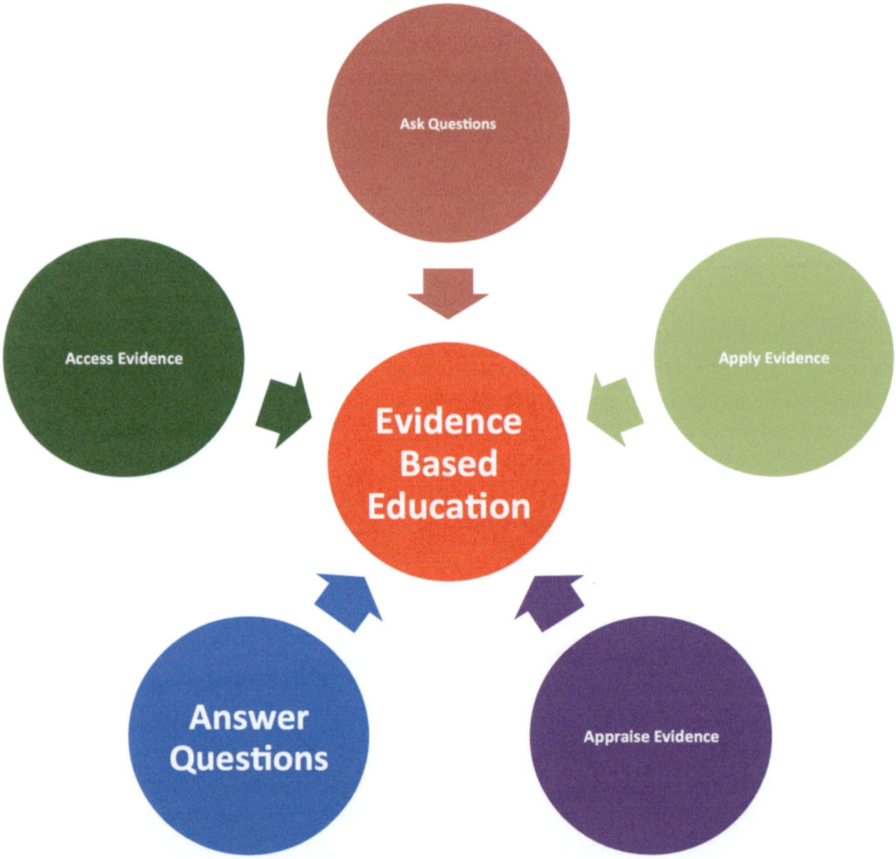
Ask Questions
Access Evidence
Evidence Based Education
Apply Evidence
Answer Questions
Appraise Evidence

Fig. 4.2 The five "As" of the scholarship of learning and teaching as a framework for evidence-based education. (Data from Saewert and Hagler [11])

Table 4.1 Advantages and disadvantages of evidence based

Evidence-based education advantages	Evidence-based education disadvantages
Student-centred outcome	Education and skill development is time-consuming
Set up education approaches based on high level of evidence	Potentially have a negative impact on educator judgement/autonomy
Ensure cross-centre level of education consistency	Lack of evidence for the less common topics
"Train the trainer": ensure better educators information and training	Lack of evidence supporting the lower-level evidence, particularly when it is the only available proof
Ability to share the outcomes supported by the evidence	
Guarantee a defined transparent education process	
Identify what is already known and what is still missing and require further research	

teaching programme setup or curriculum renewal as part of an evaluation of the education practice. A supporting example is the outcomes of a study (personal communications) done in the 1st week of year 5 school of medicine, to determine the students' attitude and preferences to medical topics to be learnt. The outcomes of that work were used to guide the curriculum setting and counteract any topics the students may feel inappropriate. This was double checked through student feedback meetings at the end of each educational round. The outcomes at the end of the educational year have been very positive in comparison with other centres who did not adopt the same approach. The evidence-based education may also form a part of an ongoing educators' educational development programmes where staff may learn and participate in local research or the evaluation of recently published studies as part of their educational process development.

It is essential for academics and practice education supervisors to be conversant with evidence-based education. Health professionals are increasingly receiving professional development in education. This is to ensure delivering high-quality educational level for the students/learners.

Student-Centred Learning Approach

Learning is a process rather than an end product [12]. The learning process encompasses a long-term and enduring change in the students' knowledge, beliefs and attitudes that is initiated by the students' contribution to their own process of learning [13]. Student-centred learning can be defined as learning that places the student at the core of the learning process [14]. This approach has an impact on teaching and service establishment. Student-centred learning curriculum requires flexible design, content sharing and interactivity between the students, activities, materials and the teachers [15].

Teaching healthcare professionals as students or postgraduates is unique. The ultimate role of the healthcare profession is taking the responsibility of caring for the others. The students should learn how to develop an awareness of the complex information they have attained and how to integrate this into their existing knowledge. Also, they should learn how to engage in higher-order thinking, self-awareness, self-monitoring and time management practices [16]. By enhancing the ability of critical thinking, the students will be able to identify their own learning needs. This engagement in professional reflective practice is mandatory for professional competence in the health sector. The ability to reflect in professional practice is a vital trait for health practitioners, allowing them to determine the appropriate action when faced with an unacquainted problem through logically deducing the possible consequences of their action and forecasting alternative possible outcomes [17]. Curricula based on student-centred learning help to promote engagement [15]. Successful engagement augments the students' knowledge, inspires them to be part of institutional culture and endorses the development of lifelong learning behaviours.

The educators have a major impact on the students' learning experience, motivation, grades and learning [18, 19]. Bloom [20] found that students supported by teaching staff (i.e. tutored) perform, on average, one to two standard deviations above those not supported (not tutored). Ideally, every student needs to receive expert teaching from education staff. This should be considered by the educational health authorities, who, under the pressure, started to provide a plethora of online teaching courses to meet the increasing learning demand, which in turn had led to minimizing the direct educational support. The input of the educators on students' progress and engagement plays an important role, not only to enhance their sense of belonging but also their academic achievement and adjustment to their professional career. The understanding of the students' experience provides important insights for course administrators, academics as well as student support services which will reflect positively on the students' learning outcomes. This endorses the student-centred learning and educators to be the most effective educational intervention. Despite cost limitations constraining the teaching hours and the availability of educators, every student should have the facility to receive expert teaching that adopts a reflective practice style.

Education as a Jigsaw

Professionalism education can be conceptualized as a "jigsaw", with smaller pieces meant to fit together to make a whole. These pieces include formal, informal and hidden curriculum [21] (Fig. 4.3). Formal curriculum is the specified and avowed curriculum. This includes professionalism codes of practice, ethics, law and humanities [22]. Informal curriculum can be described as serendipitous teaching and learning that occurs between students and teachers [21]. On another front, the hidden curriculum is about the institutional structures and cultures that communicate to students and what is and what is not valued by an institution. This involves "the norms, values and belief systems imparted to the students through daily routines, curricular content and social relationships" [23].

However, these pieces do not necessarily fit together, all the time, easily or neatly, which is, often, the case for professionalism education. Students tend to receive mixed messages about the ways things should be done as part of the formal curriculum versus the way things are done as part of the informal and hidden curriculum. Furthermore, some studies revealed that in some cases, students were infrequently supervised while on placement which reflected negatively on their practice. Such poor performance contradicts the codes taught to the students as part of their formal curriculum, reflecting a lack of neatly fitting between the informal and formal curricula. Professionalism dilemmas created by this lack of fit can cause students distress and may also have a negative impact on their further professionalism development [24].

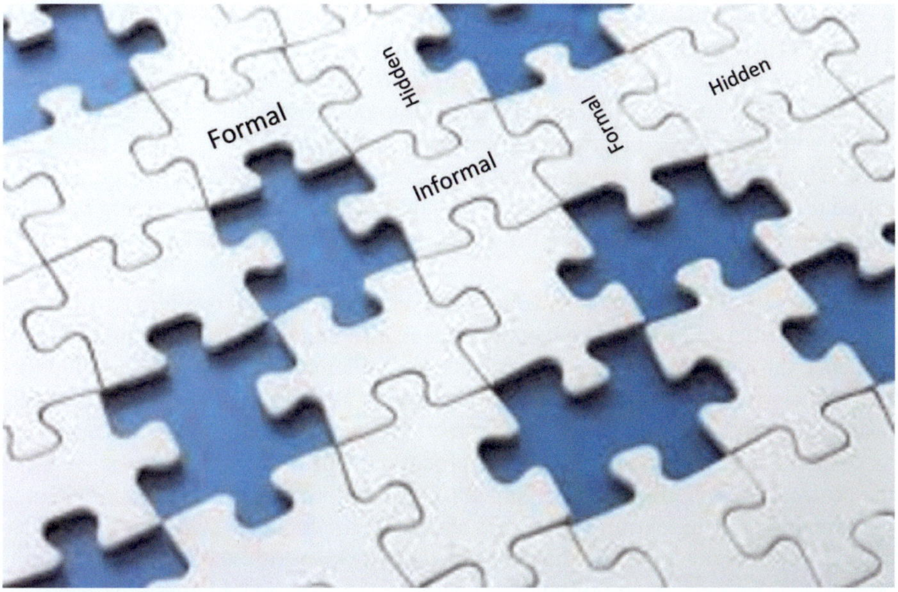

Fig. 4.3 The formal, informal and hidden curricula forming the main pieces for the jigsaw of professionalism education

Interestingly, evidence-based professionalism education can be the best solution for the professionalism puzzle. It is common for research exploring professionalism teaching and assessment (the formal curriculum) to use quantitative methods (e.g. psychometric analyses and assessment of instruments), while research investigating what professionalism is and how it is learned (informal and hidden curriculum) typically employs qualitative methods (e.g. discourse analyses of academic and grey literature and students' talk). Such research helped to understand the different pieces of the professionalism education jigsaw, particularly the informal and hidden curriculum from the students'/learners' perspective. However, while quantitative and qualitative methods abound in the healthcare education literature to explore various aspects of the formal, informal and hidden professionalism curriculum, further studies are needed to employ observational methods [25].

Best Practice in Evidence-Based Education Decision-Making

Assessing students is a key activity in health professional education programmes. Over the past years, in parallel to the increasing emphasis on teaching quality and the enhancement of the student learning experience, attention has been paid to the identification of learning outcomes. The concept of "constructive alignment" is a principle conceived by Biggs [26] for devising teaching and learning activities as well as assessment tasks which address directly the intended learning outcomes. This concept was based on four main steps: (1) Intended learning outcomes are defined; (2) Teaching learning activities likely to lead to the intended learning outcomes are selected; (3) Students' actual learning outcomes are assessed as per the match with the intended learning outcomes; (4) a final grade is derived. At the same time, Biggs has proposed the constructive alignment concept; Meyer and Land [27] introduced the principle of "threshold concept" as a way of differentiating between core learning outcomes that require students to see things differently or in a new way and those do not.

Davies [10] identified that evidence-based education should result in two actions: (1) using evidence to inform educational decisions and (2) generating high-quality evidence through research. In concordance, to implement best practice in evidence-based decision-making, Dollaghan [28] as well as Schlosser and Raghavendra [29] proposed applying the evidence-based practice cycle to evidence-based educational assessment (Fig. 4.4). Throughout this process, the primary question was: What is the desired outcome for the assessment? Ginsburg et al. [30] stated that evidence maximizing student learning outcomes should be the focus of evidence-based education. An understanding of the relevant outcomes specific to assessment within educational process is important for deciding the desired outcomes, assessment tools and the kind of evidence that should be sought to design or evaluate an assessment approach.

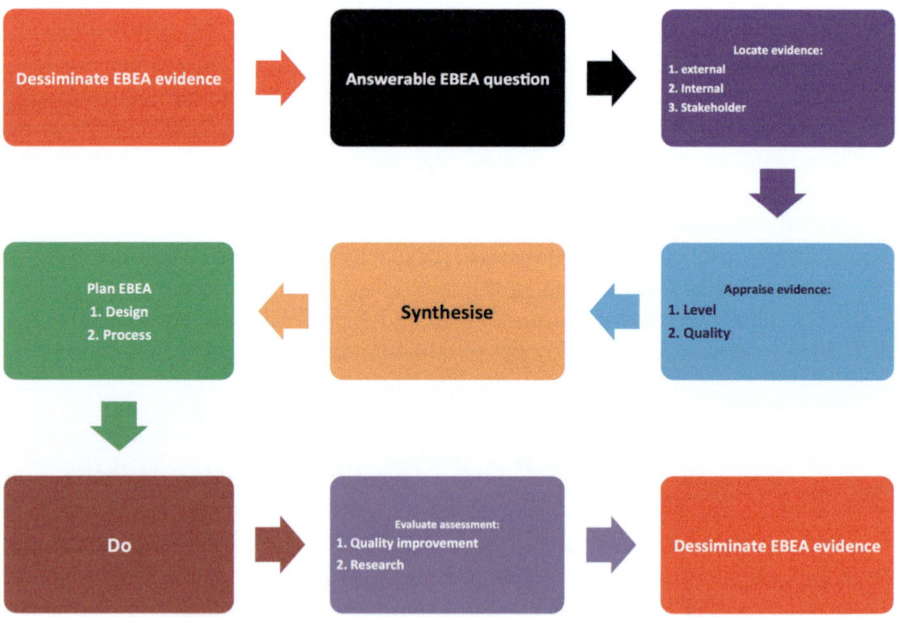

Fig. 4.4 Evidence-based educational assessment (EBEA) cycle for assessment design

Evidence-Based Rheumatology

Over the past years, there have been several advances in the field of rheumatology, leading to growing demand for rheumatology practitioners, with the expectation of a more evidence-based practice, to keep up-to-date about the research developments in their field; and to implement new findings and recommendations into clinical practice. Such evidence could be in the form of treatment guidelines, a Cochrane review or meta-analysis or original therapeutic trials published in medical journals. However, for successful patients' management, accurate diagnosis is an essential requisite. This, in turn, highlights the vital role of history taking, clinical examination and laboratory workup. Therefore, the process of evidence-based rheumatology starts right from the first point of contact between the patient and the rheumatologist and then extends through the process of establishing the diagnosis and recommending the treatment regimen. It is, however, important for making clinical decisions, to focus not only on the evidence available but also to be able to search for appropriate relevant information [31].

Why Rheumatology Is Different from Other Diseases?

The science and art of rheumatologic practice would need to follow the basic principles of clinical medicine, namely, history and examination, relevant investigations leading to a proper diagnosis, following which a treatment plan is decided. However, in contrast to many chronic diseases, where a single gold standard measure, such as blood pressure in hypertension, haemoglobin A_1C in diabetes, lipid profile in hyperlipidaemia, etc., is applicable to diagnosis, management, prognosis and analyses of outcomes in all individual patients in clinical trials, clinical care and long-term databases, in inflammatory arthritic conditions (excluding gouty arthritis), there is not a single gold standard measure to assess outcomes. This is applicable both in short-term trials such as joint and laboratory measures and in long-term studies such as radiographic progression, disability and death [32]. The absence of such a gold standard measure highlighted the need for pooled indices as a valid tool [33, 34]. However, so far, these tend to be complex, expensive and currently used in clinical trials but not in clinical care. In an attempt to standardize inflammatory arthritic conditions such as rheumatoid arthritis and spondyloarthritis, clinical practice guidelines [35–37] have been published. Similarly, a core dataset for management outcomes [38] was endorsed as a framework for all indices in rheumatology. Pharmacological and non-pharmacological treatment pathways and assessment of comorbidities and health-related quality of life measures (HrQoL), as well as lifestyle advice and patient education, have been recommended. However, as the patients' response to management and the presence of risk factors may vary from one patient to another, the treatment concept has shifted to be patient-centred [39].

On the other hand, another challenge arose, which is the fact that the patient's disease status and development of new risk factors may change over time, requiring regular screening, assessment and monitoring of disease activity as well as risk factors in standard clinical practice. Patient-reported outcome measures (PROMs) stand firmly as a valid candidate to record these changes in the standard outpatient rheumatology setting. Over the past years, the role of PROMs expanded from mere assessment of disease activity parameters to playing an active role in the diagnosis, assessment of disease activity, monitoring of comorbidities, adherence to therapy and patient self-management [40]. PROMs also progressed from the generic phase into a disease-specific era [31].

Implementing Evidence-Based Practice in Rheumatology

Implementing evidence-based practice in rheumatology is rather complex. Three factors were found to be most clearly associated with higher evidence-based practice implementation: longer experience in rheumatology practice, experience of research activities and better perceived personal ability to use research evidence in practice. In the study done by Neher et al. [41], experience in rheumatology was found to be more important than experience in profession for explaining evidence-based practice implementation. A longer exposure to the clinical problems of a specific category of patients may foster a deeper motivation to learn more and encourage interest in research. Furthermore, experience of research activities was associated with high evidence-based practice implementation, whereas perceived personal ability to use evidence in practice was an important factor for adopting evidence-based practice in standard daily practice.

Two approaches to evidence-based practice have been described in the literature: (1) evidence-based practice as a critical appraisal process, such as accessing the Cochrane Database of Systematic Reviews or the National Guidelines Clearinghouse, leading to clinical decisions informed by evidence and (2) evidence-based practice in terms of adopting and using various empirically supported interventions, including those specified in clinical guidelines, systematic review or other recommendations [42, 43]. The evidence-based practice implementation scale features mixed items and reflects both approaches to evidence-based practice. However, neither approach was favoured over the other in an earlier study [41].

Education is a strategy that may be used in attempts to facilitate evidence-based practice implementation, targeting knowledge and skills at the individual level [44]. One policy to enhance evidence-based practice in standard practice is to deviate educational efforts to tailor evidence-based practice education to work experience in the specialty. Additional implementation strategies may be needed to embed the activities related to the enactment of evidence-based practice in the organizational structure at different levels [45]. Organizational interventions to facilitate evidence-based practice implementation could include promotion of participation in research activities by healthcare professionals/rheumatologists and capitalization on opportunities for informal learning in connection with these research activities. Integration of research and practice has been shown to not only change individual behaviours but also result in a culture shift in the clinic [46]. Time for reflection and discussion with peers, and to absorb and adapt to proposed behavioural change, is important for the initiation of new behaviour, as behavioural habits may be hard to break [47]. In a larger context, being in a specialized clinic enhanced engagement in evidence-based practice activities, which may be a motive to keep specialized rheumatology units intact where possible.

Sources of Evidence

To establish clinical practice based on the available evidence, this evidence should be weighed in view of its strength and reliability. To evaluate a research study, the parameters to assess include study design, methodology and statistical analysis [48], as well as assessment of the treatment effect (effect size or numbers needed to treat for validation) [49]. On the other hand, consolidated source of evidence is considered of highest impact. Examples of consolidated source of evidence include systematic reviews and clinical practice guideline (Table 4.2). A systematic review

Table 4.2 Sources for consolidated sources of evidence

Websites which contain systematic reviews (some may require subscription to access)
The Cochrane Library
Evidence-Based Practice Evidence Reports – Agency for Healthcare Research and Quality
VA Evidence-Based Synthesis Program
Clinical practice guidelines
Clinical practice guidelines – Agency for Healthcare Research and Quality
National Guideline Clearinghouse – Agency for Healthcare Research and Quality
American College of Rheumatology's Clinical Practice Guidelines
Evaluating the evidence: levels of evidence/strength of evidence
There are many organizations that have developed systems for defining and describing levels of evidence or systematic approaches for evaluating research:
Centre for Evidence-Based Medicine – Levels of Evidence
Cochrane Collaboration – Critical Appraisal of Qualitative Research
OT Seeker
Physiotherapy Evidence Database PEDro Scale
Evaluating the evidence: critically appraised topics (CATs)
These are a systematic way of approaching and answering a clinical question:
Centre for Evidence-Based Medicine – Critical Appraisal Tools
McMaster University Evidence-Based Practice Resources
The AGREE Instrument for Guideline Evaluation
JAMA Evidence – Guidelines for Evaluating Primary Articles by Type
American College of Rheumatology Clinical Practice Guidelines

Table 4.3 Categories of evidence

Category	Evidence
1A	Meta-analysis of randomized controlled trials (RCT)
1B	At least one RCT included in the analysis
2A	At least one controlled study without randomization
2B	At least one type of quasi-experimental study
3	Descriptive studies, such as comparative studies, correlation studies or case-control studies
4	Expert committee reports or opinions and/or clinical experience of respected authorities

Table 4.4 List of some organizations that are good resources to find information regarding evidence-based practice

Agency for Healthcare Research and Quality – USA
Bandolier – Evidence-Based Thinking About Healthcare – UK
BMJ Clinical Evidence – UK
CEBM – Centre for Evidence-Based Medicine – UK
Centre for Health Evidence – CA
Centre for Reviews and Dissemination – University of York
Cochrane Collaboration – International
Evidence-Based Medicine Toolkit – CA
Health Evidence Network, World Health Organization – Europe
National Library of Medicine

is a synthesis of the primary studies that uses explicit and reproducible methods to review the literature. Thus, they consolidate the data from many studies on the same topic in an attempt to more clearly answer a research question. Guidelines for practice are prepared and published by various associations, groups and agencies with the goal of improving healthcare by providing practitioners with a consolidation of evidence related to a particular topic to guide clinical decision-making or define best practice. On evaluating reviews or meta-analysis of trials/studies, evidence can be categorized according to importance, in descending order of importance in six categories shown in Table 4.3 [50]. Thus, in considering a treatment option (e.g. use of glucosamine for osteoarthritis), a meta-analysis (category 1A evidence) would be far more relevant compared to an expert panel/committee report (category 4 evidence). Table 4.4 is a list of links to organizations that can be considered as good resources to find information regarding evidence-based practice.

Barriers to Implementing Evidence-Based Practice

Despite the availability of information, it has been observed that evidence-based practice is not as simple and straightforward process as originally thought. Controversies in the field of evidence-based practice have identified problems relating to differences

Table 4.5 Challenges to evidence-based medicine

General challenges to scientific evidence	Specific challenges to Evidence-based practice	Pseudo-challenges of evidence-based practice
1. Shortage of consistent and coherent scientific evidence	1. Need to learn and adopt new skills for searching and critical appraisal of evidence	1. Evidence-based practice degrades clinical expertise
2. Difficulties in applying available evidence to clinical care of the patients	2. Busy clinicians' schedule with lack of adequate time for to master the new skills	2. Limited to clinical research alone
3. Barriers to practice high-quality medicine	3. Evidence to support the role of the evidence-based medicine and its value has been slow to emerge	3. Ignores patients' values and preferences
		4. Indorses "cook-book" approach to medicine

in understanding research evidence as a concept and relating to how research knowledge is received and used by individuals and organizations [51].

The criticism for evidence-based practice can be stratified into three categories. The first one can be considered as universal to the practice of science in general, and the second one is fairly specific for evidence-based practice, whereas the third one includes a few "pseudo-limitations" (Table 4.5). Evidence-based practice cannot be considered as a cost-cutting tool, as the provision of evidence-based care directed at maximizing the quality of life may often result in increasing the overall cost of treatment. However, this cannot be considered as a negative aspect of evidence-based practice. In the pursuit of quality clinical care, all clinicians will need to keep abreast of new developments. The ease with which one can perform an "online search" nowadays means that evidence-based practice is not out of the reach of any practitioner. Finally, the definition that evidence-based practice involves the "use of current best clinical evidence" for a certain treatment option relieves another concern that evidence-based practice leads to therapeutic pessimism in the absence of randomized trial evidence [52].

In conclusion, evidence-based medicine trend is now infiltrating rheumatology. While clinical rheumatology practice is a mix of art and science, it is a good approach to adopt evidence-based rheumatology in the hope of offering nothing but the best to the patients living with inflammatory arthritic conditions. The development and publication of appropriate clinical guidelines by the elite organization bodies such as the American College of Rheumatology and EULAR deliver the evidence to the treating rheumatologists and help them manage their patients properly and up to the standard. However, there are grey areas in rheumatology practice where convincing evidence is not forthcoming and sometimes patients are managed on empirical bases and other time based on half-truth. All the rheumatologists are familiar with the patient who does not fit into a diagnostic category or fails to respond to treatment. In such situations, the clinician will obviously have to use appropriate clinical discretion and judgement. For the majority of patients and the bulk of clinical practice, following the principles of evidence-based practice in rheumatology will help to standardize the service and secure the best service provided based on the best evidence available.

References

1. Strauss SE, Richardson WS, Glasziou P. Evidence based medicine: how to practice and teach EBM. Edinburgh: Churchill Livingstone; 2005.
2. Cannon S, Boswell C. Evidence based teaching in nursing: a foundation for educators. Sudbury: Jones and Bartlett Learning; 2012.
3. Ginsberg SM, Friberg J, Visconti C. Scholarship of teaching and learning in speech language pathology and audiology: evidence based medicine. San Diego: Plural Publishing; 2012.
4. Petersen S. Time for evidence based medical education. BMJ. 1999;316(719):1223–4.
5. Shulman LS. Knowledge and teaching foundations of the new reform. Harvard Educ Rev. 1987;57(1):1–22.
6. Beck DE. Pharmacy educators: can an evidence-based approach make your instruction better tomorrow than today? Am J Pharm Educ. 2002;66(1):87–8.
7. Ferguson L, Day RA. Evidence-based nursing education: myth or reality? J Nurs Educ. 2005;44(3):107–15.
8. Loyola S. Evidence-based teaching guidelines: transforming knowledge into practice for better outcomes in healthcare. Crit Care Nurs Q. 2010;33(1):19–23.
9. Brown T. Chapter 4, Evidence based education and health professional education. In: Brown T, Williams B, editors. Evidence-based education in the health profession. London: Radcliffe; 2015. p. 31–46.
10. Davies P. What is evidence based education? Br J Educ Stud. 1999;47(2):108–21.
11. Saewert KJ, Hagler D. The five a's of the scholarship of teaching and learning: ask, access, answer, apprise and apply. In: Brown T, Williams B, editors. Evidence-based education in the health professions: promoting best practice in the learning and teaching of students. Abingdon: Radcliffe; 2015. CRC Press, ISBN 9781909368712.
12. Ambrose S, Bridges M, Di Pietro M. How learning works: 7 research based principles for smart teaching. San Francisco: Jossey-Bass and Wiley Publishers; 2010.
13. Korach S. You are the curriculum: participant identification of experience and practice with impact. Plan Chang. 2012;43(1–2):149–60.
14. Di Napoli R. What is student centred learning? London: Educational Initiative Centre, University of Westminster; 2004.
15. Attard A, Di Ioio E, Geven K. Student centred learning: an insight into theory and practice. Bucharest: EU Educational international; 2010.
16. Bandura A. Social foundation of thought and action: a social cognitive theory. Englewood Cliffs: Prentice-Hall; 1986.
17. Mann K, Gordon J, Mac Leod A. Reflection and reflective practice in health professions education: a systematic review. Adv Health Sci Educ Theory Pract. 2009;14(4):595–621.
18. Chi MTH, Roy M, Hausmann RGM. Observing tutorial dialogues collaboratively: insights about human tutoring effectiveness from various learning. Cogn Sci. 2008;32(2):301–41.
19. Roscoe RD, Chi MTH. Tutor learning: the role of explaining and responding to questions. Instr Sci. 2008;36:321–50.
20. Bloom BS. The 2 sigma problem: the search for methods of group instruction effective as one-to-one tutoring. Educ Res. 1984;13(6):4–6.
21. Hafferty FW. Beyond curriculum reform: confronting medicine's hidden curriculum. Acad Med. 1998;73(4):403–7.
22. Nursing and Midwifery Council (NMC). Standards for pre-registration. Nursing education. London: NMC; 2012.
23. Margolis E, Soldatenko M, Ackers S. Peekaboo: hiding and outing the curriculum. In: Margolis E, editor. The hidden curriculum in higher education. New York: Routledge; 2001. p. 1–19.
24. Monrouxe LV, Rees CE, Endacott R. Even now it makes me angry: health care students professionalism dilemma narrative. Med Educ. 2014;48(5):502–17.
25. Stern DT. In search of the informal curriculum: when and where professional values are taught. Acad Med. 1998;73(10 Suppl):S28–30.

26. Biggs JB. Teaching for quality learning at university. 2nd ed. Buckingham: Open university Press for Research into Higher Education; 2003.
27. Meyer JHE, Land R. Threshold concepts and troublesome knowledge: linkages to ways of thinking and practising. In: Rust C, editor. Improving student learning. Theory and practice ten years on. Oxford, UK: Oxford Centre for Staff and Learning Development; 2003. p. 1–15.
28. Dollaghan CA. The handbook for evidence based practice in communication disorders. Baltimore: Paul H Brookes; 2007.
29. Schlosser R, Raghavendra P. Evidence based practice in augmentative and alternative communication. Augment Altern Commun. 2004;20(1):1–21.
30. Ginsburg S, Friberg J, Visconti CF. Scholarship of teaching and learning in speech language pathology and audiology: evidence based education. San Diego: Plural publishing; 2012.
31. Rosenberg W, Donald A. Evidence-based medicine: an approach to clinical problem-solving. BMJ. 1995;310:1122–6.
32. El Miedany Y. Adopting patient-centered care in standard practice: PROMs moving toward disease-specific era. Clin Exp Rheumatol. 2014;32(Suppl. 85):S40–6.
33. Tugwell P, Bombardier C. A methodologic framework for developing and selecting endpoints in clinical trials. J Rheumatol. 1982;9:758–62.
34. Bombardier C, Tugwell P. A methodological framework to develop and select indices for clinical trials: statistical and judgmental approaches. J Rheumatol. 1982;9:753–7.
35. Singh, Furst D, Bharat A, et al. Update of the 2008 American College of Rheumatology recommendations for the use of diseasemodifying anti-rheumatic drugs and biologic agents in the treatment of rheumatoid arthritis. Arthritis Care Res. 2012;64:625–39.
36. Smolen J, Landewé R, Breedveld F, et al. EULAR recommendations for the management of rheumatoid arthritis with synthetic and biological disease-modifying antirheumatic drugs. Ann Rheum Dis. 2010. https://doi.org/10.1136/ard.2009.126532.
37. National I Nstitute For Health And Clinical Excellence. The management of rheumatoid arthritis in adults. London: NICE; 2009. www.nice.org.uk/CG79. Accessed 16 June 2017.
38. Felson DT, Anderson JJ, Boers M, et al. The American College of Rheumatology preliminary core set of disease activity measures for rheumatoid arthritis clinical trials. Arthritis Rheum. 1993;36:729–40.
39. Smolen J, Keystone E. Future of RA: building on what we know and tailoring treatment biologic therapies beyond conventional DMARDs. Rheumatology. 2012;51:v55–6.
40. El Miedany Y. PROMs in inflammatory arthritis: moving from static to dynamic. Clin Rheumatol. 2013;32:735–42.
41. Neher M, Stahl C, Festin K, Nilsen P. Implementation of evidence-based practice in rheumatology: what sociodemographic, social cognitive and contextual factors influence health professionals' use of research in practice? J Rheum Dis Treat. 2016;2:039.
42. Straus SE. Evidence-based health care: challenges and limitations. Evid-Based Commun Assess Interv. 2007;1:48–51.
43. Olsson T. Reconstructing evidence-based practice: an investigation of three conceptualisations of EBP. Evid Policy. 2007;3:271–85.
44. Yost J, Ganann R, Thompson D, Aloweni F, Newman K, et al. The effectiveness of knowledge translation interventions for promoting evidenceinformed decision-making among nurses in tertiary care: a systematic review and meta-analysis. Implement Sci. 2015;10:98.
45. Aarons A, Ehrhart MG, Farahnak LR, Sklar M. Aligning leadership across systems and organizations to develop a strategic climate for evidencebased practice implementation. Annu Rev Public Health. 2014:255–74.
46. Rycroft-Malone J, Burton CR, Harvey G, McCormack B, Graham I, et al. Implementing health research through academic and clinical partnerships: a realistic evaluation of the Collaborations for Leadership in Applied Health Research and Care (CLAHRC). Implement Sci. 2011;6:74.
47. Presseau J, Johnson M, Heponiemi T, Elovainio M, Francis JJ, et al. Reflective and automatic processes in health care professional behaviour: a dual process model tested across multiple behaviours. Ann Behav Med. 2014;48:347–58.

48. Downs SH, Black N. The feasibility of creating a checklist for the assessment of the methodological quality both of randomised and non-randomised studies of health care interventions. J Epidemiol Community Health. 1998;52:377–84.
49. Laupacis A, Sackett DL, Roberts RS. An assessment of clinically useful measures of the consequences of treatment. N Engl J Med. 1988;318:1728–33.
50. Pendleton A, Arden N, Dougados M, Doherty M, Bannwarth B, Bijlsma JWJ, et al. EULAR recommendations for the management of knee osteoarthritis: report of a task force of the standing committee for international clinical studies including therapeutic trials (ESCISIT). Ann Rheum Dis. 2000;59:936–44.
51. Bohlin I, Sager M. Evidensens många ansikten. Lund: Arkiv; 2011. (Lettland).
52. Gupta S. Evidence-based practice of rheumatology: a view-point. Indian J Rheumatol. 2007;2(2):72–5.

Chapter 5
Towards Modern Basic Science Teaching in Medical Education

Introduction

For a century, there have been repeated calls to integrate basic science into medical education. The start was in 1910, when Flexner, a high school teacher, an outsider to the practice of medicine and medical education, was commissioned to re-evaluate the medical education system in the United States and Canada [1]. He was chosen for his expertise as an educator, having critiqued the American schooling system and having explored pedagogical techniques. The landmark publication, known as *Flexner Report*, suggested that the medical school curriculum should consist of 2 years dedicated to basic sciences followed by 4 years for clinical education. The revolution of medical education, spurred by the *Flexner Report*, instilled scientific rigour into medical education, and basic science became an aid to protect and preserve professional autonomy. However, in the 1980s, instigated by the accelerated pace since that time, a new educational concept has been adopted by medical schools. The new medical curricula considered both basic and clinical sciences as complementary; hence they were integrated in the medical education model.

However, although few would argue the importance of basic sciences or that novices should be exposed to a variety of cases, clinical teachers continue to debate the role of basic sciences and biomedical knowledge in routine clinical reasoning. Whereas basic scientists may tout the importance of their discipline, some clinicians see the basic sciences as only peripherally relevant to daily practice. Proponents of such an argument can find ample support in the clinical reasoning literature, citing numerous examples of expert reasoning that is seemingly independent of basic science knowledge [1–3]. Pattern recognition [1] and other forms of non-analytic reasoning [4] can lead to accurate clinical decisions with little-to-no biomedical knowledge. A clinician simply does not need to recall the specific mechanism of a disease in order to recognize the similarities between two patients, suggesting that there is little need for basic science knowledge to play a substantial role in any model of the nature of medical expertise.

Y. El Miedany, *Rheumatology Teaching*,
https://doi.org/10.1007/978-3-319-98213-7_5

The recent developments in the management of rheumatic diseases, such as biologic therapy and small molecular medications, highlighted the vital role of basic sciences in clinical medicine, not only to understand its mechanism of action but also to evaluate its negative impact and interactions in the human body. The purpose of this chapter is to reflect on the questions regarding the relevance of basic sciences from the perspective of a clinical educator: how does basic science knowledge contribute to the competence of a physician, to what extent shall basic sciences be incorporated in the medical teaching, what are the barriers and how do basic sciences fit into the medical practice? Key supporting literature will be cited.

Basic Sciences in Medical Education: The Barriers

There have been several questions regarding whether basic science is relevant to medical education or just science needs to be taught in a different way. This paved the way to another query; given the explosion of scientific information, "what needs to be taught and when?"

While it sounds unlogical to argue about the central role of basic sciences in the practice of medicine, there have been some challenges which have risen in the last few years. One challenge came from a faculty in charge of the medical curriculum. A report published on revisiting *Flexner Report* [5] stated that "there is tension between the time needed to teach an ever-expanding knowledge base science, and the time needed for increased instruction in clinical application and it behavioural, ethical and managerial knowledge and skills needed in preparation for the clinical experiences".

Another challenge came from the fact that we are dealing with a new generation of task-oriented students. In an article about undergraduate curriculum in the twentieth century, Weatherall [6] stated that "many students still have genuine doubts about the value of basic sciences to which they had been exposed". Interestingly, the student views were in concordance with the leaders in science opinion, though reasons may appear different. The Scientific Foundations for Future Physicians from the Howard Hughes Medical Institute (HHMI) [7] reported that "In recent years the scientific knowledge important to learning and practice of medicine has changed dramatically, while the approach to science education in the premedical and medical curricula has essentially remained unchanged". This was supported by another report published by Sweeney in 1999 [8], who argued that "the curricular problem to basic scientists is that much of clinical medicine remains unnecessarily unscientific", and therefore "Until clinical medicine itself changes, the utility of science in the training of a physician will remain difficult to demonstrate".

Perhaps, such dialogue has clarified the challenge. Basic sciences are expanding as well as clinical sciences; yet, the time to teach the students is limited, and the students are expecting a new style of teaching which needs to be formalized. In their article on the role and value of the basic sciences in medical education, Finnerty and co-authors [5] posed – and answered – 5 questions on the 100th anniversary of the

Flexner report: What are the sciences that constitute the foundation for medical practice? What is the role of science in being ready for practice at different stages of training? When and how should the foundational sciences be incorporated into the medical school curriculum? What instructional methods and what assessment tools are used? What sciences are prerequisites to enter medical school *and* What are the examples of best practices?

Basic Sciences and the Physician Competency

Addressing ways of incorporating basic sciences into the medical education and how basic science fits into the physician's competency relies on the basic understanding of what the "competence" of an individual physician means. One accepted definition of competence was proposed by Epstein and Hundert: "the habitual and judicious use of communication, knowledge, technical skills, clinical reasoning, emotions, the values and reflection in daily practice for the benefit of the individual and community being served" [9]. In concordance, a similar approach was embodied in the "six general competencies" adopted by the Accreditation Council for Graduate Medical Education (ACGME) which divides competency into medical knowledge, interpersonal and communication skills, professionalism, patient care, system-based practice and practice-based learning [10]. In both models, competence is considered as a multidimensional construct in which knowledge is given a prominent role, and a knowledge of basic sciences (normal human structure and function, and mechanisms of disease and therapy) is explicit.

The Epstein definition situates competence in the specific, local context in which the physician provides care for a specific individual patient or community. These six aspects, into which competence is divided, are applied to that specific patient. An alternative to the "analytic" model suggested by Epstein and Hundert [9], in which competency entailed six domains, has been a "synthetic" model combining knowledge, skills and attitudes into: "competence is bringing to each patient in your practice what the patient requires, and nothing extraneous" [11, 12].

Since the magnitude of the science knowledge required is linked to the practice of the individual (specialty, context and scope of practice), and in view of the growing responsibility levels of medical students and residents, the problem can be framed more developmentally, and basic science education can be tailored to the physician's speciality and requirements. Another approach is changing the integration style, for example, from "preclinical/clinical" to vertical/spiral integration. This agrees with the approach of asking what students are expecting to bring to the required situations (courses and clerkships) at a specific level of their training. Additionally, as the student moves towards graduation and has chosen a specialty, this formulation fosters more flexible learning of the basic science (individual study and electives). Such concept has reflected on the common integration strategies which mandated the rearrangement of basic science and clinical curricula, early exposure to real and simulated clinical experiences, problem-based learning and shared teaching [13, 14]. While there is limited practical evidence for the value of many of these curricular integration efforts, this new concept of "cognitive integration" may reflect a new understanding where the integration of basic and clinical sciences is a cognitive activity that occurs within the learner, not in the curriculum [13]. Cognitive integration is supported through day-to-day micro-level teaching and involves specific pedagogical strategies that purposefully link the basic and clinical sciences.

How Basic Science Fits into the Medical Practice

Over the past years, there has been a growing body of literature on how basic science fits into the practice of medicine. Most of the literature focuses on the task of making a diagnosis ("diagnostic reasoning") rather than the broader concept of "clinical decision-making" which entails diagnostic and therapeutic planning, as well as shared decision-making with the patients [15]. Since, initially, students are given responsibility for thinking through problems, but not for unsupervised care of patients, this has been an appropriate first focus for educational research.

Is basic science knowledge required for developing diagnostic reasoning? This was assumed in the original "Flexner report" in which 2 years of basic science was endorsed as a prerequisite for learning clinical medicine. The domain of medical knowledge was seen as two distinct types of knowledge: one a knowledge of mechanisms (normal structure and function and derangements of these normal tissues/pathways) and the other a knowledge of clinical medicine (the disease manifestations) [16]. However, in real-life scenarios, there is not such a strict separation. Initially the treating physicians are responsible for understanding and explaining what is happening with their patients (from a point of view of mechanism). This meets the patients' curiosity of understanding what is going wrong in their body and ways to fix it. This is followed by the physician moving towards diagnostic and therapeutic planning which meets the patients' anticipation and in turn reflects the physicians' competency.

There has been a shift in terms of general principle of management towards "evidence-based medicine" and diagnostic/management guidelines, which became preferable to pathophysiologic analysis. This could be attributed to being more cost-efficient and in tune with what healthcare policy leaders see as a priority in practice and education [15]. However, large-scale, multicentre clinical trials can only give a rough approximation of a course of action, and in most of the standard day-to-day clinical practice, patients' presentations do not match the guidelines or outcomes of clinical studies. Therefore, physicians are expected to act, particularly in complex circumstances where clinical presentation might be obscure or "data" are not available, to dictate a course of action. In such cases the physician is expected to use professional skills and cognitive integration to achieve a patient-centred decision; and in such cases the treating physicians tend to verbalize the knowledge of mechanism that helped them solve problems. This supports the earlier findings [17, 18] which revealed that expert physicians, in dealing with difficult cases, uncertainty or managing complexity, do rely on the understanding of basic mechanisms.

Lastly, what separates physicians from other healthcare workers, such as physician assistants and those who must follow algorithmic care, is the ability to handle complex problems. In this respect, medical education must ensure appropriate teaching and training for those who not only follow practice guidelines but who can write such guidelines and who have the authority to deviate from or "violate" practice guidelines. This is supported by Finnerty's statement: "if physicians are to be more than technicians, then an understanding of science is essential" [5].

Which Basic Sciences Are Mandatory for Medical Practice

Out of the wide range of basic sciences, the three "Ps" are closest to the surface: physiology, pathology and pharmacology for all cases/patients, with microbiology and biochemistry dominating for diseases from the internal or external ecology, as well as from nutrition. Anatomy is essential for localized symptoms (for instance, pain and swelling) and specialities such as rheumatology and orthopaedics (Table 5.1).

Using the general definition of competence as the ability to bring to the situation (patient) what is required, the level and kind of understanding required depend on the specific problem at hand. Therefore, the competent physician must be able to move "downwards" (deeper) from a consideration of organ systems within the body to more detailed levels of mechanism and granularity (cellular and genetic mechanisms, and molecules) or "upwards" to a broader, biopsychosocial framework (such as substance dependence and family dynamics), moving from person to family and from local environment to society, and even, as required by the individual patient, to a healthcare delivery model system level. Therefore, the individual physician must have access to a wide repertory of foundational sciences available from molecular biology and genomics to physiology and organ histology, behavioural psychology as well as epidemiology and biostatistics [15].

Table 5.1 Why basic science is important for the rheumatologist

1. Rheumatology practice requires the activation and integration of both clinical and biomedical knowledge
2. To establish valuable coherence among the clinical features
3. Essential for patient education and "thinking aloud" to explain how they arrived at their conclusions
4. Inclusion of basic science facts enhances learning of novel content
5. Basic sciences form the base for all the recent rheumatology in a wide range of therapies
6. Basic science, anatomy, is important for all the procedures carried out in the standard daily practice and is vital for musculoskeletal ultrasonography

Basic Science for Postgraduates: From Understanding to Action

During medical school and after graduation, the student and later the junior doctors are gradually given more responsibility in the care of real patients; hence they acquire more "competence" for their level of training. Overall, the trainees move from understanding to action. Action takes more than knowledge and is a task that cannot easily be embraced within a cognitive model in which a trainee's understanding alone is enough. This paves the way to an important question: can basic science play a role in the formation of professional character, in which behavioural and social concepts are more fundamental?

This progression from understanding to action is even more explicit in one specific formulation, the "reporter–interpreter–manager–educator" framework [19]. In this framework basic science supports the young doctor's gathering and explaining clinical findings on their own patients. Knowledge of the anatomy of the upper limb, for instance, is essential for diagnosing shoulder/elbow or hand pain; knowledge of the normal physiology of muscle contraction is essential for understanding muscle cramps; knowledge of normal and abnormal histology supports learning to interpret patterns of muscle biopsy, whereas knowledge of immunology is important for linking the clinical findings to the most likely diagnosis and appropriate management. The knowledge is not there for its own sake but to support the responsibility that the young doctor will be given. The use of clinical vignettes, in which the basic science questions are embedded in USMLE-Step 1, reflects this linking of cognitive expertise to a potential role for students in patient care.

Motivation and Motivating Adult Learners in Medical Education

One of the early theories of motivation in medical education is that of "adult education" described by Malcolm Knowles [20]. Knowles proposed that "andragogy" (adult learning) should be distinct from "pedagogy" (child learning) because there are fundamental differences between the two groups of learners. The theory has evolved over time and is based on five fundamental principles, the fifth of which addresses motivation to learn; Knowles proposed that as a person matures, the motivation to learn shifts from external to internal.

In 2000, Ryan and Deci [21] presented a more complex model of motivation, in keeping with developments in cognitive psychology. Self-determination theory is centred on the importance of intrinsic motivation and how it drives human behaviour. Many of the studies of motivation in medical education are based on the "Self Determination Theory" [21–25]. Engaging in something because it is inherently interesting or enjoyable is deemed intrinsic motivation, while doing something because it leads to a separable outcome (e.g. grades, test scores, etc.) is extrinsic motivation. Their approach focuses on three needs: the need for competence, the need for autonomy and the need for relatedness. Self-determination theory recognizes that basic need satisfaction is partly created from engaging in activities that are interesting for the individual.

As adult learners, medical students are responsible for their own educational paths and lifelong learning. Modern medical education curricula are based on the premise that students have an inherent desire to become physicians and are motivated by internal rather than external factors [26]. Adults are autonomous and self-directed; therefore, teaching medical students should focus on facilitating learning while leaving the students free to direct themselves. Medical educators assume that as adult learners, medical students pursue medicine because it is inherently interesting and enjoyable, rather than for obtaining a separable outcome such as monetary reward or status [27].

However, while the modern teaching techniques target the internally motivated adult learner, at least some students may continue to behave as externally motivated learners. Those can be identified as being unmotivated in certain courses, not striving to meet standards, or may feel a difference between the institutions' goals and their own [26]. There are still a number of aspects of the current medical education programs that push students to behave in externally motivated patterns. It is essential to realize that motivation is a multifaceted concept. Therefore, educators should strive to find new techniques of increasing student's propensity towards self-directed learning [28]. The hope of this type of medical education is to create lifelong learners who feel a personal responsibility for their own knowledge. Consideration of different motivation patterns may result in a curriculum that motivates a greater portion of the class. Perhaps even more important is to become mindful of the characteristics of the curriculum that are robbing our students of the motivation they had.

However, enhancing motivation among the current students faces another challenge. Current generation, Generation Y (otherwise known as the millennial generation), refers to individuals born between 1982 and 2005 [29]. Generation Y has unique characteristics that affect learning in positive and negative ways. To ensure success, medical educators need to understand that Generation Y cannot be forced into the past generation's fashion. Differences are not necessarily weaknesses. On the basis of relevant literature, educators in graduate medical education should focus on four core areas: (1) interactive teaching with technology, (2) professionalism, (3) mentoring (or parenting) and (4) communication and feedback [30].

Generation Y is technology savvy and advanced in readiness to use new medical technologies [31]. Medical educators need to stay abreast of new technologies and incorporate them into teaching. Successful strategies will involve hands-on teaching with simulations and group discussion. Collaborative learning coupled with immediate feedback within a practical context is key [32]. Teachers should not rely on lectures as a primary teaching method. When lectures are used, they should

Table 5.2 Addressing motivation with computer-based resources among "millennial" learners

"Millennial" learners
Value interactivity
Are comfortable with technology
Enjoy learning by trial and error
Benefit from social connectedness
Appreciate frequent feedback

incorporate multimedia presentations or bring in live patients for case discussions with audience participation. Educators should involve residents in a project or case study that requires active problem-solving on their part (Table 5.2). Educators not as conversant with technology could use Generation Y's expertise by involving them in a technology advisory committee.

Modern Basic Sciences Teaching

How to Teach Basic Science?

The "how" is to be answered by two tests of success, which are of equal importance: one, can the students retrieve the essential facts from memory and apply them to the patient at hand; and two, is the student driven to answer the question "Why?" So, teaching methods are not aimed solely at students' memory but at their motivation and intuitive search for explanations – Is there an emotional need to explain signs and symptoms through mechanism? If not, the faculty have probably failed in this essential goal.

While differential diagnosis of clinical problems, such as rheumatoid arthritis, psoriatic arthritis or osteoarthritis, can be memorized as part of illness scripts, there is evidence that pathophysiologic understanding of mechanism supports longer-term retrieval from memory [33]. Whether in lectures, small-group teaching or one on one, the teacher probes the student's ability to unify the surface features of symptoms, signs and laboratory findings with underlying mechanisms.

As students move from understanding to action, and to the management of common problems, a knowledge of pathology and pharmacology becomes more and more essential and is essential for all training in each specialty of medical practice. But are specific learning needs the same for learners at different levels? Do students need to grasp all problems at the same level as specialists? Rheumatology fellows are more apt to be thrilled by uric acid metabolism than surgeons. Similarly, the actions of JAK kinase inhibitors are more attractive for both rheumatologists and oncologists. The problem may be resolved by deciding the specific expectations for the role of the learner at each level, i.e. what level of knowledge and competence is expected [15, 34].

Filling the Gaps

Quality teaching in medical education matters for student learning outcomes. The onus lies this time on the medical education centres. Fostering quality teaching presents education institutions with a range of challenges at a time when the education sector is coming under pressure from many different directions. Medical schools need to ensure that the education they offer meets the expectations of students as well as the requirements of medical services and patients, both today and for the future. Yet medical education schools are complex organizations where the university-wide vision and strategy need to be well-aligned with bottom-up practices and innovations in teaching and learning. Developing medical schools as effective learning communities where excellent andragogical practices are developed and shared also requires leadership, collaboration and ways to address tensions between innovators and those reluctant to change. Several aspects can help to enhance the teaching quality. One of the key factors in modern education is identifying gaps in faculty expertise and resources. Using other sources for core knowledge frees faculty to function as a facilitator (rather than a source of knowledge). Using online distribution can be a valuable tool as it allows wider dissemination of expert teaching. It not only represents a model of enhancing lifelong learning skills but also helps learners identify gaps in understanding as well as identify sources of "master teaching".

Using Narratives

Narrative learning can be a valuable tool to engage the audience and in conducting the message. There are strong theoretical arguments for the benefits of narrative learning (learning through narratives or stories) in medical education, particularly in the areas of meaning-making ("making sense") [35]. Narrative structure gets learners' attention, creates suspense, highlights important content and supports internal motivators. Figure 5.1 shows a model of the personal narrative structure [36].

There is evidence that stories are used widely outside the lecture theatre in medical training. Formal case histories (professional narratives about clinical cases) are used widely, for example, on ward rounds or in meetings, and observational studies

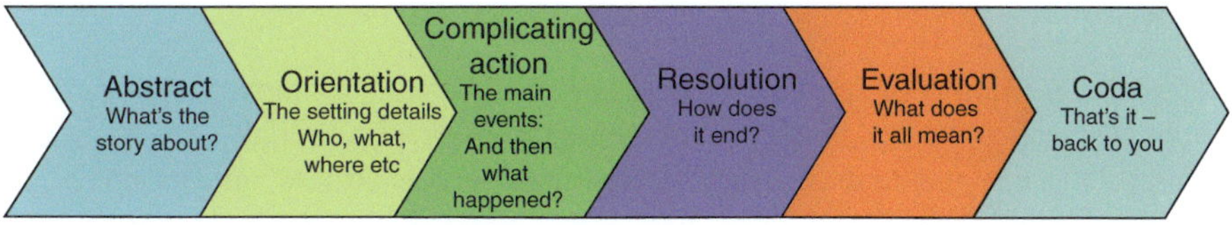

Fig. 5.1 Labov's model of the structure of the personal narratives, developed from his sociolinguistic work on the varieties of English. (Data from Labov and Waletzky [36])

have confirmed that more informal "anecdotes" are used widely in educational settings in hospitals [37, 38]. A questionnaire study has suggested that general practitioner (GP) trainers also use anecdotes frequently in teaching trainee GPs in a clinical GP setting [39]. There are many other examples of narratives being used in the curriculum, for example, in medical humanities programmes [40], significant event analysis (or critical incident analysis) [41] and reflection on practice [42].

The use of narratives in basic medical science lectures might be challenging, perhaps because the more formal and traditional setting encourages a more didactic teaching style. Educational theory suggests that tactics such as setting memorable context or encouraging the development of relevant connections or anchors may help students to get the most from their lectures [43]. Stories could be an effective way to promote understanding and embed new ideas in the narrative component of the listener's long-term memory [44]. For medical students in basic science lectures, narratives or stories may be particularly relevant in promoting the more humanistic aspects of medicine, including professional identity and empathy [45].

Using Media and Social Intelligence

Social intelligence examines the way humans are programmed to connect with one another. In his book *The New Science of Human Relationships* [46], Goleman stated his belief that emotional and social intelligence are more powerful than other intelligences. TV can give a good example of "How to tell a story". Television can be considered as the quintessential storytelling medium, though not always great art but always expert at keeping your attention! "Law and Order" can be one of the most perfect models for teaching science. Telling the story of an investigation is not that what science is; it is how we make inquiry interesting. Perhaps, this is what made it the longest running crime drama on American TV. Though it is still in syndication and has ended in 2010, it gave birth to multiple spinoffs. The core of such activity is to make a particular part or feature of the science easier to understand, define, quantify, visualize or simulate by referencing it to existing and usually commonly accepted knowledge.

Online Education

Medical education is facing various challenges in teaching tomorrow's physicians. Technological advances have become integral parts of our daily practice and changed the life standards forever, increasingly with each new generation. Such changes mean that medical schools must adopt new teaching methods while maintaining excellence in medical education. The new methods include electronic (e-learning) software programs as well as online or web-based learning. These methods shift teaching from a largely teacher-centred, product-based activity to a more student-centred, process-based activity. This strategy encourages students to be active in the experience of learning rather than being passive learners [47]. Ford et al. [48] stated that "integrating teaching, learning and technology is a mandate, not an option, and doing any less would border on professional irresponsibility". While cost is a significant barrier, such innovations can have a large impact on self-directed learning, especially when human resources are limited. Examples of implementation of online resources for teaching science include: (1) Replacing local didactics with expert presentations and group discussions. This approach mixes benefits of social learning with benefits of best-available expert teaching. However, it requires organization, identification of resources as well as supportive local community. (2) Bedside/clinic "assignments" with instructor feedback. Problem-based learning is less likely to be comprehensive in such medical education course. A good example is the "educational prescription" model. (3) Self-directed learning supported by local or national/global mentors and colleagues. Examples are online virtual learning programs. However, this depends on the resources available to individual learners and motivation to engage. Table 5.3 gives examples of web-based resources for teaching rheumatology science.

Storytelling in online education is a new style of online medical education where the "instructor" can be a software program. There are several websites already available with many examples of how clinical education may use cases to focus and highlight instructional content.

The American College of Rheumatology launched its online rheumatology e-learning module (https://www.rheumatology.org/Learning-Center/Educational-Activities/Details?meetingId=%7B8147887A-59F8-E611-A224-005056987EFD%7D). The creation of Rheum4Science modules grew out of the conviction that the teaching of science is declining in rheumatology. Rheum4Science is designed to teach the underlying biology and clinical research methodology necessary for the knowledgeable practice of rheumatology. This basic and clinical science curriculum is designed as a series of online case-based modules that can be used by trainees or practitioners working independently or with a faculty mentor. These are brief, targeted interactive modules. Each module addresses a focused topic or educational need. The interactivity module supports user engagement and reinforces learning objectives with immediate feedback available for self-assessment activities. The modules are self-paced and allow unlimited repetition as desired. To link it to the standard practice, each module starts and ends with a case, and narratives engage the learners. In general, cases illustrate the relevance of science topics to clinical practice.

Blended Learning

The method of combining electronic and face-to-face learning, known as "blended learning", is gaining popularity as increasing numbers of medical colleges use the Internet as the digital repository of teaching and learning forums [49]. E-learning provides possibilities for devising new educational tools, for learning by

Table 5.3 Web-based resources for teaching rheumatology science

Format	Examples	Link	Pros	Cons
Online books/resources	Kelly textbook of Rheumatology	https://www.sciencedirect.com/science/book/9780323316965	User-friendly, self-paced	Easier to skip "painful" areas
	UpToDate	https://www.uptodate.com/contents/table-of-contents/rheumatology	Structured and comprehensive	Less interactive
			Familiar format	
			Continuing resource	
			Easy to search online versions and easier to update	
Video or recorded lectures	ACR	www.rheumatology.org	User-friendly	Not easy to find
	EULAR	https://www.eular.org/school_of_rheumatology.cfm	Access to missed/unattended lectures	Time-consuming
			Can be viewed more than once	Quality might not be good
				Lack of interaction option
Webinar	Rheumatology toolbox	https://rheumatologytoolbox.com/registration/	User-friendly	Time-consuming
	Canadian immunology and biology research network	https://cibrn.org/2016/11/28/webinar-for-cibrn-rheumatology-subgroup-with-dr-carter-thorne-and-dr-philip-baer-thurs-dec-1-630-pm-est/	Up to date	Lack of interaction
			Availability of choosing the topic of interest	

Interactive courses	Rheum4Science	https://www.rheumatology.org/Learning-Center/Educational-Activities/Details?meetingId=%7B8147887A-59F8-E611-A224-005056987EFD%7D	User-friendly	Time-consuming
			Immediate feedback	Need subscription
			Self-paced	
			Risk taking: trial and error	
Online modules	Organization body (BSR)/university courses	www.rheumatology.org.uk	Comprehensive	Time-consuming
			User-friendly	
			Self-paced	
	Medscape	www.medscape.com	Information dissemination	Need subscription
			Creation of learners' communities and networking	

interactivity, self-paced study and easy access. To overcome the lack of a teacher in a real classroom, face-to-face teaching should be included in the course. Blended learning translates this theory into practice [50]. The term describes models of learning that combine several instructional methods, such as the use of digital resources (or e-learning) alongside traditional teaching [51]. Blended learning allows adaptive, collaborative learning and transforms the role of the teacher from a disseminator of knowledge to a facilitator. Therefore, a combination of traditional and online learning in particular or e-learning in general creates a more integrated approach for both instructors and learners. It is well suited for practice-based disciplines like the medical sciences [52]. Studies reported in both the medical and non-medical literature have consistently shown that students are satisfied with e-learning; however, they do not see e-learning as replacing traditional instructor-led training but as a complement, forming part of a blended learning strategy [53, 54]. Another benefit of e-learning for teaching medical basic and clinical sciences is that it can be delivered at any time and any place and can be tailored to individual learning needs. Although blended learning was originally promoted to save costs and increase efficiency, it was found to enhance learning, information dissemination, creation of learners' communities and networking and to support learners in choosing the ideal content [55]. A study carried out to assess the effectiveness of blended learning in studying family medicine as an example of a clinical medical science revealed that medical students, as adult learners, were open to new methods of learning. The study concluded that blended learning approach is an effective method for teaching family medicine and can be applicable to other clinical medical sciences [56].

Medical Education in the Era of Taylorized Medicine

Clinician–educators face special challenges in an era characterized by the erosion of the time allocated for reflection, for identifying new syndromes, for social contact with colleagues and for teaching [57, 58]. The pressure to see more and more patients for increasingly brief visits is of concern for clinicians, students and patients alike.

In 1911, Frederick Taylor, a son of Philadelphia aristocrats who lived at the turn of the last century, became known as the "father of scientific management" – the original "efficiency expert". He believed that the components of every job could and should be scientifically studied, measured, timed and standardized to maximize efficiency and profit. Central to Taylor's system is the notion that there is one best way to do every task and that it is the manager's responsibility to ensure that no worker deviates from it. Taylor asserted "In the past, the man has been first; in the future, the system must be first" [59]. Toyota, inspired by these principles of "Taylorism", successfully applied them to the manufacture of cars, thereby improving quality, eliminating waste and cutting costs. As healthcare comes under increasing economic pressure to achieve these same goals, Taylorism has begun permeating the culture of medicine. Advocates lecture clinicians who argued that patient care should follow standardized systems like those deployed in manufacturing cars. It is not unusual nowadays that managers are measuring the duration of the patient's visit whether in the outpatient clinic or the accident and emergency departments. The aim is to determine the optimal time for patient–doctor interactions so that they can be standardized. Meanwhile, the electronic health record, introduced with the laudable goals of making patient information readily available and improving safety by identifying dangerous drug–drug interactions, has become a key instrument for measuring the duration and standardizing the content of patient–doctor interactions in pursuit of "the one best way". Encounters have been restructured around the demands of the electronic health record: specific questions must be asked, and answer boxes filled in, to demonstrate to payers the "value" of care. Open-ended interviews, vital for obtaining accurate clinical information and understanding patients' mindsets, have become almost impossible, given the limited time allotted for visits, often only 15–20 min. Instead, patients are frequently given checklists in an effort to streamline the interaction and save precious minutes. While some are seeing the electronic as a good approach to saving time [60], other surveys revealed that nurses and doctors see that it has increased the clinical workload and, more important, taken time and attention away from patients [61].

Similarly, in teaching, standardization integral to Taylorism cannot be applied to many vital aspects of teaching medicine. The inescapable truth of medicine is that students are intellectually, psychologically and culturally diverse. Therefore, despite time constraints, it is up to the teachers and role models to reinforce the highest values of the profession, to examine the curriculum and teaching faculty, to set the teaching protocol implementing the modern technology and information technology as part of the teaching process and to remind the students of the discipline, the great calling, the passion and mystery as well as the elegant adventure that defines medicine. Reflecting on the current challenges to medical profession, a firm response is required as "there is no alternative to truth" [62].

In conclusion, although the educational strategies Flexner proposed in 1910 were daring for the time it was published, they need to be superseded by a more comprehensive set of standards to steer medical schools towards accomplishing their social mandate. There is no doubt basic sciences are vital for every medical student as well as postgraduate doctor, and its precise role as integral part of the expert knowledge base should be clarified. However, teaching these basic sciences should get the benefits of modern technology and teaching techniques to achieve the education targets. For medical educators, there is an urgent need to focus increasingly on the rigorous pathway of reason, guiding the students past the barrage of misleading signals. Incorporating computer technology, wireless and online teaching as well as blended learning to become key teaching approaches provides a relevant context for understanding, engaging learners and promoting memory. For medical students in basic science lectures, narratives or stories may be particularly relevant in promoting the more humanistic aspects of medicine, including professional identity and empathy. More research is needed to provide the evidence of the impact of modern technology on learning outcomes for students.

References

1. Duffy TP. The Flexner report – 100 years later. Yale J Biol Med. 2011;84:269–76.
2. Elstein AS, Schwartz A, Higgs J, Jones M. Clinical reasoning in medicine. Clinical reasoning in the health professions. Oxford: Butterworth Heinemann; 2000. p. 95–106.
3. Norman GR, Brooks LR. The non-analytical basis of clinical reasoning. Adv Health Sci Educ Theory Pract. 1997;2(2):173–84.
4. Patel VL, Evans DA, Groen GJ. Reconciling basic science and clinical reasoning. Teach Learn Med. 1989;1(3):116–21.
5. Finnerty EP, Chauvin S, Bonaminio G, Andrews M, Carroll RG, Pangaro LN. Flexner revisited: the role and value of the basic sciences in medical education. Acad Med. 2010;85(2):349–55.
6. Weatherall DJ. Science in the undergraduate curriculum during the 20th century. Med Educ. 2006;40:195–201.
7. Howard Hughes Medical Institute, Scientific Foundations for Future Physicians, AAMC, 2009.
8. Sweeney G. The challenge for basic science education in problem-based medical education. Clin Invest Med. 1999;22:1v–22.
9. Epstein RM, Hundert EM. Defining and assessing professional competence. J Am Med Assoc. 2002;287:226–35.
10. Accreditation Council for Graduate Medical Education. http://www.acgme.org/outcome/comp/compmin.asp. Accessed 11 Apr 2017.
11. Pangaro L. A new vocabulary and other innovations for improving descriptive in-training evaluations. Acad Med. 1999;74:1203–7.
12. Pangaro L. Investing in descriptive evaluation: a vision for the future of assessment. Med Teach. 2000;22(5):478–81.
13. Kulasegaram KM, Martimianakis MA, Mylopoulos M, Whitehead CR, Woods NN. Cognition before curriculum: rethinking the integration of basic science and clinical learning. Acad Med. 2013;88:1–8.
14. Brauer DG, Ferguson KJ. The integrated curriculum in medical education: AMEE guide no. 96. Med Teach. 2015;37:312–22.
15. Pangaro L. The role and value of the basic sciences in medical education. Acad Med. 2010;85(2):349–55.
16. Patel VL, Evans DA, Groen GJ. Reconciling basic sciences and clinical reasoning. Teach Learn Med. 1989;1:116–21.
17. Patel VL, Groen GJ, Arocha JF. Mem Cogn. 1990;18:394–406.
18. Woods NN, Brooks LR, Norman GR. The role of biomedical knowledge in diagnosis of difficult cases. Adv Health Sci Educ. 2007;12:417–26.
19. Torre DM, Daley BJ, Sebastian JL, Elnicki DM. Overview of current learning theories for medical educators. Am J Med. 2006;119:903–7.
20. Knowles M. The adult learner: a neglected species. 2nd ed. Oxford: Gulf Publishing; 1978. p. 244.
21. Ryan RM, Deci EL. Intrinsic and extrinsic motivations: classic definitions and new directions. Contemp Educ Psychol. 2000;25(1):54–67.
22. Koens F, Mann KV, Custers EJFM, Ten Cate OTJ. Analysing the concept of context in medical education. Med Educ. 2005;39(12):1243–9.
23. Sobral DT. What kind of motivation drives medical students' learning quests? Med Educ. 2004;38(9):950–7.
24. Curry L. Cognitive and learning styles in medical education. Acad Med. 1999;74(4):409–13.
25. Williams GC, Saizow RB, Ryan RM. The importance of self-determination theory for medical education. Acad Med. 1999;74(9):992–5.
26. Mann KV. Motivation in medical education: how theory can inform our practice. Acad Med. 1999;74(3):237–9.

27. Ryan RM, Frederick CM, Lepes D, Rubio N, Sheldon KM. Intrinsic motivation and exercise adherence. Int J Sport Psychol. 1997;28(4):335–54.
28. Misch DA. Andragogy and medical education: are medical students internally motivated to learn? Adv Health Sci Educ. 2002;7(2):153–60.
29. Howell LP, Joad JP, Callahan E, Servis G, Bonham AC. Generational forcecasting in academic medicine: a unique method of planning for success in the next two decades. Acad Med. 2009;84:985–93.
30. Eckleberry-Hunt J, Tucciarone J. The challenges and opportunities of teaching "Generation Y". J Grad Med Educ. 2011;3(4):458–61.
31. Pew Research Center. Millennials: a portrait of generation next. Washington, DC: Pew Research Center; 2010.
32. Mangold K. Educating a new generation: teaching baby boomer faculty about millennial students. Nurse Educ. 2007;32:21–3.
33. Pangaro LN. A primer of evaluation. In: Fincher RM, editor. Guidebook for clerkship directors. 3rd edn. North Syracuse, New York: Alliance for Clinical Education; 2005.
34. Woods NN, Neville AJ, Levinson AJ, Howley EHA, Oczkowski WJ, Norman GR. The value of basic science in clinical diagnosis. Acad Med. 2006;81:S124–7.
35. Hanninen V, Koski-Jannes A. Narratives of recovery from addictive behaviours. Addiction. 1999;94(12):1837–48.
36. Labov W, Waletzky J. Narrative analysis: oral version of personal experience. In: Helm J, editor. Essays on the verbal and visual arts. Seattle: University of Washington Press; 1967. p. 12–44.
37. Hunter K. Doctors' stories – the narrative structure of medical knowledge. Princeton: Princeton University Press; 1991.
38. Hunter K. "There was this one guy …": the uses of anecdotes in medicine. Perspect Biol Med. 1986;29(4):619–30. https://doi.org/10.1353/pbm.1986.0079.
39. Alderson TSJ, Bateman H. Doctors telling stories: the place of anecdote in GP registrar training. Med Teach. 2002;24(6):654–7.
40. Jill Gordon J, Martyn Evans H. Learning medicine from the humanities. In: Swanwick T, editor. Understanding medical education: evidence, theory and practice. London: Association for the Study of Medical Education; 2010. p. 83–98.
41. Pringle M, Bradley C, Carmichael C, Wallis H. Significant event auditing. A study of the feasibility and potential of case-based auditing in primary medical care. Occas Pap R Coll Gen Pract. 1995;70(i–viii):1–71.
42. Sandars J, Murray C, Pellow A. Twelve tips for using digital storytelling to promote reflective learning by medical students. Med Teach. 2008;30(8):774–7.
43. Ausubel DP. Educational psychology: a cognitive view. Austin: Holt, Reinehart and Winston; 1968.
44. Ellis AW, Young AW. Human cognitive neuropsychology: a textbook with readings. East Sussex/New York: Psychology Press; 2013.
45. Easton G. How medical teachers use narratives in lectures: a qualitative study. BMC Med Educ. 2016;16:3.
46. Goleman D. Social intelligence: the new science of human relationships. New York: Bantam Books; 2006.
47. Mellor C. Experiential learning through integrated project work: an example from soil science. J Geogr High Educ. 1991;15(2):135–49.
48. Ford PJ, Foxlee N, Green W. Developing information literacy with first year oral health students. Eur J Dent Educ. 2009;13(1):46–51.
49. Thakore H, McMahon T. Virtually there; e-learning in medical education. Clin Teach. 2006;3:225–8.
50. Lewin LO, Singh M. Blended learning B. Improving education in primary care: development of an online curriculum using the blended learning model. BMC Med Educ. 2009;9:33.
51. Voos R. Blended learning – what is it and where might it take us? Sloan-C View. 2003;2(1):2–5.

52. Karimzadegan D, Mojtahedzadeh R, Mohammadi A. E-learning in medical education in the world and Iran. J Med Educ. 2007;11:37–9.
53. Gibbons A, Fairweather P. Computer-based instruction. In: Tobias S, Fletcher JD, editors. Training and retraining: a handbook for business, industry, government and military. New York: McMillan Reference; 2000. p. 410–42.
54. Chumley-Jones HS, Dobbie A, Alford CL. Web-based learning: sound educational method or hype? A review of the evaluation literature. Acad Med. 2002;77(Suppl. 10):S86–93.
55. Wood BP. Blended learning in medicine: trouble in paradise? Am J Roentgenol. 2011;197:529.
56. Makhdoom N, Khoshha K, Algaidi S, Heissam K, Zolaly M. Blended learning' as an effective teaching and learning strategy in clinical medicine: a comparative cross-sectional university-based study. J Taibah Univ Med Sci. 2013;8(1):12–7.
57. Wenzel RP, Edmond MB. Academic I.D. in jeopardy: the erosion of time, professional values, and physician satisfaction. Infection. 2015;43:141–4.
58. Edmond MB. Taylorized medicine. Ann Intern Med. 2010;153:845–6.
59. Taylor FW. The principles of scientific management. New York: Harper & Brothers; 1911.
60. Palmer D, El-Miedany. EROMIA in inflammatory arthritis: the next step in standard practice. Br J Nurs. 2010;19(1):42–6.
61. Hartzband P, Groopman J. Medical Taylorism. N Engl J Med. 2016;374:106–8.
62. Wenzel RP. Medical education in the era of alternative facts. N Engl J Med. 2017;377(7):607–9.

Part III
The Art of Teaching

Chapter 6
The Art of Patient History Taking

Introduction

One of the most common aphorisms quoted in medical history is “Listen to your patients; they are telling you the diagnosis” [1]. Gaining a clear description of a clinical problem has long been recognized as the basis of a correct diagnosis and reflects good communication between doctor and patient. Reasoning and rational practice based on clinical observation was taught by Hippocrates in the fourth century BC. The value of clinical observation was further promoted by physicians such as Thomas Sydenham and William Heberden who promoted the value of clinical observation and history taking in clinical medicine [2].

In contrast to many chronic diseases, where a single “gold standard” measure, such as blood pressure in hypertension, haemoglobin A_1C in diabetes, lipid profile in hyperlipidaemia, etc., is applicable to diagnosis, management, prognosis and analyses of outcomes in all individual patients whether as part of clinical trials, clinical care or long-term databases, in inflammatory arthritic conditions, taking the patient’s history and clinical examination represent the “gold standard” for diagnosis [3]. Furthermore, identification of the earliest signs of musculoskeletal conditions is vital for improving their management, as well as prognosis [4].

This chapter will provide a standardized approach to the history taking and clinical assessment of patients presenting with musculoskeletal complaints, whether presenting to primary care, general medicine, rheumatology or orthopaedics. The aim is to help in guidance and giving a benchmark for competency. The described diagnostic strategic approach can also be used for standard clinical practice as well as a teaching aid.

Y. El Miedany, *Rheumatology Teaching*,
https://doi.org/10.1007/978-3-319-98213-7_6

The Art of Teaching

Taking a history and performing a clinical examination are core skills that are taught at an early stage of undergraduate medical education. However, at this stage, this knowledge is given usually at a basic level. After graduation, particularly on participating in a clinical attachment to a rheumatology or orthopaedics the candidates realize that their practical skills of musculoskeletal examination are lacking and that further training in taking history and clinical examination is required to achieve an optimum state in musculoskeletal medicine. When teaching clinical skills of the musculoskeletal system, it is essential that training doctors acquire a standardized approach to history taking, analysis and characteristics of the symptoms, physical examination and approach to how to interpret these clinical data [5, 6]. Musculoskeletal system is often regarded as complex in comparison to the other organ systems, therefore, appropriate history taking and examination is mandatory to identify whether the patient's symptoms represent a primary musculoskeletal disorder or secondary to another disease. An integrated musculoskeletal disease course for medical students, bringing together orthopaedics, rheumatology and physical medicine and rehabilitation, has been found to be effective [7].

It is best for one tutor to teach the basic skills to small groups (maximum ten students). History taking is an integrated part of the initial sessions, but as history is related to knowledge of the conditions, it needs to be highlighted in the context of the teaching session for each specific problem. The primary goal of the initial sessions is how to link the patients' symptoms to give a provisional diagnosis or differential diagnosis. This should be followed by another teaching phase where trainees will be able to examine a normal person, preferably coupled with a student-directed session that reviews the anatomy of the musculoskeletal system [8]. With these basic generic skills, and skills in regional examination, the students can move on to examine patients in the clinical setting and learn to recognize and characterize abnormalities. This can be done by attending outpatient clinics, by serving in the emergency room or at the admission of patients for elective procedures. Patient educators, such as the Patient Partner Program, in which people with arthritis are trained to teach students about taking a history and performing a clinical examination, have also been shown to be an effective method of teaching clinical skills [9–12].

History taking is a cornerstone and key component of patient assessment, enabling the delivery of high-quality care. Understanding the complexity of musculoskeletal system and processes involved in history taking allows the treating doctor to gain a better understanding of patients' problems and be able to make a diagnosis, hence a treatment plan. Thereafter, care priorities can be identified, and the most appropriate interventions are commenced to optimize patient outcomes. A good percentage of medical students and trainees are less comfortable with the idea of formally taking a patient history [13]. The concern is mainly focused on the style of handling a patient presenting with musculoskeletal complaint and conducting a structured assessment to generate a comprehensive picture of a patient's health and health problems. The coming section will summarize modern skills of how to take a musculoskeletal patient's history with views towards making a provisional if not a definite diagnosis.

Is Rheumatology Different?

Teaching a complex and potentially time-consuming MSK history taking and examination to medical students and young rheumatologists is fraught with difficulty. How much should they be taught? How do we get them to take it seriously, to learn the agreed skills to an optimum level of competence and to use these skills in clinical practice? The current trend in MSK teaching emphasizes the need for sound clinical skills as a fundamental part of the medical courses taught [14]. The unique character of rheumatic diseases is that it interacts with all body systems. Musculoskeletal symptoms might be the first presentation of other systemic diseases such as thyroid or diabetes mellitus. Similarly, rheumatic diseases might present initially or during its course with pulmonary, cardiac or skin symptoms. Because of the importance of patients' symptoms and clinical findings in making a diagnosis, and the lack of "gold standard" diagnostic tests, history taking in rheumatology plays a vital part of the diagnosis and management process.

Another challenge that makes rheumatology different is that, in comparison to the standard medical history taking, musculoskeletal history taking may require a unique viewing angle. In fact, there are similarities between the neurological and the musculoskeletal history taking [14]. Both are potentially very extensive with many components of the patient's history likely to be rewarding in individual patients. Because of this, in practice, experienced clinicians may modify their history taking and consequently examination according to the history and what they find on their initial encounter. The expert clinician has come to this through years of experience, but it should be possible to teach more junior clinicians in a structured way starting with a basic history-taking skills followed by examination principles and building on to it a more detailed examination that reflects the sort of patients they see and the setting they are in.

The Art of Taking History

Obtaining a true, representative account of what is troubling a patient and how it has evolved over time is not an easy task. It requires patience, practice, understanding and concentration. The history is simply a sharing of experience between patient and doctor. A consultation can allow a patient to unburden himself or herself. They may be upset about their condition or with the frustrations of life; therefore, it is important to allow patients to give vent to these feelings. This may turn the history into small pieces of information mixing between the patient's symptoms and the impact of the disease on the patient's life and his ability to carry out activities of daily living, an important aspect particularly in patients living with musculoskeletal conditions. Appreciating the patient's feelings and the negative impact on the patient's life is critical for obtaining further information from the patient. The importance of the lament and how it may be transformed from the grumbles of a heartsink patient to a useful diagnostic and therapeutic tool for both patient and physician has been discussed in an earlier published interesting paper [15].

However, it is the job of the treating physician to put the bits and pieces taken from the patient's history together. Furthermore, the doctor should be able to stratify the patient's history into those symptoms in relation to the disease, as well as duration of illness, and the others related to the impact of the disease on the patient whether physical or psychological.

Musculoskeletal history, to some extent, can be different from the general medicine history taking. Table 6.1 shows a seven-item musculoskeletal history. After listening first and listening second, giving the patients the chance to tell their story which they have been storing up for the treating doctor, it is important for the treating healthcare professional to be able to ask discriminating questions about some symptoms to verify their actual nature and give enough information to support the process of making a diagnosis. The treating doctor can go back to the overall picture and break down any aspects of the history that he feels require further clarification. This is a much better way of doing things than interrupting, and probably losing forever, the patient's initial narrative. However, in some scenarios, some patients do not come readily prepared with a proper description of their illness, and in such situation, and to be able to "draw out" the history, it is unavoidable to use questioning and clarification of the patient's symptoms. Table 6.2 shows the core competencies the healthcare professional should have in the history-taking process from patients presenting with musculoskeletal problems.

Table 6.1 The musculoskeletal seven-part history

1. Presenting complaint
2. History of the presenting complaint including all the relevant musculoskeletal questions
3. Impact on the patient functional ability and quality of life
4. History of systemic illness: whether preceding, associated or consequent
5. Past medical and surgical history
6. Drug history and allergies
7. Family history
8. Social history

Table 6.2 The art of history taking: healthcare professionals managing patients presenting with musculoskeletal problems should be able to perform several key competencies

A. *Competency of musculoskeletal history taking:* reflecting on the main characteristics of the major rheumatological conditions and able to identify:
The symptom is acute, chronic or acute on top of chronic
The condition is mechanical or inflammatory in origin
The symptoms are related to joint or soft tissue problem
The symptoms represent a primary musculoskeletal condition or secondary to another systemic disease
The impact of the condition on the patient's health-related quality of life activities (both functional ability and quality of life)
The link between the patient's symptoms, disease duration and current presentation as an outcome
B. *Analysis of the patient's symptoms*
Musculoskeletal specific
Pain: site (ask the patient to point at where he/she feels the pain), character, severity (score on VAS out of 10), radiation, what improves and what aggravates
Swelling (localized to the joint or diffuse)
Stiffness: duration of morning stiffness, history of articular gelling, localized to a joint or diffuse
Deformity: in relation to the patient's symptoms or the disease duration
Weakness: induced by pain or represent true muscle weakness
History of loss of balance, falls, slowing of the walking speed, weaker handgrip
Functional ability: better to be quantitative
Quality of life: preferred to be quantitative (mood, sleep disturbance, social, marital relations)
Work: ability to continue doing the work (absence from work because of the musculoskeletal symptoms)
General
Fatigue: severity recorded on a VAS scale 0–10
Generalized: fever, weight loss, weight gain, mouth or genital ulcers, sweating
Neurological symptoms: motor weakness, sensory deficit, tingling, numbness, difficulty in controlling passing water or bowel opening
Temple headache or pain with scalp tenderness or visual disturbance
Colour changes or coldness of digits or limbs
Other systems affection: cardiovascular, chest, endocrine

The Art of Asking the Patient Questions

In general, the questions asked by the treating doctor are vital to ensure putting the correct links between the pieces of information given by the patient and, therefore, are seen as the gold standard of historical inquiry. Subject to the case scenario, the questions can be stratified into three types.

Open Questions

They do not suggest a “right” answer to the patient, but in fact, they give the patients a chance to express what is on their mind. Open questions can be related to the patient’s particular problem that brought him to the clinic such as: “What seems to be the problem today?” “Tell me more about your joint pains.” “How has your joint pain affected your life or your ability to carry out your activities of daily living?” Open questions can be also used to obtain specific information about a particular symptom such as: “How about your bowel movement?” “Any problems with passing water, mishaps or leak?” It has to be noted that open questions may lead to more specific queries to obtain more information and discriminate features in relation to the patient’s symptoms.

Questions with Options

If open questions could not help to clarify the piece of information, then giving the patient some options would be the next step to “pin down” exactly what the patient meant by a specific statement. For example, PMR patients may present with pain in the shoulders, small joints of the hands as well as TMJ joints. Asking the patient to clarify whether the pain or the stiffness affects his arm as a whole or specifically the shoulder would help to clarify the nature of the condition. The same applies to hips and thigh pain. Similarly, pain in the “hip” can mean outer side of the hip (greater trochanter), lower back (sacroiliac joint) or referred pain from the hip joint.

This technique must be used with care as there is a possibility of getting the answer the physician wanted rather than what the patient meant. For example, buttock pain can be either due to sacroiliac joint pain or “S_1” nerve root impingement referred pain. It is advisable to avoid using specific medical terms such as “sacroiliac joint or greater trochanter”. Alternatively, the patient can be asked to point at where he/she feels the pain, rather than giving names or suggesting options. This approach is more likely to give a true picture of what the patient is suffering from [16].

Leading Questions

These questions, most likely, tend to lead the patient down an avenue that is framed by the treating physician assumptions. Therefore, they are best avoided if at all possible. An example is a 55-year-old male patient presenting with episodic chest pain. He is an overweight, known smoker; hence, angina would be a strong possibility. Questions like these should be avoided: “Does it get worse when you’re walking?” “Does cold or windy weather make it worse?” The patient may not be sure of the answer, not having thought of the influence of exercise or the weather on his/her pain, but answers yes, remembering a cold day when walking the dog when the pain was bad. This moves the whole dialogue between the patient and the treating doctor off to the wrong track, and it could be hard to get back from there. It is much better to ask an open question such as: "Have you noticed anything that might aggravate your pain or make it worse?" If the patient answered "chilli or fatty food", this may direct the treating doctor's attention to the suggestion that this chest pain may be of gastrointestinal origin.

The Art of Patient Symptom Analysis

The proper analysis of the patient's symptoms is the best way to guide the treating physician towards a diagnosis. Associating joint pain to morning stiffness would indicate chronic inflammatory arthritic condition, whereas identifying the pain site would help to identify whether the cause of the pain is joint or soft tissue. Table 6.3 shows a guide to the clinical patterns and how it differs in patients presenting with joint pains versus those having soft tissue pain. Furthermore, the characteristics of the pain, duration, site and distribution of these symptoms, as well as their chronology, are important as it differentiates between acute from chronic conditions. Recognizing whether symptoms are generalized, localized or referred would help in identifying whether the symptoms can be attributed to a focal pathology or systemic illness and also whether the symptoms are localized to one joint (e.g. gout/pseudogout or septic arthritis) or multiple joints (inflammatory or degenerative arthritis). Table 6.4 shows a guide to correlate site of joint pain to the systemic pathology whether it was monoarticular or polyarticular joint pain. When did the symptoms start and what pattern has developed over time? And lastly, are there any other systemic diseases in association with the current musculoskeletal pains? In contrast to joint pain, bone pain owing to metastatic bone disease is usually persistent day and night, whereas neuralgic pain is deep and might be associated with paraesthesia.

Response to previous treatment can also be informative. Prompt response to steroid therapy can be diagnostic of polymyalgia rheumatic or inflammatory arthritis. Good response to NSAIDs is one of the diagnostic criteria of spondyloarthritis.

Table 6.3 Joint vs soft tissue

Joint pain	Soft tissue pain (tendon, muscle, ligament)
Localized to a joint	More diffuse covering a wider area
Pain localized to the joint region	Pain radiates up or down along the tendon or muscle
Pain at rest and on movement	Pain on movement
Pain on passive mobilization in all directions	No pain at all on passive mobilization in all directions
Pain on active mobilization in all directions	Pain on active mobilization in one direction
Difficult to do resisted movement in all directions	Pain aggravated on resisted movement in one direction only
Swelling: synovial hypertrophy and possible effusion	Swelling: tenosynovitis, localized bleeding (if traumatic)

Table 6.4 Frequent joint affection in different arthritic conditions

	Common with	
Monoarticular arthritis		
Wrist joint	Gout, pseudogout	
Knee joint	Infection, haemarthrosis, OA, trauma, gout, CPPD, osteochondritis	
Ankle and mid foot	Gout, gonococcal, reactive arthritis, Charcot joint, sarcoid, tuberculosis	
Sternoclavicular joint	Infection (TB), haemarthrosis, inflammatory	
Cricoarytenoid joint	Rheumatoid arthritis	
Hip joint	Avascular necrosis	
Polyarticular arthritis		
	Common with	*Less likely to be seen in*
Polyarticular joint pain		
TMJ	RA, JIA, psoriasis, PMR	Gout, myalgias
Elbows/wrists/MCP	Bilateral wrist joints: rheumatoid arthritis (RA)	
	Any synovitis	
Hips	Any synovitis	Gout
Ankles only	Erythema nodosum	
Talonavicular	RA	
Cervical spine	RA, JIA, PsA, OA	Gout, gonococcal arthritis
Thoracolumbar	Spondyloarthritis	Gout, RA

Adjustment of the thyroid hormone level in patients with hypothyroidism can improve frozen shoulder or pseudogout symptoms.

Analysis of the preceding factors, associated symptoms and risk factors can give clues to the cause of the original problem. Whilst nonspecific symptoms such as fatigue and lethargy can be one of the dominant manifestations in inflammatory conditions, significant weight loss, night fever or night sweat can direct the attention to specific infections or the possibility of having a space-occupying lesion. Septic arthritis is associated with generalized symptoms, whereas preceding diarrheal illness, urethritis or conjunctivitis can be linked to reactive arthralgia or arthritis. If back pain is the main problem, presence of paraesthesia, loss of sensation or numbness in the limbs, motor weakness or difficulty to control sphincters would attract the attention to a focal pathology in the spine, whereas low back pain in association with anaemia and elevated inflammatory markers (ESR) may attract the attention to space-occupying lesion, particularly multiple myeloma.

Analysis of associated comorbidities or other recognized risk factors which could be linked to patient's musculoskeletal condition is also important. These include comorbidities such as diabetes mellitus, thyroid dysfunction, cardiovascular disorders and liver and kidney problems. Similarly, risk factors such as obesity, lack of physical activity, vitamin D deficiency or insufficiency, inadequate dietary calcium, smoking, excess alcohol and activities that expose the person to sprains, strains and trauma (such as certain physical-demanding occupations or sports) are important to be clarified. The impact of the illness on the patient's ability to carry out activities of daily living as well as quality of life (e.g. sleep, social life, get going in the morning or stiffness) is important for the assessment of the severity of the disease and monitoring its progression and response to therapy. Absence from work, inability to do light work, depression, low educational level, poor sleep and fatigue can be considered as "yellow flags" which need to be considered in patients with chronic low back pain [16]. Table 6.5 shows the yellow and red flags to be considered on taking a musculoskeletal history.

The Art of Interpreting Patient Clinical Manifestations

The aim of the diagnostic process is to build up a picture of what is happening to the patient. Interpreting the patient's narrative, clinical record and biographical data, in combination with the investigations outcomes, is vital for any structured proficient approach to decision-making. However, musculoskeletal medicine differs from other acute or chronic medical conditions, in some aspects which might impact on the expected outcomes. Examples are:

- Reducing pain and disability rather than achieving a complete cure could be the goal of treatment.
- The concept of "yellow flags" in musculoskeletal disease should be considered, and treating physician should be aware of the tools that can be used to stratify those at risk of progression to long-term pain and disability (The term "yellow flags" encompass psychological and social/environmental risk factors

Table 6.5 Yellow vs red flags in rheumatology

Yellow flags	Red flags
Adults	
Persistent joint pain >6 weeks	Progressive and significant weight loss in short time
Joint swelling	Fever
Abdominal pain	Temporal headache/tenderness or visual affections
Absence from work	Sensory loss
Difficulty to do job	Motor weakness
Disturbed/poor sleep	Inability to control passing water (mishaps or leak) or bowel opening
Unexplained fatigue	Fingernail infarcts or colour changes fingers or toes
Loss of balance, repeated falls	Haemoptysis, haematuria
Recurrent mouth or genital ulcers	Low trauma fracture
Children	
Absence from school, bone tenderness to palpation, inability to stand up from the floor or low chair, persistent or recurrent joint swelling	Fever, rest pain better with activity, night pain refractory to paracetamol/ibuprofen, fall in height or weight growth curve, morning stiffness

for prolonged disability and failure to return to work as a consequence of musculoskeletal symptoms) [16, 17].

- Understand the limitations of blood tests for diagnosing musculoskeletal conditions where "negative" tests may not rule out disease and where diagnostic criteria are often not clear-cut. This is particularly the case with inflammatory arthritis (e.g. rheumatoid arthritis) where early referral should be initiated on clinical suspicion rather than based on the results of tests [15].
- Identify "red flags" that relate to infection (e.g. septic arthritis or osteomyelitis), cancer (e.g. bony metastases and osteogenic sarcoma), fracture (e.g. fragility fracture in osteoporosis), neurological compromise (e.g. cauda equina syndrome) and inflammatory arthritis (e.g. rheumatoid arthritis, ankylosing spondylitis).
- Managing medical complexity: multi-professional management of comorbidity and polypharmacy, as well as uncertainty and risk. It also covers appropriate referral, planning and organizing complex care, promoting recovery and rehabilitation.

The diagnosis (or diagnostic formulation) may have to include prediction about past, present and future causes, consequences, interactions and other independent processes. As well as internal medical processes, it should also include external factors such as circumstances at home and the effects on self-care, employment and leisure. An open-mind approach is important to reach a final diagnosis. This can be done by covering the list of diagnoses, looking at the diagnostic lead above the list and then reading the suggestive and confirmatory findings. The next section will discuss an approach to patients presenting with mono- or polyarthritis manifestations and how to work out the most likely diagnosis.

Augmenting History Taking: Clinical Examination

The medical examination complements the history in characterizing the problem. It is an exercise in applied anatomy and requires knowledge of surface and functional anatomy, such as the normal ranges of movement and function. After taking full musculoskeletal history and before moving to do the clinical examination, the rheumatologist should have figured out what is the problem or at least have considered a differential diagnosis in his/her mind. The key questions of examination aim to identify and characterize the abnormality, to look for any pattern and any other abnormalities that will augment the conclusions made after the history taking and contribute to the decision-making of a specific diagnosis and also to identify the structures where the pathology is and the possible reasons. There are two main approaches to musculoskeletal examination; these are screening and regional musculoskeletal examination. The screening musculoskeletal examination is designed to provide an introduction to the physical assessment of musculoskeletal structures and will enable the examining rheumatologist to recognize normal joint appearance and alignment and the spectrum of normal joint range of motion and will help recognize basic abnormalities of musculoskeletal structure and function. As a screening examination, it is brief yet systematic, easily performed, and increases examiner confidence that no important musculoskeletal findings have been overlooked. With practice, the screening musculoskeletal examination can be performed in about 3–4 min. Furthermore, the screening examination provides the foundation for learning a more complete examination, the general musculoskeletal examination, at a later point in your training. The screening musculoskeletal examination is clinically useful as the musculoskeletal component of an athletic preparticipation physical examination, as part of a complete physical examination or as the initial examination in an individual with a local or regional musculoskeletal complaint with possible musculoskeletal symptoms in other sites. GALS examination (gait/arms/legs/spine; Table 6.6) is the most common examination approach often used as a quick screening tool to detect locomotor abnormalities and functional disability in a patient. Regional examination of the musculoskeletal system (REMS) refers to the more detailed examination that would be expected once an abnormality has been detected through either the history or screening examination. Regional examination (Table 6.7) refers to a group of joints linked together by function, examination of which may require detailed neurological and vascular examination including examination of all joints within that region. It is intended to provide a comprehensive assessment of structure and function combined with special testing to permit the examining physician to evaluate and diagnose the underlying musculoskeletal problem(s) and set up a pathway for investigation and treatment.

Approach to Monoarthritis

One of the important challenges in dealing with a patient presenting with a monoarticular pain is to assess whether the disorder is actually within the joint or is periarticular, involving the associated ligaments, tendons or other structures. A detailed history and clinical examination can help in identifying whether the primary pathology is in the joint or a periarticular lesion. Table 6.3 summarizes ways to differentiate between the two problems.

A primary intra-articular problem can involve the entire joint or be localized to a part of the joint (an example is meniscal tear in knee joints). Care should be directed to the patient's presenting complaint and the involved joins. Diagnostic clues can be obtained by analysis of events that may have precipitated the problem, such as onset type, the patient's age and sex and the nature of pathological findings within or around the affected joints.

Anatomic localization of the joint disease might play a vital role in the diagnosis-making process. Certain joints have the reputation of being associated with specific arthritic conditions. Table 6.4 shows joints of predilection for diseases which cause chronic monoarthritis. However, it should be remembered that whilst identifying specific site of arthritis might be helpful, it remains a suggestion and not a final diagnosis, which requires further confirmation.

Table 6.6 GALS screening examination

Screening questions
Do you feel stiff or pain in your arms or leg muscles, neck or the back?
Have you noted swelling in any of your joints?
Any difficulty in dressing yourself or cutting the food?
Do you feel pain or find it difficult to go up and down the stairs?
Screening examination
Patient standing 1. General inspection: view from front, sides and back, looking at
Bulk and symmetry of these muscles
Shoulder
Gluteal
Quadriceps
Calf
Full elbow extension
Spinal alignment
Abnormal lordosis/kyphosis
Knee flexion and popliteal swellings
Gross foot abnormalities
2. *Gait:* Observe the patient standing from sitting position, walking forwards for a few meters, turning and walking back again. Recognize abnormalities of the different phases, considering
Smooth
Symmetrical
Turns quickly
Heel strike—toe off
3. Arms: ask the patient to place both hands behind their head and then move elbows right back, then straighten the arms down the side of the body and bend elbows to 90° with palms down and fingers straight
Arms
Hands behind the head
Shoulder abduction, external rotation
Elbow flexion
Hands
Thenar and hypothenar muscle bulk
Joint deformity and swelling
Palpate MCP joints for tenderness
Make a fist, and then splay out fingers. Assess both movements
Grip two of your fingers
Oppose each of their own fingers
4. *Spine*: ask the patient to flex the neck laterally to each side. Place several fingers on the lumbar spinous processes, and ask the patient to bend forward and attempt to touch their toes whilst standing with legs fully extended; examine patient from side as they touch their toes for any curvature problems and observe
Spine
Slide their hand down the side of their leg to the knee level

(continued)

Table 6.6 (continued)

Tilt head to place ear on shoulder		
Look up at the ceiling and down at the floor		
Jaw		
Move side to side to examine TMJ		
Patient lying down		
5. *Legs:* Get the patient to recline on a couch, and then flex, in turn, each hip and knee while holding and feeling the knee; check for		
Crepitus: flex knee and hip passively, with hand on the kneecap		
Pain: whilst bending the knee, rotate the hip joint both internally and externally		
Effusion/swelling: patellar tap		
Squeeze metatarsophalangeal joints for tenderness—observe the patient's face		
An example of recorded GALS outcomes		
	Appearance	*Movement*
Gait	√	Not applicable
Arms	√	√
Legs	√	X
Spine	√	X
Restricted movement left hip		
Restricted movement lumbar spine with crepitus		

In addition to the clinical interview, immediate laboratory studies might also be of great help in the decision- and management-making process. Patients with monoarthritis may present with joint effusion. Aspiration and microscopic examination of the synovial fluid for crystals and pus cells can give clues towards the nature of the underlying pathology. Table 6.8 shows diagnostic findings from joint fluid examination in monoarthritic patients. Urine, blood and other body fluid examinations as well as conventional laboratory tastings may provide valuable information which can direct the physician's attention towards the appropriate diagnosis. Figure 6.1 shows an algorithm for the diagnosis of monoarthritis.

Approach to Polyarthritis

Being the most common symptom bringing patients for rheumatology consultation, polyarticular pain represents the true face of rheumatology. In majority of the cases, it is the skilled and experienced physician, able to implement the tolls of history and physical examination, who can formulate a correct diagnosis and treatment plan. Although radiologic investigations as well as lab tests can be helpful, they are used mainly as adjuncts, and musculoskeletal medicine remains one of the few areas in medicine where the bedside skills of the physician are important for the diagnosis-making process. This may give the rheumatologist the joy of being able to use one's experience and intellectual abilities for the patient's benefit. In most of the

Table 6.7 Musculoskeletal regional examination of the locomotor system

Regional examination	
Upper limb joints	Lower limb joints
Shoulder	*Shoulder*
Look: ask the patient to point at the painful site, and look for muscle wasting, asymmetry of the scapula or scoliotic list of the mid-dorsal spine *Feel*: tender sites (joint line/soft tissue attachment), crepitus over acromioclavicular joint, tenderness or swelling in the sternoclavicular joint, interscapular muscle spasm *Move*: passive range of motion (pain, limited), active range of motion, resisted movement	*Look*: site of pain (anterior, groin, outer hip, pack of the hip, ischial tuberosity, sacroiliac joint), levelling of ASIS, for muscle wasting (buttock/thigh), spinal scars, gait *Feel*: tender sites (joint line/soft tissue attachment, ischial tuberosity, sacroiliac joint), Trendelenburg's test, localized swelling (articular/lymph nodes) *Move*: passive range of motion (pain, limited), active range of motion, resisted movement. Thomas' test, SLR, femoral stretch test
Elbow:	*Knee:*
Look: painful site (joint line/inner or outer side of the elbow), swelling whether localized or diffuse	*Look*: painful site (joint line/supra-patellar, collateral ligament attachment/back of the knee/front of the thigh back of the leg, tibial tuberosity), quadriceps muscle wasting, swelling (whether joint, suprapatellar or Baker's cyst)
Feel: tender sites (joint line/medial or lateral epicondyle/soft tissue attachment)	*Feel*: tender sites (joint line/collateral ligament attachments/tendon-bone attachments), hypermobility, crepitus, soft tissue swelling (joint/bursa/other), patella stability
Move: passive range of motion (pain, limited), check for hypermobility, active range of motion, resisted movement	*Move*: passive range of motion (pain, limited), check for hypermobility, active range of motion, resisted movement, meniscal and cruciate ligament testing
Wrist *Look*: painful site (dorsal/palmar, joint line or dorsum of the hand), muscle wasting, swelling whether localized or diffuse, deformity *Feel*: tender sites (joint line whether wrist joint or first CMC joint/collateral ligaments/palmar side) *Move*: passive range of motion (pain, limited), active range of motion, resisted movement	*Ankle* *Look*: painful site (dorsal/back of the ankle, inner or outer sides); check for flat feet, lower limb oedema, muscle wasting, swelling whether localized or diffuse, deformity and gait *Feel*: tender sites (joint line/collateral ligaments/behind malleoli, tendons), swelling, tendo-Achilles *Move*: passive range of motion (pain, limited), active range of motion, resisted movement (arthritis/tendinitis)

Table 6.7 (continued)

Regional examination	
Upper limb joints	Lower limb joints
Hand *Look*: painful site (joints or interphalangeal/ dorsum of the hand); look for muscle wasting, deformity, swelling whether localized or diffuse and finger nail infarcts; check the nails and the skin *Feel*: tender sites (joint line/soft tissue), swellings (Heberden, Bouchard's, soft tissue), squeeze test MCP and PIP joints *Move*: passive range of motion (pain, limited), active range of motion, resisted movement, hypermobility, specific tests (De Quervain, carpal tunnel, gripping and pinching)	*Foot* *Look*: painful site (top of the foot, metatarsophalangeal joints or heel); look for muscle wasting, deformity, swelling whether localized or diffuse, toe nail infarcts, toes discoloration, callosity(ies) at the metatarsal heads and deformities; check the nails, skin and gait (heel strike-toe off) *Feel*: tender sites (joint line/soft tissue/heel), swellings (joints, soft tissue), squeeze test MTP joints, planter fascia *Move*: passive range of motion (pain, limited; joint/soft tissue), active range of motion, resisted movement, hypermobility, specific tests (De Quervain, carpal tunnel, gripping and pinching)
Spine	
Cervical spine *Look*: painful site, radiation, posture, shoulder pathology, look for shoulder or hand muscle wasting and swelling whether localized or diffuse *Feel*: tender sites (vertebrae/trapezius muscle), trapezius muscle spasm, trigger points, fibromyalgia tender points, distribution of tingling or motor weakness	*Lumbar spine* *Look*: levelling of ASIS, abdominopelvic crease, dorsolumbar scoliotic list/scoliosis, increased lumbar lordosis, painful site, paramedian tenderness/sacroiliac joint pain, radiation *Feel*: tender sites (vertebrae/paraspinal muscle/renal angle), paraspinal muscle spasm, trigger points, fibromyalgia tender points, distribution of tingling or motor weakness
Move: active range of motion (pain, limited, clicking); to be avoided in cases with past history of trauma or instability	*Move*: active range of motion (pain, limited, clicking); hypermobility; test for abdominal muscle weakness. To be avoided in cases with past history of trauma or instability

rheumatology cases, applying general medical rules, do not work perfectly well in musculoskeletal cases; therefore, musculoskeletal teaching must be adapted to meet the expected targets.

In concordance with the monoarticular approach, in evaluating patients presenting with polyarticular symptoms, the initial decision is to determine whether one is dealing with either (1) polyarticular (inflammatory) synovitis, (2) multiple structural lesions (non-inflammatory or degenerative) or (3) diffuse myalgia. Table 6.9 shows a list of inflammatory as well as structural common causes of polyarthritis seen in the standard musculoskeletal practice.

Polyarticular pain is characterized by having different patterns which, if put together, can help in making a final diagnosis. These patterns can be anatomic, inflammatory (synovitis), soft tissue or skin manifestations, evolution of the condition whether acute or chronic, involvement of other systems or therapeutic responses.

Table 6.8 Diagnostic findings from joint fluid examination in mono-articular arthritis

Test	Finding	Possible diagnosis
Appearance	Clear	Degenerative arthritis, mechanical derangement
	Bloody	Traumatic, bleeding/clotting pathology, pigmented villonodular synovitis, neuropathic, septic
	Turbid	Inflammatory arthritis, septic arthritis
White cell count	$<2000/\text{mm}^3$	Degenerative arthritis, amyloidosis, osteochondritis dissecans, haemochromatosis, Gaucher's disease, osteochondromatosis
	$2000–100,000/\text{mm}^3$	Juvenile inflammatory arthritis, inflammatory arthritis, familial Mediterranean fever, gout, pseudogout, septic arthritis
	>100,000	Septic arthritis
Microscopy	Urate	Gout
Crystals	Calcium pyrophosphate	Pseudogout
	Lipid droplets	Traumatic arthritis, arthritis with pancreatic disease
Glucose (no diabetes)	<20 mg%	Septic arthritis
	>20 mg%	Septic arthritis, non-specific inflammatory arthritis
Fat droplets	Large fat droplets	Possible fracture (need X-ray or MRI)
Stained smear	Congo red	Amyloidosis
	Gram stain	Septic arthritis
	Acid-fast bacilli	Tuberculosis
	PAS-positive fungal bodies	Fungal arthritis

Table 6.10 summarizes these patterns. An approach to the patient presenting with polyarticular joint pain should implement the outcomes of the clinical interview, arthritic patterns and radiologic or sonographic findings in addition to laboratory outcomes.

The Art of Recording the Patient's Data

Involving the patients in the history-taking process has attracted the attention of many researchers. Literature abounds on the prevalent nature of self-reported musculoskeletal symptoms. This can vary from self-reported survey to patient-reported outcomes. These also can be done online using computers or on paper format.

Self-report heath survey data is a major source of information for epidemiological studies and other health research [18, 19]. Use of self-reported health data is feasible because health survey data are often routinely collected by government departments and/or agencies (especially in developed countries) and are readily available and accessible [18–20]. Self-reported diagnosed arthritis is among the most commonly used case definition for prevalence and other epidemiological

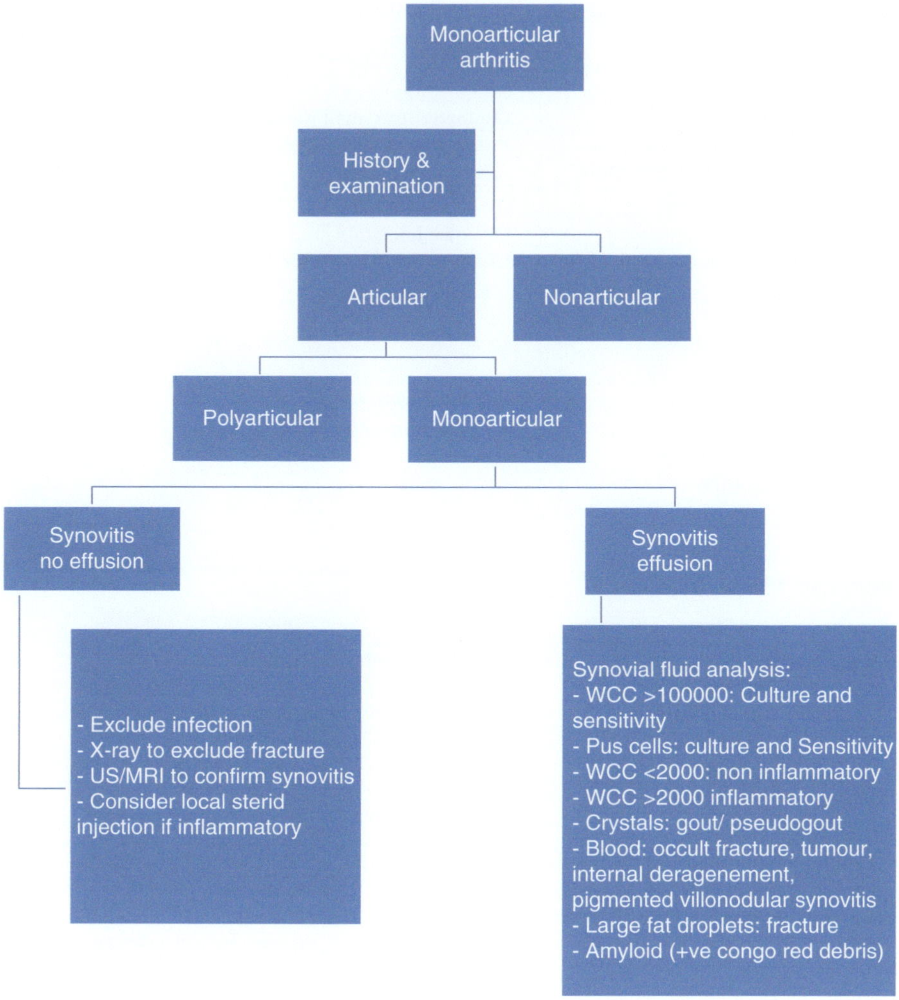

Fig. 6.1 An algorithm for the diagnosis of monoarthritis

studies of arthritis burden [21–31]. Although it has been argued that self-reported diagnosis of chronic conditions may suffer from recall bias, which could lead to under-reporting of conditions and underestimation of prevalence [21, 32–34], some researchers have justified the use of self-reported arthritis as it has good agreement with medical records [24–26] and an adequate level of sensitivity and specificity in previous validation studies [28]. However, it is acknowledged that generalization of the findings of validation studies from one population to another may be inappropriate due to the differences in sociodemographic, lifestyle and health characteristics which may affect the willingness of individuals to report medical conditions and/or seek healthcare [27–31]. For example, there is evidence indicating women tend to

Table 6.9 Classification of polyarthritis

Inflammatory polyarthritis	Non-inflammatory polyarthritis
Peripheral polyarticular	*Hereditary*
Rheumatoid arthritis Systemic lupus erythematosus Subacute bacterial endocarditis	Osteoarthritis (small joints of the hands) Primary generalized osteoarthritis
Peripheral pauciarticular	*Traumatic osteoarthritis*
Psoriatic arthritis Sexually acquired reactive arthritis Rheumatic fever Polyarticular gout Enteropathic arthritis Behcet's disease	OA knee joints/hip joint (local injury or obese patients) Chondromalacia patellae
Spondyloarthritis	*Metabolic disorders*
Psoriatic arthritis Ankylosing spondylitis Enteropathic arthritis Sexually acquired reactive arthritis	Haemochromatosis Ochronosis Acromegaly

Table 6.10 Patterns of polyarticular arthritis

Pattern	Additive	Migratory	Palindromic
Description	Inflammatory arthritis tends to add on as it flares and subtract as it gets quiescent	Initial inflamed joints totally remit, while simultaneously other joints get actively inflamed	Repetitive attacks of polyarticular synovitis which completely remit without sequelae or spread to other joints
Manner	Sequential	Drifting	Remittent
Specificity	Non-specific	Specific	Non-specific
Examples	Rheumatoid arthritis, lupus, psoriasis, reactive	Acute rheumatic fever, gonococcal arthritis	Early rheumatoid arthritis, sarcoidosis, familial Mediterranean fever, Whipple's disease, Behcet's disease, sickle cell anaemia, gout, polyarthritis associated with intestinal bypass

overreport (i.e. instead of under-report) arthritis in health survey compared to men [35]. Nonetheless, previous validation studies of self-reported arthritis have mostly been based on a non-gender-specific sample and/or have not performed stratified analysis by gender [36–39]. Since women are most at risk of arthritis, a study with a particular focus on women represents an important step to the better understanding of the validity of self-reported arthritis and its application in large epidemiological studies.

Electronic data recording has recently booked its place in standard clinical practice [40]. Patient self-reported outcome measures, completed online and emailed to the treating physician, were found to be equivalent to standard paper PROM format. Further, it enabled the patients to personally monitor how they are doing regarding their disease activity and helped to optimize their adherence to their treatment. This was tried in rheumatoid arthritis patients as well as in patients with systemic lupus erythematosus [41–44]. Electronic health records in rheumatology started to book its place in rheumatology research with emphasis on automated scoring and use in day-to-day practice. Reports have documented that electronic health records and other applications provided by health information technology may be associated with better outcomes (e.g. reductions in mortality, complications), adherence to therapy as well as cost-effectiveness [42, 45]. Electronic health record enhances the patients' active involvement in their disease management. Health information applications can help record patient's reported outcomes, automatic calculation of disease as well as comorbidity scores as well as the patients' motivation towards their disease management [43, 44]. However, relevant legal and regulatory aspects in the context of electronic health records and their data processing are still required [46].

In conclusion, musculoskeletal history taking is one of the most important skills for any rheumatologist or rheumatology nurse to acquire, and this can only be achieved through proper teaching program as well as regular practice. Musculoskeletal teaching is characterized by being interactive rather than one-way teaching approach. The interaction between teaching rheumatologists and students or junior colleagues in the setting of a consult offers an important learning opportunity. Enhanced teaching not only improves communication and management skills but also fosters a multidisciplinary approach to rheumatological care. Clinical approaches, as well as taking history and communication skills, are valuable tools enabling the rheumatologist to make the correct patient diagnosis.

References

1. Smith R. Thoughts for new medical students at a new medical school. BMJ. 2003;327(7429):1430–3.
2. Woolf A, Kristina Åkesson K. Primer: history and examination in the assessment of musculoskeletal problems. Nat Clin Pract Rheumatol. 2008;4(1):26–32.
3. El Miedany Y. Adopting patient-centered care in standard practice: PROMs moving toward disease specific era. Clin Exp Rheumatol. 2014;32(suppl 85):S40–6.
4. European Action Towards Better Musculoskeletal Health. 2004. http://europa.eu.int/comm/health/ph_projects/2000/promotion/fp_promotion_2000_exs_15_en.pdf. Accessed 10 Sept 2017.
5. Bub B. The patient's lament: hidden key to effective communication: how to recognise and transform. J Med Ethics Med Humanit. 2004;30:63–9.
6. European Action Towards Better Musculoskeletal Health. 2004. http://europa.eu.int/comm/health/ph_projects/2000/promotion/fp_promotion_2000_exs15_en.pdf. Accessed 13 Sept 2017.
7. Saleh K, et al. Development and evaluation of an integrated musculoskeletal disease course for medical students. J Bone Joint Surg Am. 2004;86-A:1653–8.
8. Badcock LJ, et al. Meeting the needs of increasing numbers of medical students—a best practice approach. Rheumatology (Oxford). 2006;45:799–803.
9. Bideau M, et al. Benefits of a programme taking advantage of patient-instructors to teach and assess musculoskeletal skills in medical students. Ann Rheum Dis. 2006;65:1626–30.

10. Hendry GD, et al. Patients teach students: partners in arthritis education. Med Educ. 1999;33:674–7.
11. Smith MD, et al. Evaluation of patient partners in the teaching of the musculoskeletal examination. J Rheumatol. 2000;27:1533–7.
12. Woolf AD, et al. Improving patient care by involving people with arthritis as educators of primary care physicians: the revised patient partner programme. Ann Rheum Dis. 2006;65(Suppl 2):620.
13. Woolf A, Åkesson K. Primer: history and examination in the assessment of musculoskeletal problems. Nat Clin Pract Rheumatol. 2008;4(1):28–33.
14. General Medical Council. Tomorrow's doctors: recommendations on undergraduate medical education. London: Education committee, General Medical Council; 1993.
15. Walker D, Kay L. Musculoskeletal examination for medical students: the need to agree what we teach. Rheumatology. 2002;41:1221–3.
16. El Miedany Y, El Gaafary M, Youssef S, Almedany S, Palmer D. Using simulation in clinical education: psoriasis area and severity index (PASI) score assessment. Curr Rheumatol Rev. 2016;12(3):195–201.
17. Miller A, Mahtani KR, Waterfield MA, Timms A, Misbah SA, Luqmani RA. Is rheumatoid factor useful in primary care? A retrospective cross-sectional study. Clin Rheumatol. 2013;32(7):1089–93.
18. Kendall N, Burton K, Main C, Watson P. Tackling musculoskeletal problems: a guide for the clinic and workplace – identifying obstacles using the psychosocial flags framework. London: The Stationery Office (TSO); 2009.
19. Hill JC, Dunn KM, Lewis M, Mullis R, Main CJ, Foster NE, et al. A primary care back pain screening tool: identifying patient subgroups for initial treatment. Arthritis Rheum. 2008;59(5):632–41. http://onlinelibrary.wiley.com/doi/10.1002/art.23563/abstract
20. Centers for Disease Control Prevention (CDC). 2013. About the Behavioral Risk Factor Surveillance System (BRFSS). http://www.cdc.gov/brfss/about/about_brfss.htm. Accessed 16 Mar 2018.
21. Beland Y. Canadian community health survey–methodological overview. Health Rep. 2002;13(3):9–14.
22. Australian Bureau of Statistics. National health survey: user's guide. 2009. http://www.abs.gov.au/ausstats/abs@.nsf/ProductsbyReleaseDate/2851D0FD9C52AB56CA257ACC000E3DE1?OpenDocument. Accessed 7 Jan 2018.
23. Busija L, Buchbinder R, Osborne RH. Quantifying the impact of transient joint symptoms, chronic joint symptoms, and arthritis: a population-based approach. Arthritis Care Res. 2009;61(10):1312–21.
24. Badley EM, Ansari H. Arthritis and arthritis-attributable activity limitations in the United States and Canada: a cross-border comparison. Arthritis Care Res (Hoboken). 2010;62(3):308–15.
25. Dominick KL, Golightly YM, Jackson GL. Arthritis prevalence and symptoms among US non-veterans, veterans, and veterans receiving Department of Veterans Affairs Healthcare. J Rheumatol. 2006;33(2):348–54.
26. Stang PE, Brandenburg NA, Lane MC, Merikangas KR, Von Korff MR, Kessler RC. Mental and physical comorbid conditions and days in role among persons with arthritis. Psychosom Med. 2006;68(1):152–8.
27. van't Land H, Verdurmen J, Ten Have M, van Dorsselaer S, Beekman A, de Graaf R. The association between arthritis and psychiatric disorders; results from a longitudinal population-based study. J Psychosom Res. 2010;68(2):187–93.
28. Globe DR, Varma R, Torres M, Wu J, Klein R, Azen SP. Self-reported comorbidities and visual function in a population-based study: the Los Angeles Latino Eye Study. Arch Ophthalmol. 2005;123(6):815–21.
29. Ferucci ED, Schumacher MC, Lanier AP, Murtaugh MA, Edwards S, Helzer LJ, et al. Arthritis prevalence and associations in American Indian and Alaska native people. Arthritis Care Res. 2008;59(8):1128–36.

30. Busija L, Hollingsworth B, Buchbinder R, Osborne RH. Role of age, sex, and obesity in the higher prevalence of arthritis among lower socioeconomic groups: a population-based survey. Arthritis Rheum. 2007;57(4):553–61.
31. Lee S, Tsang A, Huang Y-Q, Zhang M-Y, Liu Z-R, He Y-L, et al. Arthritis and physical-mental comorbidity in metropolitan China. J Psychosom Res. 2007;63(1):1–7.
32. Vuković D, Bjegović V, Vuković G. Prevalence of chronic diseases according to socioeconomic status measured by wealth index: health survey in Serbia. Croat Med J. 2008;49(6):832–41.
33. Lima MG, De Azevedo Barros MB, César CLG, Goldbaum M, Carandina L, Ciconelli RM. Impact of chronic disease on quality of life among the elderly in the state of Sao Paulo, Brazil: a population-based study. Rev Panam Salud Publica. 2009;25(4):314–21.
34. Balluz LS, Okoro CA, Mokdad A. Association between selected unhealthy lifestyle factors, body mass index, and chronic health conditions among individuals 50 years of age or older, by race/ethnicity. Ethn Dis. 2008;18(4):450–7.
35. Ng TP, Niti M, Chiam PC, Kua EH. Prevalence and correlates of functional disability in multiethnic elderly Singaporeans. J Am Geriatr Soc. 2006;54(1):21–9.
36. Niti M, Ng TP, Kua EH, Ho RCM, Tan CH. Depression and chronic medical illnesses in Asian older adults: the role of subjective health and functional status. Int J Geriatr Psychiatry. 2007;22(11):1087–94.
37. Kriegsman DM, Penninx BW, van Eijk JT, Boeke AJ, Deeg DJ. Self-reports and general practitioner information on the presence of chronic diseases in community dwelling elderly. A study on the accuracy of patients' self-reports and on determinants of inaccuracy. J Clin Epidemiol. 1996;49(12):1407–17.
38. Singh JA. Discordance between self-report of physician diagnosis and administrative database diagnosis of arthritis and its predictors. J Rheumatol. 2009;36(9):2000–8.
39. Bombard JM, Powell KE, Martin LM, Helmick CG, Wilson WH. Validity and reliability of self-reported arthritis: Georgia senior centers, 2000–2001. Am J Prev Med. 2005;28(3):251–8.
40. March LM, Schwarz JM, Carfrae BH, Bagge E. Clinical validation of self-reported osteoarthritis. Osteoarthr Cartil. 1998;6(2):87–93.
41. Kvien TK, Glennas A, Knudsrod OG, Smedstad LM. The validity of self-reported diagnosis of rheumatoid arthritis: results from a population survey followed by clinical examinations. J Rheumatol. 1996;23(11):1866–71.
42. Palmer D, El Miedany Y. EROMIA in inflammatory arthritis: the next step in standard practice. Br J Nurs. 2013;9(1):42–6.
43. El Miedany Y, El Gaafary M, Youssef S, Bahlas S, Almedany S, Ahmed I, Palmer D. Toward electronic health recording: evaluation of electronic patient-reported outcome measures system for remote monitoring of early rheumatoid arthritis. J Rheumatol. 2016;43(12):2106–12.
44. El Miedany Y, El Gaafary M, El Aroussy N, Bahlas S, Hegazi M, Palmer D, Youssef S. Toward electronic health recording: evaluation of electronic patient reported outcome measures (e-PROMs) system for remote monitoring of early systemic lupus patients. Clin Rheumatol. 2017;36(11):2461–9.
45. Amarasingham R, Plantinga L, Diener-West M, Gaskin DJ, Powe NR. Clinical information technologies and inpatient outcomes: a multiple hospital study. Arch Intern Med. 2009;169:108–14.
46. Richter J, Chehab G, Schneider M. Electronic health records in rheumatology: emphasis on automated scoring and additional use. Clin Exp Rheumatol. 2016;34(Suppl. 101):S62–8.

Chapter 7
The Art of Teaching Undergraduates

Introduction

Musculoskeletal (MSK) conditions are common in healthcare practices and have been identified as the leading cause of chronic health problems, long-term disability and consultations with health professionals [1, 2]. MSK conditions are also associated with significant healthcare expenditures and population morbidity. In a survey of eight countries, including Denmark, France, Germany, Italy, Japan, the Netherlands, Norway and the United States, arthritis had the greatest negative impact on health-related quality of life [3]. MSK care is delivered by a spectrum of medical specialists, including internists, orthopaedic surgeons, paediatricians, family physicians and general practitioners; yet they usually work with limited multi-specialty focus. Despite the high prevalence of MSK disorders in all fields of clinical practice, patients with MSK complaints are often ignored, and mostly their problems are overlooked. Studies reported almost full documentation of cardiovascular, respiratory, gastrointestinal and neurology system examinations but almost a major neglect of MSK examination [4, 5]. Such overlook of MSK examination and delay of diagnosis mostly have led to serious complications. Limitations of the essential MSK competencies among medical trainees and physicians were attributed to the inadequate exposure to appropriate musculoskeletal teaching and training during the undergraduate period.

The MSK clinical assessment is essentially a set of different actions that must be executed in a sequential or step-like fashion. This form of "complex learning" is referred to as a procedure [6]. The MSK clinical skill procedure includes both motor and intellectual skills. The common characteristic of a motor skill is the development of smoothness of asking, action, precision and timing. An intellectual skill involves the learner's ability to interact with the environment, make decisions about a variety of events and reach a diagnosis. The feature of the motor skill that sets it apart from other varieties of learning (i.e. attitudes) is that it improves through practice, whereas the intellectual skill improves through interaction and application to a

Y. El Miedany, *Rheumatology Teaching*,
https://doi.org/10.1007/978-3-319-98213-7_7

range and variety of different situations and contexts. Bearing in mind this "theoretical base", learning MSK clinical skills is very much like learning how to drive a car. It would not be logic to assume that 10 h of both theoretical and practical driving learning, in a large-group format, would be sufficient to absorb such a complex task [7].

There are several challenges in undergraduate musculoskeletal education which need tackling. This chapter will enlighten the readers about the current situation of undergraduate teaching, the science and art of teaching the undergraduates and the new concepts in this field. It aims to serve as a resource guide for students and experts alike and provide a review of new innovative strategies to improve musculoskeletal undergraduate teaching. The chapter will conclude with discussing what should be done regarding the future of undergraduate rheumatology teaching.

Undergraduate Education: Current Situation

The average number of hours devoted to teaching MSK clinical skills at medical schools has been reported to be restricted, particularly when compared to the prevalence of MSK complaints in the population. In a cross-sectional survey of 297 primary care physicians, about 80% of participants reported a low level of confidence in performing a musculoskeletal physical examination [8]. Another study indicated that 79% of respondents including medical students, residents and staff physicians failed the essential MSK cognitive examination [9]. Investigators also reported overlooking of essential physical examination of MSK in residency education and undergraduate programmes [10, 11]. Medical students from 1st to 4th years at Johns Hopkins failed musculoskeletal evaluations, and confidence in musculoskeletal physical examination remains low there as well as elsewhere [12–14]. While confidence increases through the 4th year [15], overall musculoskeletal competence is still lacking, especially given the frequency with which physicians encounter musculoskeletal presentations [16–18]. A survey indicated that new medical graduates had lower competence in demonstrating physical examination especially for MSK and cardiovascular system [19]. Furthermore, about 50% of the United State medical schools had no obligatory MSK basic sciences course or clinical clerkships [20]. Harvard medical students considered MSK medicine as the third most important topic in a physician's career, yet they presented low levels of confidence in MSK examination [21]. Medical school curricula represent scant attention for MSK medicine: it is estimated that only 3% of most US undergraduate curriculum is devoted to MSK medicine [22]. The underrepresentation of MSK in medical curricula was highlighted by the Association of American Medical Colleges which recommended the essential competencies for medical graduates including MSK skills and knowledge [23]. This concurred with the US Bone and Joint Initiative that announced Project 100, which recommended that 100% of US medical schools begin requiring a musculoskeletal course by the end of the decade. Accordingly, medical schools developed their MSK curriculum. However, most of these initiatives did not meet the expected results of improving medical students' competencies of MSK [24, 25].

In the United Kingdom (UK), Nammari et al. [26] highlighted that the UK Foundation Programme provided inadequate training in MSK medicine. The MSK training exposure was limited; about 15% of the 112 respondents had any exposure to orthopaedics during the foundation programme, and only 13% felt they had adequate exposure to MSK medicine.

Similarly, undergraduate education in rheumatology in Argentina, Bolivia, Brazil, Chile and Uruguay has been considered insufficient, and graduates were reported to become general practitioners without having the necessary knowledge for adequate management of patients with the most common rheumatic disorders [27]. Inadequacies in undergraduate education have similarly been noted in South African medical schools [28] and in several Asia-Pacific countries [29], attributed in part to the lack of an appropriate faculty. This concurred with a Nigerian study which revealed inadequate musculoskeletal competency of the pre-internship Nigerian medical school graduate, according to the Freedman and Bernstein test for musculoskeletal competency [30]. Despite the opportunity for paediatric residents to participate in rheumatology rotations, a minority partakes, and as a result, paediatricians tend to rely heavily on serologic tests and specialist referrals [31].

The Science of Teaching Undergraduates: Principles and Challenges and Solutions

Basic Principles

Setting up agreed standards for undergraduate medical education represents the cornerstone of the undergraduate education. Establishing standards with clearly defined outcomes is the most positive approach to enhance the future doctors' competence in assessing and managing patients presenting with musculoskeletal conditions. One of the key actions is to increase awareness of musculoskeletal conditions, not only among the faculty putting the curricula but also among the educating physicians. As education is the most important method of providing sustainable and long-term effects in the healthcare community, organization bodies like the American College of Rheumatology and EULAR have started to pay attention to undergraduate educational issues with the aim of ensuring global standards adaptable to local needs. In addition to the promotion of undergraduate electives and self-selective components in rheumatology for undergraduates, the "Arthritis Research Council", UK, has also developed a range of literature and electronic resources for undergraduates [32].

Undergraduate Curriculum

In developing an undergraduate curriculum, a structured plan of content from the basic science (the preclinical) teaching to the clinical competencies defined as the ultimate outcome of the programme must be identified and agreed upon by the faculty concerned. A clear strategy for each component and consecutive building of knowledge and skills will ensure that students have the ability to recognize and evaluate patients with musculoskeletal complaints at the end of their medical school training. The enormous expansion of knowledge in medicine and the additional roles of doctors as leaders, administrators and team workers are also relevant to musculoskeletal conditions and affect demands on training [33].

In order to avoid overloading the curriculum, it is vital to agree on outcomes defined by core knowledge and core skills. Musculoskeletal history taking and examination should be essential core skills for all undergraduates. Spiral learning, whereby musculoskeletal learning opportunities as well as associated assessments are provided throughout the undergraduate curriculum rather than simply at one or two time points, is the best educational curriculum strategy to enhance musculoskeletal learning. As general goals, upon graduating from medical school, every new doctor should be able to assess (by appropriate history taking and examination) a patient with locomotor symptoms by differentiating normal from abnormal in terms of structure and function, determining relevant investigations and interpreting the results, formulating a limited differential diagnosis, recognizing the impact of the problem on the individual and making an appropriate management plan for medical, surgical and rehabilitation services [34].

Preclinical Education

The preclinical teaching of basic science should include cell biology, anatomy and pathophysiology of bones, joints and muscles and form the foundation for the clinical training phase. Applied anatomy and pharmacology can help the student link between the basic science and clinical application. Also learning anatomy will form a good base for understanding musculoskeletal ultrasonography. This makes the locomotor system serve as a useful model including a range of aspects from cell regulation and tissue repair to biomechanics and linking it to real-life clinical practice.

Clinical Education

The focus of a clinical undergraduate course in musculoskeletal medicine should be on clinical skills, interpreting patient's data and knowledge of the common conditions. In addition, since many patients suffer from long-term chronic pain, it is imperative to understand its impact on the patients' lives and to have an attitude that is appropriate to treating patients with such chronic inflammatory disorders in a broader spectrum. Chronic musculoskeletal conditions require interdisciplinary teamwork. For example, it is important for a gynaecologist to know whether a patient with a hip replacement can sit in the examination chair, for a gastroenterologist to be able to balance the needs of a person with rheumatoid arthritis for anti-inflammatory analgesics against their risk of gastrotoxicity, for a cardiologist to know about joint replacement procedures so as to estimate the cardiac demands during surgery and for the chest physician to be aware of the possibility of aggravating the asthma if the patient took anti-inflammatory medication [35].

The key message is thus that all doctors need a minimum competence in evaluating patients with musculoskeletal conditions, combined with basic knowledge. The exact content of any curriculum needs to be defined in the context of local needs, the relative prevalence and incidence of various conditions and the local resources. In general, most common conditions are the same around the world, including fractures caused by high-energy trauma or related to bone fragility; low back pain; joint conditions such as osteoarthritis, chronic inflammatory arthritis and gout; as well as septic arthritis. The minimum competence is to be reached by all students at the end of their undergraduate education. Competence includes development of an appropriate attitude in managing patients with chronic conditions, which most often involves chronic pain. Additional levels of competence are added depending on future postgraduate specialty training.

Earlier studies revealed that there appears to be a correlation between the amount of time spent in preclinical musculoskeletal education and musculoskeletal knowledge. Study outcomes revealed that increasing the amount of time spent studying musculoskeletal medicine resulted in higher exam scores [25, 36, 37]. Integration of musculoskeletal subjects is one way to increase mastery. At Harvard Medical School, a new integrated curriculum that involved more time in gross anatomy and laboratories and more emphasis on orthopaedic pathophysiology resulted in higher levels of clinical confidence and cognitive mastery among students [37]. Integrating orthopaedics, rheumatology and physical medicine and rehabilitation has shown to be effective in increasing knowledge and retention of physical examination skills [21]. Interactive small groups are also popular among students in learning musculoskeletal medicine, and one can use such a setting to help students by breaking tasks down so that students can fully learn the physical examination first and then explore clinical correlates [21, 38, 39]. Computer-based instruction has shown positive outcomes, with some evidence of higher student satisfaction and skill gained [40, 41] and students preferring computer-based learning to be combined with bedside teaching [42].

Teaching Methods

The majority of medical schools have curricula with varying degrees of vertical or horizontal integration between preclinical and clinical training. Traditional teaching methods (such as lectures and apprenticeship) are widely complemented with problem-based learning from the 1st year of study. Teaching methods should, however, be regarded as tools, the precise method within each module to be determined by the specific objectives for each training session, whether it is an element of knowledge, examination of a joint or reduction of a fracture. Clinical skills are best learnt in the real-life situations of outpatient clinics, emergency services or primary care, but clinical teaching alone does not give sufficient competence without formal instruction as well [13].

A number of methods are suitable for teaching musculoskeletal conditions. Problem-based learning is useful in the preclinical phase, preferably complemented by case studies of the more complex problems in the clinical phase, with inclusion of social aspects of management.

Competence in clinical examination gives confidence, and a simple screening examination has been developed with the "GALS" (gait–arms–legs–spine) screen [40]. Students who had formal instruction in the GALS screen were as proficient in examining the locomotor system as they were regarding other organ systems [41].

Another challenge in teaching locomotor medicine is the lack of confidence in teaching among non-musculoskeletal specialties and poor communication among specialties [28]. It is prudent to remember that mastery of a test or assessment does not necessarily yield clinical competence. True competency includes proficiency in both taking history and physical exam. A new physical examination decision-making test has recently been developed that educators can utilize, which may more effectively assess student knowledge in musculoskeletal medicine [43]. Further tests that are developed should ideally account for multiple competencies, including physical exam skills in addition to assessments of knowledge and diagnostic acumen.

On the other hand, "Teaching the Teachers" workshops are important to encourage rheumatologists and MSK tutors to develop their skills as clinical teachers. Through direct teaching involvement as well as by becoming champions and role models, teachers and rheumatologists within the specialty can have a significant impact on the undergraduate curriculum.

On another front, a study was carried out at the University Of Nebraska College Of Medicine to obtain student feedback regarding best teaching modalities from the students' point of view in order to improve undergraduate rheumatology education moving forward [44]. Results were obtained through a voluntary survey which included 114 students. Outcomes revealed that in addition to the standard lecture format, students were receptive and positive towards the novel educational methods employed. Blending both traditional and novel teaching methods was very well received as the student found it highly effective in engaging medical students. Other teaching modalities employed, which were well perceived, too, included faculty-led live patient encounters (these appear to be particularly appealing to trainees early in rheumatology learning), problem- and case-based learning, student- and faculty-led case discussion including pathognomonic rheumatology findings, video game on gout and independent time in the simulation lab for joint injections. With ongoing threats to a sustainable rheumatology workforce, it is vital that training curricula engage students early with goals of knowledge acquisition and learner satisfaction.

Assessment

Assessment of students is a matter of continuing concern for medical teachers as it is supposed to steer student learning. It drives learning in four ways, through its content, its format, its timing and subsequent feedback given to the examinee. The most important point is that examination should promote strategic and deep learning over memory recall [42]. Examination of the student with regard to the musculoskeletal system must use reliable and validated tests and should be consistent with the objectives and priorities set for the course. In order to determine if competence has been achieved in all three areas (practical skills, theoretical knowledge and attitude), more than one test should be used. The various modes of assessment are written and oral examinations. The existing written examinations, which traditionally were the most common approach to assessment, have been subject to bias and are dependent on a number of extraneous variables such as student's handwriting legibility, content, way of presenting the content, teacher's appreciation of written matter, etc. On the whole, the actual knowledge of the student is not judged in a fair and valid manner.

Assessment of Clinical Competence

The Consensus Statement from the 2010 Ottawa (Assessment in Medicine) conference published criteria for assessment in 2011 [45]. The report highlights the wide range of assessment tools which have been developed for the assessment of competency in medicine and the breadth of teaching and learning strategies employed. The statement acknowledges the increasing use of advanced psychometrics to test reliability and validity of assessment, together with the need to take into account other factors which determine the utility of an assessment.

Educators who are involved in assessment should be clear in the differentiation of formative assessment (which is used to help drive learning and provide feedback on performance against learning goals) and summative assessment (which uses assessment tools with appropriate reliability/validity to pass, fail or rank participants in high-stakes assessment) [46]. Epstein [47] reported three main goals of assessment in medical education, which are (1) identifying learning needs including knowledge, skills and professionalism in order to drive future learning, (2) setting professional standards of competence and performance to safeguard the public and (3) ranking applications to recruitment to postgraduate training posts. The first of these goals encapsulates the formative purpose of assessment, sometimes referred to as "assessment for learning", while the last two describe the summative purpose of assessment or "assessment of learning" in making judgement about the standards that learners have achieved. Figure 7.1 shows Miller's pyramid of learning [48] with examples of assessment modalities for each level.

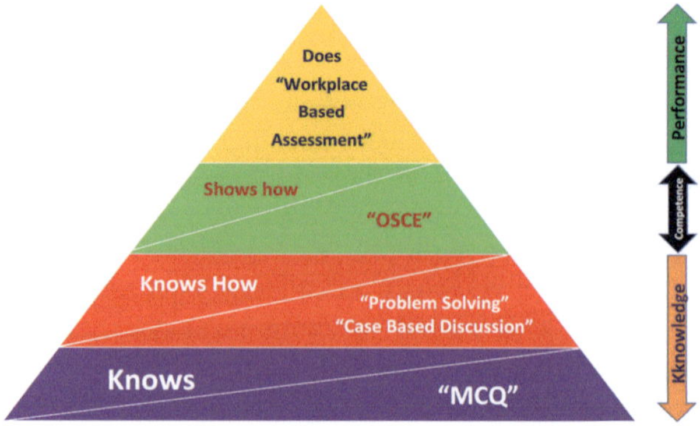

Fig. 7.1 Miller's pyramid of learning with examples of assessment modalities for each level. OSCE objective structured clinical examination, MCQ multiple-choice question

The modified (matched) essay question (MEQ) method of assessing reasoning as well as factual knowledge is particularly useful for musculoskeletal conditions. This form of examination has the advantage of testing knowledge at different levels but also allowing for the use of modified authentic clinical problems in the test situation. In addition, it is relatively easy to administer and grade. Multiple-choice questions (MCQs) are the most common form of written assessment, being both reliable and valid by broad coverage of subject content. They are probably the most widely used components of objective examinations and are used for formative and summative assessment as well as for various entrance examinations, where ranking of students is of paramount importance [49]. However, a study carried out to assess multiple-choice questions (MCQs) as a tool for formative assessment indicated that MCQs alone are not sufficient to assess the learning and should be mixed with objective/subjective tests [50]. Another study by Frederiksen showed that MCQs have limitations like difficulty in framing MCQs that are rich in context. MCQs can also create situations in which an examinee can answer a question by recognizing the correct option, but could not have answered it in the absence of option. This effect is called cueing effect. Extended matching items can minimize cueing. Another study revealed that MCQs emphasize recall of factual information rather than conceptual understanding and integration of concepts [51].

Portfolio is another tool used to evaluate the student's performance over an extended period of time. By nature, a portfolio is a storybook capturing a student's progression of learning as they move through the year. It includes a collection of the student's works that are associated with the required learning standards. This collection of work is often gathered over a long period of time to reflect what the students have been taught as well as what they have learned. Each piece in the portfolio is selected because it is an authentic representation of what the students have learned and is meant to demonstrate their current knowledge and skills. The portfolio assessment provides an opportunity for the students to, individually, self-assess and reflect on their learning, as well as formulate a deeper understanding for the concepts they are learning beyond a simple surface explanation.

The portfolio can be used to document the student's development over time, to promote the student's abilities or to assess the student's learning within a specific course. Its purpose may also be combination of all the three areas. In comparison to the standardized testing which provides a snapshot of what a student can do on a particular day, portfolios are indicative of what a student's true abilities over certain period. Eventually, the guiding teacher helps determine the purpose of the final portfolio. Portfolio assessment requires a great level of individual interaction between the student and teacher wherein they are always collaborating about the requirements and components going into the portfolio [52–55].

Challenges to using the portfolio as an assessment tool are that it is a very subjective approach of evaluation. For students or tutors who feel uncomfortable to work without a grading key or answer sheet, subjective evaluation can be a relatively difficult task. Secondly, teachers often are unsure themselves of the purpose of a portfolio and its uses in the classroom. Thirdly, there is a question of how the portfolio can be most effectively used to assess student learning [56]. Two students working on the same learning standard may have two totally different approaches; thus, learning reflection and outcomes may not be the same. Table 7.1 shows suggestions to facilitate the utilization of student's portfolio in order to evaluate the learning outcomes.

Table 7.1 Suggestions to facilitate the utilization of student's portfolio in order to evaluate the learning outcomes

Goal	Characters
Tutor: set a goal	What kind of data does the tutor want to collect and how he/she plans to use it
	Goal should be tied to how it is planned to use the portfolio
	One of two goals: (1) recording the scope of student's learning over time or (2) ticking the boxes by collecting samples of student work before passing the portfolio along to the next level
Approach: define how	Efficient way to grade a portfolio is through a rating scale
	Consider a checklist, including all the required items, if a specific skill is targeted
	Example of rating guidelines:
	The work completed correctly (mechanics)
	Completely (information)
	Comprehensively (depth)
	Each area is marked on a scale of 1–5. Scale is 1 = not at all; 2 = somewhat; 3 = mostly; 4 = entirely; 5 = innovative
Student: ensure correct student involvement	Tutor takes time at the beginning of the unit to explain the type of evaluation it is and what is expected in terms of work product
	Student understands
	The aims of the portfolio
	How it will be used to evaluate the work
	How grades for it will be determined
	Students are given the checklist of what is expected in the portfolio before they begin submitting work
	Students have the ability of adding one or two pieces of their choice in their portfolios
	Students have the opportunity to reflect about the work included in the portfolio

Practical Skills

To test practical skills, an objective structured clinical examination (OSCE) is the most commonly implemented approach. OSCE is a form of multi-station examination for clinical subjects first described by Harden et al. from Dundee and Glasgow [57]. It was firstly adopted in North America in a widespread manner, followed by the United Kingdom in the 1990s. Shortly after, it became the principle method for clinical skills assessment in medical schools and licensure bodies across the United States, Canada, the United Kingdom, Australia, New Zealand and other countries. OSCE is a form of performance-based testing used to measure candidates' clinical competence. During an OSCE, candidates are observed and evaluated as they go through a series of stations in which they interview, examine and treat standardized patients who present with some type of medical problem.

The hallway of OSCE exam rooms, each occupied by a uniquely challenging patient, is a familiar milieu to the physician or other healthcare professional. When standardized patients are utilized in OSCE exams, the linear sequence of the multiple station and skill challenges bears remarkable similarity to that real environment. This examination can also, to a certain extent, test attitude, which is the most difficult area to evaluate [58]. Objective structured clinical examination (OSCE) has proved to be so effective that it is now being adopted in disciplines other than medicine, like dentistry, nursing, midwifery, pharmacy and event engineering and law. Table 7.2 shows characters of the OSCE session and targeted outcomes.

In general, assessment drives learning. If the assessment system can be made fair, then students more likely intend to study the subject rather than only prepare for the examinations. "The assessment tail wags the curriculum dog"; or grab the student by the tests, and their heart and mind will follow [59]. All the methods of assessment have strength and intrinsic flaws. Subjective test alone is also not sufficient to assess the students learning as they have been criticized for being highly subjective and inadequate for covering the full range of topics studied. It has also been linked to several subjective factors, such as the students' script, its clarity, the teacher's perception and views of the written matter,

Table 7.2 Characters of the OSCE session and targeted outcomes

Characters	Targeted outcomes
Stations are short	What candidates can do rather than what they know
Stations are numerous	The application of knowledge rather than the recall of knowledge
Stations are highly focused	Ensure competency: mix of station types
Candidates are given very specific instructions	Adequate reliability: 18–20 stations/2 h
A pre-set structured mark scheme is provided	Standardized: checklists provided. Random independent examiners
Reduce examiner input and discretion	
Ensure rest stations are provided	

etc.; the whole the actual knowledge of the students is not judged in a fair and valid manner [53]. The use of multiple methods of assessment can overcome many of the limitations of individual assessment formats [60–62]. Van der Vleuten [60] described five criteria for determining the usefulness of a particular method of assessment; there are reliability, validity, impact on future learning and practice, acceptability to learners and faculty and costs (to the individual trainee, the institution as well as society at large).

Time

The vast increase in medical knowledge has raised the demand for inclusion of new subjects in the curriculum. However, curriculum time in medical schools is not expandable, so it is necessary to consider redistributing the available curricular hours and increasing the efficiency of their use. Nevertheless, a certain amount of time is needed to master practical skills and to assess a sufficient number of patients in order to gain experience. It is also necessary to allow time to digest, reflect on and incorporate the new knowledge and experience for long-term retention. Several approaches can be adopted to tackle this problem. Early introduction of the clinical component of the medical education programme with vertical integration of musculoskeletal examination, with gradual levels of complexity, as part of the medical education can be the start to raise the students' awareness of the different forms of rheumatologic presentations. This can start as early as the 1st year of medical education, when students are learning applied musculoskeletal anatomy/physiology and links can be introduced to clinical correlations whether articular or soft tissue rheumatism, as a way of basic science-to-clinical integration. In the consequent 2 years, learning activities are focused in development of semiological skills, including history taking, physical examination and clinical reasoning. In the last years, students should be introduced to most of the prevalent rheumatic diseases through theoretical and practical activities. Rheumatology is an excellent specialty for medical education because locomotor disorders are often multisystem and consistently require the application of the principles of professionalism. This stimulates broad-based thinking and improves problem-solving. The learner therefore acquires skills in both general internal medicine and rheumatology. Integration of basic sciences and clinical medicine is another time-effective learning approach. Implementation of applied anatomy, physiology and history in the case-based learning and radiology modules will help to facilitate the competency-based curriculum. Utilization of modern learning techniques including lecture, discussion, small group sessions, online learning, standardized patent encounters, simulators and case-based learning will enable fitting musculoskeletal education within the curriculum. While finding a dedicated time for musculoskeletal education might represent a challenge, by utilizing modern teaching tools other than lectures, and by eliminating redundancies, extra time can be generated to include musculoskeletal care not only for adults but also for paediatrics and older adults.

In contrast, dedicating enough time for clinical practice is vital for the students to master the musculoskeletal practical skills and to assess/share in management of a sufficient number of patients. It is also necessary to allow time to incorporate the new knowledge and experience for long-term retention. A course of 6–8 weeks at the undergraduate level is required to require the minimum level of musculoskeletal competence.

Time challenge is not only confined to the learning students and the curriculum but also the educators. It is well appreciated that the effective teaching of clinical medicine is not easy. There are many competing demands for a clinician educator's time that distract from teaching, including the need for clinical and administrative productivity, personal and family expectations as well as the required involvement with educational oversight committees [63]. Allocating time in the educators' job plan, sharing internal education resources, providing educational facilities, identifying and helping to sort out problems and providing useful feedback to educators are items that can help educators having dedicated time for teaching, develop their educational skills and adopt a time-effective approach in handling their teaching activities.

Enhancement of undergraduate rheumatology teaching through the use of musculoskeletal ultrasound has been studied and recommended. Review of the literature indicated that the integration of ultrasound in undergraduate medical education is both feasible and beneficial to medical students [64]. Musculoskeletal US helps to provide the students with a spatial and 3D structure of joints, refresh the students' memory of basic and surface MSK anatomy, provide an insight into the pathological process of inflamed joints and tendons, boost the students' learning curve in musculoskeletal medicine and allow appreciation of usefulness and limitations of musculoskeletal ultrasonography as a diagnostic imaging modality. These advantages endorsed the suggestion to employ musculoskeletal ultrasound as a teaching topic in the curriculum (i.e. anatomy, physical examination, physiology, invasive procedures).

The Art of Rheumatology Undergraduate Teaching

Continuous innovation and creativity in medical education have revitalized the art of teaching and given it a new makeover. Creative education is defined as the process of education and learning that employs interactive student-oriented techniques. The creative educational setup encourages critical thinking and learning as well as facilitates the recalling and application processes. The aim is to improve MSK teaching in a student-friendly style. The key elements of improvement of MSK creative education include (1) refinement, dissemination and broad acceptance of clearly defined goals and objectives, (2) continued lobbying for time and resources and (3) continued development of novel teaching methodologies and dissemination of existing successful teaching methodologies [65].

New strategies implemented to progress MSK teaching include standardized clinical instruction modules (SCIM) and the Patient Partners in Arthritis (PPIA) Program. Standardized clinical instruction modules are similar in structure to an objective structured clinical examination (OSCE) but are designed to teach medical students and provide formative feedback. With the standardized clinical instruction modules, an MSK specialist teaches a clinical skill and then supervises students during practice and provides immediate feedback. This approach led to significant improvement in the students' evaluations, self-confidence and satisfaction [66].

The Patient Partners in Arthritis (PPIA) Program involves training patient with arthritis to teach and evaluate MSK clinical examination skills, however studies on the effectiveness of the Patient Partners in Arthritis Program have been conflicting. Utilizing student OSCE examinations as the outcome measure, teaching superiority of rheumatology faculty over trained patient educators was found in one study [63], whereas similar results between the two groups were found in another one [67]. A combined programme of the Patient Partners in Arthritis Program and an integrated expert MSK clinician would be an optimal approach, although likely limited by resources.

The availability and vast expansion of Internet use have changed the educational scene. Most of the universities now have their medical undergraduate curriculum available online. This is usually supplemented by large number of online lectures, available for asynchronous learning and review. The limited number of hours devoted to teaching MSK clinical skills was another factor that enforced implementing online teaching modules for undergraduate education. Computer-assisted learning is defined as supplementing regular lecture and lab activities with computer activities during or surrounding class time [68]. Computer activities may range from interactive CD-ROM programs in the classroom as part of lectures, labs, student assignments or self-study materials to Internet search activities using the computer during class. Web-based, or online, instruction may include portions or entire classes conducted via the Internet. Students can access a class through a website and participate in lectures and group discussions in real time. Materials may also be provided asynchronously such that students access the website and hear lectures or complete assignments according to their own schedule [69].

Several educational goals have been proposed that could be achieved by using computer-assisted learning. Computer-assisted learning has the potential to increase the efficiency and productivity of teaching and learning [70–73]. Computer-assisted learning can also enable more self-directed learning, promote contemporary technological skills and enhance critical thinking and problem-solving skills [74]. A large variety of cases can be presented through computer-assisted learning, a practice that is difficult within conventional clinical lectures [75].

Live video streaming is a technique where patients can be evaluated and treated in the clinical setting, while students simultaneously observe from the classroom. By having a video camera in both facilities, the experience becomes interactive, as students could direct the evaluation or treatment [76]. The video clips of patient–doctor interaction also provide students with a reference for actual treatment time devoted to a particular activity and the intensity and variety of cueing provided by the treating healthcare professional. Schittek-Janda et al. [71] created a virtual patient for students of dentistry to "reflect a real scenario as much as possible and to put the student in the role of a professional". The results demonstrated that students who experienced the virtual patients performed a more complete history interview and had more empathy for the patients. By creating virtual clinical experiences, student interaction with patients can be evaluated, while the issue of protecting patient confidentiality disappears [72, 73]. Computer-assisted learning products can also offer access to interdisciplinary education [75, 77].

The usefulness and effectiveness of using an online module for teaching MSK examination was assessed in a study [78]. Three groups of students were exposed to a web-based module, tutorial-based learning or independent study of a standard textbook, respectively. Test results revealed that the students using the module had significantly higher scores than the students using either of the other study methods. These results are encouraging in that many online evaluations generally report equivalent results between face-to-face learning and web-based learning.

In a case study of student satisfaction, So [20] reported that blended learning was an effective teaching method. Key elements of a successful programme were integration of technology components and instructional design strategies. So explains further: "To be more learner-centered, the learning environment needs to be designed to allow individual learning, as well as to create opportunities for interaction with other classmates and the instructors". For effective online communication, it is important to provide channels for both synchronous (e.g. face-to-face meetings) and asynchronous (e.g. online discussion forums) interactions. Finally, the online learning environment should include a place where students can receive socioemotional support to reduce their feeling of frustration, isolation, and dissatisfaction, as well as to provide content-related support for "cognitive learning" [79, 80].

Using musculoskeletal US in undergraduate education has taken another step further. Over the past 10 years, medical schools have begun to implement ultrasound into their curricula, and point-of-care ultrasound training was reported to enhance student education in physical examination, basic sciences as well as on clinical rotations [81–84]. Medical schools that provide point-of-care ultrasound training have shown that students find it useful in various aspects of medical education and expressed interest in obtaining further education using ultrasonography [85, 86].

The value of point-of-care ultrasound in modern medicine is becoming evident [87]. Ultrasound allows physicians to quickly assess patients' anatomic and physiologic characteristics at the bedside [83, 85]. Ultrasound is also becoming the standard of care for safely and accurately performing invasive procedures as well as evaluating unstable patients [88–93]. Recently, point-of-care ultrasound has been shown to have diagnostic equivalence to computed tomography. As ultrasound technology becomes more portable and affordable, its use will become increasingly widespread and accessible [94, 95]. Given the applicability, portability and patient-centred benefits of point-of-care ultrasound, it seems reasonable that this technology should be introduced during undergraduate medical education [96–98].

Virtual education refers to a new style of education in the learning environment where teacher and student are separated by time or space, or both, and the teacher provides course content through the course management applications, multimedia resources, Internet as well as video conferencing. Several virtual educational systems have been developed and more in the pipeline. Virtual education represents the future of e-learning. New systems take the education standards to another level as it offers interactive holographic lessons. 3D images can pop off the screen thanks to lightweight glasses, and the student can manipulate them with a stylus. Such softwares can be viewed on computers, on tablet and perhaps in the future on smartphones using apps. Students can view them at school and the library at a time that suites them.

What Should Be Done Regarding Undergraduate Teaching in Rheumatology?

The aim of undergraduate medical training is to deliver a graduated doctor who would be able to implement all the key clinical skills and knowledge he/she has learnt in real-life practice and to be able to demonstrate the readiness to handle all the duties and responsibilities of a fully registered doctor [99]. Applying this to rheumatology, a student should have learnt core knowledge and key skills about the locomotor system and should be able to put this into practice in regard to clinical musculoskeletal work. The EULAR standing committee on education and training [100] was among the first authorities to outline the expected musculoskeletal skills expected from a newly graduated doctor. The committee stated that at the end of the medical course, students should be able to assess, by appropriate history taking and clinical examination (adopting a problem-orientated approach), an adult patient with locomotor symptoms in terms of descriptive symptoms and signs, impact on the patient's functional ability and quality of life including psychological status, state a limited differential diagnosis, consider relevant investigations and outline an appropriate management plan (medical/surgical/rehabilitation). Dealing with chronic and debilitating arthritic conditions, rheumatology represents an excellent model for enhancing the generic skills necessary for a good doctor–patient relationship. Rheumatologist should have extra good communication and motivation skills to be able to manage this cohort of patients [100, 101]. It is suggested that attaining these should be an additional objective of undergraduate training in rheumatology.

How can these educational targets and objectives best be achieved? Perhaps the first step is to ensure uniformity in core teaching. A core curriculum for rheumatology with principal domains and learning objectives should be agreed [101]. There are a number of components within each of these domains that have been listed, and this could provide the basis upon which individual medical schools can build. It is envisaged that the content of the curriculum would contain certain common conditions that are universal, such as trauma, low back pain, osteoarthritis, inflammatory arthritis, infections and gout, but there would be a further development of the curriculum dependent upon local needs. There are also needs for an agreement on what are the expected skills and procedures to be taught in the examination of the locomotor system. One of the steps in that direction was made with the development and validation of a screening examination, the *GALS* (gait, arms, legs, spine) [102]. This screening examination is a simple valuable tool for the recognition of important abnormalities in the locomotor system. It has been suggested by Walker and Kay [103] that there should be a two-level approach to the examination of the locomotor system. The first level would be a GALS screening examination, which distinguishes normal from abnormal and localizes abnormality to a region of the body. This is then followed by a more targeted and detailed regional examination if an abnormality is found. An alternative diagnostic strategy is the "pathobiology approach" where assessment starts first by reviewing the anatomy and pathophysiology of the affected skeletal tissue/structure. Targeted history taking and examination are expected to identify the pattern of predominant tissue involvement and can direct attention towards the disease primarily associated with that tissue [104]. Regardless of the approach, in general, there is a need for agreement as to what should be taught at the level of regional examination which should be included in the core curriculum for rheumatology training. Such an agreement needs to be at national level and should be underpinned by the approval of the professional bodies.

Ideally, the elements of the core curriculum should be spread over the whole undergraduate course. Longitudinal integrated clerkships are good example of how learners spend an extended time in a clinical setting (or a variety of interlinked clinical settings). In this way, the learning experience of each year cannot only be reinforced but can also build incrementally upon that of the previous years to endorse deeper, and more effective, learning. Though traditionally rheumatologists or orthopaedic surgeons would be the best role model for teaching musculoskeletal disorders, many of the components of the core curriculum can be taught by teachers from other specialties. In fact, over the past years, there has been a shift towards greater community-based locomotor teaching through primary care physicians [105].

The team-based learning is a teaching model which adopts group learning, emphasizes collaboration and coordination in learning and advocates classroom tests and previews of study content. It was proposed by Michaelsen et al. [106], an educator at the University of Oklahoma, in 2002, with an initial intention of coping with the teaching pressure resulting from the surge of student numbers in the 1970s. The operating feature of the team-based learning is that students are the main actors who engage in group discussions under the guidance of teachers to promote the students' self-motivated learning and teamwork [107–109]. Compared with the traditional teaching method that is dominated by a teacher's lectures, the team-based learning underscores primarily the students' main actor role in the learning process, while teachers act as guides and advisers. The team-based learning cornerstone is the students' participation taking the initiative in the teaching process [110, 111]. Currently, although its teaching effectiveness and applicability remain controversial, the team-based learning teaching method has been recognized and adopted by medical schools in most countries [112–116]. According to a systemic review by Fatmi et al. [115], most existing studies have demonstrated that the team-based learning significantly improves students' knowledge level. However, some investigators found that compared with other teaching methods, the team-based learning exhibited no advantage. In addition, students' attitudes towards team-based learning teaching have been mixed. Although the team-based learning has been applied for many years, its impact on teaching effectiveness and recognition by teachers and students still requires more studies to provide more definitive evidence for validation and support [117].

To date, there have been no large-scale initiatives involving professions allied to medicine in the teaching of undergraduate medical students in rheumatology or for the examination of the locomotor system. However, with the growing role of specialist rheumatology nurses, it is expected that rheumatology nurse specialists as well as specialist physiotherapists and occupational therapists may provide a valuable pool of teachers. Patients living with chronic inflammatory arthritic conditions have also given a role in teaching the undergraduate students some of the musculoskeletal skills. These approaches represent an opportunity to improve the ratio of teachers to learners, as well as provide the student with a wider exposure to experiences of healthcare delivery that is not restricted by arbitrary professional boundaries.

Having conferred objectives and strategies of the educational process, the third step to be addressed is assessment. In George Miller's proposed classification of skills and performance, methods of assessment in medical education were set up in a pyramid, where "knows" (knowledge) is at the lowest level of the pyramid followed by "knows how" (competence), "shows how" (performance) and "does" (action) [48]. These four levels of the pyramid correspond broadly to knowledge base, skills, competence and performance. Miller specifically distinguished between the top two levels of the pyramid and the lower two levels. The higher levels are considered as "testing situation" as they focus on what actually happens in practice rather than what happens in an artificial testing situation. Work-based assessment methods target the higher levels, whereas the two lower levels are targeted mainly by the more conventional forms of assessment. In a model in which undergraduate rheumatological training is a single longitudinal program, it is expected that in the early years, the student might focus on a knowledge base which could be assessed using multiple-choice questions or the short answer question format. As teaching progresses through the years, clinical skills are expected to be developed, and the student will need to demonstrate that they know what to do and how to do it. OSCEs [58, 118] and objective structured long examination records (OSLERs) [119] should feature much more prominently in this sort of assessment. Towards the end of the training and as a junior doctor, the learner will need to be assessed against competence: "Can the candidate do it?" For an established practitioner, the assessment is against performance: "Is it actually done?"

There is a subtle, but important, difference between skills and competence. Skill is the ability to do something. Competence is the ability to do something effectively and well. The crucial difference lies in the word "effectively". The relevance of this in clinical practice is that a skill may be learned by rote and repeated practice. However, competence requires the addition of attitudes, behaviour and responsiveness to the application of a skill in a particular clinical situation. A useful definition of competence has been provided by Epstein and Hundert as "the habitual and judicious use of communication, knowledge, technical skills, clinical reasoning, emotions, values and reflection in daily practice for the benefit of the individual and the community being served" [61]. Competence is an integrative function that builds on the foundation of basic clinical skills and scientific knowledge. It requires the use of knowledge, moral development, effective communication with patients and colleagues and willingness and emotional awareness to use such skills judiciously and humanely in order to solve real-life problems [120].

Performance assessment, which provides a measure of the individual competence, is an essential component of any physician management process. As the physician performance is actually a complex process, which measures the outcomes that are achieved through the application of both clinical and affective skills, it is argued that a variety of measures and instruments are required to provide an overall assessment of performance. Therefore, the assessment of competence requires an assessment of knowledge, technical skills, problem-solving, understanding attitudes and ethics [121]. Direct observation of the consultation can be one possible approach to competency-based assessment in rheumatology practice. The clinical consultation is an integral part of the rheumatology practice, and the subsequent part of patient management is driven based on it. Direct observation of the consultation would reliably assess whether the competencies attained from the rheumatology core curriculum components have been successfully achieved. Vital to the consultation assessment process is to identify and use the appropriate evaluation tool. A possible instrument that could be used for the consultation assessment is the Leicester Assessment Package (LAP). The LAP, developed in Leicester, was designed for both formative and summative purposes. There are seven prioritized categories of consultation competence with a number of individual components in each category. The seven categories include history taking, physical examination, patient management, problem-solving, relationship with patients, anticipatory care and record-keeping. The Leicester Assessment Package has been used in general practice, in the postgraduate setting in ENT surgery and for the assessment of medical students at the Leicester Warwick Medical School for the intermediate clinical examinations and the final clinical examinations. It is suggested that using the Leicester Assessment Package (LAP) for direct observation of the consultation would be a useful tool to assess whether the student has successfully acquired the necessary competencies expected at the end of an undergraduate training in rheumatology. It is suggested that using the Leicester Assessment Package (LAP) or another direct observation assessment method would allow assessment of whether the student has successfully acquired the necessary competencies and also address the more complex psychosocial and attitudinal issues involved in a rheumatology consultation [122].

Another emerging tool in assessing performance includes 360-degree evaluation [114]. This method is extremely helpful in assessing professionalism and communication. A 360-degree performance assessment provides the physicians with an opportunity to obtain feedback on their effectiveness as clinicians. Feedback is gathered from the physician colleagues, admin staff, allied professionals, nurses as well as patients. It should help the rheumatologists/physicians reflect on how they work and identify ways they can improve their practice.

In conclusion, undergraduate medical students need to develop a minimum level of competence in evaluating patients, and this needs to be combined with basic knowledge of the locomotor system, which should include cell biology and the anatomy, physiology and pathology of bones, joints and muscles. It is envisaged that the content of the curriculum would contain certain common conditions that are universal, such as acute and chronic inflammatory arthritic conditions, mechanical joint and spine pains, degenerative changes as well as sepsis, but there would be a further development of the curriculum dependent upon local needs. Clinical skills are usually best acquired in outpatient clinics, specialist wards, emergency services, primary care and clinical skills centres. However, this needs to be combined with formal instruction and problem-based learning which are a useful adjunct, especially for more complex problems and those that have a large social aspect to their management. Assessment should be by the use of reliable and validated tests, and the desired competence should include the acquisition not only of the skills necessary for the assessment and diagnosis of musculoskeletal conditions but also of an appropriate attitude in managing patients with chronic conditions. An integrated musculoskeletal core curriculum in the undergraduate years could provide a powerful tool to achieve this [33].

References

1. Cividino A. The challenges of developing online learning. J Rheumatol. 2009;36:3–4.
2. Walker JG, Littlejohn GO. Measuring quality of life in rheumatic conditions. Clin Rheumatol. 2007;26:671–3.
3. Alonso J, Ferrer M, Gandek B, Ware JE Jr, Aaronson NK, Mosconi P, Rasmussen NK, Bullinger M, Fukuhara S, Kaasa S, Leplege A. Health-related quality of life associated with chronic conditions in eight countries: results from the International Quality of Life Assessment (IQOLA) project. Qual Life Res. 2004;13:283–98.
4. Almoallim H, Khojah E, Allehebi R, Noorwali A. Delayed diagnosis of systemic lupus erythematosus due to lack of competency skills in musculoskeletal examination. Clin Rheumatol. 2007;26:131–3.
5. Beattie KA, Bobba R, Bayoumi I, Chan D, Schabort I, Boulos P, Kean W, Obeid J, Mccallum R, Ioannidis G, Papaioanno A, Cividino A. Validation of the GALS musculoskeletal screening exam for use in primary care: a pilot study. BMC Musculoskelet Disord. 2008;9:115.
6. Gagne R. The conditions of learning. New York: Holt, Rinehart and Winston; 1977.
7. Thompson A. Improving undergraduate musculoskeletal education: a continuing challenge. J Rheumatol. 2008;35:2298–9. https://doi.org/10.3899/jrheum.080972.
8. Abou-Raya A, Abou-Raya S. The inadequacies of musculoskeletal education. Clin Rheumatol. 2010;29:1121–6.
9. Matzkin E, Smith MEL, Freccero CD, Richardson AB. Adequacy of education in musculoskeletal medicine. J Bone Joint SurgAm. 2005;87:310–4.

10. Beran MC, Awan H, Rowley D, Samora JB, Griesser MJ, Bishop JY. Assessment of musculoskeletal physical examination skills and attitudes of orthopaedic residents. J Bone Joint Surg. 2012;94:e36.
11. Comer GC, Liang E, Bishop JA. Lack of proficiency in musculoskeletal medicine among emergency medicine physicians. J Orthop Trauma. 2014;28:e85–7.
12. Hull P, Chaudry A, Prasthofer A, Pattison G. Optimal sequencing of bedside teaching and computer-based learning: a randomised trial. Med Educ. 2009;43:108–12.
13. Vioreanu MH, O'Daly BJ, Shelly MJ, Devitt BM, O'Byrne JM. Design, implementation and prospective evaluation of a new interactive musculoskeletal module for medical students in Ireland. Ir J Med Sci. 2013;182:191–9.
14. Day CS, Yeh AC. Evidence of educational inadequacies in region specific musculoskeletal medicine. Clin Orthop Relat Res. 2008;466:2542–7.
15. Skelley NW, Tanaka MJ, Skelley LM, LaPorte DM. Medical student musculoskeletal education: an institutional survey. J Bone Joint Surg Am. 2012;94:1–7.
16. Modica RF, Thundiyil JG, Chou C, Diab M, Von Scheven E. Teaching musculoskeletal physical diagnosis using a web-based tutorial and pathophysiology-focused cases. Med Educ Online. 2009;14:13.
17. Lynch JR, Gardner GC, Parsons RR. Musculoskeletal workload versus musculoskeletal clinical confidence among primary care physicians in rural practice. Am J Orthop (Belle Mead NJ). 2005;34:487–91.
18. Matzkin E, Smith EL, Freccero D, Richardson AB. Adequacy of education in musculoskeletal medicine. J Bone Joint Surg Am. 2005;87:310–4.
19. Ramani S, Ring BN, Lowe R, Hunter D. A pilot study assessing knowledge of clinical signs and physical examination skills in incoming medicine residents. J Grad Med Educ. 2010;2:232–5.
20. Di Caprio MR, Covey A, Bernstein J. Curricular requirements for musculoskeletal medicine. J Bone Joint Surg Am. 2003;85:565–7.
21. Day CS, Yeh AC, Franko O, Ramirez M, Krupat E. Musculoskeletal medicine: an assessment of the attitudes and knowledge of medical students at Harvard Medical School. Acad Med. 2007;82:452–7.
22. Craton N, Matheson GO. Training and clinical competency in musculoskeletal medicine. Identifying the problem. Sports Med. 1993;15:328–37.
23. AAMC. Report VII contemporary issues in medicine: musculoskeletal medicine education, medical school objectives project no. VII. Washington, DC: Association of American Medical Colleges; 2005.
24. Wise EM, Walker DJ, Coady DA. Musculoskeletal education in general practice: a questionnaire survey. Clin Rheumatol. 2014;33:989–94.
25. Day CS, Ahn CS, Yeh AC, Tabrizi S. Early assessment of a new integrated preclinical musculoskeletal curriculum at a medical school. Am J Orthop. 2011;40:14–8.
26. Al-Nammari SS, James BK, Ramachandran M. The inadequacy of musculoskeletal knowledge after foundation training in the United Kingdom. Bone Joint J. 2009;19:1413–8.
27. Onetti CM. Undergraduate education in rheumatology in Latin America. J Rheumatol. 1999;26(Suppl 55):22–3.
28. Kalla AA. Undergraduate rheumatology teaching in Africa. J Rheumatol. 1999;26(Suppl 55):26–8.
29. Lien IN. Undergraduate education in rheumatology in Asian Pacific countries (APLAR). J Rheumatol. 1999;26(Suppl 55):19.
30. Nottidge TE, Ekrikpo U, Ifesanya AO, Nnabuko RE, Dim EM, Udoinyang CI. Pre-internship Nigerian medical graduates lack basic musculoskeletal competency. Int Orthop. 2012;36:853–6.
31. Praemer A, Furner S, Rice D. Musculoskeletal conditions in the United States. Rosemont: American Academy or Orthopaedic Surgeons; 1999.

32. Adebajo A, Windsor K, Hassell A, Dacre J. Rheumatology. 2005;44(9):1202–3. https://doi.org/10.1093/rheumatology/keh677.
33. Åkesson K, Dreinhöfer K, Woolf A. Improved education in musculoskeletal conditions is necessary for all doctors. Bull World Health Organ. 2003;81:677–83.
34. Woolf AD, Walsh N, Akesson K. Global core recommendations for a musculoskeletal undergraduate curriculum. Ann Rheum Dis. 2004;63(5):517–24.
35. Coxib and traditional NSAID Trialists' (CNT) Collaboration, Bhala N, Emberson J, Merhi A, Abramson S, Arber N, Baron JA, Bombardier C, Cannon C, Farkouh ME, FitzGerald GA, Goss P, Halls H, Hawk E, Hawkey C, Hennekens C, Hochberg M, Holland LE, Kearney PM, Laine L, Lanas A, Lance P, Laupacis A, Oates J, Patrono C, Schnitzer TJ, Solomon S, Tugwell P, Wilson K, Wittes J, Baigent C. Vascular and upper gastrointestinal effects of non-steroidal anti-inflammatory drugs: meta-analyses of individual participant data from randomised trials. Lancet. 2013;382(9894):769–79.
36. Schmale GA. More evidence of educational inadequacies in musculoskeletal medicine. Clin Orthop Relat Res. 2005;437:251–9.
37. DiGiovanni BF, Chu JY, Mooney CJ, Lambert DR. Maturation of medical student musculoskeletal medicine knowledge and clinical confidence. Med Educ Online 2012;17:17092.
38. Day CS, Ahn CS, Yu Y. The addition of an upper-extremity curriculum in medical school education and its assessment. J Hand Surg Eur. 2009;34:797–9.
39. Queally JM, Kiely PD, Shelly MJ, O'Daly BJ, O'Byrne JM, et al. Deficiencies in the education of musculoskeletal medicine in Ireland. Ir J Med Sci. 2008;177:99–105.
40. Clawson DK, Jackson DW, Ostergaard DJ. It's past time to reform the musculoskeletal curriculum. Acad Med. 2001;76:709–10.
41. Henrickson M. Policy challenges for the pediatric rheumatology workforce: Part I. Education and economics. Pediatr Rheumatol Online J. 2011;29:23.
42. Monrad SU, Zeller JL, Craig CL, Diponio LA. Musculoskeletal education in US medical schools: lessons from the past and suggestions for the future. Curr Rev Musculoskelet Med. 2011;4:91–8.
43. Lynch JR, Schmale GA, Schaad DC, Leopold SS. Important demographic variables impact musculoskeletal knowledge and confidence of academic primary care physicians. J Bone Joint Surg Am. 2006;88:1589–95.
44. Cannella AC, Moore GF, Mikuls TR, O'Dell JR, McBrien SB, Hearth-Holmes M, Klassen LW, Snow MH, Feely MG, Fowler ZD, Burchell M, Erickson AR. Teaching rheumatology in undergraduate medical education: what are the students saying? [abstract]. Arthritis Rheumatol. 2015;67(suppl 10). http://acrabstracts.org/abstract/teaching-rheumatology-in-undergraduate-medical-education-what-are-the-students-saying/. Accessed 7 Mar 2018.
45. Norcini J, Anderson B, Bollela V. Criteria for good assessment: consensus statement and recommendations from the Ottawa 2010 conference. Med Teach. 2011;33:206–14.
46. Harlen W, James M. Assessment and learning differences and relationships between formative and summative assessment. Assess Educ Princ Policy Pract. 1997;4:365–79.
47. Epstein RM. Assessment in medical education. N Engl J Med. 2007;356(4):387–96.
48. Miller GE. The assessment of clinical skills/ competence/performance. Acad Med. 1990;65(Suppl. 9):S63–7.
49. McCoubrie P. Improving the fairness of multiple choice questions: a literature review. Med Teach. 2004;26(8):709–12.
50. Gupta M, Sharma G, Pal R, Thaman R, Tikoo D. Strategic use of MCQs in undergraduate medical students to improve objectivity of formative assessment. NJIRM. 2012;3(2):113–8.
51. Srivastava A, Dhar A, Aggarwal CS. Why MCQ? Indian J Surg. 2004;66:246–8.
52. Frederiksen N. The real test bias influences of testing on teaching and learning. Am Psychoanal. 1984;39:193–202.
53. Schuwrith LW, Van der Vleuten CP, Donkers HH. A closer look at cueing effects in multiple choice questions. Med Educ. 1996;30:44–9.

54. Schuwirth LW, Van der Vleuten CP. Different written assessment methods: what can be said about their strengths and weaknesses? Med Educ. 2004;38:974–9.
55. McDonald E. The new teacher advisor: student portfolios as an assessment tool. Educ World. http://www.educationworld.com/a_curr/columnists/mcdonald/mcdonald025.shtml. Accessed 9th Mar 2018.
56. Van Der Vleuten CPM. The assessment of professional competence: developments, research and practical implications. Adv Health SciEduc. 1996;1:41–67.
57. Singh T. Evaluation of knowledge. In: Singh T, Singh D, Paul VK, editors. Principles of medical education. 2nd ed. New Delhi: IAP Education Centre; 2000. p. 54.
58. Harden RM, Gleeson FA. Assessment of clinical competence using an objective structured clinical examination (OSCE). Med Educ. 1979;13(1):41–54.
59. Swanson DB, Case SM. Assessment in basic science instructions: direction for practice and research. Adv Health Sci Educ. 1997;2:71–84.
60. Van Der Vleuten CP, Norman GR, De Graaff E. Pitfalls in the pursuit of objectivity: issue of reliability. Med Educ. 1991;25:110–8.
61. Epstein RM, Hundert EM. Defining and assessing professional competence. JAMA. 2002;287:226–35.
62. Epstein RM, Dannefer EF, Nofziger AC, et al. Comprehensive assessment of professional competence: the Rochester experiment. Teach Learn Med. 2004;16:186–96.
63. Mandell B. Energizing rheumatology training: put teaching back into the academic limelight. J Rheumatol. 2013;40:2. https://doi.org/10.3899/jrheum.120935.
64. Birrane J, Misran H, Creaney M, Shorten G, Nix C. A scoping review of ultrasound teaching in undergraduate medical education. Med Sci Educ. 2017; https://doi.org/10.1007/s40670-017-0491-4.
65. Oswald A, Bell M, Snell L, Wiseman J. The current state of musculoskeletal clinical skills teaching for pre-clerkship medical students. J Rheumatol. 2008;35:2419–26.
66. Miedany YE, Gaafary ME, Arousi NE, et al. Flipped learning: can rheumatology lead the shift in medical education? Ann Rheum Dis. 2017;76:431.
67. Raj N, Badcock LJ, Brown GA, Deighton CM, O'Reilly SC. Undergraduate musculoskeletal examination teaching by trained patient educators—a comparison with doctor-led teaching. Rheumatology (Oxford). 2006;45:1404–8.
68. Kosmahl E. Instructional use of computers for entry-level physical therapy education. J Phys Ther Educ. 1994;8:25–31.
69. Simpson B. Web-based and computer-assisted instruction in physical therapy education. J Phys Ther Educ. 2003;17:45–9.
70. Barzak M, Ball P, Ledger R. The rationale and efficiency of problem-based learning and computer assisted learning in pharmaceutical education. Pharm Educ. 2001;1:105–13.
71. Schittek-Janda M, Mattheos N, Nattestad A, Wagner A, Nebel D, Farbom D, Le D, Attstrom R. Simulation of patient encounters using a virtual patient in periodontology instruction of dental students: design, usability, and learning effect in history taking skills. Eur J Dent Educ. 2004;8:111–9.
72. Velan G, Killen M, Dziegielewski M, Kumar R. Development and evaluation of a computer-assisted learning module on glomerulonephritis for medical students. Med Teach. 2002;24:412–6.
73. Vichitvejpaisal P, Siithikongsak S, Preechakoon B, Kraiprasit K, Parakkamodom S, Manon C, Petcharatana S. Does computer-assisted instruction really help to improve the learning process? Med Teach. 2001;35:983–9.
74. Humphrey-Murto S, Smith CD, Touchie C, Wood TC. Teaching the musculoskeletal examination: are patient educators as effective as rheumatology faculty? Teach Learn Med. 2004;16:175–80.
75. Roesch A, Gruber H, Hawelka B, Hamm H, Arnold N, Popal H, Segerer J, Landthaler M, Stolz W. Computer assisted learning in medicine: a long-term evaluation of the Practical Training Programme Dermatology 2000. Med Inf Internet Med. 2003;28:147–59.

76. Stow RC. A study of students' attitudes, perceptions, and satisfaction regarding the use of video streaming for patient assessments in the athletic training and physical therapy classroom [Dissertation]. Bowling Green State University; 2003.
77. Veneri D. The role and effectiveness of computer-assisted learning in physical therapy education: a systematic review. Physiother Theory Pract. 2010;26(6):1–12. https://doi.org/10.3109/09593985.2010.493192.
78. Averns H, Maraschiello M, van Melle E, Day A. Evaluation of a web-based teaching module on examination of the hand. J Rheumatol. 2009;36:623–7.
79. So HJ. Is blended learning a viable option in public health education? A case study of student satisfaction with a blended graduate course. J Public Health Manag Pract. 2009;15:59–66.
80. Cividino A. The challenges of developing online learning. J Rheumatol. 2009;36:470–1. https://doi.org/10.3899/jrheum.090007.
81. Fodor D, Badea R, Poanta L, Dumitrascu DL, Buzoianu AD, Mircea PA. The use of ultrasonography in learning clinical examination: a pilot study involving third year medical students. Med Ultrasonogr. 2012;14:177–81.
82. Hoppmann RA, Rao VV, Poston MB, et al. An integrated ultrasound curriculum (iUSC) for medical students: 4-year experience. Crit Ultrasound J. 2011;3:1–12.
83. Afonso N, Amponsah D, Yang J, et al. Adding new tools to the black bag: introduction of ultrasound into the physical diagnosis course. J Gen Intern Med. 2010;25:1248–52.
84. Brown B, Adhikari S, Marx J, Lander L, Todd GL. Introduction of ultra-sound into gross anatomy curriculum: perceptions of medical students. J Emerg Med. 2012;43:1098–102.
85. Dreher SM, DePhilip R, Bahner D. Ultrasound exposure during gross anatomy. J Emerg Med. 2014;46:231–40.
86. Dinh V, Fu J, Lu S, Chiem A, Fox C, Blaivas M. Integration of ultrasound in medical education at United States Medical Schools. J Ultrasound Med. 2016;35:413–9.
87. Moore CL, Copel JA. Point-of-care ultrasonography. N Engl J Med. 2011;364:749–57.
88. Anderson KL, Jenq KY, Fields JM, Panebianco NL, Dean AJ. Diagnosing heart failure among acutely dyspneic patients with cardiac, inferior vena cava, and lung ultrasonography. Am J Emerg Med. 2013;31:1208–14.
89. Kirkpatrick AW. Clinician-performed focused sonography for the resus-citation of trauma. Crit Care Med. 2007;35(suppl):S162–72.
90. Wu SY, Ling Q, Cao LH, Wang J, Xu MX, Zeng WA. Real-time two-dimensional ultrasound guidance for central venous cannulation: a meta-analysis. Anesthesiology. 2013;118:361–75.
91. Mercaldi CJ, Lanes SF. Ultrasound guidance decreases complications and improves the cost of care among patients undergoing thoracentesis and paracentesis. Chest. 2013;143:532–8.
92. Nicolaou S, Talsky A, Khashoggi K, Venu V. Ultrasound-guided interventional radiology in critical care. Crit Care Med. 2007;35(suppl):S186–97.
93. Perera P, Mailhot T, Riley D, Mandavia D. The RUSH exam: rapid ultrasound in SHock in the evaluation of the critically ill. Emerg Med Clin N Am. 2010;28:29–56. vii
94. Smith-Bindman R, Aubin C, Bailitz J, et al. Ultrasonography versus computed tomography for suspected nephrolithiasis. N Engl J Med. 2014;371:1100–10.
95. Shmueli H, Burstein Y, Sagy I, et al. Briefly trained medical students can effectively identify rheumatic mitral valve injury using a hand-carried ultra-sound. Echocardiography. 2013;30:621–6.
96. Mollenkopf M, Tait N. Is it time to include point-of-care ultrasound in general surgery training? A review to stimulate discussion. ANZ J Surg. 2013;83:908–11.
97. Beggs AD, Thomas PR. Point of use ultrasound by general surgeons: review of the literature and suggestions for future practice. Int J Surg. 2013;11:12–7.
98. Duvall WL, Croft LB, Goldman ME. Can hand-carried ultrasound devices be extended for use by the non-cardiology medical community? Echocardiography. 2003;20:471–6.
99. General Medical Council. The new doctor. Recommendations on general clinical training. London: GMC; 1997.
100. Zeidler H. Methods in undergraduate education in rheumatology. J Rheumatol. 1999;26(Suppl. 55):35–7.

101. Doherty M, Woolf A. Guidelines for rheumatology undergraduate core curriculum. Ann Rheum Dis. 1999;58:133–5.
102. Doherty M, Dacre J, Dieppe M, Snaith M. The 'GALS' locomotor screen. Ann Rheum Dis. 1992;51:1165–9.
103. Walker DJ, Kay LJ. Musculoskeletal examination for medical students: the need to agree what we teach. Rheumatology. 2002;41:1221–3.
104. El Miedany Y, El Aroussy N, Youssef S, Almedany S, Palmer D. Teaching the millennials: using Youtube for teaching rheumatology in the standard educational settings. Ann Rheum Dis. 2018;77:1782.
105. Doherty M, Lanyon P. Rheumatology: what should all doctors know? Ann Rheum Dis. 2000;59:409–13.
106. Michaelsen LK, Bauman KA, Fink LD. Team-based learning: a transformative use of small groups in college teaching. Sterling: Stylus Publishing Press; 2004.
107. Burgess AW, Mcgregor DM, Mellis CM. Applying established guidelines to team-based learning programs in medical schools: a systematic review. Acad Med. 2014;89(4):678–88.
108. Michaelsen LK, Parmelee DX, McMahon KK, Levine RE. Team-based learning for health professions education: a guide to using small groups for improving learning. Sterling: Stylus Publishing Press; 2008.
109. Kilgour JM, Grundy L, Monrouxe LV. A rapid review of the factors affecting health-care students' satisfaction with small-group, active learning methods. Teach Learn Med. 2016;28(1):15–25.
110. Thompson BM, Schneider VF, Haidet P, et al. Team-based learning at ten medical schools: two years later. Med Educ. 2007;41(3):250–7.
111. Gray J, Fana GT, Campbell TB, Hakim JG, Borok MZ, Aagaard EM. Feasibility and sustainability of an interactive team-based learning method for medical education during a severe faculty shortage in Zimbabwe. BMC Med Educ. 2014;28(1):14–63.
112. Hunt DP, Haidet P, Coverdale JH, Richards B. The effect of using team learning in an evidence-based medicine course for medical students. Teach Learn Med. 2003;15(2):131–9.
113. Nieder GL, Parmelee D, Stolfi A, Hudes PD. Team-based learning in a medical gross anatomy and embryology course. Clin Anat. 2005;18(1):56–63.
114. Wiener H, Plass H, Marz R. Team-based learning in intensive course format for first-year medical students. Croat Med J. 2009;50(1):69–76.
115. Fatmi M, Hartling L, Hillier T, Campbell S, Oswald AE. The effectiveness of team-based learning on learning outcomes in health professions education: BEME Guide No.30. Med Teach. 2013;35(12):1608–24.
116. Yang LH, Jiang LY, Xu B, et al. Evaluating team-based, lecture-based, and hybrid learning methods for neurology clerkship in China: a method comparison study. BMC Med Educ. 2014;20(1):14–8.
117. Zeng R, Xiang LR, Zeng J, Zuo C. Applying team-based learning of diagnostics for undergraduate students: assessing teaching effectiveness by a randomized controlled trial study. Adv Med Educ Pract. 2017;8:211–8.
118. Petrusa ER, Blackwell TA, Ainsworth MA. Reliability and validity of an objective structured clinical examination for assessing the clinical performance of residents. Arch Intern Med. 1990;150:573–7.
119. Gleeson F. Assessment of clinical competence using the objective structured long examination record (OSLER). Med Teach. 1997;19:7–14.
120. Goh L, Samanta A, Cavendish S, Heney D. Rheumatology curriculum: passport to the future successful handling of the musculoskeletal burden? Rheumatology. 2004;43:1468–72.
121. McKinley RK, Fraser RC, Van der Vleuten C, Hastings AM. Formative assessment of the consultation performance of medical students in the setting of general practice using a modified version of the Leicester assessment package. Med Educ. 2000;34:573–9.
122. Pritchard L. Lifelong lessons in competence. Med Educ. 2003;37:848–9.

Chapter 8
The Art of Teaching Primary Care Physicians

Introduction

There is an international trend among different health managing authorities towards shifting the locus of care from inpatient to outpatient. This necessitated a relook at the roles of different specialties in both primary and secondary care. Considering rheumatology, outpatient care by specialists is important as rheumatology is broadly an outpatient specialty, and rheumatologists provide "principal care" (i.e., the patient identifies the physician as his or her "doctor") for many of their patients [1–3]. This paved the way for the recommendation endorsed by the Executive Group of the American College of Rheumatology who recommended that rheumatologists should pursue the dual role of consultant and primary care physician for about one-half of their patients [4]. To do so, rheumatologists need to be trained in the knowledge base and skills of primary care.

One might ask, what is the scope of the primary care training? General internal medicine and family medicine educators have more than 20 years' experience in developing primary care residency programmes. Insights into what can be done for rheumatology can be gleaned from that experience. Primary care programmes have some features in common as the primary care service run mostly as community-based practice. An organized curriculum is adopted. It not only covers clinical problems but also preventive medicine and issues important to "doctoring" that are the social, organizational, psychological and communicative aspects of medicine [5]. Their teachers are mostly primary care physicians who have expertise in these areas.

General practitioners (GP)/family medicine residency programmes often develop practice centres in the community [6]. The important principle is that high-quality patient care meets criteria for continuity, accessibility and comprehensiveness. At these sites, there are organized systems to provide laboratory results in a timely, reliable manner, easy access to patients' medical records and adequate support staff for the practitioners. Almost all sites nowadays also include

Y. El Miedany, *Rheumatology Teaching*,
https://doi.org/10.1007/978-3-319-98213-7_8

nurse practitioners and/or physician's assistants, social workers, nutritionists and other allied health professionals so that residents can learn to work on a team. These practices are therefore "good role models" [7].

Why Teaching Rheumatology in Primary Care Is Important?

General practitioners, as their title inform, are trained to be generalists. They have an extremely broad knowledge base, and, in the course of a standard clinic, they are expected to manage different conditions, with a wide age range from the newborn to the elderly and clinical problems in every specialty from gynaecology to psychiatry. Complaints may vary from minor self-limiting problems to terminal illness. They are also expected to manage difficult social problems, drug dependency conditions, as well as absence from work. It would, therefore, be nearly impossible for all GPs to have specialist abilities in all subjects. In fact, many primary care physicians do have in-depth knowledge of certain diseases. However, although GPs cannot be expert in all specialities, they should have basic competencies in all the major illnesses and on how to manage them in a day-to-day service.

In primary care daily practice, patients presenting with musculoskeletal complaints represent a real challenge. Firstly, as they represent the third commonest cause for patients seeking a consultation in general practice, these problems account for 15% of all consultations in primary care [8]. Secondly, if such patients could be adequately diagnosed and treated by the primary care physicians and with the resources within the community, this would reduce some of the pressure on secondary care and leave rheumatologists free to deal with inflammatory and connective tissue disease. Thirdly, bearing in mind the importance of early diagnosis of inflammatory arthritic conditions and the new concept of "window of opportunity", the major role of primary care physicians shifted to be focused on early identification of these patients and referring them to the secondary care to be reviewed in specialized clinics [9].

The Primary Care Needs

Many primary care physicians have reported inadequate training and consequently lack the competency, skills and confidence to manage musculoskeletal disorders in their daily practice [10]. This may reflect in difficulty or inability to recognize musculoskeletal conditions or be aware of what can be achieved by appropriate care. Table 8.1 summarizes the needs met as well as the unmet needs for rheumatology education in the primary care.

In elective programmes only 3.5% of rotating postgraduate interns selected orthopaedic surgery, and less than 1% had training in rheumatology, sports medicine and physical medicine combined [11, 12]. Only 10% of the vocational training schemes for GPs in the United Kingdom include orthopaedics [13]. A survey of

Table 8.1 The met as well as unmet needs for rheumatology education in the primary care

Met needs	Unmet needs
Regional musculoskeletal examinations	Adequate training
Managing specific conditions	Confidence to manage musculoskeletal disorders in their daily practice
Use of analgesics/anti-inflammatory drug therapy	When to refer to the secondary care
	How to manage patients waiting for or in between specialist appointments
	Joint injections/aspirations
	Radiographic and laboratory evaluation

general practice trainees [14] demonstrated that 35% had not received any tutorials on rheumatological topics; 65% of trainees had tutorials for about 2 h instead of the recommended 280 h per year of total teaching in their GP training [15]. The majority of GP trainees in the United Kingdom felt confident in performing regional musculoskeletal examinations and managing specific conditions, but not in injection techniques. Overall, they perceived the amount of rheumatology education during their vocational training as inadequate [14].

In the United States, family practice graduates reported a lower level of confidence in their physical examination, radiographic evaluation, diagnosis and treatment of musculoskeletal patients compared with their confidence levels in dealing with other patients, despite training rotation on an orthopaedic service during their residency [16, 17]. Those with training periods of 8 weeks or longer, however, reported higher confidence in all areas [16].

Primary care physicians in Canada have also been shown to be significantly more confident with a cardiovascular examination than with a musculoskeletal examination [18] and, in particular, lack confidence in joint injections and aspirations and more rarely encountered problems.

The highest level of confidence was observed for using non-steroidal anti-inflammatory drugs (NSAIDs) and managing common/specific musculoskeletal disorders, but the unnecessary use of diagnostic tests, inappropriate prescription of NSAIDs, low use of patient-centred options and lack of diagnostic suspicion of uncommon but dangerous conditions were cause for concern [19]. With the introduction of "window of opportunity" and the need to identify those patients presenting with early inflammatory arthritic conditions [19], primary care physicians faced another unmet need of identifying those patients who need to be referred to the specialized secondary care centres and how to manage these patients in the transition period before being seen in the secondary care.

Examination is known to drive learning. In examinations, students and trainee GPs are seldom assessed for their competency to take an appropriate history and to examine the musculoskeletal system. A change has been reported in the United Kingdom, however, with clinical skills being tested in 64% of medical schools in 1997 compared with 22% in 1990 [20]. Lack of assessment means that graduate physicians may enter clinical practice with deficient knowledge and skills needed to assess and treat these conditions. This was supported by the outcomes of a recent report [21] where students and newly graduated doctors reported that musculoskeletal specialty-led teaching has been inconsistent and bears little resemblance to the curricula.

What Needs to Be Done?

Perhaps the first action need to be taken is to agree standards for undergraduate and postgraduate medical education. Table 8.2 summarizes main tasks to be handled to ensure meeting the standards required by the primary care physicians to manage musculoskeletal conditions. Establishing standards with clearly defined outcomes is the most powerful way of influencing the competence of future doctors in assessing patients with musculoskeletal conditions. The preclinical teaching of basic science should form the foundation for the clinical training phase and include cell biology, anatomy and pathophysiology of bones, joints and muscles. In fact, the locomotor system can serve as a good model for preclinical education as it includes a range of aspects from anatomy, physiology, biomechanics, cell regulation and tissue repair. The focus of a clinical musculoskeletal medicine education should be focused on clinical skills, interpretation of clinical findings and knowledge of common conditions. Since many patients suffer from long-term chronic pain, it is imperative to consider this in the curriculum set-up and the time dedicated to teaching and training to treat patients with such conditions. In its new 2020 curriculum, King's College School of medicine in London dedicated specific time for management of long-term condition for their stage 3 level of teaching (years 4 and 5 students) [22].

Primary care programmes do not include regular rotations in rheumatology, orthopaedics or rehabilitation, which is a gross under provision for the health needs of the population. To make a difference, present and future training programmes should include training at units within these specialties and proactively participate in continuing medical education programmes in musculoskeletal medicine. The latter approach has been successfully tested in Canada, where orthopaedic and rheumatology specialists participated in an injection-skills acquisition programme [23]. Development of collaborative programmes is required, with shared care and assigned contact persons between primary and secondary care.

Table 8.2 Requirements for primary care musculoskeletal education and training

Establishing standards with clearly defined outcomes
Preclinical education
Clinical education and training
Teaching methods
Curriculum/time
Reminders/feedback: promote strategic and deep learning over memory recall
Continuous professional development

General Practitioners with Special Interest (GPSI)

Primary care physicians with expert knowledge in specific disease areas are often influential in improving knowledge and education in primary care. General practitioners (GPs) working in practice are much more accepting of educational activities arising from within primary care itself, rather than those imposed by secondary care. Gillian Hosie [24] reported several reasons for this:

- Primary care GPs understand the nature of general practice, with its specific pathways, protocols, opportunities and stresses.
- If a primary care physician can undertake specialist treatments and educational activities while still working as a GP, other primary care physicians can accept that such activities are both possible and reasonable to perform.
- GPs with specialist knowledge usually have a good working relationship with secondary care staff, thus facilitating improved working of the primary care/secondary care interface.
- There is a greater sense of ownership and partnership, rather than being seen as a "second-rate" practitioner by some members of secondary care.
- Some secondary care practitioners, while decrying the knowledge and skills of GPs, nevertheless fear GPs becoming too skilled, as they may then represent a threat. There is no doubt, however, that the better doctors are educated, in both primary and secondary care, and the more aware they are of each other's strengths and expertise, the better care will be given to the patients, which is the ultimate aim of medical care.

Who to Teach?

When considering who to teach rheumatology in primary care, it is important to include several different target groups:

- GP trainees/registrars who are training in vocational training schemes with a mixture of hospital and GP rotations
- GP principals who are established in a practice
- GP assistants, locums and retainer scheme doctors
- The practice team, including practice nurses, health visitors, district nurses and other practice support staff

Each group has different needs at different times, and educational activities must be sufficiently flexible to deliver what is needed at the appropriate time.

Rheumatology training is largely delivered by the local postgraduate centre and by the GP trainers. Therefore, the quality of this training depends on the interests and enthusiasms of the people involved. Many postgraduate centres concentrate heavily on the quality of the teaching offered and run courses on "teaching the teachers". The old-fashioned standard lecture format has been superseded by short talks, with more small workshops or group work, including practical demonstrations and case history-based presentations. Meetings often concentrate on a particular disease and require input from hospital consultants as well as general practitioners. As a result, such meetings have had the potential for improving the interface between primary and secondary care locally. This, however, does not ensure that rheumatology is well taught until it becomes a core subject with a recognized curriculum and vocational training. Unfortunately, till this is achieved, musculoskeletal training will remain of variable quantity and quality.

The Art of Primary Care Physicians Teaching

For education to be successful, it should be (1) relevant to the doctor's daily work, (2) help to improve patient care and (3) produce an outcome which the individual doctor can see.

Over the past few years, postgraduate centres have looked closely at the kind of educational activities provided for primary care and have devised many interesting and challenging programmes. Those relevant to rheumatology include such topics as:

- GP guide to specific musculoskeletal conditions
- Workshops on referral pathways and treatment protocols/alternative treatments
- Cognitive approach to pain management
- Soft tissue and joint injection workshops using models

In addition to the different types of educational activities, there has been also a shift of the musculoskeletal teaching style from the standard disease-specific to GP-specific approach. This means that instead of focusing on the specific disease standard symptoms, signs, investigations and management teaching style, the GP is taught how to elicit findings, red flags and ways of assessment in standard practice. In order to build an accurate picture of the patient's symptoms and attain a hypothesis of the underlying cause, it is important to assess the pattern of musculoskeletal pain in line with the patient's history. Table 8.3 gives an example of questions which may help the primary care physician to determine if the patient has, or has had, some of the clinical signs associated with inflammatory musculoskeletal condition. Distinguishing inflammatory from non-inflammatory musculoskeletal conditions requires some extra supportive questions. There are several key questions to help further classify if the patient's symptoms are mechanical or inflammatory. Table 8.4 gives an example of how to distinguish between inflammatory and non-inflammatory joint pain, whereas Table 8.5 gives a guide towards differentiating between inflammatory and non-inflammatory back pain. Interpreting simple laboratory or radiology results can be also valuable to stratify the patients suffering from inflammatory arthritic conditions from those who have mechanical musculoskeletal symptoms (Table 8.6).

Table 8.3 Subjective examination and management: the importance of interpreting patient's history, prognostic features and management strategy in the primary care setting

Patient's history	
Joint or soft tissue pain?	
Inflammatory or non-inflammatory joint pain?	
Is there any poor prognostic features?	
Are there extra-articular manifestations?	
How to manage in the primary care setting?	
What are the investigations to do?	
Who to refer to the secondary care?	
Leading questions	
What hurts as you get out of bed in the morning?	
Does the pain wake you up from sleep?	
How long does it take to feel as limber as you are going to feel for the day?	
When is your pain the worst (when you wake up or by the end of the day)?	
Do you smoke?	
Does any member of your family have rheumatoid arthritis/inflammatory arthritis?	
Functional abilities	
Turn faucet/tap handles	Hold a hairbrush/toothbrush
Dress/bath independently	Fix your own breakfast
Walk outdoors on a flat ground	
Poor prognostic features [29]	
Functional limitation (e.g. health assessment questionnaire score or similar valid tools)	
Extra-articular disease (e.g. presence of rheumatoid nodules, RA vasculitis, Felty's syndrome)	
Positive rheumatoid factor or anti-CCP antibodies	
Bony erosions by radiograph	
Treatment in the primary care setting	
NSAID (short term)	
Assess CV, renal, chest and GI risks	
Consider GI protectives (PPI, misoprostol)	
Consider Cox-2 selective agents when indicated	
Paracetamol (<4 gm/day)	
Screen for other over-the-counter paracetamol agents to avoid toxicity	
Steroids	
Intra-articular steroid injection might reduce a flare	
Use steroids as bridge therapy with DMARs while waiting for DMARDs to kick in	
Should not be used as solo therapy	

Table 8.4 Distinction between mechanical and inflammatory arthritic joint pain

Non-inflammatory/mechanical joint pain	Inflammatory arthritis
Subjective manifestations	
Symptoms with use only	Symptoms at rest on and on movement
Pain worse by the end of the day	Pain and stiffness worse in the morning
Morning stiffness <30 min	Morning stiffness >30 min
	Variable course
Progressive worsening course	Variable course
Flares not common	Flares: common
Minimal response to medical treatment	Patient often benefit from medical treatment
Patient symptomatically well	Patient often systemically ill
Objective features	
Swelling: bony	Swelling: soft tissue
Erythema: uncommon	Erythema: common
Warmth: uncommon	Warmth: common
Palpable crepitus	Soft tissue swelling

Table 8.5 Distinction between mechanical and inflammatory back pain

Non-inflammatory back pain	Inflammatory back pain
Age of onset: any age	Age of onset <40 years
Variable onset; may be acute	Insidious onset; less likely to be acute
Less likely to feel stiff in the morning	Morning stiffness >30 min
Pain may worsen with movement	Pain improves with exercise
Pain often improves with rest	Pain does not improve with rest
	Pain at night which may wake patient during second half of the night
Patient systemically well	Psoriasis, uveitis, enthesitis, mouth ulcers, IBD

Analysis of delayed treatment trials (extensions of placebo-controlled investigations in which the placebo group is switched to active treatment at the end point of the initial study) showed the efficacy of early DMARDs treatment for early inflammatory arthritic conditions. In each trial the group treated at presentation with DMARDs showed significantly more improvement in efficacy parameters than the groups whose treatment was delayed. Early intervention improved patient function (reduced HAQ score) and reduced or slowed radiographic disease progression, as well as decreasing swollen joint counts in ~50% of the trials. Criswell et al. showed evidence of systematic differences between rheumatologists and non-rheumatologists in initiating the use of DMARDs for the treatment of RA [25]. Non-rheumatologists generally delay treatment, which can result in substantial differences in the long-term outcome of the disease. Other investigations [26–28] have shown that patients with RA managed by rheumatologists maintained greater functional status over the duration of the disease and had better health outcomes. In addition, newer treatments require specialized administration and monitoring for maximal efficacy and safety.

Therefore, primary care should be taught the identification criteria for those who might have active inflammatory conditions [29]. Table 8.7 gives a list of the referral

Table 8.6 Interpreting investigations in the primary care setting

	Non-inflammatory arthritis	Inflammatory arthritis
Laboratory		
Inflammatory markers (ESR/CRP)	Usually within normal	Commonly elevated
Immunological markers (rheumatoid factor, anti-CCP, ANA)	Negative	Positive
Systemic affection (diabetes mellitus, thyroid functions)	Could be abnormal	Usually within normal
Synovial fluid	White cell count <2000	White cell count >2000
X-ray		
X-ray changes	Usually positive	Negative early in the disease course
Cartilage loss	Focal cartilage loss	Diffuse/symmetrical cartilage loss
Osteophyte formation	Often new bone formation	No new bone formation
Joint distribution	Weight bearing joints involved	Any joint involved (commonly symmetrical)
Presence of erosions	No erosions	More common to find erosions

Table 8.7 Early referral criteria of inflammatory arthritic conditions

Rheumatoid arthritis [30]	Early spondyloarthritis [31]	SLE [32]
1. Persistent joint inflammation >6 weeks 2. Tenderness over the joint line joint 3. Swelling painful limited RoM	Inflammatory back pain in <40 years old Chronic LBP ≥3 months Moring stiffness >30 min Improvement of pain with exercise No improvement with rest Pain at night with improvement upon getting up	Acute/chronic cutaneous lupus
Morning stiffness >30 min	Sacroiliitis (clinical and/or X-ray)	Arthritis
The above two criteria plus one of the following	The above two criteria plus one of the following	Renal disorder
Positive squeeze test MCP and/or MTP joints	HLA-B27	Serositis
Positive rheumatoid factor or anti-CCP	Arthritis	Non-scarring alopecia
Elevated inflammatory markers (ESR or CRP)	Uveitis/enthesitis/dactylitis	Mouth ulcers
	Psoriasis/Crohn's disease	Neurological manifestations
	Good response to NSAIDs	ANA
	Family history of Spondyloarthritis	Anti-dsDNA/anti-sm, anti-phospholipid
	Elevated CRP	Leucopenia, thrombocytopenia
		Direct Coombs' test/low complement

criteria for patients suspected to have early inflammatory musculoskeletal conditions [30–32]. The purpose of the referral recommendation is to provide a tool based on clinical evidence that summarizes the essential and basic diagnostic criteria, allowing early identification of the patient, with suspected inflammatory arthritic condition, in the primary care setting for referral to a rheumatologist. A relatively brief opportunity may exist for initiating the DMARD treatment that can substantially improve the long-term outcome of the disease, as well as the overall quality of life for patients with active inflammatory arthritic conditions. Such referral pathway should be paralleled by specialized clinics in the secondary case able to review these patients within 1–2 weeks. Assessment and management pathways should be clear, published and available for share with the primary care as well as secondary healthcare professionals.

How Can We Improve Education in the Primary Care?

Learning is lifelong, and continuous medical education should extend throughout the physician's professional career. Advances in medicine are rapid and cannot be learnt during initial training, and there is natural public and political concern that the highest standards of care are consistently delivered. Indeed, it turns out it is not enough to solely rely on experience. Although it is generally assumed that an increase of professional experience, knowledge and skills through the years of practical exercise leads to a higher quality of care, research demonstrated an inverse relationship [33–35].

Primary care physicians have been required to gain a certain number of postgraduate education points every year, spread between disease management, health promotion and service management. In most areas, the older-fashioned standard lecture format has been superseded by short talks, with smaller group work, including practical demonstrations and case history-based presentations. Educational meetings are usually organized by the local secondary care hospitals or the primary care trusts and often concentrate on a particular disease. These scientific meetings often require input from hospital consultants as well as general practitioners. As a result, such meetings have had the potential for improving the interface between primary and secondary care locally.

With the publication of different management guidelines, and treatment protocols, more innovative ways have evolved by which GPs can gain educational competencies or five points. These activities have included (1) practice-based meetings, (2) audit, (3) personal learning plans, (4) clinical attachments and (5) critical incidents review. Audit is an objective evaluation comparing the local service provided to a gold standard. It is a good way of monitoring processes and outcomes to identify and subsequently investigate differences in care that require education to overcome. More recently, a formal assessment of performance, appraisal and revalidation have been introduced and become compulsory in many countries. The medical royal colleges and faculties in England have produced guidance to help doctors in all the main specialties, including primary care, to collect their supporting information [36]. Every doctor is expected to bring a portfolio of supporting information to their appraisal which shows how they are meeting the professional values set out in good medical practice. Appraisers will be interested in what doctors think the supporting information says about their practice and how they plan to develop or modify their practice as a result. There are six types of supporting information that doctors will be expected to provide and discuss at their appraisal. They are (1) continuing professional development, (2) quality improvement activity, (3) significant events, (4) feedback from colleagues, (5) feedback from patients and (6) review of complaints and compliments.

Recertification is becoming a requirement in an increasing number of countries. Revalidation of the physician will be considered in view of the appraisal outcomes each 5-year cycle.

Clinical Evaluation: The Way Forward

The way forward in evaluating clinical outcome should include an appraisal of how all patients with musculoskeletal disease are treated at present and should consider the best way forward to improve their care. This should involve close cooperation between primary and secondary care together with community services such as physiotherapy, occupational therapy and social services and with input from relevant patient organizations, to provide the best care possible within the existing limitations of staffing, time constraints and financial restrictions. Primary care groups have the potential to deliver this kind of service, especially in the field of chronic musculoskeletal disease. Over the past few years, some chronic diseases, such as diabetes, asthma and hypertension, have been targeted for increased attention, with most GPs now running clinics for monitoring the care of such patients. With these conditions, it is possible to measure definite end points such as HbA1C in diabetes, peak flows in asthma and blood pressure in hypertension. Although it is possible to monitor patients with chronic musculoskeletal disease using disease activity indices, this is much more difficult and time-consuming than with many other diseases. With a chronic condition such as osteoarthritis, good management requires practical help and advice, repeated patient education and encouragement and support by all members of the practice team during times of disabling and painful flares of disease. The ability to provide such management over many years is one of the attributes of a caring primary care physician.

Caring for chronic inflammatory musculoskeletal conditions require special care similar to other long-term condition. The patients should not only be monitored for their disease activity status but also regularly monitored for their comorbidity and side effects linked to their medications. Recent studies revealed comorbidity indices which can help the primary as well as the secondary care professionals calculate the comorbidity risk [37, 38] or fracture risk [39, 40].

In conclusion, teaching the primary care physicians is a multi-faceted task which requires a dynamic innovative teaching approach. Over the course of a GP's professional life, huge changes will occur owing to advances in medicine, organizational changes in the way primary care is delivered, increasing emphasis on cost effectiveness and changes in society itself. Therefore, it is essential that a primary care physician should take part in a lifelong learning programme; otherwise, he/she won't be able to maintain and continue to improve patient care. As medicine becomes ever more complex, it is increasingly important that all involved in patient care continue, whether primary or secondary care, to work together to provide continuing education and support.

References

1. Council on Graduate Medical Education. Improving access to health care through physician work force reform: directions for the twenty-first century (third report). Washington, DC: United States Department of Health and Human Services, Public Health Service, Health Resources Services Administration; 1992.
2. Colwill JM. Where have all the primary care applicants gone? N End J Med. 1992;326:387–93.
3. Aiken LH, Lewis CE, Craig J. The contribution of specialists to the delivery of primary care: a new perspective. N Engl J Med. 1979;300:1363–70.
4. Sergent JS, Kaplan H, Ruddy S, Weaver A, Koopman W. Managed competition and the rheumatologist. Bulletin on healthcare reform from the ACR executive group. Atlanta: American College of Rheumatology; 1993.
5. Branch WT. Teaching models for ambulatory training programs. J Gen Intern Med. 1990;5(suppl):S15426.
6. Ende J. Feedback in clinical medical education. JAMA. 1983;250:777–81.
7. Branch W. Primary care practice and training in rheumatology. Arthritis Rheum. 1994;37(3):305–6.
8. Office of Population Censuses and Surveys. Morbidity statistics from general practice – 4th national study 1991/92. London: HMSO; 1995.
9. El Miedany Y, Youssef S, Mehanna A, El Gaafary M. Development of a scoring system for assessment of outcome of early undifferentiated inflammatory synovitis. Joint Bone Spine. 2008;75(2):155–62.
10. Åkesson K, Dreinhöfer KE, Woolf AD. Improved education in musculoskeletal conditions is necessary for all doctors. Bull World Health Organ. 2003;81:677–83.
11. Cantillon P, Jones R. Does continuing medical education in general practice make a difference? BMJ. 1999;318:1276–9.
12. Craton N, Matheson GO. Training and clinical competency in musculoskeletal medicine. Identifying the problem. Sports Med. 1993;15:328–37.
13. Booth A, Wise DI. General practice training in musculoskeletal disorders. Br J Gen Pract. 1990;40:390.
14. Lanyon P, Pope D, Croft P. Rheumatology education and management skills in general practice: a national study of trainees. Ann Rheum Dis. 1995;54:735–9.
15. Crawley HS, Levin JB. Training for general practice: a national survey. BMJ. 1990;300:911–5.
16. Matheny JM, Brinker MR, Elliott MN, Blake R, Rowane MP. Confidence of graduating family practice residents in their management of musculoskeletal conditions. Am J Orthop. 2000;29:945–52.

17. Saywell RM Jr, O'Hara BS, Zollinger TW, Wooldridge JS, Burba JL, McKeag DB. Medical students' experience with musculoskeletal diagnoses in a family medicine clerkship. Med Teach. 2002;24:186–92.
18. Glazier RH, Dalby DM, Badley EM, Hawker GA, Bell MJ, Buchbinder R, et al. Management of common musculoskeletal problems: a survey of Ontario primary care physicians. Can Med Assoc J. 1998;158:1037–40.
19. Kay LJ, Deighton CM, Walker DJ, Hay EM. Undergraduate rheumatology teaching in the UK: a survey of current practice and changes since 1990. Arthritis Research Campaign Undergraduate Working Party of the ARC Education Sub-committee. Rheumatology. 2000;39:800–3.
20. KUMEC Curriculum Change 2020. Curriculum Kings College 2020. https://www.kcl.ac.uk/lsm/research/divisions/hscr/study/undergradops/kumec/MBBS-2020.aspx.
21. Blake T. Teaching musculoskeletal examination skills to UK medical students: a comparative survey of rheumatology and orthopaedic education practice. BMC Med Educ. 2014;14:62.
22. Miedany YE, Gaafary ME, Arousi NE, et al. THU0597 Flipped learning: can rheumatology lead the shift in medical education? Ann Rheum Dis. 2017;76:431.
23. Bellamy N, Goldstein LD, Tekanoff RA. Continuing medical education driven skills acquisition and impact on improved patient outcomes in family practice setting. J Contin Educ Heal Prof. 2000;20:52–61.
24. Hosie G. Teaching rheumatology in primary care. Ann Rheum Dis. 2000;59:500–3.
25. Criswell LA, Such CL, Yelin EH. Differences in the use of second-line agents and prednisone for treatment of rheumatoid arthritis by rheumatologists and non-rheumatologists. J Rheumatol. 1997;24:2290.
26. Yelin EH, Such CL, Criswell LA, Epstein WV. Outcomes for persons with rheumatoid arthritis with a rheumatologist versus a non-rheumatologist as the main physician for this condition. Med Care. 1998;36:513–22.
27. Ward MM, Leigh JP, Fries JF. Progression of functional disability in patients with rheumatoid arthritis. Associations with rheumatology subspecialty care. Arch Intern Med. 1993;153:2229–37.
28. Solomon DH, Bates DW, Panush RS, Katz JN. Costs, outcomes, and patient satisfaction by provider type for patients with rheumatic and musculoskeletal conditions: a critical review of the literature and proposed methodologic standards. Ann Intern Med. 1997;127:52–60.
29. Singh J, Furst D, Bharat A, Curtis J, Kavanaugh A. 2012 update of the 2008 American College of Rheumatology recommendations for the use of disease-modifying antirheumatic drugs and biologic agents in the treatment of rheumatoid arthritis. Arthritis Care Res. 2012;64(5):625–39.
30. El Miedany, Palmer D, El Gaafary M. Diagnosis of early arthritis: outcomes of a nurse-led clinic. Br J Nurs. 2006;15(7):394–9.
31. El Miedany Y, Palmer D. Early referral of ankylosing spondylitis patients: results of one year outcome of a specialized early ankylosing spondylitis clinic. Rheumatology (Oxford). 2011;50(S3). Abstract number 263. https://academic.oup.com/rheumatology/article/50/suppl_3/iii137/1789320.
32. Gladman D, Ginzler E, Goldsmith C, Fortin P, Liang M, Urowitz M, et al. The development and initial validation of the systemic lupus international collaborating clinics/American College of Rheumatology Damage Index for systemic lupus erythematosus. Arthritis Rheum. 1996;39(3):363–9.
33. Price D. Continuing medical education, quality improvement, and organizational change: implications of recent theories for twenty-first-century CME. Med Teach. 2005;27:259–68.
34. Rhee SO. Factors determining the quality of physician performance in patient care. Med Care. 1976;14:733–50.
35. Choudhry NK, Fletcher RH, Soumerai SB. Systematic review: the relationship between clinical experience and quality of health care. Ann Intern Med. 2005;142:260–73.

36. GMC. Supporting information for appraisal and revalidation. http://www.gmc-uk.org/doctors/revalidation/revalidation_information.asp.
37. Miedany YEI, Gaafary EIM, Youssef S, Almedany S, Bahlas S, et al. Rheumatoid arthritis comorbidity index (RACI): development and validation of a new comorbidity index for rheumatoid arthritis patients. J Arthritis 2017. 2017;6:244. https://doi.org/10.4172/2167-7921.1000244.
38. El Miedany Y, El Gaafary M, Youssef S, Bahlas S, Hegazi M. Psoriatic arthritis comorbidity index: development and validation of a new specific tool for classifying prognostic comorbidity in psoriasis and psoriatic arthritis patients. Rheumatol Orthop Med. 2017;2:1–7. https://doi.org/10.15761/ROM.1000117.
39. Miedany YE, Gaafary ME, Yassaki AE, Youssef S, Nasr A, Ahmed I. Monitoring osteoporosis therapy: can FRAX help assessing success or failure in achieving treatment goals? World J Rheumatol. 2014;4(2):14–21.
40. El Miedany Y, Toth M. Osteoporosis, fracture prevention and falls risk assessment – closing the gap between treatment guidelines and clinical practice. Eur Musculoskelet Rev. 2011;6(1):7–14.

Chapter 9
The Art of Teaching Nurses

Introduction

The past decades have seen significant changes in nursing education turning it more practically focused, with the purpose of preparing the nurses for their duties as nursing care professionals. Nurse education integrates today a broader awareness of other disciplines allied to medicine, often involving inter-professional education, and the utilization of research when making clinical and managerial decisions. Orthodox training can be argued to have offered a more intense practical skills base but emphasized the handmaiden relationship with the physician. This is now outmoded, and the impact of nurse education is to develop a confident, inquiring graduate who contributes to the care team in a partnership style.

Understanding the continuum of developments in nursing education endorses a mindfulness of the diversity that exists within nursing education and the common purposes that bind it together. It also encourages shared understandings of the various pathways that exist within nursing education and recent approaches to help nurse educators address the complexities surrounding nursing practice. This chapter will provide a descriptive account of nursing education including a contemporary understanding of the art and science in educating nurses, the modern concept of rheumatology nursing as well as the current change in the anatomy of the clinic visits and the nurses' educational needs. It will expand to discuss teaching strategies for nurses' education and current challenges to specialist nursing education and will conclude with a reflection on how future services are likely to be delivered and a vision towards nurse's education in the year 2030.

Y. El Miedany, *Rheumatology Teaching*,
https://doi.org/10.1007/978-3-319-98213-7_9

Understanding the Modern Rheumatology Nurses' Role

Over the past few decades, there have been significant advances in the rheumatology nursing career. Early in the 1980s, the rheumatology nurse's role was limited to data collection (e.g. vital signs, symptoms), drug therapy monitoring, patient and staff education and patient counselling [1]. The introduction of new lines of therapy and the regularly updated diagnostic and management guidelines mandated similar developments in the nurses' role and job responsibilities. In addition to the thorough in-depth patient evaluation (detailed history and physical findings, review of laboratory studies, disease activity assessment and scoring), the rheumatology nurses became in charge of advice (help) lines; ordering, administering and monitoring biologic therapy [2]; patient self-management; care coordination assistance; referral facilitation; as well as patient education and support [3]. The nurses' clinical role also expanded to include nurse-led early arthritis service, disease and treatment risk management, assessment of comorbidities, compliance/adherence counselling regarding the treatment regimen and medical record (paper and electronic) documentation [4–9].

However, specific nurse activities vary tremendously because of several factors, including education requirements, level of training, experience in patients' care, practice setting, support from the senior rheumatologists within the team, attitudes of affiliated healthcare professionals, geographic location, practice regulations, professional societies and the cultural context and policies of their administrators [9]. Similar to all specialist nurses, rheumatology nurses tend to work better within an agreed and defined job responsibilities. Rheumatology nurses have proven their ability to absorb, understand and implement all the recent developments in rheumatology over the past 20 years. Their role even has shifted from a "collaborative caregiver", playing their role within the ordering direction of physicians, to a "decision-making partnership" nurse-led care. However, this is subject to the team they are working with, the set-up of the service as well as meeting their educational targets [10].

Changing the Anatomy of the Clinic Visit and the Nurses' Educational Needs

Nursing education has expanded to advanced degrees and specialization, with the registered nurse's role including more comprehensive gathering of clinical information, patient-reported outcomes measurement, interdisciplinary care coordination, focusing on patient engagement and self-management, in-depth treatment education and monitoring. This development in the nurse's role was paralleled by another change in the anatomy of the clinic visit which becomes increasingly complex and time-consuming. The elements in a typical visit now include the following: the patients registers and checks in; rooming the patients and obtaining their chief complaint, interval history, medication review, assessment and recording of the patient reported outcomes, measurement of the vital signs; assessment of disease activity score, review the lab results and radiology reports, engages in discussion and joint decision making with the patient, provides documentation in the electronic or paper medical record, and creates referral communication whenever required; and the patients checking out, schedules follow-up, as well as dictate a visit outcome report. Completing all these activities in average of 30-min session is challenging [11].

Rheumatology nurse's education should aim at the development of the nurse's skills, knowledge and attitudes relevant to the advanced level of nursing practice in rheumatology. This will include the engagement of rheumatology nurses in aspects of drug therapy, clinical assessment, psychosocial issues and appraisal of the existing service versus the guidelines and treatment recommendation so that they may be able to analyse, reflect on, evaluate and develop the existing clinical practice and enhance their own professional capabilities. At the same time the nurses should be equipped with the necessary skills to appraise and evaluate research and to design and undertake their own research projects [12].

Educational rheumatology nurses' courses should encourage an analytical and questioning approach to the care of people living with inflammatory musculoskeletal conditions. They should lead the students to evaluate their current practice and to adopt innovative practice, based on critical appraisal of research and development of evidence-based practice developing from such evaluation of research. The ability to reflect on the present management approach and being amenable to changes in healthcare system while preserving the quality of the service provided prove attractive to employers who are seeking high-quality trained rheumatology nurses.

The Science of Nursing Education

Nurses are educated over a minimum 3-year period to a degree level (some diploma-level courses for nurses still exist). While the nurses' education is organized in the university campus, where the theoretical component is delivered, the required clinical experience is obtained during the nurses' placements in hospitals or the community. Clinical placements may last from 6 weeks to 6 months, during which time students are generally supernumerary to the workforce [13].

Education includes theoretical and practical elements designed to give nurse students appropriate knowledge, skills and attitudes for their future roles. University courses follow guidelines from the professions' governing bodies [14, 15], who also participate in course validation. The nursing profession face two problems in providing musculoskeletal nurses' education. Firstly, there is pressure on time for theoretical input. Similar to undergraduate medical students, the nursing curricula become increasingly overcrowded, with rheumatology having to compete with other specialties for timetable space. Research into rheumatology education revealed that the total time spent teaching rheumatology in 2000 was half that reported in 1992 [16]. Secondly, there are limitations in clinical exposure to inpatients with chronic illness, as inpatient facilities became concentrated on acute illness [17], leading to closure of dedicated rheumatology inpatient wards. Paradoxically, this threat to the availability of rheumatology theoretical and clinical experience comes at a time when the role of the rheumatology specialist nurses is expanding. Consequently, rheumatology nurses' education became dependent on apprenticeship or mentoring. However, with the current pressure on the service and the shortage of the specialist rheumatology nurses, this, by itself, is also facing several challenges.

Little has been published about the rheumatology content of nursing courses. A study of health professionals' undergraduate rheumatology education in the United States and Canada 25 years ago showed that, while programme directors believed the rheumatology theory content to be adequate (irrespective of the actually delivered amount), they generally believed clinical exposure to rheumatology was insufficient [18, 19]. A more recent survey of Canadian physiotherapy undergraduate courses showed an average 22.5 h instruction, with clinical placements in rheumatology offered on 77% of courses [20]. The only UK study which explored the teaching of general rehabilitation, disability and chronic illness issues to undergraduate nurses showed teaching to be both limited and superficial [21].

The Association of Rheumatology Health Professionals (USA) has published competencies for entry- and advanced-level nurses [22]. Similarly, the arthritis research campaign (UK) has produced consensus standards for qualified health professionals entering into extended clinical roles in rheumatology [23]. These recommendations outline the required rheumatology knowledge and skills as well as attitude needed to be achieved by the rheumatology nurse specialist. However, these recommendations apply to qualified staff who wish to make a career in rheumatology and do not necessarily reflect the minimum rheumatology knowledge that would be appropriate for undergraduate students.

On another front, one of the major advantages in modern rheumatology nursing is the significant development of evidence-based care. Evidence-based healthcare promotes the collection, interpretation and integration of valid important and applicable patient-reported, nurse-/clinician-observed and research-derived evidence. The diagnostic and management guidelines paved the way for rheumatology nurses to implement science into their day-to-day practice [24]. Moreover, the Internet and other sources of research evidence have increased exponentially, facilitating the availability of treatment recommendations and disease activity score calculators at the nurses' fingertips while they are reviewing the patient. However, evidence-based practice is a way of thinking which requires discipline and practice. The nurse should be able to weigh the evidence against the validity and reliability of daily practice activities. The ability to implement the available up-to-date information and shift the standard nursing practice to be evidence based results in care decisions that are more concordant with current recommendations, better tailored to the individual patient's condition, and is ultimately associated with improved clinical as well as patient-reported outcomes [25, 26].

The Art of Nursing

Aesthetics, or the art of nursing, is the type of knowledge underlying the performance of nursing practice or "knowing how". Aesthetic knowledge lies beneath the skilful performance of the manual and technical procedures in nursing, as well as the ability to grasp the significance of a patient's symptoms or behaviour immediately and respond insightfully to it [27]. Learning the art of nursing requires nurses to master the ability to put together several information about a patient's behaviour into a holistic understanding of what is significant in that behaviour. Through empathy, the nurse gains understanding of the patient's experience, and based on the nurse's collection of choices, she/he can design and provide nursing care that is effective and satisfying. Aesthetic knowledge is action- oriented and includes both the technical skills of the profession and the intellectual skill necessary for grasping a situation, making a care plan and then intervening in a clinical encounter.

Aesthetic knowledge is more complex than empirical knowledge and requires both motor skills and strategies which enable the nurse to make sense of information. This practical knowledge is what was described earlier as "knowing how" [28] and is gained through experience, when one's frame of reference about what can be expected is somehow altered or challenged in an actual, real-life situation, not just mere passage of time. The complex acquisition of skills sometimes escapes our expectations to describe even simple activities theoretically. As a result, some practical knowledge will not be easily reduced to step-by step explanation [29].

An example is that when people find out that they have arthritis, they often feel a sense of shock, disbelief or helplessness. After they learn more about arthritis and its treatment, they may feel overwhelmed or angry. At some point most people with arthritis realize that the disease is, indeed, a fact of their lives. With this awareness, they may become depressed [30–32]. The role of the rheumatology specialist nurse should be responsive, dynamic and give a good example about the art of nursing. Patients need a point of contact when they feel ill, anxious or depressed. The rheumatology nurse specialist within the hospital and the community is seen to be the professional who is able to coordinate and support the patients, by networking and linking with all the extended multidisciplinary teams and trying to deal with the psychological impact of the disease [33].

The Art of Nursing Education

When it comes to the nurses and nursing education, the expression "art of education" would have a special flavour. Art has been considered as understanding the person and seeing it from their point of view. Unfortunately, over the past years, it has been suggested that there is too much emphasis on the science and not enough focus on the aesthetic which nature of care. This reflects the mutual concept of nurse education, where the main emphasis is focused on fitness for practice and the statutory competencies. Putting the art back into nursing education would have a significant impact on the career, not only as a specialist nurse but as a nurse practitioner.

Adding "art" to nursing education gives the education process a "3-D" experience. Table 9.1 shows a guide to successful nursing education. These principles provide insight on the infrastructure and capacities that educators should have in place to improve their teaching skills and ensure conducting the message. The first nurse education principle, away from the crude science, is to "get the theory across". Nurses, like many people, tend to be practical or experiential learners [34], i.e. they learn best from doing something rather than reading about it. This can make understanding theory or retaining facts more difficult. To dilute this challenge, it is important to link the theory to everyday life activity and use practice or real-life scenarios to bring facts and theory alive, and allowing apprenticeship or setting up workshops to pool ideas and learn from each other is helpful to get over the hurdle. Feeding back to the larger group and facilitator can help to rectify the anomaly. Furthermore, letting the nurses or learning nurses explore "what if" situations or case histories where a problem can be solved using the information they've been learning would have a positive feedback on the nurses' learning and self-confidence. The "what if" scenario exercises can help learning become real and applicable to reality. Asking questions encourage the nurses to actively engage in the learning process and enables them to take responsibility for their answers. Using visual media such as video, pictures and diagrams is expected to simplify the difficulty of the subject.

Another approach is "practical learning". Psychomotor skills like setting up a biologic therapy infusion suite and learning intravenous or subcutaneous injection skills will enhance practical learning while a new neural pathway is formed in the brain. The "see one, do one, teach one" model of learning is useful as it encourages the nurse to learn as if she were going to be a teacher. This encourages greater mental involvement in the knowledge-gaining process. So in a group setting it might be advantageous to let learners work in monitored trios, with a teacher, student and observer each participant taking a role in turn and the observer feeds back.

On another front, most of the nurses' learning relies on lectures, and presentations play an important role in nursing education. Giving a talk is an art by itself. Enhancing

Table 9.1 Guide to nursing education: what do the nurses like when attending an educational activity

Get theory across (learn from doing rather than reading)
Link theory to everyday practice
A framework, written guidance, handouts
Apprenticeship / workshop work positively
Explore "what if" situations or case history
Visual aids (simplifying videos, pictures, diagrams)
See one, do one, teach one
Eye contact ("gathering friends") technique
Implementing new education strategies, e.g. simulation, role play, games
Cost-effective

presentation skills is the key towards effective and positive outcome. In groups, it is always advisable to make eye contact while speaking and holding pauses. Ron Hoff [35] called this "gathering friends" in the audience. Smiling while talking and speak as if the speaker is addressing each person individually. Confident and relaxed body language plays an important role in delivering the message. Up to 55% of the message given is non-verbal, 38% is the tone of voice, and 7% is the actual words (Fig. 9.1) [36]. It is always advisable to breathe and speak more slowly during giving a talk. It's easier to project the speaker's voice and make it heard when speaking more slowly.

The art also goes beyond the talk to the presentation itself. Preparing PowerPoint slides for teaching is an art by itself. It is always advisable to make one point/argument on one slide, keep the text big –font 26 points or above – so that is it is visible to everyone, use the "KISS" principle (keep it short and sweet), use pictures in place of words, use plain font without a distracting slide design and use bullet points and headings that can be expanded on. Giving handouts of the slides will give the nurses the security that they have the scientific content and help them to focus on the content of the presentation (Table 9.2).

In short, *educating nurses requires the art to implement the science.* The best nurse educators are the nurses themselves. Nurses do have the art of educating and are uniquely placed as educators in the clinical and classroom settings. This is simply based on their excellent communication skills with both patients and peers. Nurses often underestimate how effective they are in passing on the skills they do every moment of every working day, because someone (student nurse, colleague or patient) is watching and learning.

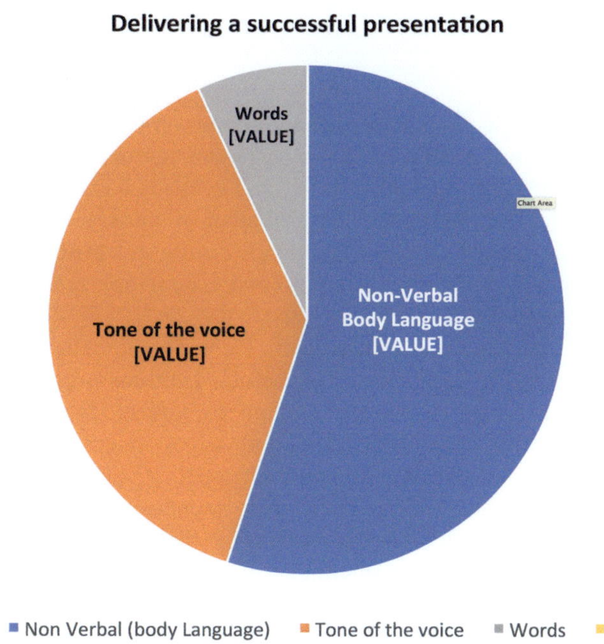

Fig. 9.1 Presentation skills: delivering the message in a given talk. Up to 55% of the message given is non-verbal and relies mainly on the body language, 38% is the tone of voice, 7% the actual words

Table 9.2 The art of nurse education. Tips for presentation skills and using PowerPoint presentations

Tips on using PowerPoint for teaching	Presentation tips
Make one point/argument on one slide	Make eye contact as you speak and hold pauses
Keep the text big – 26 points or above – so that it's visible to everyone	Smile as you talk, and speak as if you're addressing each person individually
Use the KISS principle – keep it short and sweet	Make your body language confident and relaxed
Use pictures with or in place of words	Breathe and speak more slowly during your talk
Use plain font without a distracting slide design	
Use bullet points and headings that you can expand on	

Teaching Strategies in Nursing Education

There are a variety of teaching strategies that educators can use to improve the nurses learning. It is of great importance to select appropriate teaching strategy in nurse education to make the training more appealing and more effective. In fact, selecting the proper teaching strategy is the fundamental component of instructional design (Fig. 9.2). The goal is to help the learners process information more deeply, which allows them to relate new information to existing ideas or experiences [37, 38]. There are several useful teaching strategies, these include:

Lecturing

Lecturing is the oldest and most common teaching strategy that is widely used up until now. Lecturing is a direct smooth approach to deliver the message and export knowledge to students efficiently. Lecturing has some advantages: (1) the facility to provide information to a big number of students and cover a whole topic quickly while managing the class time efficiently in a cost-effective style and (2) a way to present new subjects, open discussion on a topic and sum up course content, as well as teach complex material [39].

However, on the other hand, some people believe that lecturing is no more an effective educational tool as before. Lectures impart the students a passive, non-thinking, receiving mode. Though the students listened to the explanation from the tutor, they did not have the opportunity to discuss any queries they might have, the study outcomes and ways to implement it. Some lecturers may sound monotonous or boring and students tend to lose attention in 15–20 min [40].

Despite that, lecturing remains the most common and basic teaching strategy for trainers. With the development of technology, the lecture can be combined with a variety of other techniques, for example, PowerPoint presentations, video clips as well as the facility of having a voting system. Not only can this kind of combination attract students' attention, but it can also make the lecture a lot more fun [41, 42].

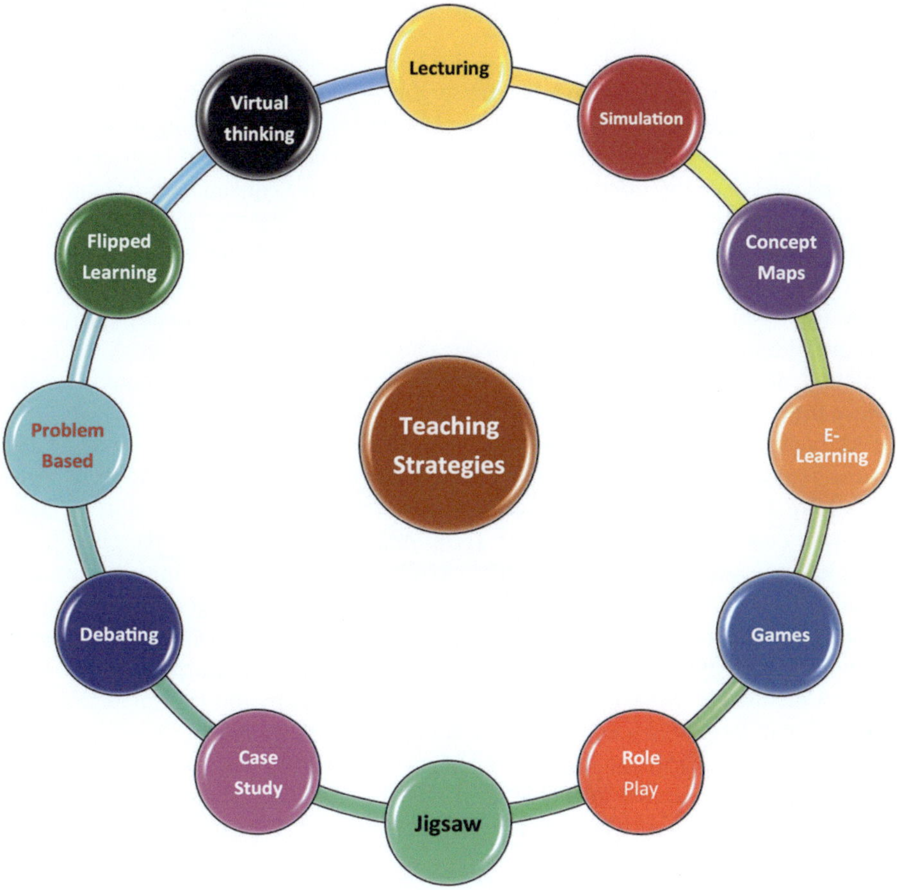
Lecturing
Simulation
Concept Maps
E-Learning
Games
Role Play
Jigsaw
Case Study
Debating
Problem Based
Flipped Learning
Virtual thinking
Teaching Strategies

Fig. 9.2 Teaching strategies in nursing education

Simulated Teaching

Simulation, the art and science of recreating a clinical scenario in an artificial setting, has been an important item in the nursing educational curricula for decades. High-fidelity simulation is useful for creating realistic scenarios that mimic the patient care environment and facilitates simple and direct application of theoretical knowledge in comparison to the other traditional teaching methods [43].

Simulation delivers an innovative educational approach which help nurses achieve clinical competency, indorse teamwork, and improve patient's care in a realistic and safe environment without any potential negative impact on the patients [44]. Simulated teaching often emphasizes the application and integration of knowledge, skills and critical thinking [45]. In a study carried out by Smith and Roehrs [46], they demonstrated that using high-fidelity simulation has a positive impact and in fact improves student satisfaction and self-confidence. A debriefing session is imperative after simulation to improve critical thinking and clinical reasoning.

Concept Maps

Concept maps are graphical tools for organizing and representing knowledge. Teaching and learning using concept maps relies on the tutor setting up a diagram that depicts suggested concepts (enclosed in circles or boxes) and the relationship between the concepts (indicated by lines connecting two concepts) to organize and structure knowledge. Therefore, this technique allows learners to understand the relationships between ideas by creating a visual map of the connections [47]. Concept maps help students organize and structure their thoughts to further understand information and the connections between ideas that they already have, connect new ideas to their existing knowledge and organize ideas in a logical, not rigid, structure which facilitates new information or viewpoints to be included in the future [48].

Mapping technique was reported to enhance motivation among the students and to characterise ideas visually, thus enabling them to analyse, assess and think critically [49]. The target of this approach is to teach the students through actively linking new concepts to existing ones [50]. Accordingly, concept mapping helps complete missing knowledge, clarify existing knowledge and improve critical thinking. In terms of nursing education, concept mapping is a good technique for teaching clinical care planning. Concept mapping of clinical problems allows learning nurses to identify the interrelationships in clinical data and grasp a patient's total clinical picture. In this case, students do not need to copy the care plan from the textbook any more. They will be able to set up a specific care plan for every patient by using concept mapping. Particularly, many concept mapping applications, which are convenient to use, are available on mobile devices, (e.g. the online brainstorm and mind map, bubll.us, which can be also downloaded as an app) [37].

E-Learning

E-learning platform is a flexible, convenient and effective method of learning new skills and knowledge. Online courses do not have scheduled on-campus class meetings. It is an integrated learning program entirely accessible at any time and any place via a computer with an Internet connection. Online education endorses the new concept of student-centred education. The effectiveness of the online learning environment should be ensured. This can be achieved by the instructor setting up a full course design, including the content and discussion topics in addition to the activities [51]. Online education provides increased flexibility, access and cost-effectiveness, factors that are highly required in nursing education. This is attributed to the facts that attending classes on campus is often difficult for nurses due to their work schedules, family duties as well as other commitments. Online courses are an effective strategy for continuing education for nurses in clinical settings. The instructor should prepare diverse e-learning materials, such as literature, videos, websites and discussion forums. Upon completion, an online test is required to evaluate comprehension. In this case, nurses are able to control their study time, and they also have time to absorb the materials.

Games

Games, and the entertainment value of play, have the ability to teach and transform [52]. The use of games as a teaching strategy inspires involvement and enhances both the interest as well as motivation of the learner. Games can turn learning into an enjoyable experience. Nursing literature highlighted the value of using games as a teaching strategy in nursing education. This was attributed to the endorsement of active learning, inspiration of critical thinking, the mix of fun and excitement in learning as well as imitation of real-life scenarios [53]. Using a game to teach content that may be considered boring or tough can generate a pleasant and entertaining atmosphere. Moreover, games combined with lectures are more effective than lectures alone in improving the learners' knowledge [54]. Educational apps which can be downloaded on mobile gadgets can facilitate playing games and can turn nursing education more fun and engaging. Examples are Nobelprize, CyberNurse, Blood Flow Through the Heart, Learning Nurse, Free Nurse Tutor, EnglishMed, Casualty Challenge Nurse Game, Medical Abbreviations and Nursing Learning Games and Activities.

Role Play

Role play is a very flexible teaching approach because it requires no special tools, technology or environments. Simply role play is a dramatization of an event or situation. The situation usually presents a problem or opinion conflict between two or more people or situation that incites anxiety [55]. It differs from simulation-based learning activities in that it is unscripted. The learners interact in a completely spontaneous manner. In role playing the student represents and experiences a character known in everyday life. Role playing is a particularly useful strategy for practicing clinical communication skills and dealing with conflict in nursing educational curses [56]. Role playing can also be very effective for experiencing cultural principles and awareness as it gives the students the opportunity to become emotionally involved in cross-cultural learning and reflect upon cultural differences [57]. At the beginning of a role playing activity, the activity's goal should be established. Also, the instructor should make the students aware of the situation or background for the interaction that will occur. Finally, debriefing is imperative for the instructor and students to discuss the situation and various perspectives of the individual characters. Debriefing also allows time to provide feedback to students.

Jigsaw Teaching Technique

The jigsaw technique is a method of organizing classroom activity that makes students dependent on each other to succeed. It breaks classes into groups and breaks assignments into pieces that the group assembles to complete the (jigsaw) puzzle. The jigsaw classroom is a great teaching strategy for cooperative learning [58]. This strategy, developed by Elliot Aronson, involves the formation of home groups to resolve a task [59]. The home groups allocate one member to each expert or research group, who gather data to bring back to the home group. This cooperative learning technique reduces racial conflict among students, promotes better learning, improves student motivation and increases enjoyment of the learning experience. The jigsaw process encourages listening, engagement and empathy by giving each member of the group an essential part to play in the academic activity [60]. Concerning nursing education, the jigsaw technique can be used to teach the content of many topics in the classroom as well as in the workplace. The instructor needs to manage the process and provide a summary and debriefing session after study.

Case Study

Case studies are stories. They present realistic, complex and contextually rich situations and often involve a dilemma, conflict or problem that one or more of the characters in the case must negotiate [61]. Case studies bridge the gap between theory and practice and between the classroom and the workplace [62]. They also enable the learners to practice identifying the parameters of a problem, recognizing and articulating positions, evaluating courses of action and arguing different points of view [61]. Hayward and Cairns state that the use of cases allow students to integrate and apply clinical and basic science knowledge and skills such as clinical reasoning, critical thinking, problem-solving and interpersonal ability to hypothetical or real-case scenarios [63]. The case study is a helpful strategy in nursing education. It can be used both in the classroom and online courses. It is also suitable for teaching about clinical diseases, culture competence, communication skills and other topics. A summary or suggestion from the instructor is essential after study.

Debating

Debating is presenting the "pro" and "con" arguments of a specific situation, proposal or solution to a problem [64]. This teaching/learning strategy offers students an opportunity to learn new content in an exciting way. Debating permits students to become actively involved in learning the course content while it promotes critical thinking and enhances verbal communication skills [65]. Also, debating triggers higher-order learning, such as analysis, synthesis and evaluation [66]. It can help students learn both critical reading and writing. Bradshaw and Lowenstein claimed that debating is a useful teaching/learning activity for nursing students at all levels [67]. Debating can be used when teaching a controversial issue or discussing a trend in nursing education. All students are responsible for researching the issue being proposed. Debaters need to examine relevant literature, analyse the data, develop a solution or hypothesis and present their ideas clearly during the debate. After the debate, the students in the audience evaluate the debaters' presentations and participate in postdebate discussion. This type of debate with feedback engages all the students to learn, improves team collaboration and develops critical thinking.

Problem-Based Learning

The teaching method that uses patient situations or scenarios to stimulate students to acquire and apply information to solve problems is known as problem-based learning [68]. Educators present realistic patient scenarios, ask questions and require students to search for holistic answers. Problem-based learning encourages active learning through self-directed learning, self-appraisal, clinical problem-solving skills, teamwork, discipline and integration of information. Problem-based learning also improves clinical reasoning skills, increases the retention of learned material and enhances self-directed study [69]. Problem-based learning is widely used for teaching a relatively complex or messy problem that has a broad association with basic science and clinical experience, such as heart failure or pneumonia. The instructor should manage the discussion process, give positive feedback and conduct a summary.

Flipped Learning

"Flipping the classroom" is contrary to the traditional class where lecture is given in class and assignments are sent as homework. Instead; with the flipped classroom, lecture is sent as homework and class time is devoted to active learning assignments [70, 71] Nurse educators are in a prime position to implement curricular changes to better prepare the future generation of nurses. Employing new teaching strategies to enhance clinical reasoning skills was embraced by the faculty of two medical–surgical courses at a University in the Southern United States. Using "flipping the classroom" strategy, students were able to view prerecorded lecture videos prior to class and use class time for simulation activities, case study analysis, question and answer sessions as well as discussions. These active learning approaches were designed to make the medical–surgical content more engaging and meaningful while helping students "make connections" from theory to practice [72, 73].

Virtual Thinking

Observational skills and the ability to pay close attention to detail are fundamental nursing skills that can improve patient outcomes. Equally important is the ability to accurately and effectively communicate these findings to other members of the healthcare team. These skills are not always intuitive, and students often lack opportunities for practice. At the same time, nurse educators are called upon to provide innovative teaching strategies that are student-centred [74, 75]. Visual Thinking Strategies is a teaching technique that uses art to engage students through discussion to increase observational and communication skills [76]. Art can be used to develop observational skills in students and can provide an innovative mechanism for students to develop higher levels of awareness and sensitivity to change [77]. Art has been used to improve observational skills in several ways in nursing education. Frie et al. [78] found when nursing students viewed and described artwork at different distances, the students developed a broadened understanding of the role of perception and an awareness of the need to make accurate, precise observations. In a master's degree accelerated program, Pellico et al. [79] found students exposed to an art-based intervention generated more alternative diagnoses for patients in photographs. Art was used by Inskeep and Lisko [80] in a fundamentals nursing course and found it helped students refine their ability to formulate nursing diagnoses and developed their critical thinking skills.

Challenges to Specialist Nursing Education

National and international reports described the potential for specialist nurses and advanced nurse practitioners to contribute to the provision of high-quality healthcare as part of comprehensive healthcare reform [81–83]. Preparing these specialist nurses for practice and fostering their role in a variety of educational, clinical and research settings are necessary steps towards achieving this vision. However, success may be elusive. At present, a shrinking number of nurse educators carry an increasingly large responsibility for educating a declining number of specialist nurses [84, 85]. In many settings, outdated regulations, policies and biases prevent them from practicing to the fullest extent of their education, skills and competencies [86–88]. Some US-based physician organizations have mounted campaigns aimed at discrediting advanced nurse education and practice and decrying the potential of specialist nurses to provide cost-effective and clinically efficient care [89, 90]. The challenges associated with providing effective specialist nurses clinical education, particularly in clinical practice settings, are summarized in Table 9.3. They could be stratified into internal as well as external challenges [91]. Radical transformation in the nursing education is the key to conquer such challenges. Therefore, it is imperative that nurse educators work with all stakeholders to improve the education of

Table 9.3 Challenges to effective specialist nurse education

Internal challenges
Increasing demand for nurse educators
Non-competitive educational salaries
Increasing faculty workloads
Difficulties accessing education in rural communities
Diversity of the required clinical skills
External challenges
Limited options of apprenticeship and mentoring
Concentration of educational programs in urban areas
Limited national funding for clinical education research
Demographic mismatch between nursing and populations served
Seniority politics and power relationships

specialist nurses through the identification and implementation of best practice clinical education strategies designed to overcome the current barriers to the provision of high-quality clinical experiences.

Educating Nurses at 2030

The rapid pace of the technological advances has not shown any abatement signs and has already impacted significantly on the nursing education curricula. Nurses' education, whether they were students, practitioners or specialist nurses, has always required a balance between teaching for present needs and anticipating future demands. What challenges and opportunities await the nurses of 2030? It has been less than a decade since their introduction, and yet for many nurses, practice without the use of a smartphone or tablet device may already be a distant memory. There are planned, and perhaps yet unpredicted, technological innovations that will have a similar profound influence in the next 10 years (Table 9.4). Studies on remotely monitoring patients with inflammatory arthritis have already been published [92–94] and big chunk of this responsibility lies in the nurses' hands. A careful look at what technology trends are likely to influence the healthcare transformation in the next decade and its impact on the current teaching policies particularly informatics education is mandatory now. Similarly, a critical reflection on what nursing educators would currently consider as teaching material should be carefully evaluated with views towards amending the present informatics curriculum to accommodate such developments.

Change is a familiar feature of nursing landscapes, but the technological advancements of the next decade may cause greater shifts than have previously been navigated. In North America significant work has been done in providing curricular support for nursing educators in informatics. The Technology Informatics Guiding Education Reform or TIGER initiative in the United States and the Canadian

Table 9.4 Recent healthcare technology trends impacting on the nursing education: a comparison of its current state, existing aims, expectations, challenges and required nurses' education skills

	Electronic health records, interoperability and the cloud	Wearable technology	Big data	Patient engagement and empowerment
Current state	Electronic health record and/or electronic medical records is a current practice[100]	Wearable devices are reality	Electronic healthcare occupied space is massive (around 500 petabytes) [101]	Increase sense of ownership for patients with the hopes that improved outcomes
Existing targets	Meet stringent meaningful use standards [102] A mean to strengthen communication between healthcare providers [103] Existing algorithms can be used to generate automatic clinical alerts [104]	Acute care: Monitoring devices (heart rate, blood pressure, weight, activity level, blood glucose and calorie intake [105] Chronic care: people collect electronic data such as pain score, functional ability, sleep pattern, quality of life [106]	Predictive analytics which can support medical decision and triage of care [107]	Opportunity for the patients to access and contribute to their own healthcare data [108]
Expectation	By using cloud-based systems improve interconnectivity which can offer care teams working, provide real-time integrated care and improved collaborative access to data [109] The use of artificial intelligence in decision support tools [110] Future inter-professional teams may be robotic members [111]	Aggregate and deliver key data to both patients and practitioners [104] Use new adhesive sensors for patient data collection and contact lenses, body implants and sensor-embedded fabric in hospital gowns The future of Google Glass in health education and practice is blooming and may transform medical education as well as clinical practice Nurses will likely be equipped with their own wearable technology in future practice and serve as primary instigators of technological connection and data transfer between patients and clinicians [112]	Prospects of pairing massive data reservoirs with predictive analytic tools and identifying healthcare crises before they even begin	Patient electronic health record portals, one-note or other shared provider patient data collection, and increased e-visits or other electronic communication with healthcare team members with the hopes that improved outcomes will follow

Table 9.4 (continued)

	Electronic health records, interoperability and the cloud	Wearable technology	Big data	Patient engagement and empowerment
Advantages	Electronic integrated care planning and increased availability of clinical decision aids for both patients and providers [110] Improved connection of interdisciplinary team members [113]	Existing adhesive sensors are being used for patient data collection in some care settings, and these technologies will continue to expand	Data mining and predictive analytics are presented as opportunities to forecast patient demand for service, such as emergency department visits [114] To tailor diagnosis and patient interventions [101] To discover patterns that may have otherwise gone unnoticed in particular patient populations [101] or potentially in epidemic situations and in tracking and providing automated responses to collected patient data to their care providers [115]	Formal and informal online patient networks and the use of tools, such as hashtags, provide streamlined opportunities to share experiences, questions and concerns Social media is used by the patients as a health information tool [116] Nurses can make benefits of these social media tools such as the creation of personal learning networks [99]

(continued)

Table 9.4 (continued)

	Electronic health records, interoperability and the cloud	Wearable technology	Big data	Patient engagement and empowerment
Challenge	Technical issues such as access speeds, content lag and the inevitable interruptions related to malfunction Nurses should be equipped to advocate for improvement in "areas of integrated practice registries, care management software integration, whole-person-orientated care plans and longitudinal tracking of individual patients" [117] Require training on enhanced data management and specific data extraction skills Training on interoperability or integration of systems and data Concerns regarding security, workability, privacy and ultimately user acceptance and use [109]	Nurse educators must be prepared to support students in a future practice that may include numerous biometric sensor types and data delivery mechanisms It seems increasingly likely that nurses will need to become astute data analysts as opposed to primary data collectors as the use of these technologies advances	Ethical concerns abound in these applications, with calls for additional research and training in this area The ever-present issue of patient privacy and data security must also be considered [101] There is urgent need for additional healthcare personnel with specific data management or analytic skills as well as further collaborations between informed clinicians and computer science teams [118]	Patients will present with great differences in digital literacy and even basic computer skills, and nurses should take the lead in either providing the needed patient education or making referrals to community resources that will allow all patients to get connected, digitally speaking Current patient education skills related to accessing health information online should be expanded to allow for further assessment of patients' digital literacy skills and networked connections
Nursing requirement	Nursing curriculums should include detailed digital best practice content covering all the legal, and additional ethical, concerns	How algorithms are used to shape data and what influence the results may have on patient and practitioner decisions are an urgent curricular priority	Establishing or expanding dedicated informatics courses in nursing curriculums to manage the new specific learning needs	Nurses must have an in-depth understanding of how information is aggregated and distributed through social media [99] Social media will emerge as significant factor in nursing practice in the coming years

Association of Schools of Nursing (CASN) Entry-to-Practice Nursing Informatics Competencies and accompanying toolkit have already considered features of the curricular landscape for several years [95–97]. However, educators should do their best to apply and promote these advances. The National League for Nursing [98] issued a recent call for further action in preparing students for a technological healthcare future highlighting a clear need for nursing education "to teach with and about technology to better inform healthcare interventions that improve healthcare outcomes and prepare the nursing workforce" [98]. The need is urgent, as much of what was anticipated as part of a technological future have already been materialized in the existing healthcare landscapes [99].

Transforming Nurses' Curricula for the Future

Future nurse practitioners should be prepared for such technology-infused healthcare future. In their recent research, van Houwelingen et al. [100] have identified several unique technological competencies that should be demonstrable by nursing graduates today. Many of these skills align with key informatics competencies identified by groups such as TIGER and CASN [95, 97] and include a basic familiarity with a host of varying digital tools and information formats. The use of computers and smart gadgets (phones or tablets), electronic communication, multimedia presentations such as podcasts or blogs and computer software for creating and sharing professional documents and an understanding of social networking applications such as Twitter and LinkedIn have all been identified as vital for future nursing professionals [97]. However, in addition to hi-tech skills, nurses also need to maintain their clinical knowledge, skills, communication, critical thinking and problem-solving abilities which are essential to support the expected technology-based practice.

In conclusion, although the art of caring has its roots far back in history, there has been significant shift in the nursing career which become more formal and modernized. The new patient-centred care concept, modern nursing role in partnership with the treating doctor and the introduction of the specialist nurses' category have mandated that nursing education must advance in order to prepare future nurses for effective and collaborative clinical practice. There is a growing expectation that the twenty-first-century nurses should not only be equipped with the basic skills to function in a hospital but also armed with the ability to rapidly learn and teach the new information relevant to their speciality practice. Several teaching approaches have shown efficacy in the nurses' educational approach, and it is up to the instructor to choose the educational strategy he/she feels appropriate. Nurse educators, both in practice and education, will be essential in leading a successful technological evolution for nursing. Educators may need to increase their own comfort and knowledge of technology and be a role model for the critical importance of embracing these changes.

References

1. Hill J. Rheumatology nurse specialists—do we need them? Rheumatology (Oxford). 2007;46:379–81.
2. Palmer D, El Miedany Y. Rheumatology helpline: challenges in the biologic therapy era. Br J Nurs. 2011;20(12):728–32.
3. Palmer D, El Miedany Y. PROMs: a novel approach to arthritis self-management. Br J Nurs. 2012;21(10):601–2. 605–7
4. Palmer D, El Miedany Y. EROMIA in inflammatory arthritis: the next step in standard practice. Br J Nurs. 2010;19(1):42–6.
5. Brady T. Strategies to support self-management in osteoarthritis: five categories of interventions, including education. Orthop Nurs. 2012;31:124–30.
6. Goh L, Samanta J, Samanta A. Rheumatology nurse practitioners' perceptions of their role. Musculoskelet Care. 2006;4:88–100.
7. Swanson KI, Pfenning S. The nurse practitioner's role in the management of rheumatoid arthritis. J Nurs Pract. 2011;7:858–62. 870
8. Juhola H, Kukkurainen ML, Suominen T. Rheumatology nurses' work-related empowerment. Musculoskelet Care. 2007;5:91–7.
9. van Eijk-Hustings Y, van Tubergen A, Boström C, EULAR, et al. EULAR recommendations for the role of the nurse in the management of chronic inflammatory arthritis. Ann Rheum Dis. 2012;71:13–9.
10. Schlenk E, Starz T, Levesque M, Baker N, Rogers J. Understanding function in RA: the nurse's role in patient evaluation. Rheumatology network 2012. http://www.rheumatologynetwork.com/rheumatoid-arthritis/understanding-function-ra-nurses-role-patient-evaluation.
11. Keele University. Postgraduate diploma/master in rheumatology nursing. http://haywoodrheumatology.org.uk/documents/2011_MSc_Info_Pack.pdf.
12. Almeida C, Clarke B, O'Brien A, Hammond A, Ryan S, Kay L, Hewlett S. Current provision of rheumatology education for undergraduate nursing, occupational therapy and physiotherapy students in the UK. Rheumatology. 2006;45:868–73.
13. Nursing and Midwifery Council. Standards of proficiency for preregistration nursing education. London: NMC; 2004.
14. College of Occupational Therapists. Standards for education: pre-registration education standards. London: COT; 2003.
15. Chartered Society of Physiotherapy. The curriculum framework. London: CSP; 2002.
16. Kay L, Deighton C, Walker D, Hay E. Undergraduate rheumatology teaching in the UK: a survey of current practice and changes since 1990. Rheumatology. 2000;39:800–3.
17. Nolan M, Nolan J. Rehabilitation, chronic illness and disability: the missing elements in nurse education. J Adv Nurs. 1999;29:958–66.
18. Hill J, Bird H, Lawton C, Harmer R, Wright V. An evaluation of the effectiveness, safety and acceptability of a nurse practitioner in a rheumatology outpatient clinic. Br J Rheumatol. 1994;33:283–8.
19. Jette AM, Becker MC. Nursing, occupational therapy and physical therapy preparation in rheumatology in the United States and Canada. J Allied Health. 1980;9:268–75.
20. Westby MD. Rheumatology instruction in physical therapy undergraduate programs: a survey of Canadian universities. Physiother Can. 1999;51:264–7.
21. Jones A, Maddison P, Doherty M. Teaching rheumatology to medical students: current practice and future aims. J R Coll Phys. 1992;26:41–3.
22. Association of Rheumatology Health Professionals. Standards of practice. Available at: www.rheumatology.org/arhp/practice/standards. Accessed 22 Feb 2018.
23. Carr A, Gordon T. Defining the extended clinical role for allied health professionals in rheumatology. ARC Conference Proceedings 12. Chesterfield, 2001.

24. El Miedany Y, Palmer D. Can standard rheumatology clinical practice be patient-based? Br J Nurs. 2008;17(10):673–5.
25. Palmer D, El Miedany Y. From guidelines to clinical practice: cardiovascular risk management in inflammatory arthritis patients. Br J Commun Nurs. 2013;18(9):424–8.
26. Palmer D, El Miedany Y. Treat-to-target: a tailored treatment approach to rheumatoid arthritis. Br J Nurs. 2013;22(6):308. 310, 312-8
27. Stein K, Corte C, Colling K, Whall A. A theoretical analysis of Carper's ways of knowing using model of social cognition. Sch Inq Nurs Pract Int J. 1998;12:43–60.
28. Benner P. From novice to expert: excellence and power in clinical nursing practice. Menlo Park: Addison-Wesley; 1984. p. 13–34.
29. Kuhn T. The structure of scientific revolutions (2nd ed). University of Chicago Press; 1970.
30. Dickens C, Creed F. The burden of depression in patients with rheumatoid arthritis. Rheumatology. 2001;40(12):1327–30.
31. Sheehy C, Murphy E, Barry M. Depression in RA-underscoring the problem. Editorial Rheumatol. 2006;5(11):1325–7.
32. Palmer D, El Miedany Y. Self-helplessness in arthritis: an important but overlooked index. Br J Nurs. 2010;19(15):965–71.
33. Royal College of Nursing (2002). A charter for rheumatology nursing. Publication number 000 762. http://www.rcn.org.uk/__data/assets/pdf_file/0011/78491/000762.pdf. Accessed 5 Feb 2017.
34. Hoff R. I can see you naked. Kansas City: Andrews and McMeel; 1992.
35. Kolb DA. Experiential learning: experience as the source of learning and development. New Jersey: Prentice-Hall; 1984.
36. Professor Mehabrian's work 1960s. Accessed 24 Feb 2018 at http://www.businessballs.com/mehrabiancommunications.htm.
37. Xu J-h. Toolbox of teaching strategies in nurse education. Chin Nurs Res. 2016;3:54–7.
38. Kemp JE, Morrison GR, Ross SM. Developing evaluation instruments. In: Designing effective instruction. New York: MacMillan College Publishing. p. 1994.
39. Morgan RL, Whorton JE, Gunsalus C. A comparison of short term and long term retention: lecture combined with discussion versus. J Instr Psychol. 2000;27:53.
40. Johnson JP, Mighten A. A comparison of teaching strategies: lecture notes combined with structured group discussion versus lecture only. J Nurs Educ. 2005;44:319e322.
41. Goodin HJ, Stein D. Deliberative discussion as an innovative teaching strategy. J Nurs Educ. 2008;47:272e274.
42. Gomez GE, Gomez EA. Learning of psychomotor skills: laboratory versus patient care setting. J Nurs Educ. 1987;26:20e24.
43. Nagle BM, McHale JM, Alexander GA, French BM. Incorporating scenario-based simulation into a hospital nursing education program. J Contin Educ Nurs. 2009;40:18e25.
44. Reese CE, Jeffries PR, Engum SA. Learning together: using simulations to develop nursing and medical student collaboration. Nurs Educ Perspect. 2010;31:33e37.
45. Kaddoura MA. New graduate nurses' perceptions of the effects of clinical simulation on their critical thinking, learning, and confidence. J Contin Educ Nurs. 2010;41:506e516.
46. Smith SJ, Roehrs CJ. High-fidelity simulation: factors correlated with nursing student satisfaction and self-confidence. Nurs Educ Perspect. 2009;30:74e78.
47. Carnegie Mellon University. Innovative teaching strategies; 2006. 2015.10.9. http://www.cmu.edu/teaching/assessment/howto/assesslearning/conceptmaps.html.
48. All AC, Huycke LI, Fisher MJ. Instructional tools for nursing education: concept maps. Nurs Educ Perspect. 2003;24:311e317.
49. All AC, Havens RL. Cognitive/concept mapping: a teaching strategy for nursing. J Adv Nurs. 1997;25:1210e1219.
50. Harpaz I, Balik C, Ehrenfeld M. Concept mapping: an educational strategy for advancing nursing education. Nurs Forum. 2004;39:27e30. 36

51. Karaman S, Kucuk S, Aydemir M. Evaluation of an online continuing education program from the perspective of new graduate nurses. Nurse Educ Today. 2014;34:836e841.
52. Masters K. Development and use of an educator-developed community assessment board game. Nurse Educ. 2005;30:189e190.
53. Glendon K, Ulrich D. Using games as a teaching strategy. J Nurs Educ. 2005;44:338e339.
54. Royse MA, Newton SE. How gaming is used as an innovative strategy for nursing education. Nurs Educ Perspect. 2007;28:263e267.
55. University of New Mexico. Teaching and Learning Strategies. 2015.10.9. http://nursing.unm.edu/resources/teaching-and-learning-strategies.html.
56. Shearer R, Davidhizar R. Educational innovations: using role play to develop cultural competence. J Nurs Educ. 2003;42:273e276.
57. Kodotchigova MA. Role play in teaching culture: six quick steps for classroom implementation. Internet TESL J. 2002;8:10e12.
58. Lai C, Wu C. Using handhelds in a Jigsaw cooperative learning environment. J Comput Assist Learn. 2006;22:284e297.
59. Jigsaw Classroom. The Jigsaw classroom overview. 2015.10.19. https://www.jigsaw.org.
60. Jigsaw strategy. Pennsylvania State University; 2007. 2015.10.19 https://www.schreyerinstitute.psu.edu/pdf/alex/jigsaw.pdf.
61. Case Studies. Carnegie Mellon University. 2015.10.19. https://www.cmu.edu/teaching/designteach/teach/instructionalstrategies/casestudies.html.
62. Barkley EF, Cross KP, Major CH. Collaborative learning techniques: a handbook for college faculty. San Francisco: Jossey-Bass; 2005.
63. Hayward L, Cairns M. Physical therapist students' perceptions of and strategic approaches to case-based instruction: suggestions for curriculum design. J Phys Ther Educ. 1998;12:33e42.
64. Garrett M, Schoener L, Hood L. Debate: a teaching strategy to improve verbal communication and critical-thinking skills. Nurse Educ. 1996;21:37e40.
65. Darby M. Debate: a teaching-learning strategy for developing competence in communication and critical thinking. J Dent Hyg. 2007;81:78.
66. Park C, Kier C, Jugdev K. Debate as a teaching strategy in online education: a case study. Can J Learn Technol. 2011;37:17e20.
67. Bradshaw MJ, Lowenstein AJ. Innovative teaching strategies in nursing and related health professions. Sudbury: Jones and Bartlett Publishers; 2011.
68. Problem-based learning. Stanford University; 2001. 2015.10.19 http://web.stanford.edu/dept/CTL/cgibin/docs/newsletter/problem_based_learning.Pdf.
69. Baker CM. Problem-based learning for nursing: integrating lessons from other disciplines with nursing experiences. J Prof Nurs. 2000;16:258e266.
70. Post J, Deal B, Hermanns M. Implementing of a flipped classroom: nursing students' perspectives. J Nurs Educ Pract. 2015;5(6):25–30.
71. Keene K. Blending and flipping distance education. Dist Learn. 2013;10(4):63–9.
72. DeMaio DN, Oakes CE. Flipping the classroom with screencasts. Radiol Technol. 2014;85(3):340–2. PMid:24395903
73. Schwartz TA. Flipping the statistics classroom in nursing education. J Nurs Educ. 2014;53(4):199–206.
74. Moorman M. The meaning of visual thinking strategies for nursing students. Humanities. 2015;4:748–59.
75. Benner P, Sutphen M, Leonard V, Day L. Educating nurses: a call for radical transformation, vol. 15. Hoboken: Wiley; 2009.
76. Housen A. Eye of the beholder: research, theory and practice. Lisbon: Visual Understanding in Education; 2005.
77. Reilly JM, Ring J, Duke L. Visual thinking strategies: a new role for art in medical education. Fam Med. 2005;37:250–2.
78. Frei J, Alvarez SE, Alexander MB. Ways of seeing: using the visual arts in nursing education. J Nurs Educ. 2010;49:672–6.

79. Pellico LH, Friedlaender L, Fennie KP. Looking is not seeing: using art to improve observational skills. J Nurs Educ. 2009;48:648–53.
80. Inskeep SJ, Lisko SA. Alternative clinical nursing experience in an art gallery. Nurse Educ. 2001;26:117–9.
81. Institute of Medicine. The future of nursing: leading change, advancing health. Washington, DC: The National Academies Press; 2011.
82. Sargen M, Hooker RS, Cooper RA. Gaps in the supply of physicians, advance practice nurses, and physician assistants. J Am Coll Surg. 2011;212(6):991–9.
83. Wilson JF. Primary care delivery changes as nonphysician clinicians gain independence. Ann Intern Med. 2008;149(8):597–600.
84. Aiken LH, Cheung RB, Olds DM. Education policy initiatives to address the nurse shortage in the United States. Health Aff. 2009;28(4):w646–56.
85. Buerhaus PI, Staiger DO, Auerbach DI. The future of the nursing workforce in the United States: data, trends, and implications. Boston: Jones and Bartlett; 2009.
86. Hansen-Turton T, Ritter A, Valdez B. Developing alliances: how advanced practice nurses became part of the prescription for Pennsylvania. Policy Polit Nurs Pract. 2009;10(1):7–15.
87. Ritter A, Hansen-Turton T. The primary care paradigm shift: an overview of the state-level legal framework governing nurse practitioner practice, Health Lawyer: National Nursing Centers Consortium. Chicago: American Medical Association; 2008. http://www.policyarchive.org/handle/10207/bitstreams/11855.pdf
88. Safriet B. State legislative requirements for prescriptive authority for nurses, Specialty Nursing Forum, Park Ridge, 1991.
89. American Medical Association. The AMA scope of practice data series: nurse practitioners. Chicago: American Medical Association; 2009.
90. American Academy of Family Practitioners. Primary health care professionals: a comparison. 2011. http://www.aafp.org/online/en/home/media/kits/fp-np.html.
91. Fitzgerald C, Kantrowitz-Gordon I, Katz J, Hirsch A. Advanced practice nursing education: challenges and strategies. Nurs Res Pract. 2012;12:1–8.
92. El Miedany Y, El Gaafary M, Youssef S, Bahlas S, Almedany S, Ahmed I, Palmer D. Toward electronic health recording: evaluation of electronic patient-reported outcome measures system for remote monitoring of early rheumatoid arthritis. J Rheumatol. 2016;43(12):2106–12.
93. El Miedany Y, El Gaafary M, El Aroussy N, Bahlas S, Hegazi M, Palmer D, Youssef S. Toward electronic health recording: evaluation of electronic patient reported outcome measures (e-PROMs) system for remote monitoring of early systemic lupus patients. Clin Rheumatol. 2017;36(11):2461–9.
94. El Miedany Y. Telehealth and telemedicine: how the digital era is changing standard health care. Smart Homecare Technol TeleHealth. 2017;4:43–51. https://doi.org/10.2147/SHTT.S116009.
95. Amarasingham R, Patzer RE, Huesch M, Nguyen NQ, Xie B. Implementing electronic health care predictive analytics, electronic health care predictive analytics: considerations and challenges. Health Aff. 2014;33:1148e1154.
96. Byrne MD, Lang N. Examination of nursing data elements from evidence-based recommendations for clinical decision support. Comput Inf Nurs. 2013;31:605e614.
97. Canadian Association of Schools of Nursing, CASN. Nursing informatics: entry-to-practice competencies for registered nurses. Toronto: NLN (Vision Series); 2015.
98. National League for Nursing. A VISION for changing faculty role: preparing students for the technological world of health care. Washington, DC: NLN (Vision Series); 2015.
99. Risling T. Educating the nurses of 2025: technology trends of the next decade. Nurse Educ Pract. 2017;22:89–92.
100. van Houwelingen CTM, Moerman AH, Ettema RGA, Kort HSM, Cate OT. Competencies required for nursing telehealth activities: a delphi-study. Nurse Educ Today. 2016;39:50e62.
101. Roski J, Bo-Linn GW, Andrews TA. Creating value in health care through big data: opportunities and policy implications. Health Aff. 2014;33:1115e1122.

102. Luchenski SA, Reed JE, Marston C, Papoutsi C, Majeed A, Bell D. Patient and public views on electronic health records and their uses in the United Kingdom: cross-sectional survey. J Med Internet Res. 2013;15
103. Krist AH. Electronic health record innovations for healthier patients and happier doctors. J Am Board Fam Med. 2015;28:299e302.
104. Rodgers MM, Pai VM, Conroy RS. Recent advances in wearable sensors for health monitoring. IEEE Sensors J. 2015;15:3119e3126.
105. Williamson B. Algorithmic skin: health-tracking technologies, personal analytics and the biopedagogies of digitized health and physical education. Sport Educ Soc. 2015;20:133e151.
106. El Miedany Y. e-Rheumatology: are we ready? Clin Rheumatol. 2015;34(5):831–7.
107. Cohen IG, Amarasingham R, Shah A, Xie B, Lo B. The legal and ethical concerns that arise from using complex predictive analytics in health care. Health Aff. 2014;33:1139e1147.
108. Giardina TD, Menon S, Parrish DE, Sittig DF, Singh H. Patient access to medical records and healthcare outcomes: a systematic review. J Am Med Inform Assoc. 2014;21:737e741.
109. Hsieh PJ. Healthcare professionals' use of health clouds: integrating technology acceptance and status quo bias perspectives. Int J Med Inform. 2015;84:512e523.
110. Liao PH, Hsu PT, Chu W, Chu WC. Applying artificial intelligence technology to support decision-making in nursing: a case study in Taiwan. Health Inf J. 2015;21:137e148.
111. Sharts-Hopko NC. The coming revolution in personal care robotics: what does it mean for nurses? Nurs Adm Q. 2014;38:5e12.
112. Sultan N. Reflective thoughts on the potential and challenges of wearable technology for healthcare provision and medical education. Int J Inf Manag. 2015;35:521e526.
113. Kuhn L, Reeves K, Taylor Y, Tapp H, McWilliams A, Gunter A, Cleveland J, Dulin M. Planning for action: the impact of an asthma action plan decision support tool integrated into an electronic health record (EHR) at a large health care system. J Am Board Fam Med. 2015;28:382e393.
114. Ekstrom A, Kurland L, Farrokhnia N, Castren M, Nordberg M. Forecasting emergency department visits using internet data. Ann Emerg Med. 2015;115;65:436e442.
115. Grossglauser M, Saner H. Data-driven healthcare: from patterns to actions. Eur J Prev Cardiol. 2014;21:14e17.
116. Fernandez-Luque L, Bau T. Health and social media: perfect storm of information. Healthc Inf Res. 2015;21:67e73.
117. O'Malley AS, Draper K, Gourevitch R, Cross DA, Scholle SH. Electronic health records and support for primary care teamwork. J Am Med Inform Assoc. 2015;22:426e434.
118. Honavar VG. The promise and potential of big data: a case for discovery informatics. Rev Policy Res. 2014;31:326e330.

Chapter 10
The Art of Patient Education

Introduction

The relationship between patients and physicians has received attention since the Hippocratic times [1]. It is undoubtedly a relationship that has changed and matured over the years. In early years, the patient's role, while recognized as crucial, has been largely passive, and the patients' consultations tended to adopt the monologue style, with the treating doctor teaching and the patient trying to absorb and remember all, or most of, what is being said. Since the 1980s, the patients' role in the contemporary healthcare has become one of the key underlying elements of reform and modernization. Involving people actively in healthcare has shifted the patient-doctor contact into a new phase, with the emphasis now on the patient talking and the physician listening and considering the patient's notes, the physician giving opinion and information and the patient making a choice together with the physician and the patient asking and the physician answering. The communication between physicians and patients in the majority of the communities has progressively evolved into an open dialogue, transforming patients from passive recipients of information and instructions to active participants in the management of their disease. The shift towards more patient-centred healthcare has necessitated important changes in the infrastructure and the way healthcare is delivered. This is, not surprisingly, more suited and more appealing to the targeted cohort of patients living with chronic, rheumatic musculoskeletal diseases often in the setting of many other coexisting comorbid conditions [2]. Interestingly in the most recent treatment guidelines for inflammatory rheumatic disorders released by the European League Against Rheumatism (EULAR), one of the overarching principles is that treatment should be based on a shared-decision process between the patient and the physician [3, 4]. Patient empowerment through tailored education and information became therefore a crucial aspect of healthcare. This chapter will discuss the patient education

Y. El Miedany, *Rheumatology Teaching*,
https://doi.org/10.1007/978-3-319-98213-7_10

concept and its difference from health education, evidence for the effectiveness of patient education, the art and science of patient education and strategies to implement it, as well as the use of technology to enhance patient education.

Patient Education Versus Health Education

Patient education is a significant component of modern healthcare. Patient education can be divided into two large categories: clinical patient education and health education. Clinical patient education is a planned, systematic, sequential and logical process of teaching and learning provided by the healthcare professional to the patient in the standard daily practice [5]. It is also a continuous teaching and learning process involving the healthcare provider and the patient (sometimes extend to involve the patient's family if appropriate). The goal of the clinical teaching and learning is based on the patient's assessment, evaluation, diagnosis, disease activity and severity, presence of comorbidities as well as prognosis. Modern patient education is usually tailored to the patient's requirements as well as disease status.

Health education is also a teaching and learning process, similar to patient education. However, its focus is mostly wellness, prevention and health promotion. Furthermore, health education can be provided to individuals, groups and communities. The basic focus of health education is to develop and improve social health behaviour. This new active approach to health education can be linked to new terms that started to book its place in the modern medical practice such as adherence to therapy, cost-effectiveness, window of opportunity, treat to target and risk assessment. The disease-centred thinking has changed to a risk-based model, which involve the patient as a collaborator and partner of care, with commitment and responsibilities to share with the clinician [6]. The level of success is directly linked to the degree to which risky behaviours are reduced, which in turn reflects the patients' understanding of the significance of the risk and the importance of changing. In this context, the primary role of the healthcare provider is that of patient's expert guide and educator.

The Science of Patient Education

Patient empowerment has gone through several phases to reach its current state of partnership. Patient participation in healthcare initial phase was limited to knowledge transfer and information about the disease and medications. Patient education, then, moved to the next level of patient-reported outcomes. Patient-reported outcomes are measures assessed directly from the patient, without interpretation from the physician. It contrasts with the main information used in the past based on the doctor's evaluation. Patient-reported outcomes reflect the impact of the disease on the patient both physically and psychologically in addition to self-reported joint tenderness and swelling as well as disease activity parameters [7, 8]. By sharing the patient's recorded disease activity measures, through a visual feedback process, this has enabled the patients to see how they are doing regarding their disease activity and helps to optimize their adherence to their treatment. Visual feedback also had a positive and significant impact on the disease activity control [9]. The next phase is that of shared decision-making, where this resource is provided to support discussions between patients and their healthcare professionals concerning the available treatment options and to assist the process of the decision-making [10]. The principle of shared decision-making is allowing patients and their providers to make healthcare decisions together, based on the best scientific evidence available, as well as the patient's values and preferences. A recent study [11] underscored the variability in the patients' treatment preferences and that different patients find different aspects of concerns about medication use. Decision aids are evidence-based tools designed to inform people of the potential benefit and harm of the treatment options, clarify their preferences and provide a shared decision-making structure for discussion at a clinic visit [10, 12, 13]. The last phase is developing a specific patient educational programme tailored to the patient's needs. This step ensures that the human nature of healthcare has not been lost and highlights the importance to understand what aspects of individuality and service responsiveness are important and valued by each patient. To achieve treatment targets and minimize the risk of comorbidities, patient education and health services must be tailored to recognize patients as individuals and to respond to their needs, disease activity, preferences and values, taking into account functional abilities, quality of life, shared requirements, personal goals and individual characteristics (such as individuals' expectations of service, their cultural background and gender) [14]. This approach has reflected positively on the disease control as well as adherence to therapy [15].

The Benefits of Patient Education in Healthcare

Healthcare centres have recognized the benefits of implementing patient education in improving patients' adherence to therapy, disease control, patient experience as well as satisfaction. In modern healthcare, patient education has shown the potential to be cost-effective and combat the risk in the health service, by reducing expenses and helping patients manage pricey chronic conditions [10]. Furthermore, adopting patient education programmes can help healthcare providers and organizations produce better outcomes and enhance quality of care. Effective educational tools can help patients understand medical complexities and enhance their motivation while reducing anxiety and increasing compliance to instructions. Patient education has the power of changing communication into action with consequent improvement in health status. Keeping the patient in the heart of the management process has ensured coordinated and efficient teaching and learning between healthcare professionals and providers involved in each patient's management [16]. Table 10.1 summarizes the benefits of patient education.

Table 10.1 Benefits of clinical patient education

Enhance patient empowerment and responsibility for their own health
Gives the patient the opportunity to share in the decision-making process and choose the appropriate approach of management
Ensure better patient satisfaction and quality of life
Enhance better adherence to therapy
Ensure better disease management outcome and achieving the targeted goals
Promotes patient-centred care concept and as a result, the patients active involvement in their healthcare plan
Endorse continuity of care and reduce the likelihood of comorbidity occurrence
Maximizes the patient's independence and ability to manage his condition in between visits to the treating doctor

Techniques of Delivering Patient Education

Effective patient education programmes are based on psycho-behavioural theories and incorporate techniques designed to actively engage patients in their care and to enhance their problem-solving skills (Fig. 10.1) [17]. They can be provided by one or more individuals involved in the patients' care and may occur in variable settings (Table 10.2).

Nowadays, patient education starts even before the clinical encounter. Patients today are information seekers with a plethora of knowledge available at their fingertips. Most of the patients surf the net, looking for a possible explanation of their symptoms. This may deviate the patient's attention to certain diagnosis, which the patient feels it fit well with their symptoms [18]. During the clinic visit, the clinician should establish rapport with the patient, listen to the patient's ideas and concerns, ensure successful exchange of information and discuss the treatment options aiming at meeting the patient's expectations or goals. At the conclusion of the clinic visit, a plan of care acceptable to both parties should be established.

After the clinic encounter, patient education starts a new phase. The clinician may give the patient a printed material or link to a website for further reading and understanding of the illness and ways of treatment. Strategies such as having pre-set patient education services for fatigue or sleep self-management, patients' groups and YouTube specialized channels are different approaches for the continuum of successful indirect communication and education [19].

The Art of Patient Education

Traditionally, educating adults follow the same approach and philosophy developed for the youth. However, when adults approach learning, they have different perspectives and requirements that have to be considered when developing instructional courses or materials. In their book, *The Adult Learner: The Definitive*

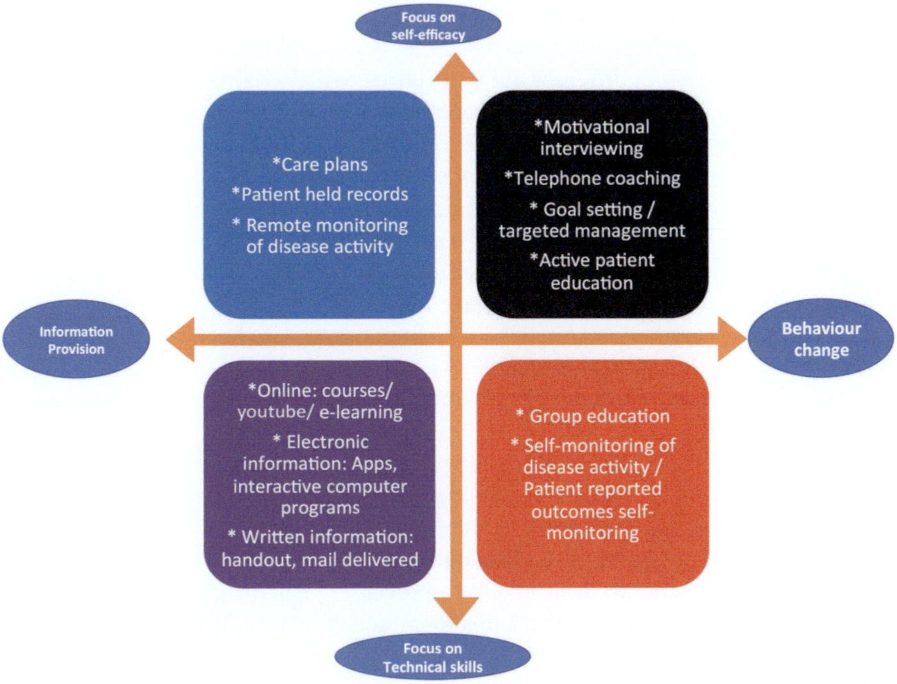

Fig. 10.1 Continuum strategies to support self-management: several styles have been assessed for its role to support self-management. One way to theorize self-management is to split the interventions into those focussing on building self-efficacy (confidence in self-care) versus those which aim at building knowledge and technical skills. Another approach is that it ranges from more passive information provision tactic at one side to more active behavioural change interventions at the other side

Table 10.2 Settings of patient education in standard daily practice

Setting	Who to deliver	Type of patient education
Hospital	Doctors, specialist nurses Conducted individually	Clinic: patient education delivered as part of the medical consultation Preoperative, e.g. joint surgery or other conditions
Outpatient/ community	Occupational therapy, physiotherapy, nurses Conducted in groups	Self-management, fatigue, sleep, sexual health
Media	YouTube, Social media, Organizations, brochures, internet, videos	Nature of the disease, mechanism of action of medication, side effects, importance of taking the medication
Population-based	Patients' groups, charities, societies, national centres	Group therapy, storytelling/narrative of disease progression, consequence of stopping or not taking therapy

Classic in Adult Education and Human Resource Development [20], the authors provided policies for how adult education can be accomplished. Basically, as people get older, they adopt different life trajectories, with variable educational levels, life experiences, acceptance to learn, goals, motivation and learning styles. In contrast to the young learners, adult education is driven by the need to learn and the priority of information that will be instantly helpful. "Hands-on" or "Active Learning" are the most successful learning strategies, particularly, if they match the learner's readiness to learn. "Teach-back", is another tactic to achieve effective learning. Educator ask learners to describe how will they respond if they faced similar scenario, based on what they have learnt [21]. An example of how to initiate the dialogue with the patient, the clinician may ask, "we have discussed several points today, would you tell me what you learnt from today's visit and how will you take the new medication?" The patient's reply will convey the outcome of today's education.

In self-management patient education programs, practice is the best approach to endorse skills learning. Strategies include group problem-solving, modelling and interactive discussions. Peer leaders often give the example of role-model behaviour. Small-group programs usually include six to ten people to permit time for individual requirements as well as group processes. Patient groups composed of people living with similar medical disorders and needs facilitate discussion and cross-fertilization of thoughts and skills [22]. Programme duration, learning objectives and goals as well as choice of the leaders are vital considerations. Short-term self-management programs endorse knowledge and skills, although these skills may lessen over time. Periodic reinforcement is recommended to maintain abilities and apposite behaviour. A mix of caregiver-based individual counselling and small-group education is optimal [23].

E-learning and interactive computer-based patient education are starting to book its place as a tool for patient education. The number of people turning to the Internet to search for a diverse range of health-related subjects continues to grow. In the United States, 80% of Internet users have searched for a health-related topic online, according to a study released by the Pew Internet and American Life Project. That's up from 62% of Internet users who said they went online to research health topics in 2001, the Washington research firm found [24]. Using online facilities to teach patients require certain characteristics. An interactive computer-based education programme has been defined as a computer-based programme that employed video, still pictures and audio presentations that interact with the user. The principle of e-learning is to be user centric with attention grabbing multimedia learning tools that are proven to engage and inform. Other tactics include simulating medical procedures with animation, assessing user comprehension with interactive quizzes and tracking enrolment and performance. The aim is to help patients and their families understand health conditions, aims and approaches to management and facilitate communication.

Advanced Technology and Patient Education

One of the biggest changes in patient education is the acceptance that it is no longer appropriate to just give a leaflet to a patient and send them away. The use of technology has revolutionized the way patients are educated about health. A major pharmaceutical company working in diabetes launched an innovative first person simulation using 3D headsets for patients, healthcare professionals and the general public. The simulation showed the high impact of mild hypoglycaemia (low blood sugar) on a patient; it made the viewer "feel" the symptoms of hypoglycaemia in various scenarios through a typical day for a person with type 2 diabetes. While this also increased empathy in healthcare professionals, for newly diagnosed patients, it acted as an effective tool to give them greater understanding of symptoms to be aware of, which allows them to take action earlier to address low blood sugar. No amount of written text could realistically give the same level of impact or information as this 3D simulation. It has since been translated into 9 languages and used in 26 countries across the world, demonstrating how effective patient education tools can be used globally [25].

Automated delivery of patient education can be both efficient for the patient and free up physician time. In 2008, Northeastern University developed a virtual nurse ("Louise"), which provides an interactive discussion with the patient about home care, and this takes place before the patient is discharged, and the conversation is composed based on the patients' medical records. The aim of this initiative is to free physician time, and any unanswered questions are included in a report which can be handled by a human nurse. The reduced physician time was calculated to save the hospital $145 per patient; interestingly 74% of interviewed hospital patients preferred to get the information from "Louise" rather than the doctor [26]. Not all technology has to be completely revolutionary; the simple use of iPads has also been shown to enhance conversations between patients and clinicians through quick access to illustrations and videos [27].

The rapid expansion of smartphone use has opened a route for patient education to be used as and when a patient requires. This was very successfully demonstrated by the United Kingdom's largest men's health charity, the Men's Health Forum [28]. During Men's Health Week 2011, they launched the smartphone app "Bloke Noises" which allowed men to play a simple game and be directed to trusted information on the Internet where they could become informed about health issues they may previously have been reluctant to discuss. In fact, apps are almost ubiquitous, with many disease-specific apps available on both iPhone and android devices. The relative simplicity of producing an app has been demonstrated by a study carried out in Bournemouth University showing how people with type 1 diabetes can participate effectively in the design of an app for their use [29]. Interactive technology has also proved particularly effective in general communication with patients, with a report showing a 42% increase in patient satisfaction with hospital educational materials when interactive technology was used [30]. An interesting trend in measuring whether patient education is effective is remote monitoring. For instance, in cardiology, this allows doctors to monitor the heart rhythm and any potential problems [31]. Such remote monitoring of specific or general health has the potential to allow doctors to see if a patient has been implementing the education they've received. Remote monitoring has also been used in rheumatology. "Rheumote" service for e-monitoring of inflammatory arthritis patients was studied in recent research [32, 33]. Results revealed that electronic remote monitoring was equivalent to standard format. Further, it enabled the patients to personally monitor how they are doing regarding their disease activity and helped to optimize their adherence to their treatment.

Education Programs for Patients

Patient education programs range from provision of information to the use of cognitive-behavioural strategies, exercise prescriptions and psychosocial support. Many different patient education programmes have been developed for health conditions including arthritis. These have been subclassified into categories based on the targeted patient cohort, the underlying disorder as well as the format (Table 10.3) [34]. In addition to increased knowledge and patient empowerment, these programmes also aim at changing health behaviour, by teaching patients how to solve problems, manage flare up and set individual goals [35]. Reviews indicated that patient education programmes can improve knowledge, change behaviour and improve health outcomes in some chronic conditions, but the magnitude of effect varies [36–40]. However, though the overall effect size for improving pain and functioning on a short-term basis is at best small (0.06, 95%CI 0.02–0.10) [41], the long-term changes in health status have not been convincingly demonstrated. In addition to the effects on health status, it has also been shown that patient education and self-management programmes can improve psychological outcomes [42]. Table 10.4 shows a list of the most famous education programs for arthritis patients. The most widely known example of patient educational programmes for arthritis is the Chronic Diseases and Arthritis Self-Management programmes (ASMP) developed at Stanford University in the United States. The ASMP has been generally

Table 10.3 Sub-classification of patient education programs

Program	Education programme category
Disease based	Disease specific or generic approach
Patient based	Group-based, and some are individually targeted, including spouse
Tutor based	Health professionals or lay tutors
Format	Workshop, paper-format, e-learning, telephone based, mail delivered
Content	Behaviour education, behaviour and exercise, behaviour and exercise and flare up management (Fig. 10.2)

Table 10.4 Characteristics of the most commonly used ten patient education programs for arthritis and other rheumatic conditions

Education program	Characteristics		
Group self-management	Target patients	Trainer(s)/training period	Methods and duration
Arthritis Self-Help Course (ASHC)	People with chronic arthritis and their significant others (SO)	Two-person team (laypersons or health professionals)/2.5 days of training	Weekly 2-h group sessions for 6 weeks (total 12 h)
SLE Self-Help Course (SLESH)	People with systemic lupus erythematosus and their SO	Two- to three-person team (at least one person with SLE and a health professional)/ 2.5-day training	Weekly 2-h group sessions for 7 weeks (total 17 h)
Fibromyalgia Self-Help Course (FSHC)	People with fibromyalgia and SO	Two- to three-person team (at least one person with fibromyalgia and a health professional)/2.5 day training	Weekly 2-h group sessions for 7 weeks (total 17 h)
Individual education programs			
Bone Up on Arthritis (BONE UP)	People with arthritis in rural areas or with low literacy	Mail-delivered instruction; support personnel	Self-paced six lessons on audiocassettes and workbook
Self-Management Arthritis Treatment (SMART)	People with multiple forms of arthritis	Mail-delivered instruction and quarterly questionnaires	Individualized, computer-tailored program, books, relaxation audiotape and exercise videotape
Exercise interventions			
People with Arthritis Can Exercise (PACE)	People with arthritis	Health and fitness professionals/12-h training	One to three times per week; 1-h sessions; 8 weeks—ongoing
Joint Efforts	Sedentary people with arthritis	Senior centre and nursing home activity directors/4 h training	One to five times weekly for 1-h group for 6–8 weeks or ongoing
Arthritis Foundation Aquatics Programme (Aquatics)	People with arthritis	Health and fitness professionals and lifeguards/ 8- to 10-h training for instructors	One to three times weekly 1-h group sessions for 6–10 weeks or ongoing
EDUCIZE	People with arthritis	Trained health or fitness professionals as instructors	Two times per week for 6 weeks
Joint Fitness Programme (Fig. 10.2)	People with arthritis	Health professional/ rheumatology nurse/ occupational therapist/ 2.5 days	One to three times per week, 1-h sessions, 8 weeks—ongoing

tested with positive results [35], but a randomized controlled trial investigating the effectiveness of the programme for patients with arthritis did not demonstrate any significant benefits at 4-month follow-up [43]. ASMP is given in groups, often led by lay tutors, and they have a generic approach, and the groups are not disease specific [44]. Other patient education programmes combine exercise and patient education [45], include the spouse with the aim of increasing coping skills [46], describe mail delivered leaflets [47] or individual telephone-based [47] programmes. The group size and description of the educational content is often not reported in detail, and the length of the programmes varies. Table 10.5 shows examples of patient education courses [48–53]. Figure 10.2 shows the components of the joint fitness program, which is a patient-based self-management programme that is dedicated to all patients with different types of rheumatic diseases such as osteoarthritis, rheumatoid arthritis, psoriatic arthritis and lupus. The process of the programme was based on the integration of the patient-reported outcome measures and patient education. The programme includes four main components: educational, i.e. Joint

Table 10.5 Examples of patient education courses

Managing symptoms such as pain and tiredness
Dealing with anger, fear and frustration
Coping with stress, depression and low self-image
Eating healthily
Learning relaxation techniques and taking regular exercise
Improved communication with family, friends and health professionals
Cooking and handling
Sexual health problems
Planning for the future

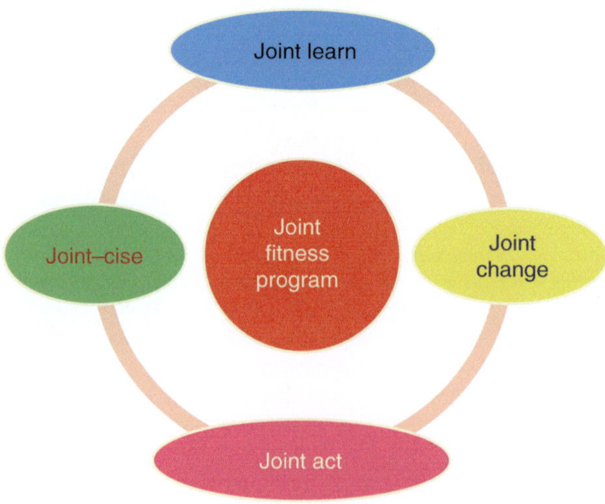

Fig. 10.2 Joint Fitness Program: The four components of the Joint Fitness Program. The programme can be undertaken by the patient in any sequence to meet his/her specific needs at the time of assessment based on the completed patient-reported outcome measures questionnaire

Learn; behavioural, i.e. Joint Change; information, i.e. Joint Act; and self-efficacy, i.e. Joint-cise (Joint-exercise) [53].

Core concepts of patient self-management have been described as engagement in activities which promote health; monitoring physical and emotional status, appropriate interaction with healthcare providers; and management of the effects of illness on emotions, self-esteem and relationships with others [49, 50]. Patients and health professionals may view patients' needs differently [51]. With these concepts in the essence of patient management, patient education will give the standard patient's care a 3D dimension.

In summary, though current patient education programmes may vary in form and content, the majority of these interventions are led by health professionals in a group setting where most participants are affected by a similar condition. While the intervention components can be tailored to specific needs of the group, there is, so far, no evidence that longer programmes with extended meeting points are more effective or feasible than brief patient education programmes.

The Patients' Teaching Role

The patients have always been central to medical education, but their role has been always passive and considered as a part of the students' or junior doctors' experiential learning, in clinical setting. The term "patient" is commonly used as a matter of brevity, to describe "people with health problems". Other words to describe these people are clients, service users, consumers, survivors, etc.; their carers (including parents and families) are healthy people (also described as community members, lay people) [54].

The active patient involvement in teaching was recorded as early as 1960s [55]. Patients acted as clinical skills instructors as they taught medical students how to conduct physical examinations and provide feedback [56]. To be qualified for that role, training about anatomy, examination techniques and how to teach and evaluate students was provided to the patients. The long-lasting programmes are found in North America where many medical schools have a cadre of healthy women who used to teach the intimate examinations, e.g. pelvic, breast and rectal. Another long-lasting intervention is the "arthritis educator" programmes in which highly trained patients used to teach the musculoskeletal examination to enhance the pool of clinical teachers [57].

Over the last two decades, the patients' expertise has been implemented in standard medical teaching to augment the learning process. A wide variety of patients were invited to share their experiences of living with illness or disability. The standard is to invite one or more patients into the classroom or a small group tutorial to share their stories and answer questions from students. Examples include people with HIV/AIDS [58, 59], cancer [60], dementia [61] and mental illness [62].

Other programmes aim to sensitize trainees to the underserved population requirements. These include older adults or complex conditions such as childhood chronic illness. Examples include workshops run by professional actors with learning disabilities [63] or teaching by parents of children with developmental disabilities or chronic illness [64].

The objectives of such patient teaching approach include validating patient experiences, understanding the importance of the patients' needs when therapeutic interventions is designed and learning the principles of equality, patient empowerment and service user involvement [65]. Some initiatives have used specific strategies to promote partnerships between patients and learners, for example, "facilitated dialogue", a technique used to provide an arena for meaningful dialogue between two groups that are unequal in power and position.

The extent of the expertise that patients can offer healthcare professional education continues to expand. At the University of British Columbia, two doctors (William Godolphin and Angela Towle) [66] worked with patients on topics that were identified as important by the patient educators. Their work included patients with mental health problems, arthritis and epilepsy and their caregivers, as well as HIV/AIDS. Patient-led workshops were developed about a diverse range of topics, including living with chronic disease, both day to day and over time, the diversity of the illness experience, impact on partners and families, physical examination skills, diagnostic challenges, stigma and stereotyping, peer support, practical aids to daily living, advice about what health professionals can do and information about support groups in the community. The ongoing publication of new initiatives in the literature indicates that patient involvement in teaching continues to be explored.

Other Educational Roles

Although involvement in curriculum delivery is the commonest role, patients have the potential to make a major contribution to all aspects of the educational process. The most comprehensive list is provided by Tew et al. [67]. They gave examples of patient involvement in (1) direct delivery of teaching and learning: practice learning/student assessment (global rating of the student's performance from the patient's point of view in the clinical exams)/course evaluation/courses as participants and to less extent curriculum planning. (2) Academic: In medical education patients are mainly involved in curriculum delivery, curriculum development and course planning, programme management and student assessment [68]. The patients' role expanded to rating of medical services provided by the individual departments as well as the hospital in general. Several approaches have been implemented including gaining consumers' views through surveys and sharing it on the medical organization website, example is friends and family survey, reference groups who help in making decisions regarding services provided and future plans, conferences and invitation onto existing groups as well as involvement in the production of learning materials.

In nursing and social work, a greater range of patient involvement has been reported. Examples of inclusion are input into curriculum planning, involvement in the design and delivery of a Diploma of Higher Education in Nursing [69], the development of a new preregistration nursing course [70], the design of continuing education and higher education in cancer care nursing [71] and the production of an Open University course on mental health [72]. Table 10.6 shows examples of patient education role in medical education.

Table 10.6 shows examples of patient education role in medical education

Patient role	Format	Setting	Duration of contact with learner	Training for the patient	Patient autonomy during the encounter
Volunteering patient in standard clinical setting	Standard patients serves as an example to illustrate or reinforce learning Student writing patient's story	Standard in or outpatient setting: enhance clinical and communication skills Patient volunteer may get involved in teaching and giving feedback	Encounter based	None	None
Patients get involved in preparing learning resources to be used by the university	Paper based Electronic based Course material Pictures or videos	Problem-based learning: real patient problem Virtual patient education: may involve video or pictures about a patient Implement patient narratives	None	Not applicable	Not applicable
Patient contribution in university-directed curriculum	Personal patient contribution (faculty members plan the encounter, but the patient determines level of participation)	Mentor programs In-classroom sharing of personal experience with the illness Community-based patient/family attachment program	Encounter based	Simple, short	None – low
Patient teachers	Personal, patient given a specific teaching role	Teaching and assessment of specific clinical skills Feedback to students regarding their communication skills	Variable	Structured, extensive	Moderate
Partnership in medical education	A true partnership in which patients make meaningful and valued contributions to decision-making Personal involvement in student education, evaluation and development of the curriculum	Patients are involved in many aspects of educational delivery, development and evaluation, beyond specific courses to the curriculum as a whole Collaboration of patient educators in educational decision-making (e.g. curriculum objectives, assessment criteria)	Moderate to extensive	Extensive	High

(continued)

Table 10.6 (continued)

Patient role	Format	Setting	Duration of contact with learner	Training for the patient	Patient autonomy during the encounter
Formal position in the institution (e.g. consumer academic)	Persons with expertise and experience in health, illness or disability and understand their designated role in education	Patients involved in institutional education, curriculum, assessment and decision-making (e.g. student selection criteria)	Extensive	Extensive	High

Outcomes of the "Teaching Patient" Involvement

A consistent theme in the reviews on patient involvement in teaching is the lack of clear and measurable educational outcomes. Towle et al. [57] have identified a variety of limitations to the literature. Most studies are descriptive and few interventions have been rigorously evaluated. Some evaluation of short-term outcomes for a small subset of initiatives has been reported (primarily teaching of clinical skills), but few of these studies had rigorous experimental designs. In a small study, a group of 11 patient educators, trained to teach musculoskeletal examination, were involved in a study where learning outcome of teaching undergraduate students (50 students) was assessed using an objective structured clinical examination (OSCE). Results revealed that students rated the patients' teaching acceptable for their needs in the setting of initial core examination skills teaching, as long as subsequent faculty teaching allows for supervised assessment and instruction on disease management [73]. To make patients' education meaningful, clear learning objectives are required and to inform the learners precisely what to expect from that session; this will ensure that the patient educators can practice within their range of competency.

Overall, the quality of the literature regarding outcomes of patient teaching is generally low as assessed by accepted criteria such as those of Best Evidence Medical Education (BEME) for quantitative studies or Côté and Turgeon for qualitative studies [74, 75]. Methodological weaknesses and the lack of specificity of objectives or intended outcomes, as well as their diversity, make it difficult to draw strong general conclusions about the effectiveness of patient involvement in teaching.

The Future

Thanks to technology innovations, it is very likely the future of patient education will feature fast and extensive use of apps, in particular those helping the patients living with complex "lifestyle diseases" such as arthritis or type 2 diabetes. While there is concern that the field of medical apps is somewhat unregulated [76], there can be no doubt that apps provide a fantastic opportunity to provide information, conveniently, to the patients. With the expanding use of the Internet, e-learning will also facilitate providing patients with increasingly useful resources. While cutting edge innovation is more likely to be driven by the private sector, the pharmaceutical industry often competes in a very crowded market; as such they are always seeking a new way to stand out from their competitors. The use of technology and innovation should seek to drive enhanced patient experience and improve outcomes both on an individual and an economic level.

In conclusion, patient education is at the core of modern healthcare, and its importance has been demonstrated in many diverse disease and treatment areas. Providing quality information and education will ultimately empower the patients, give them greater control over their disease and increase their compliance to therapy, all of which can lead to improved outcomes and reduced healthcare burden. Health policy analysis in the mid-1990s demonstrated the effectiveness of patient education, showing that for every $1 spent, between $3 and 4 were saved [77].

There is a persuasive rationale for the active involvement of patients in health professional education, and the evidence suggests that patients remain willing to take part in medical education provided that they are treated with respect. There is promise and some evidence of benefits to students, patients, teachers and communities. For patients, involvement in the education of those who will care for them is an intrinsically attractive idea. However, little is known regarding how to do it and how to optimize its impact.

Technology plays a crucial role in patient education, and its importance is only likely to increase. It is no longer appropriate to just give a leaflet to a patient and send them away. The use of technology has revolutionized the way patients are educated about health. Automated delivery of patient education can be both efficient for the patient and free up physician time. More innovations are expected in the future, which will make patient education attractive and promising.

References

1. Dorr Goold S, Lipkin M. The doctor-patient relationship: challenges, opportunities, and strategies. J Gen Intern Med. 1999;14(Suppl (1)):S26–33.
2. Nikiphorou E, Alunno A, Carmona L, Kouloumas M, Bijlsma J, Cutolo M. Patient–physician collaboration in rheumatology: a necessity. RMD Open. 2017;3:e000499. https://doi.org/10.1136/rmdopen-2017-000499.
3. Strehl C, Bijlsma JW, de Wit M, et al. Defining conditions where long-term glucocorticoid treatment has an acceptably low level of harm to facilitate implementation of existing recommendations: viewpoints from an EULAR task force. Ann Rheum Dis. 2016;75:952–7. http://ard.bmj.com/lookup/doi/
4. Smolen JS, Landewé R, Breedveld FC, et al. EULAR recommendations for the management of rheumatoid arthritis with synthetic and biological disease-modifying antirheumatic drugs. Ann Rheum Dis. 2017;0:1–18.
5. Riemsma R, Taal E, Kirwan J, Rasker J. Systematic review of rheumatoid arthritis patient education. Arthritis Care Res. 2004;51(6):1045–59.

6. Basic concepts of patient education. Jones and Bartlett (Pub). https://www.jblearning.com/samples/0763755443/55447_CH01_Dreeben.pdf. Accessed 28 February 2018.
7. El Miedany Y, El Gaafary M, Youssef S, Palmer D. Towards a multidimensional patient reported outcome measures assessment: development and validation of a questionnaire for patients with ankylosing spondylitis/spondyloarthritis. Joint Bone Spine. 2010;77(6):575–81.
8. El Miedany Y, El Gaafary M, Youssef SS, Palmer D. Incorporating patient reported outcome measures in clinical practice: development and validation of a questionnaire for inflammatory arthritis. Clin Exp Rheumatol. 2010;28(5):734–44.
9. El Miedany Y1, El Gaafary M, Palmer D. Assessment of the utility of visual feedback in the treatment of early rheumatoid arthritis patients: a pilot study. Rheumatol Int. 2012;32(10):3061–8. Epub 2011 Sep 11
10. Yasser EM, Gaafary ME, Sayed S, Palmer D, Ahmed I. Implementing shared decision making in clinical practice: outcomes of a new shared decision making aid for chronic inflammatory arthritis patients. J Patol Care. 2016;2:117. https://doi.org/10.4172/2573-4598.1000117.
11. Fraenkel L, Nowell WB, Michel G, Wiedmeyer C. Preference phenotypes to facilitate shared decision-making in rheumatoid arthritis. Published online ahead of print December 15, 2017. Ann Rheum Dis. https://doi.org/10.1136/annrheumdis-2017-212407.
12. Palmer D, El Miedany Y. Shared decision making for patients living with inflammatory arthritis. Br J Nurs. 2016;25(1):31–5.
13. Li L, Adam P, Townsend A, Lacaille D. Usability testing of ANSWER: a web-based methotrexate decision aid for patients with rheumatoid arthritis. BMC Med Inform Decis Mak. 2013;13:131.
14. NICE Clinical Guidelines, No. 138. Patient experience in adult NHS services: improving the experience of care for people using adult NHS services: patient experience in generic terms. https://www.ncbi.nlm.nih.gov/books/NBK115239/.
15. El Miedany Y, El Gaafary M, El Arousy N, Ahmed I, Youssef S, Palmer D. Arthritis education: the integration of patient-reported outcome measures and patient self-management. Clin Exp Rheumatol. 2012;30(6):899–904.
16. Towle A, Bainbridge L, Godolphin W, Katz A, Kline C, Lown B, Madularu I, Solomon P, Thistlethwaite J. Active patient involvement in the education of health professionals. Med Educ. 2010;44(1):64–74.
17. De Silva D. What works to support self-management. Chapter 3 in helping people helping themselves. The Health Foundation (pub). 2011. https://www.health.org.uk/sites/health/files/HelpingPeopleHelpThemselves.pdf.
18. El Miedany Y. Telehealth and telemedicine: how the digital era is changing standard health care. Dove Medical Press. 2017;4:43–5.
19. El Miedany Y, El Aroussy N, Youssef S, Almedany S, Palmer D. Teaching the millennials: using youtube for teaching rheumatology in the standard educational settings. Ann Rheum Dis. 2018; (in press).
20. Knowles MS, Holton EF III, Swanson RA. The adult learner: the definitive classic in adult education and human resource development. 6th ed. St. Louis: Elsevier; 2005.
21. Lorenzen B, Melby CE, Earles B. Using principles of health literacy to enhance the informed consent process. AORN J. 2008;88:23–9.
22. Iversen MD, Hammond A, Betteridge N. Self-management of rheumatic diseases state of the art and future perspectives. Ann Rheum Dis. 2010;69:955–63.
23. Iversen MD, Sharby N. Arthritis patient education health promotion and team approach to management. Principles of management. Chapter 46. 396–5.
24. Fox S. Online Health search 2006. Pew Research Center 2006. http://www.pewinternet.org/2006/10/29/online-health-search-2006/.
25. How technology is shaping patient education. PMLive.com. PMHub 2013. http://www.pmlive.com/pmhub/medical_communications/fti_consulting/white_papers_and_resources/how_technology_is_shaping_patient_education.

26. Jack BW, et al. A reengineered hospital discharge program to decrease rehospitalization: a randomized trial. Ann Intern Med. 2009;150(3):178–87.
27. Patient Education Management. "Don't get left behind: iPads making strong inroads with patient education" 2011.
28. New Media Trend Watch. http://www.newmediatrendwatch.com/markets-by-country/18-uk/154-mobile-devices.
29. Pulman A, Hill J, Masding MG. The development of an innovative mobile phone app for type 1 diabetes alcohol education. In: Diabetes UK professional conference, 13–15 March 2013, Manchester; 2013.
30. The Beryl Institute. Enhancing the patient experience through the use of interactive technology. 2011.
31. Acosta-Lobos A, Riley JP, Cowie MR. Current and future technologies for remote monitoring in cardiology and evidence from trial data. Futur Cardiol. 2012;8(3):425–43.
32. El Miedany Y, El Gaafary M, El Aroussy N, Bahlas S, Hegazi M, Palmer D, Youssef S. Toward electronic health recording: evaluation of electronic patient reported outcome measures (e-PROMs) system for remote monitoring of early systemic lupus patients. Clin Rheumatol. 2017;6(11):2461–9.
33. El Miedany Y, El Gaafary M, Youssef S, Bahlas S, Almedany S, Ahmed I, Palmer D. Toward electronic health recording: evaluation of electronic patient-reported outcome measures system for remote monitoring of early rheumatoid arthritis. J Rheumatol. 2016;43(12):2106–12.
34. Moe R, Haavardsholm E, Grotle M, Steen E, Kjeken I, Hagen K, Uhlig T. Development of a brief multidisciplinary education programme for patients with osteoarthritis. BMC Musculoskelet Disord. 2011;12:257.
35. Coleman S, Briffa NK, Carroll G, Inderjeeth C, Cook N, McQuade J. Effects of self-management, education and specific exercises, delivered by health professionals, in patients with osteoarthritis of the knee. BMC Musculoskelet Disord. 2008;9:133. https://doi.org/10.1186/1471-2474-9-133.
36. Superio-Cabuslay E, Ward MM, Lorig KR. Patient education interventions in osteoarthritis and rheumatoid arthritis: a meta-analytic comparison with nonsteroidal antiinflammatory drug treatment. Arthritis Care Res. 1996;9(4):292–301. 10.1002/1529-0131(199608)9:4<292::AID-ANR1790090414>3.0.CO;2-4
37. Lorig KR, Sobel DS, Ritter PL, Laurent D, Hobbs M. Effect of a self-management program on patients with chronic disease. Eff Clin Pract. 2001;4(6):256–62.
38. Ofman JJ, Badamgarav E, Henning JM, Knight K, Gano AD, Levan RK, Gur-Arie S, Richards MS, Hasselblad V, Weingarten SR. Does disease management improve clinical and economic outcomes in patients with chronic diseases? A systematic review. Am J Med. 2004;117(3):182–92. https://doi.org/10.1016/j.amjmed.2004.03.018.
39. Devos-Comby L, Cronan T, Roesch SC. Do exercise and self-management interventions benefit patients with osteoarthritis of the knee? A metaanalytic review. J Rheumatol. 2006;33(4):744–56.
40. Chodosh J, Morton SC, Mojica W, Maglione M, Suttorp MJ, Hilton L, Rhodes S, Shekelle P. Meta-analysis: chronic disease self-management programs for older adults. Ann Intern Med. 2005;143(6):427–38.
41. Zhang W, Nuki G, Moskowitz RW, Abramson S, Altman RD, Arden NK, Bierma-Zeinstra S, Brandt KD, Croft P, Doherty M, Dougados M, Hochberg M, Hunter DJ, Kwoh K, Lohmander LS, Tugwell P. OARSI recommendations for the management of hip and knee osteoarthritis: part III: changes in evidence following systematic cumulative update of research published through January 2009. Osteoarthr Cartil. 2010;18(4):476–99. https://doi.org/10.1016/j.joca.2010.01.013.
42. Jamtvedt G, Dahm KT, Christie A, Moe RH, Haavardsholm E, Holm I, Hagen KB. Physical therapy interventions for patients with osteoarthritis of the knee: an overview of systematic reviews. Phys Ther. 2008;88(1):123–36. https://doi.org/10.2522/ptj.20070043.

43. Solomon DH, Warsi A, Brown-Stevenson T, Farrell M, Gauthier S, Mikels D, Lee TH. Does self-management education benefit all populations with arthritis? A randomized controlled trial in a primary care physician network. J Rheumatol. 2002;29(2):362–8.
44. Warsi A, Wang PS, LaValley MP, Avorn J, Solomon DH. Self-management education programs in chronic disease: a systematic review and methodological critique of the literature. Arch Intern Med. 2004;164(15):1641–9. https://doi.org/10.1001/archinte.164.15.1641.
45. Hopman-Rock M, Westhoff MH. The effects of a health educational and exercise program for older adults with osteoarthritis for the hip or knee. J Rheumatol. 2000;27(8):1947–54.
46. Keefe FJ, Caldwell DS, Baucom D, Salley A, Robinson E, Timmons K, Beaupre P, Weisberg J, Helms M. Spouse-assisted coping skills training in the management of knee pain in osteoarthritis: long-term followup results. Arthritis Care Res. 1999;12(2):101–11. 10.1002/1529-0131(199904)12:2<101::AID-ART5>3.0.CO;2-9
47. Fries JF, Carey C, McShane DJ. Patient education in arthritis: randomized controlled trial of a mail-delivered program. J Rheumatol. 1997;24(7):1378–83.
48. Allen KD, Oddone EZ, Coffman CJ, Datta SK, Juntilla KA, Lindquist JH, Walker TA, Weinberger M, Bosworth HB. Telephone-based self-management of osteoarthritis: a randomized trial. Ann Intern Med. 2010;153(9):570–9.
49. Osborne RH, Spinks JM, Wicks IP. Patient education and self-management programs in arthritis. Med J Aust. 2004;180(5 Suppl):S23–6.
50. Osborne RH, Buchbinder R, Ackerman IN. Can a disease-specific education program augment self-management skills and improve health-related quality of life in people with hip or knee osteoarthritis? BMC Musculoskelet Disord. 2006;7:90. https://doi.org/10.1186/1471-2474-7-90.
51. Hewlett SA. Patients and clinicians have different perspectives on outcomes in arthritis. J Rheumatol. 2003;30(4):877–9.
52. Brady T, Kruger J, Helmick C, Callahan L, Boutaugh M. Intervention programs for arthritis and other rheumatic diseases. Health Educ Behav. 2003;30(1):44–63.
53. Palmer D, El Miedany Y. PROMs: a novel approach to arthritis self-management. Br J Nurs. 2012;21(10):601–7.
54. British Medical Association, Medical Education Subcommittee. Role of the patient in medical education. 2008. http://www.bma.org.uk/images/roleofthepatient_ tcm27–175953.pdf. Accessed 28 Feb 2018.
55. Barrows HS, Abrahamson S. The programmed patient: a technique for appraising student performance in clinical neurology. J Med Educ. 1964;39:802–5.
56. Stillman PL, Ruggill JS, Rutala PJ, Sabers DL. Patient instructors as teachers and evaluators. J Med Educ. 1980;55:186–93.
57. Towle A, Bainbridge L, Godolphin W, Katz A, Kline C, Lown B, Madularu I, Solomon P, Thistlethwaite J. Active patient involvement in the education of health professionals. Med Educ. 2010;44:64–74. Available from. https://doi.org/10.1111/j.1365-2923.2009.03530.x.
58. Vail R, Mahon-Salazar C, Morrison A, Kalet A. Patients as teachers: an integrated approach to teaching medical students about the ambulatory care of HIV infected patients. Patient Educ Couns. 1996;27:95–101.
59. Solomon P, Guenter D, Stinson D. People with HIV as educators of health professionals. AIDS Patient Care STDs. 2005;19:840–7.
60. Plymale MA, Witzke DB, Sloan PA, Blue AV, Sloan DA. Cancer survivors as standardized patients: an innovative program integrating cancer survivors into structured clinical teaching. J Cancer Educ. 1999;14:67–71.
61. Skog M, Grafstrom M, Negussie B, Winblad B. The patient as "teacher": learning in the care of elderly persons with dementia. Nurse Educ Today. 2000;20:288–97.
62. Coodin S, Chisholm F. Teaching in a new key: effects of a cotaught seminar on medical students' attitudes toward schizophrenia. Psychiatr Rehabil J. 2001;24:299–302.
63. Hall IS, Hollins S. The Strathcona theatre company: changing medical students' attitudes to learning disability (mental handicap). Psychiatr Bull. 1996;20:429–30.

64. Hanson JL, Randall VF. Patients as advisors: enhancing medical education curricula. Bethesda: Uniformed Services University of the Health Sciences; 2007. p. 156.
65. Langton H, Barnes M, Haslehurst S, Rimmer J, Turton P. Collaboration, user involvement and education: a systematic review of the literature and report of an educational initiative. Eur J Oncol Nurs. 2003;7:242–52.
66. Spencer J, Godolphin W, Karpenko N, Towle A. Can patients be teachers? The Health Foundation (pub). 2011. https://www.health.org.uk/sites/health/files/CanPatientsBeTeachers.pdf. Accessed on 28 Feb 2018.
67. Tew J, Gell C, Foster S. Learning from experience. Involving service users and carers in mental health education and training. Nottingham: Higher Education Academy/National Institute for Mental Health in England/ Trent Workforce Development Confederation; 2004.
68. Jha V, Quinton ND, Bekker HL, Roberts TE. Strategies and interventions for the involvement of real patients in medical education: a systematic review. Med Educ. 2009;43(1):10–20.
69. Masters H, Forrest S, Harley A, Hunter M, Brown N, Risk I. Involving mental health service users and carers in curriculum development: moving beyond 'classroom' involvement. J Psychiatr Ment Health Nurs. 2002;9:309–16.
70. Ingham M. How patients can contribute to nurses' education. Nurs Times. 2001;97:42–3.
71. Flanagan J. Public participation in the design of educational programmes for cancer nurses: a case report. Eur J Cancer Care. 1999;8:107–12.
72. Seden J, Reynolds J, Henderson J, Kubiak C. Managing care and joined up thinking in the curriculum. Soc Work Educ. 2005;24:841–56.
73. Raj N, Badcock LJ, Brown GA, Deighton CM, O'Reilly SC. Student and patient educators' (PE) attitudes to PE led undergraduate musculoskeletal examination training. Rheumatology Oxford 2007; i115.
74. BEME: Best Evidence in Medical Education. Guidelines and coding sheets. www. bemecollaboration.org. Accessed 28 Feb 2018.
75. Côté L, Turgeon J. Appraising qualitative research articles in medicine and medical education. Med Teach. 2005;27(1):71–5.
76. Buijink AW, Visser BJ, Marshall L. Medical apps for smartphones: lack of evidence undermines quality and safety. Evid Based Med. 2013;18(3):90–2.
77. Bartlett E. Cost-benefit anaylysis of patient education. Patient Educ Couns. 1995; 26(1–3):87–91.

Chapter 11
The Art of Teaching Postgraduates and Future Learners

Introduction

Rheumatology incorporates the investigation, diagnosis, management and rehabilitation of patients with disorders of the musculoskeletal system (bone, muscles, joints, ligaments and connective tissue), i.e. the locomotor apparatus. The rheumatological disorders thus include diverse conditions such as inflammatory arthritis, autoimmune connective tissue disorders, inflammatory spine disorders and soft tissue conditions including injuries, osteoarthritis, spinal pain and other chronic pain syndromes as well as metabolic bone disease.

While rheumatologists appreciate that musculoskeletal problems are a very common cause of pain and disability, both in hospital [1] as well as the community [2, 3], patients with bone and joint complaints are often taken lightly, and their problems are underestimated by junior training doctors or general practitioners. This is, partly, a reflection of inadequate education at the undergraduate level and partly the result of the common notion that all will have aches and pains at some stage which people have to live with, and there is nothing that can be done about them. Furthermore, the psychological, social and impairment dimensions of "chronic" illness tend to be less frequently studied than the technical aspects of musculoskeletal disorder management [4, 5]. On another front, the consequences of musculoskeletal disorders are usually high with the direct costs that constitute only a quarter of the indirect costs. Examples of the indirect costs include sick leave, sick pensions, early retirement and the inability to support oneself. The consequences of this inability may be even more serious in developing countries. Furthermore, worldwide, up to 15 million injured persons survive road traffic accidents, most of whom will suffer sequelae of musculoskeletal trauma [6].

Surveys show that undergraduate medical students spend very few hours learning basic science and in clinical training of the musculoskeletal system [7, 8]. Currently, rheumatology modules are relatively short and mainly hospital based, and specific assessment of locomotor history taking and examination skills is not a priority [9].

Y. El Miedany, *Rheumatology Teaching*,
https://doi.org/10.1007/978-3-319-98213-7_11

While it would be considered negligent for a medical graduate to be incompetent at adequately assessing any of the four "core" bodily systems, cardiovascular, respiratory, abdominal and neurological, it is quite common for students to leave medical school without being able to make a general assessment of the musculoskeletal system. Furthermore, training in orthopaedics and rheumatology are rarely mandatory in systems with rotating internships or in family practice training programmes, with examination frequently overlooked in routine clinical practice, despite the high prevalence of musculoskeletal symptoms in the general population [10–12].

In order to truly improve the assessment and management skills for musculoskeletal conditions, it is vital that education at all levels pays proper attention to musculoskeletal training and ways to interpret the patient history and identify those patients who require early referral to the secondary care and those who can be managed in the primary care setting. This chapter will discuss the present situation regarding musculoskeletal training, particularly the challenges to the rheumatology education at the postgraduate level, the art and science of teaching postgraduates and future learners. It will expand to discuss competency-based medical education, the milestones, where are we now in postgraduate training and what need to be done. It will conclude by discussing the use of innovations in postgraduate medical teaching.

Challenges to the Rheumatology Education at the Postgraduate Level

Educational Setting

Following the shift in the rheumatology service from the inpatient to the outpatient setting, fewer patients are admitted to hospital, and there is a reduction in the length of in-patient stay, whereas most of the patients are seen in the outpatient setting [9]. They will reduce the opportunities of training doctors to view and assess patients presenting with acute musculoskeletal problems while on hospital attachments. Unfortunately, this also is not always counterbalanced by the availability of outpatient teaching facilities or dedicated time for the training doctors to attend the outpatient rheumatology clinic.

Another challenge is that most of the patients presenting with musculoskeletal symptoms are seen in general practice, where they cause a significant workload. While this could be a good opportunity for the trainees to assess and manage these patients during their general practice modules, the aims of this part of the curriculum are biased towards the teaching of general practice technique, not rheumatology. In addition, many of the general practitioners (GPs), lacking the proper training in musculoskeletal medicine, may not feel competent or confident enough to teach either on patient assessment or on diseases of the locomotor system; hence a learning opportunity is missed [13].

Thirdly, as rheumatology is such an active research area with rewarding pharmaceutical interest and support, rheumatology academics paid full attention to research in preference to teaching. On another front, teaching, in general, is not recognized as an important area of expertise, equivalent to research and fund raising. However, the lack of recognition of teachers is not unique to rheumatologists and has been reported in most other specialities of clinical medical education [14].

The Learners

The medical profession is highly diverse and is changing. General medical council report about medical service in the United Kingdom [15] revealed that the average age of doctors is falling (overall distribution peaked at approximately 33 years). The changing age demographic has implications for the profession and service delivery. A younger doctor profile is likely to affect the balance of inexperienced to experienced doctors, which may have implications both for service delivery and for maintaining enough opportunities for high-quality training for all.

This generation of younger training doctors have distinctive learning needs and characteristics that are different from the older teaching style. Training doctors of today generally have a deeper level of critical thinking and have more educational resources available to them compared to a decade or two ago. Today's learners also prefer multi-linked information coming from many sources and are multitaskers; are highly visual learners, preferring to process pictures and sounds rather than text; and are experiential learners who learn by discovery rather than being "told". They like to interact with content to explore and draw their own conclusions. Simulations, games and role playing are used for learning [16]. In addition, they have short attention spans and therefore prefer small packets of information, preferably online (e.g., on a personal computer, smartphone or tablet) [17, 18]. In order to capitalise on these and to meet their learning needs with the aim of optimizing their future clinical acumen as residents and specialists, medical education has to be evolved significantly to meet these requirements.

Effective Educators

Teachers are one of the key elements in any educational system, and effective teaching is one of the key propellers for improving the learning process. However, it has been acknowledged that teaching per se is not enough; hence a new term was introduced "effective teaching". Effective teaching requires criteria for effectiveness. These criteria refer to the objectives of education in general and of teaching in particular. Teacher effectiveness is generally referred to in terms of the focus on student outcomes [19]. One of the main challenges in the postgraduate education process is the teaching approach adopted by tutors. As most of the teachers represent an older generation than the students, the teachers usually adopt the old informative education approach which relay on knowledge delivery, e.g. lectures or workshops, where the students' role is passive in general. This comes in contrast to the learners'

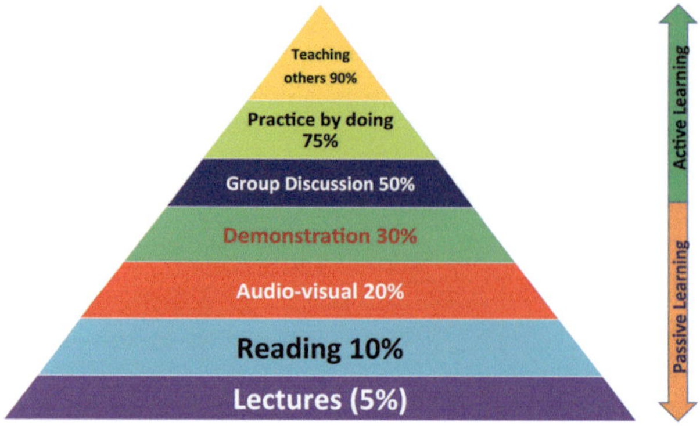

Fig. 11.1 The learning pyramid: There are several methods a learner can engage in which will allow him/her to learn information at various percentages of retention. The pyramid of average learning retention rates, researched and created by the National Training Laboratories in Betel, Maine, illustrates the percentage of what learner can recall in association with various approaches. The first four levels (lecture, reading, audio–visual and demonstration) are passive learning methods. In contrast, the top three levels (discussion group, practice by doing and teaching others) are active (participatory) learning methods. As shown in the pyramid, the active participation in the learning process leads to a higher retention of learning

characteristics mentioned above. The pyramid of average learning retention rates (Fig. 11.1) are lectures 5%, reading 10%, audio–visual 20%, demonstration 30%, group discussion 50%, practice by doing 75% and teaching others 90%. Lectures have been criticized as "spoon-feeding" and being overloaded with information that may not be relevant. Tutorials, expected to supplement learning in small groups, help only if the students come prepared with prior study [20]. To handle this challenge, "teaching the teachers" courses delivered by educational supervisors are highly required. Training educational programmes can be produced by the regional training committees. The educational role of each doctor should be recorded in the doctor's annual appraisal. Doctors also have been encouraged to include their educational scientific activities among their continued professional development certificate.

The Science of Teaching Postgraduates

Education Theories

Postgraduate training and education in the hospital specialities have undergone a major restructuring, with a considerable shift towards structured training programmes and away from reliance on learning by "osmosis", whereby time spent exposed to clinical practice was taken to be synonymous with learning and proficiency. Though there are many theories that explain how adults learn and each has its own merits, none of the individual theories fully explain what is happening when an aspiring health professional is engaged in learning. Looking at all the published educational theories, it became clear that the authors held a broadly constructivist view (Fig. 11.2). Constructivists, like Vygotsky [21], considered that learning is the process of constructing new knowledge on the foundations of what you already know, whereas Malcolm Knowles [22] considered that adults learn in different ways from children. He introduced the term "andragogy" to differentiate adult learning from pedagogy; this differentiation now seems to be artificial. Many of the principles of andragogy can be applied equally to children's learning. It is probably more appropriate to think in terms of a learning continuum, which stretches throughout life, with different emphases, problems and strategies at different times. The transformative learning theory developed by Mezirow [23] explored the way in which critical reflection can be used to challenge the learner's beliefs and assumptions. Transformative learning involves experiencing a deep, structural shift in the basic premises of thought, feelings and actions, where "We Accommodate new in our open system of value, paradigm by voluntary changing our own self according to new information, situation, experiences, insights etc.". This comes in contrast with the standard information system where "We Assimilate new in our close system of value, 'box', paradigm, etc. without changing our own self according to new information, situation, experiences, insights, etc." (Fig. 11.3) [24].

In 1984, David Kolb's presented his experiential learning model (Fig. 11.4) [25]. In Kolb's scheme, the learner has a concrete experience, upon which they reflect. Through their reflection they are able to formulate abstract concepts and make appropriate generalizations. They then consolidate their understanding by testing the implications of their knowledge in new situations. This then provides them with a concrete experience, and the cycle continues. Learners with different learning preferences will have strengths in different quadrants of the (Kolb) cycle. In Kolb's terminology "activists" feel and do, "reflectors" feel and watch, "theorists" watch and think and "pragmatists" think and do (Fig. 11.2). Experiential learning may begin at any of the four steps. Each step allows the learner to reflect and form new principles to guide future situations. From the educator's point of view, it is

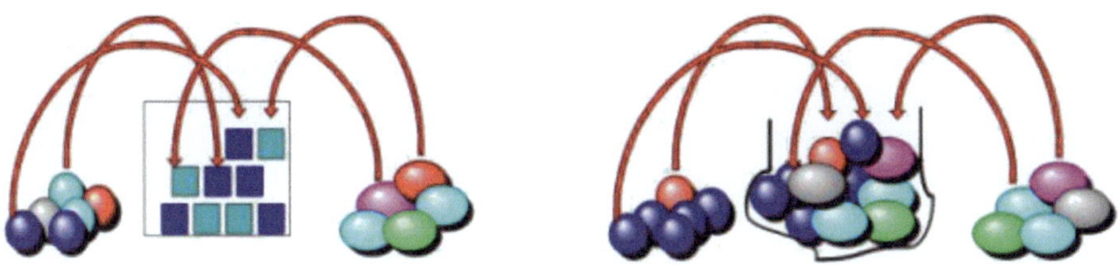

Fig. 11.2 Informative learning–teaching strategy (to the left) vs transformative learning method. Informational learning is teachers talking, students listening, taking notes, putting the boxes neatly and in order as the student was told, taking tests and getting that ever important "letter" grade at the end. It's about memorization and regurgitation. Whoever can master that can master the schooling system. Transformational learning on the other hand is all about letting individuals figure out the answer on their own. It's a much slower way of learning, but it triggers more creativity, empowerment, problem-solving and real-world applicability. Boundaries are more open, and the mind is able to collect, gather and create as it wants

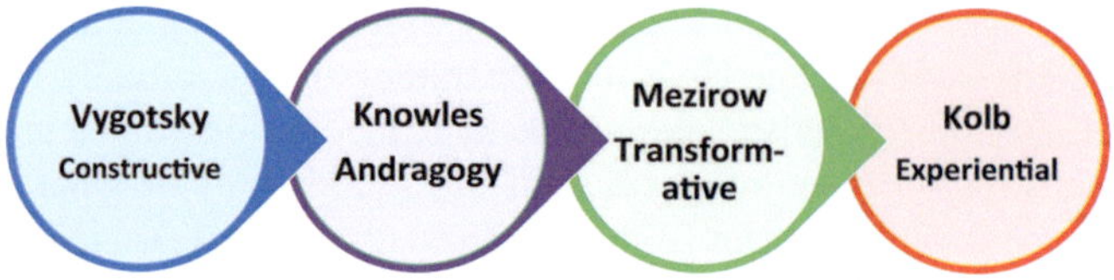

Fig. 11.3 Education theories: Vygotsky considered that learning is the process of constructing new knowledge on the foundations of what you already know, whereas Malcolm Knowles considered that adults learn in different ways from children. He introduced the term "andragogy" to differentiate adult learning from pedagogy. The transformative learning theory developed by Mezirow explored the way in which critical reflection can be used to challenge the learner's beliefs and assumptions, whereas Kolb's presented his experiential learning model

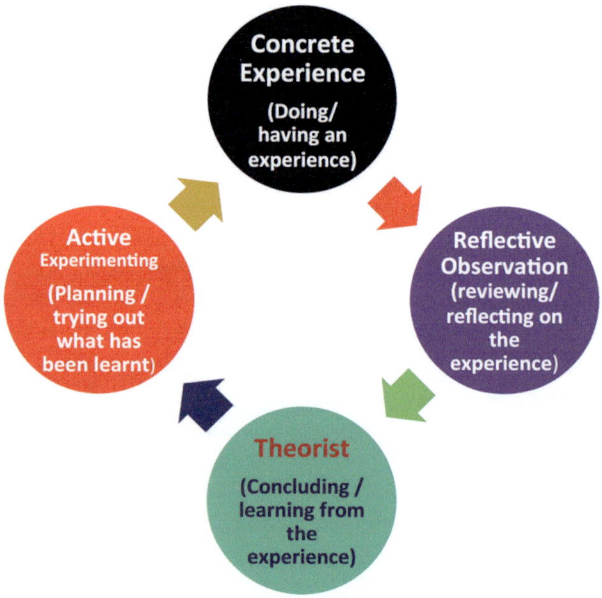

Fig. 11.4 Kolb's education cycle. In Kolb's terminology "activists" feel and do, "reflectors" feel and watch, "theorists" watch and think and "pragmatists" think and do (Fig. 11.2). Experiential learning may begin at any of the four steps. Each step allows the learner to reflect and form new principles to guide future situations

important to design learning activities that allow the cycle to be followed, engaging each of the quadrants. Although it is often quoted and easily understood, the learning style inventory developed from the Kolb cycle has poor reliability and validity [26]. Interestingly, despite the new generation of learners having different learning characteristics, these established education theories still hold true until now.

Teaching Rheumatology to Postgraduates

Many medical school curriculums are directly or indirectly associated with these educational theories. Principles of adult learning that emerge from the theories mentioned above form the basis of rheumatology curriculum design and are as follows: (1) learning is an active process, whereby learners determine when and how to modify their knowledge; (2) emphasis is on the developing of their own understanding through self-directed learning; (3) learners should be encouraged to seek easily available guidance for complex tasks; (4) learners should aim to complete the full experiential learning cycle; (5) learners should be given opportunities and support for practice with self-assessment and constructive feedback from their learning community that includes peers and faculty; and (6) learning should be closely related to the understanding and solution of real-world problems [16]. These principles form a major portion of rheumatology teaching in that the emphasis on curriculums should be based on interaction with peers, senior medical staff, allied health and self-directed learning. The faculty facilitates the learning process through small and large group teaching as well as bedside clinical teaching. Faculty serve as role models of knowledge and professionalism to inspire students.

The Postgraduate Rheumatology Curriculum

Traditionally, the standard curriculums for teaching rheumatology, commonly used prior to 1990, were consisted of didactic lectures and clinical teaching in the ward. Assessments were usually in the form of multiple-choice questions (MCQ) and written examinations. Clinical skills were tested using traditional short and long case examinations. A study by Kay et al. of 26 medical schools in the United Kingdom in 1999 [27] revealed that while the majority of medical schools included rheumatology clinical teaching in the curriculum for all their students, up to about 50% of the students in five schools received no clinical rheumatology teaching whatsoever. In some medical schools, rheumatology was found to be an elective rather than a core component in some schools. Rheumatology was generally taught in conjunction with other specialties, usually orthopaedic surgery, whereas in other schools, rheumatology was taught with general medicine and rehabilitation medicine. Furthermore, not all schools tested students on their rheumatology clinical skills. Only a minority of schools had the rheumatology examination counted towards the final degree.

Over the past two decades, medical education in general including the teaching of rheumatology has undergone a paradigm shift and has become recognized as required to be a lifelong process [28, 29]. Learners would need to acquire learning skills that will take them from their undergraduate experience, through their general training and specialist training. Another theme is the shift from a teacher-centred approach, where the emphasis is on the teachers and what they do, to a learner-centred approach, where the emphasis is on what the students learn (Fig. 11.5) [30]. This is achieved by the replacement of the traditional didactic teacher by a "learning facilitator", and traditional didactic teaching methods are replaced by interactive teaching in smaller groups. Current curriculum designs to teach rheumatology recommend the introduction of student-selected modules and to use more additional teaching sites, including general practice if applicable [31].

Learner-centred teaching and self-directed learning are most effective in small groups. The principles of self-directed learning are that the student defines their

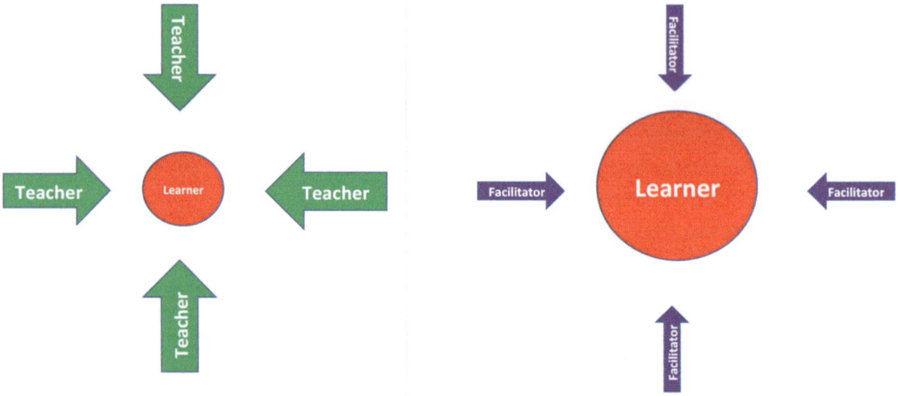

Fig. 11.5 Change strategy of teaching from informative style implementing teacher-centred approach into interactive facilitator style adopting learner-centred approach

own learning needs, sets their own objectives, identifies necessary resources to enhance learning and then is able to evaluate the outcome. Learner-centred teaching and self-directed learning method of teaching stimulate adult-type learning characteristics of deep learning and develop the learners' reasoning and problem-solving skills, a necessary quality for clinicians to excel. The most common example of learner-centred teaching methods is "problem-based learning", in which learning is centred around clinical problems [32–34]. Although there is some evidence that problem-based learning reduces acquisition of basic science knowledge, it promotes several key features of learning. These include deep learning, enhancing self-directed skills and provision of a more stimulating and safe learning environment free of intimidation and ridicule. PBL also improves interaction between students and staff.

Another example of learner-centred teaching methods is "portfolio-based learning". Portfolio-based learning encourages "reflective practice", a term used to describe the process of internally examining and exploring experiences. A common portfolio in medical education is the log book. This method of learning requires intensive supervision by the teacher to discuss with the learner the learning objectives and to monitor their progress [35].

While didactic lectures have had bad impression because there is good evidence to show that learners remember very little (5–10%) of what they hear during lectures, large group teaching will remain a component of rheumatology curriculums. Instead of being a "transmitter" of knowledge, the lecturer should aim to achieve "active learning". It would be advisable to plan a lecture in 10–15 min blocks with 5-min breaks for exercises or notetaking. Audience response systems, brainstorming of ideas written onto a whiteboard, flipchart for discussion and bringing patients to a lecture are a few examples of the ways in which active learning is encouraged during lectures [16].

One of the methods of standardizing the teaching of clinical skills is the development of centres that are purpose-built areas. They are designed to enhance the teaching of clinical skills in a safe environment for the learner. They have access to databases of real and simulated patients who can be invited for teaching [36]. Ideally, the centre would have facilities to simulate a ward or other clinical environments. Computer facilities should be available with Internet access for interactive learning [37, 38]. Manikins and models are more lifelike to enable the student to practice a skill, such as joint examination and joint injection.

Assessment drives learning and is an important component of a curriculum. It should carefully match the teaching that occurs. End of rheumatology rotation assessments to test mainly theoretical knowledge is discouraged because students would spend a large proportion of their time on learning facts that involve mainly superficial "rote" learning. Instead, combining MCQs with objective structured clinical examinations (OSCE) is a reliable and valid measure of a student's performance. OSCE encourages students to spend more time learning patient interaction and allows their clinical skills to be directly observed [39].

Competency-Based Medical Education

Internationally, competency-based medical education has been around for over 60 years. Dr. J. Frank was the lead researcher who published research studies on competency-based medical education curriculum being an outcome-based method of training [40]. A competency-based medical education curriculum deemphasizes training time and puts focus on trainees' skill. In his earlier published reports, Dr. Frank noted that this type of training is able to assess whether graduates of medical education training programmes can practice quality medicine.

The history of competency-based medical education was engrained in the history of the medical profession of Britain. In the United Kingdom, the General Medical Council (GMC) used to adopt structure-based competency tools and tests to assess primary care physicians in training and out of practice. This testing system has been utilized for years. A similar system was used in New Zealand and Australia, where a council would review a physicians' medical record to make sure written documentation is done correctly [41].

From a developmental standard, trainees' abilities develop at different times and stages. Competency-based assessments are used to distinguish between the skills and knowledge that trainee already has and those for which the trainee needs more education and training. In contrast to time-based educational methods, competency-based medical education is a learner-centred, active and lifelong experience that incorporates feedback between the teacher and the learner to fulfil the desired competency outcomes. In a competency-based educational program, the trainee does not just acquire knowledge and then spit it back at the time of a final exam. Instead, the method of assessment is formative rather than summative, and the learners are evaluated on how they apply their knowledge to clinical situations that physicians often face. While summative exams, such as certification exams, play an important role in gauging levels of acquired knowledge, formative assessments are equally important.

With a competency-based medical education curriculum, the "Learner centeredness encourages trainees to take responsibility for their progress by mapping out a transparent pathway to competence" [40]. This type of educational model also takes into account the fact that different competencies are needed in different geographical areas. If a resident is trained in a location of the United States that is medically underserved, there is a need for training in specific procedures and skills and that training can be tested and assessed using a competency-based medical education model.

The Milestones

In 1999, the Accreditation Council for Graduate Medical Education (ACGME) and the American Board of Medical Specialties (ABMS) endorsed six domains of core competencies, and the outcome initiative (the Outcome Project) was soon launched.

The Six ACGME Core Competencies

Patient care
Medical knowledge
Professionalism
Interpersonal and communication skills
Practice-based learning and improvement
System-based practice

Even though there was standardized language around the core competencies of medical education, there were still no standardized assessment methods to determine if a learner had achieved all of the core competencies prior to completion of residency training. This deficiency ultimately led to the creation of milestones (Table 11.1) to operationalize and implement the competencies. These milestones described the performance levels residents and fellows are expected to demonstrate for skills, knowledge and behaviours in the six clinical competency domains and are significant points in development that are unique to each specialty. Table 11.2 gives an example of the basic anatomy of a musculoskeletal milestone.

Table 11.1 General description of milestone levels

Milestone description				
Level 1	Level 2	Level 3	Level 4	Level 5
What are the expectations for a beginning resident?	What are the milestones for a resident who has advanced over entry but is performing at a lower level than expected at mid-residency?	What are the key developmental milestones mid-residency? What should they be able to do well in the realm of the speciality at this point?	What does a graduating resident look like? What additional knowledge, skills and attitude have they obtained? Are they ready for certification?	Stretch goals – exceed expectations
Comments				

Table 11.2 Example of the basic anatomy of a milestone of a musculoskeletal case

Milestone description				
General competency	Sub-competency		Developmental progression or set of milestones	
Level 1	Level 2	Level 3	Level 4	Level 5
Take a general medical/ musculoskeletal history	Acquire a basic speciality specific medical history including medical, functional and psychological elements (E.g. complaint, pain, morning stiffness, functional ability, quality of life, other systemic illnesses, history of medication and response to treatment)	Acquire a comprehensive medical history integrating medical, functional and psychosocial elements Seek and obtain data from secondary sources when needed (E.g. integrate patient's data trying to identify underlying pathology and possible diagnosis/ differential diagnosis)	Efficiently acquires and presents a relevant history in a prioritized and hypothesis driven fashion across a wide spectrum of ages and impairments Specific milestone Elicit information that may not be readily volunteered by the patient (E.g. comorbidity history, self-helplessness, motivation)	Gathers and synthesizes information in a highly efficient manner Rapidly focusses on presenting problem and elicits key information in a prioritized fashion Models the gathering of subtle and difficult information from the patient
Comments				

In 2014, the Accreditation Council for Graduate Medical Education (ACGME) required the reporting of milestones as part of the next accreditation system (NAS) for all ACGME-accredited residency and fellowship programmes. In undergraduate medical education, there are two AAMC-defined performance levels: novice performance and performance expected of a graduating medical doctor (MD). In graduate medical education, there are five performance levels for each competency: novice, advanced beginner, competent individual, proficient individual and expert physician.

Postgraduate Training: Where Are We Now

Musculoskeletal complaints are the second most common reason for consultation, exceeded only by disorders of the respiratory system. In average, this constitutes 14–28% of primary care workload [42] as well as visits to emergency services [43]. A study in Australia revealed that only 10% of 166 medical inpatients underwent a musculoskeletal examination, despite the fact that 40% had a documented history of musculoskeletal symptoms on admission [44]. In another survey, 80% of nearly 400 Australian interns failed in assessing the patient's disability and handicap [4].

Many general practitioners (GPs) and family doctors do not have adequate musculoskeletal training and consequently lack the competency, skills and confidence to manage rheumatologic disorders in their daily practice: they may not recognize conditions or be aware of what can be achieved by appropriate care.

In elective programmes only 3.5% of rotating postgraduate interns selected orthopaedic surgery, and less than 1% had training in rheumatology, sports medicine and physical medicine combined [45]. Only 10% of the vocational training schemes for GPs in the United Kingdom include orthopaedics [46]. A survey of general practice trainees [47] demonstrated that 35% had not received any tutorials on rheumatological topics; 65% of trainees had tutorials for about 2 h instead of the recommended 280 h per year of total teaching in their GP training [48]. In the United States, family practice graduates reported a lower level of confidence in their physical examination, radiographic evaluation, diagnosis and treatment of musculoskeletal patients compared with their confidence levels in dealing with other patients, despite training rotation on an orthopaedic service during their residency [47, 48]. Those with training periods of 8 weeks or longer, however, reported higher confidence in all areas [49].

The majority of GP trainees in the United Kingdom felt confident in performing regional musculoskeletal examinations and managing specific conditions, but not in injection techniques. Overall, they perceived the amount of rheumatology education during their vocational training as inadequate [47]. Primary care physicians in Canada have also been reported to be significantly more confident in cardiovascular examination than with a musculoskeletal examination and, in particular, lack confidence in joint injections and aspirations and more rarely encountered problems. The highest level of confidence was observed for using nonsteroidal anti-inflammatory drugs (NSAIDs) and managing common musculoskeletal disorders, but the unnecessary use of diagnostic tests, inappropriate prescription of NSAIDs, low use of patient-centred options and lack of diagnostic suspicion of uncommon but dangerous conditions were cause for concern [50].

Examination is known to drive learning. In examinations, students and trainee GPs are seldom assessed for their competency to take an appropriate history and to examine the musculoskeletal system. A change has been reported in the United Kingdom, however, with clinical skills being tested in 64% of medical schools in 1997 compared with 22% in 1990 [51]. Curriculum 2020 adopted by King's college (started in the year 2017) has dedicated 8-week period for chronic long-term medical condition. Rheumatology and orthopaedics were given a week out of the 8 weeks. However, in real-life practice, the musculoskeletal training is limited maximum to 4–5 h/8 weeks (the author personal contact). Lack of assessment means that graduate physicians may enter clinical practice with deficient knowledge and skills needed to assess and treat patients presenting with musculoskeletal complaints.

What Needs to Be Done?

Curriculum

The main task is to set agreed standards for undergraduate and postgraduate medical education. Establishing standards with clearly defined outcomes is the most powerful way of influencing the competence of future doctors in assessing patients with musculoskeletal conditions. One of the key actions for the Bone and Joint Decade was to increase awareness of musculoskeletal conditions, including awareness among physicians. As education is the most important method of providing sustainable and long-term effects in the healthcare community, a task force focusing on educational issues has been set up through a global network, with the aim of ensuring global standards adaptable to local needs [16].

In many countries, graduation from medical school is followed by an internship, often rotating, in order to be exposed to the major prevailing conditions. Rotation may often include internal medicine and general surgery but not specialties dealing with musculoskeletal conditions. Considering the frequency of consultations for these conditions, those in an advisory capacity should strongly promote rotations in orthopaedics or rheumatology during this important phase of professional development.

Family Practice

Most patients with musculoskeletal complaints will be assessed and treated within primary care settings. Many, even most, primary care or family practice programmes do not include rotations in rheumatology, orthopaedics or rehabilitation, which is a gross under provision for the health needs of the population. To make a difference, several approaches may be used: (1) increase training at the undergraduate level leading to a higher standard at the time of graduating, influence present and future training programmes to include training at units within these specialties, and (2) proactively participate in continuing medical education programmes in family practice. The latter approach has been successfully tested in Canada, where orthopaedic and rheumatology specialists participated in an injection-skills acquisition programme [52, 53]. (3) Development of collaborative programmes is required, with shared care and assigned contact persons between family practice and specialist units.

Specialist Training

The robust developments in the diagnosis and management of rheumatic disease [54, 55], the importance of early diagnosis and management adopting a treat to target approach [56] and the importance of regular assessment and management of comorbidities following a management holistic approach [57, 58], all highlighted the importance of implementing a multi-professional treatment approach. There is therefore a clear need for more interaction and overlap: specialists in orthopaedics, rheumatology, gastroenterology, radiology and rehabilitation should have cross-specialty rotations in order to foster a greater understanding of the respective conditions, early diagnostic approaches and treatment options. A person with back pain may present to a rheumatologist, orthopaedic surgeon or physiatrist; having a pathway for referral criteria, assessment and investigations is vital to ensure a common understanding and approach to management of the condition even if the specific interventions used by the specialists differ. Similarly, different specialists may share the management of a patient with inflammatory arthritis or osteoarthritis. There is no reason for differences in the basic understanding of the conditions, the problems they cause, pathogenesis and the principles of management, but there is a need for a better understanding of what each specialty can offer, when to continue the conservative management approach and when to proceed to the surgical option. Increased interaction during training is likely not only to improve the combined care of the patient but also to lead to a more integrated approach to research in order to improve future knowledge and treatment.

Continuing Professional Development

Considerable progress has been made in the treatment and management of inflammatory arthritic conditions in the past two decades, with rheumatologists now able to manage the effects of this chronic, debilitating condition for most of their patients. With better understanding about the process of inflammation and its applications for therapy, continuing professional development became essential for the rheumatologist. Continuing professional development is important because it ensures the professionals continue to be competent in their profession. It is an ongoing process and continues throughout a professional's career. The ultimate outcome of well-planned continuing professional development is that it safeguards the public, the employer, the professional and the professional's career. At its core it is a personal responsibility of professionals to keep their knowledge and skills current so that they can deliver the high quality of service that safeguards the public and meets the expectations of customers and the requirements of their profession.

It is important that such continuing professional development activity is also multidisciplinary, including clinical and nonclinical activities, external and internal scientific meetings attended. It should also be able to accommodate some personal activities such as reading scientific manuscripts, reviewing and/or writing articles. Continuing professional development activities should aim to maintain and improve the standards of the professional own practice as well as the other members of the team in which the professional work. Identification of needs helps in shaping the continuing professional development activities to meet the professional's requirement, the needs of the service and the people who use it. Reflection plays an important role in assessment of the continuing professional development outcomes. The professional must reflect on what he/she has learnt through the continuing professional development and record any impact (or expected future impact) on his/her performance and practice.

Continuing professional development became compulsory in many countries, with a minimum requirement: usually defined in terms of time spent pursuing educational activities such as meetings or courses and using some system of credits. Regular annual appraisal ensures recording of the professional's educational and scientific activities. Audit is a way of monitoring processes and outcomes to identify and subsequently investigate differences in care that require education to overcome. Revalidation/recertification is becoming a requirement in an increasing number of countries. Standards for appraisal/continuing professional development are being established for the various musculoskeletal professional disciplines [59].

In the United States, the mandates of "Maintenance of Licensure and Maintenance of Certification" are competency based [60]. In the American education model, this occurs after the trainee has finished residency and during their continuing medical education requirements. This certification process includes peer reviews, tests and lifelong learning models. This requirement was enacted to ensure a physicians' competency throughout their career. There has been a recent push against standardized testing in medical education, as some research has shown it is not a reliable predictor of how a trainee does on his or her clinical rotation. Much more emphasis has been placed on competence in a trainee's communication skills and level of professionalism [61].

The Art of Postgraduate Teaching

Technological advances in information technology (IT), simulation and medical technology have had a profound effect on the lives of today's medical trainees. As these technological innovations have become increasingly pervasive and indispensable in our everyday lives, they have changed the nature of how medical trainees work, learn and even think. Consequently, these technologies will also continue to drive and direct innovations in postgraduate medical education. With the current changes in the learners as well as teaching gadgets landscape, there is a room for implementing "*modern art*" of teaching the future learners.

Today's residents are more connected than ever to an increasingly diverse pool of resources, with a multitude of choices as to where and how they implement them. E-resources such as online discussion forums, technology-enhanced problem-based learning tools, email, apps like what's app, social media, electronic library resources, as well as adaptive education systems (adaptive learning systems endeavour to transform the learner from passive receptor of information to collaborator in the educational process. Adaptive learning systems' primary application is in education and aims at creating an instructionally sound and flexible environment that supports learning for students) [62] are just some examples of how information technology have dramatically changed the way learners access knowledge.

For example, e-resources have improved the breadth of knowledge accessible to learners, helping to overcome many of the limitations of traditional face-to-face teaching such as logistical barriers, access to collaboration and expertise and the implementation of longitudinal educational programmes [63, 64]. Furthermore, e-resources have given learners a myriad of new tools through which they can interact with their instructors, colleagues and educational material.

Along with improving the range and types of educational material available to today's residents, information technology such as personal digital assistants (PDAs), tablets/iPads as well as smartphones has made such material both instantly and constantly available. Over 70% of today's residents have reported daily clinical use of these devices for applications such as lab data retrieval, referencing pharmacology guides and accessing treatment protocols. Answers to clinical problems or questions posed during rounds are now accessible within seconds, allowing trainees to both acquire and apply knowledge immediately within the same clinical setting.

Video-conferencing technology has addressed the distance barrier to educational resources through technologies such as telemedicine, tele-mentoring and tele-simulation. Expanding on the concept of e-resources, tele-mentoring provides an effective means for real-time guidance and instruction to trainees in remote locations [65]. Tele-simulation represents an even further evolution of this technology combining the remote proctoring benefits of tele-mentoring with the deliberate practice and patient safety profile of simulation-based medical education [65, 66]. Interactive educational resources and training that was once restricted to a single institution can now be easily shared on a global scale [66–69].

Simulation-based medical education (SBME) is another technology that has had a significant impact on trainees access to knowledge and skills. The details of the various types, limitations,and benefits of SBME are discussed in a separate commissioned paper [70]. However, the common attribute among these various manifestations of SBME is that they have fundamentally changed how and where trainees acquire certain skills and knowledge. Training doctors are no longer reliant on their preceptors and the clinical setting in the same way as previous generations were [71].

In spite of the vast array of technological innovations and implementations, there are common themes among them: improved access to educational material in breadth, timing and distance. Some may consider these technologies, timely given that current economic limitations, have restricted working hours [72]. Furthermore, it has placed increasing pressure on educators to develop more efficient and effective methods of teaching residents. However, improved accessibility to medical information should not be equated to improved medical education [73]. For example, while these mobile gadgets have been shown to provide trainees with additional time for other education practices, how the trainees have used this additional time is unknown [74]. Additionally, learners were reported to prefer electronic resources for referencing previously learned material and that they preferred media for initial learning [75]. On the other hand, studies have demonstrated that the knowledge retention from passive electronic information retrieval is inferior to the retention gained from more traditional self-directed educational activities [76, 77], exemplified by the so-called palmomental reflex of trainees' use of smartphones and PDAs [78]. Similarly, research in SBME has also emphasized that simulators alone were not as effective as those that are combined with instructor training and an educational and professional context [79, 80].

These examples, however, do not mean that technological advances do not have a place in postgraduate medical education. Rather, they illustrate that these technologies should supplement and be integrated within the existing educational framework. It appears that the question of how trainees use this technology is just as important, if not more so, than if trainees use this technology. Therefore, educators must look at ways to discourage passive use of information technology as simple portals to information and find ways to integrate and leverage their potential within the broader learning programmes. While successful innovations in postgraduate medical education recognize and respect the complex interplay among workplace, learner and patient, educational innovations must be implemented with consideration for the impact they will have on the ultimate goal of medical practice, which is optimal patient care. Through thoughtful consideration of the educational impact of a proposed programmatic change, future innovations will continue to evolve the pedagogy signature of postgraduate medical education.

In conclusion, patients with complaints about bones and joints are often ignored, and their problems are underestimated by doctors. This is partly a reflection of inadequate education at undergraduate level or lack of skill/knowledge at the postgraduate level. Assessment of the current situation regarding musculoskeletal training at the postgraduate level revealed some challenges that require tackling both at the curriculum as well as training levels.

The core competencies are now the basic language for defining physician competence and are also the principles used in the training of physicians. The next goal of competency-based medical education is to link education in the competencies and to improved quality of patient care. This ambitious step will require standardized methods to securely collect patient data and stratify for various clinical variables including disease specificity, overall patient health and the multitude of healthcare professionals who care for each patient.

References

1. Wright V. The epidemiology of disability. R Coll Phys Lond. 1982;16:178–83.
2. Morbidity statistics from general practice 1981–1982. Third National Study. Series MB5 No. 1. London: HMSO.
3. Arthritis and Rheumatism Council Field Unit. Digest of data on the rheumatic diseases. 1. Morbidity in industry, and rheumatism in general practice. Ann Rheum Dis. 1974;33:93–105.
4. Crotty M, Ahern MJ, McFarlane AC, Brooks PM. Clinical rheumatology training of Australian medical students; a national survey of 1991 graduates. Med J Aust. 1993;158:119–20.
5. McCredie M, Brooks PM. Rheumatology teaching in Australia: the need for review. Med J Aust. 1985;143:492–5.
6. Åkesson K, Dreinhöfer K, Woolf A. Improved education in musculoskeletal conditions is necessary for all doctors. Bull World Health Organ. 2003;81(9):677–83.
7. Pinney SJ, Regan WD. Educating medical students about musculoskeletal problems. Are community needs reflected in the curricula of Canadian medical schools? J Bone Joint Surg (Am Vol). 2001;83:1317–20.
8. Williams JR. The teaching of trauma and orthopaedic surgery to the undergraduate in the United Kingdom. J Bone Joint Surg Br Vol. 2000;82:627–8.
9. Jones A, Maddison P, Doherty M. Teaching rheumatology to medical students: current practice and future aims. R Coll Phys Lond. 1992;26:41–3.
10. Dequeker J, Esselens G, Westhovens R. Educational issues in rheumatology. The musculoskeletal examination: a neglected skill. Clin Rheumatol. 2007;26(1):5–7.
11. Sirisena D, Begum H, Selvarajah M, Chakravarty K. Musculoskeletal examination–an ignored aspect. Why are we still failing the patients? Clin Rheumatol. 2011;30(3):403–7.
12. Jordan KP, Kadam UT, Hayward R, Porcheret M, Young C, Croft P. Annual consultation prevalence of regional musculoskeletal problems in primary care: an observational study. BMC Musculoskelet Disord. 2010;11:144.
13. Dacre J, Griffith S, Jolly B. Rheumatology and medical education in Great Britain. Br J Rheumatol. 1996;35:269–74.
14. Bjcllc A. European medicine. Training. Br J Rheumatol. 1993;32(suppl. 4):14–7.
15. The state of medical education and practice in the UK. General medical council 2011. https://www.gmc-uk.org/State_of_medicine_Final_web.pdf_44213427.pdf.
16. Yoong J, Lui NA. Educating future learners of rheumatology. Proc Singap Healthc. 2013;22(1):15–20.
17. Hart J. Understanding today's learner. Learning solutions magazine. 2008. Cited 2012 Nov 22. Available at http://www.learningsolutionsmag.com/articles/80/understanding-todays-learner.
18. Asthana A. They don't live for work, they work to live. The Observer. 2008. Cited 2018 March 1st. Available at http://www.guardian.co.uk/money/2008/may/25/workandcareers.worklifebalance.
19. Day C. Change agendas: the roles of teacher educators. Teach Educ. 2004;15(2):145–58.
20. Haranath P. Integrated teaching in medicine – Indian scene. Indian J Pharmacol. 2013;45(1):1–3.
21. Vygotsky LS. Mind in society: the development of higher psychological processes. Cambridge, MA: Harvard University Press; 1978. p. 79–81.
22. Knowles M. The adult learner: a neglected species. Houston: Gulf; 1988.
23. Mezirow JE. Transformative learning: theory to practice. In: Welton MR, editor. In defense of the lifeworld. New York: Suny Press; 1995. p. 36–70.
24. Janaka das BVG. Comparison between transformative and informative learning methods. 2011. https://bhls.wordpress.com/2011/06/17/comparison-between-transformative-and-informative-learning-methods/.
25. Kolb D. Experiential learning. Englewood Cliffs: Prentice-Hall; 1984.
26. Coffield F, Moseley D, Hall E, Ecclestone K. Learning styles and pedagogy in post-16 learning: a systematic and critical review. London: The Learning and Skills Research Centre; 2004.

27. Kay LJ, Deighton CM, Walker DJ, Hay EM. Undergraduate rheumatology teaching in the UK: a survey of current practice and changes since 1990. Rheumatology (Oxford). 2000;39:800–3.
28. Dacre JE, Fox RA. How should we be teaching our undergraduates. Ann Rheum Dis. 2000;59:662–7.
29. Spencer JA, Jordan RK. Learner centred approaches in medical education. BMJ. 1999;318:1280–3.
30. Newble D, Cannon R. A handbook for medical teachers, vol. 1994. Boston: Kluwer Academic Publishers; 1994. p. 38–53.
31. General Medical Council Education Committee. Tomorrow's doctors. Recommendations on undergraduate medical education London, UK. General Medical Council, 2009. https://www.gmc-uk.org/7___Tomorrow_s_Doctors_Project_Evaluation.pdf_29622932.pdf.
32. Dolmans D, Schmidt. The advantages of problem based curricula. Postgrad Med. 1996;72:535–8.
33. Finucane PM, Johnson SM, Prideaux DJ. Problem based learning: its rationale and efficacy. Med J Aust. 1998;168:445–8.
34. Wilson AS, Goodall JE. Development of an interactive learning tool for teaching rheumatology: a simulated clinical case studies program. Rheumatology. 2006;45:1158–61.
35. Challis M, Mathers NJ, Howe AC, Feild NJ. Portfolio based learning: continuing medical education for general practitioners-a mid-point evaluation. Med Educ. 1997;31:22–6.
36. Dacre J, Nicol M, Holroyd D, Ingram. The development of a clinical skills centre. J R Coll Physicians Lond. 1996;30:318–24.
37. McCrea JD, McCredie MR, McSherry DM, Brooks PM. A controlled evaluation of diagnostic criteria in the development of a rheumatology expert system, Br J. Rheumatology. 1989;28:13–7.
38. Armstrong R. Interactive rheumatology tutor CD rom. Port Chester: Cambridge University Press; 1997. ISBN 0521629144
39. Newble DI, Jaegger K. The effect of assessments and examinations on the learning of medical students. Med Educ. 1983;17:165–71.
40. Frank J, Snell LS, Ten Cate O. Competency-based medical education: theory to practice. Med Teach. 2010;32:638e45.
41. Leung W. Competency based medical training: review. BMJ. 2002;325:693–6.
42. Rasker JJ. Rheumatology in general practice. British J Rheumatol. 1995;34:494–7.
43. De Lorenzo RA, Mayer D, Geehr EC. Analysing clinical case distributions to improve an emergency medicine clerkship. Ann Emerg Med. 1990;19:746–51.
44. Ahern MJ, Soden M, Schultz D, Clark M. The musculo-skeletal examination: a neglected clinical skill. Aust NZ J Med. 1991;21:303–6.
45. Craton N, Matheson GO. Training and clinical competency in musculoskeletal medicine. Identifying the problem. Sports Med. 1993;15:328–37.
46. Booth A, Wise DI. General practice training in musculoskeletal disorders. Br J Gen Pract. 1990;40:390.
47. Lanyon P, Pope D, Croft P. Rheumatology education and management skills in general practice: a national study of trainees. Ann Rheum Dis. 1995;54:735–9.
48. Crawley HS, Levin JB. Training for general practice: a national survey. BMJ. 1990;300:911–5.
49. Matheny JM, Brinker MR, Elliott MN, Blake R, Rowane MP. Confidence of graduating family practice residents in their management of musculoskeletal conditions. Am J Orthop. 2000;29:945–52.
50. Saywell RM Jr, O'Hara BS, Zollinger TW, Wooldridge JS, Burba JL, McKeag DB. Medical students' experience with musculoskeletal diagnoses in a family medicine clerkship. Med Teach. 2002;24:186–92.
51. Kay LJ, Deighton CM, Walker DJ, Hay EM. Undergraduate rheumatology teaching in the UK: a survey of current practice and changes since 1990. Arthritis research campaign undergraduate working party of the ARC education sub-committee. Rheumatology. 2000;39:800–3.

52. Bellamy N, Goldstein LD, Tekanoff RA. Continuing medical education driven skills acquisition and impact on improved patient outcomes in family practice setting. J Contin Educ Health Prof. 2000;20:52–61.
53. Woolf AD. Specialist training in rheumatology in Europe. Rheumatology (Oxford). 2002;41:1062–6.
54. Aletaha D, Neogi T, Silman AJ, et al. 2010 rheumatoid arthritis classification criteria: an American college of rheumatology/European league against rheumatism collaborative initiative. Rheumatic. 2010;62:2569–81.
55. van der Heijde D, Ramiro S, Landewé R, et al. 2016 update of the ASAS-EULAR management recommendations for axial spondyloarthritis. Ann Rheum Dis Published Online First. 2017; https://doi.org/10.1136/annrheumdis-2016-210770.
56. Smolen JS, Breedveld FC, Burmester GR, et al. Treating rheumatoid arthritis to target: 2014 update of the recommendations of an international task force. Ann Rheum Dis Published Online First. 2015; https://doi.org/10.1136/annrheumdis-2015-207524.
57. El Miedany Y. Psoriatic arthritis comorbidity index: development and validation of a new specific tool for classifying prognostic comorbidity in psoriasis and psoriatic arthritis patients. Rheumatol Orthop Med. 2017;2:1. https://doi.org/10.15761/ROM.1000117.
58. Miedany YEI, Gaafary EIM, Youssef S, Almedany S, Bahlas S, et al. Rheumatoid arthritis comorbidity index (RACI): development and validation of a new comorbidity index for rheumatoid arthritis atients. J Arthritis. 2017;6:244. https://doi.org/10.4172/2167-7921.1000244.
59. Continuing professional development. Guidance for all doctors. General Medical Council. 2012. https://www.gmc-uk.org/Continuing_professional_development___guidance_for_all_doctors_0316.pdf_56438625.pdf.
60. Heffron M, Simpson D, Kochar MS. Competency-based physician education, recertification, and licensure. Wis Med J. 2007;106:215e8.
61. Riley B, Riley G. Innovation in graduate medical education e using a competency based medical education curriculum. Int J Osteopath Med. 2017;23:36–41.
62. Clouder DL. Technology-enhanced learning: conquering barriers to interprofessional education. Clin Teach. 2008;5(4):198–202.
63. Moulton C-A, Dubrowski A, MacRae H, Graham B, Grober E, Reznick R. Teaching technical skills: what kind of practice makes perfect?: a randomized controlled trial. Ann Surg. 2006;44:400–9.
64. Pashler H, Rohrer D, Cepeda NJ, Carpenter SK. Enhancing learning and retarding forgetting: choices and consequences. Psychon Bull Rev. [Research Support, U.S. Gov't, Non-P.H.S. 2007;14(2):187–93.
65. Sebajang H, Trudeau P, Dougall A, Hegge S, McKinley C, Anvari M. The role of telementoring and telerobotic assistance in the provision of laparoscopic colorectal surgery in rural areas. Surg Endosc. 2006;20(9):1389–93.
66. Panait L, Rafiq A, Tomulescu V, Boanca C, Popescu I, Carbonell A, et al. Telementoring versus on-site mentoring in virtual reality-based surgical training. Surg Endosc. 2006;20(1):113–8.
67. Sebajang H, Trudeau P, Dougall A, Hegge S, McKinley C, Anvari M. Telementoring: an important enabling tool for the community surgeon. Surg Innov. 2005;12(4):327–31.
68. Choy I, Okrainec A. Simulation in surgery: perfecting the practice. Surg Clin North Am. 2010;90(3):457–73.
69. Okrainec A, Henao O, Azzie G. Telesimulation: an effective method for teaching the fundamentals of laparoscopic surgery in resource-restricted countries. Surg Endosc. 2010;24(2):417–22.
70. Scott DJ, Dunnington GL. The new ACS/APDS skills curriculum: moving the learning curve out of the operating room. J Gastrointest Surg. 2008;12:213–21.
71. Grantcharov TP, Reznick RK. Training tomorrow's surgeons: what are we looking for and how can we achieve it? ANZ J Surg. 2009;79:104–7.
72. What is the European Working Time Directive? : Department of Health; 2009. [Cited 2009 September 15, 2009]; Available from: http://www.dh.gov.uk/en/Managingyourorganisation/Humanresourcesandtraining/Modernisingworkforceplanninghome/Europeanworkingtimedirective/DH_077304.

73. Tempelhof MW. Personal digital assistants: a review of current and potential utilization among medical residents. Teach Learn Med. 2009;21(2):100–4.
74. Mazloomdoost D, Embi PJ. Impacts of PDA-based access to clinical data in a teaching hospital: perceptions of housestaff physicians. AMIA Annu Symp Proc. 2006;1025
75. Briscoe GW, Fore Arcand LG, Lin T, Johnson J, Rai A, Kollins K. Students' and residents' perceptions regarding technology in medical training. Acad Psychiatry. 2006;30(6):470–9.
76. Bero LA, Grilli R, Grimshaw JM, Harvey E, Oxman AD, Thomson MA. Closing the gap between research and practice: an overview of systematic reviews of interventions to promote the implementation of research findings. The cochrane effective practice and organization of care review group. BMJ .[Review. 1998;317(7156):465–8.
77. Barwick MA, Boydell KM, Strasiulis E, Ferguson HB, Blase K, Fixsen D. Knowledge transfer and evidence-based practice in children's mental health. Toronto: Children's Mental Health Ontario; 2005.
78. Crelinsten GL. The intern's palmomental reflex. N Engl J Med. 2004;350(10):1059.
79. McGaghie WC, Issenberg SB, Petrusa ER, Scalese RJ. A critical review of simulation-based medical education research: 2003–2009. Med Educ. [Research Support, Non-U.S. Gov't Review. 2010;44(1):50–63.
80. Gallagher AG, Ritter EM, Champion H, Higgins G, Fried MP, Moses G, et al. Virtual reality simulation for the operating room: proficiency-based training as a paradigm shift in surgical skills training. Ann Surg. 2005;241(2):364–72.

Part IV
Innovations in Medical Education

Chapter 12
Reflective Learning, Reflective Teaching

Introduction

Reflection is about students becoming aware of their own thinking processes and being able to make those transparent to others. It enables assessment of the "why" and "how" of the learning, and what needs to be done as a result. Reflection readily follows on from self or peer assessment. When students become reflective about the teaching and learning process, they are strengthening their own capacity to learn. Central to this is the principal of reflection as metacognition (awareness and understanding of one's own thought processes), where students are aware of and can describe their thinking in a way that allows them to "close the gap" between what they know and what they need to learn. Therefore, reflective learners assimilate new learning, relate it to what they already know, adapt it for their own purposes and translate thought into action. Over time, they develop their creativity, their ability to think critically about information and ideas and their metacognitive ability (i.e. their ability to think about their own thinking) [1].

Reflective practice is not a new concept. More than 30 years ago, Boud et al. [2] state that it features the individual and his or her experiences, leading to a new conceptual perspective or understanding. Their definition of reflective practice as "Reflection is a forum of response of the learner to experience" has been based on both the element of learning, as well as involvement of the self. Johns and Freshwater [3] also describe the value of reflective practice as a means of learning. There is no doubt that "reflection" is a complex concept that has defied consensus on definition although some commonalities exist. It involves the self and is triggered by questioning of actions, values and beliefs. An understanding of the purpose of reflective practice and its components can also be gained by considering some of the definitions provided in the literature. A few useful definitions include the following: "Reflection is a process of reviewing an experience of practice in order to describe, analyse, evaluate and so inform learning about practice" [4].

Y. El Miedany, *Rheumatology Teaching*,
https://doi.org/10.1007/978-3-319-98213-7_12

"Reflective practice is something more than thoughtful practice. It is that form of practice that seeks to problematise many situations of professional performance so that they can become potential learning situations and so the practitioners can continue to learn, grow and develop in and through practice" [5]. In reflective thought, a person examines underlying assumptions, core beliefs and knowledge, while drawing connections between apparently disparate pieces of information. Brain science, popularized in Daniel Kahneman's book, has shown that this type of "slow thinking" is negatively correlated with "fast thinking", which might be employed when driving a car or solving a simple sum. In other words, reflective thinking (slow and deliberative) and reactive thinking (fast and instinctual) effectively exist at opposite ends of a switch. When one is "on", the other is "off". This chapter will discuss the art and science of reflection, characters of reflective learning, reflecting on one's own practice, reflective teaching and how to become a reflective learner.

The Forgotten Role of Reflection

The standard teaching style is based mainly on the "passive learning" method. This involves reading textbooks and journal review articles, listening to lectures and answering exams questions dependent on rote memory. However, in the learning process, some situations may arise on daily bases where, frequently, there are unanswered queries, reaching a status of no right or wrong answers, no procedures or clear pathways to follow and no time or opportunity to consult with supervising staff or colleagues. Perhaps, this could be one of the reasons why students adopt surface, rather than deep, approaches to learning. Also, this might explain the shift in the students target from appropriate learning into just study to pass the exam, regardless of the content and understanding. In the core of this "passive learning" teaching style stands the teacher whose role is central being the only active part of the band. In that way teachers are more like farmers than anything else; their job is to properly prepare the ground, plant ideas at the right time and with the right spacing from each other and then nurture, troubleshoot and supplement as the tiny tendrils of understanding slowly turn into solid stalks rich with the fruit of knowledge [6]. However, do all the implanted trees grow look alike? Though this might be the farmer's expectations, definitely this is not the case in real-life scenarios. This is similar to the teacher's role in the standard teaching pattern. For example, when students do an assignment, the person who reflects on it the most in a lot of classrooms is the teacher, not the student. That is a problem, as in view of this fact; it is only one person reflecting, who is the teacher; and therefore the outcomes of the students' tasks will be similar without any differences. This in turn will kill the creativity and inspiration among the students. On the other hand, it is the student, not the teacher, who needs to learn the lessons; here comes the role of reflection which has been missed for long time.

Over the past decade, there has been growing interest in this forgotten role of reflection, its concept, theory, forms as well as its role in developing the learning process. The core argument is that reflection is a practice that facilitates the exploration, examination and understanding of what the learners are thinking, feeling and learning. It is a thoughtful consideration of academic material, personal experiences and interpersonal relationships. Reflection is a form of internal inquiry that extends the relevance of theory and deepens the learners' understanding of the practice of their day-to-day practice as well as work. Therefore, it emerged that reflection is an incredibly potent learning tool and students at the very least should be reflecting as much as the teachers concerning their learnt topics, given tasks and probably a whole lot more in an ideal world.

Through reflection the learners can challenge their assumptions, ask innovative questions and try to make sense of their experiences. Instead of being passive receivers of external expert knowledge, the learners become active creators (and cocreators) of their own knowledge. As reflective learners, the informal theories (developed through their practices) are tested against the formal theories (developed by researchers and academics). Thus, the theory and practice are integrated. This can be achieved through either a process of reflection-on-action, i.e. trying to make sense of experience after the fact, or reflection-in-action, i.e. trying to make sense of experience while it is occurring [7].

The Science of Reflection

The term "reflective practice" derives from the work of Dewey [8] and Schon [9]. Dewey [8] writes that reflective practice refers to "the active, persistent and careful consideration of any belief or supposed form of knowledge in the light of the grounds that support it". This means that a person may have a questioning approach; he/she will consider why things are as they are, and how they might be. Dewey goes on to say that being reflective "enables us to direct our actions with foresight … It enables us to know what we are about when we act". This is extremely important in teaching. What the teachers do in the classroom and how they behave should have been carefully planned and informed by theory and experience and be purposeful.

Schon [10] presents a slightly different view. He regarded reflection as having two aspects: reflection-in-action and reflection-on-action. Reflection-in-action refers to the quick thinking and reaction that occur as things are being done, for example, in the classroom while teaching a topic which the teacher can see the pupils are not understanding well. The reflection-in-action allows the teacher to see this, consider why it is happening and respond by doing it differently. This could involve reframing the explanation given by the teacher or approaching the topic from a different perspective.

Reflection-on-action is what occurs outside the classroom when the situation is reconsidered; deep thinking about why the students did not understand, what caused the situation, what were the available options, why certain option was chosen and not another. The responses are usually linked to the person's knowledge and experience levels, as well as the person's understanding of theories and values.

Kolb and Fry [11] look at the constituent parts of reflection and from these created a learning cycle framework. Kolb [12] identifies four parts to the learning cycle. To make Kolb's model (Fig. 12.1a) more understandable, Pedler et al. [13] simplify the terminology. Both models are shown in Fig. 12.1b.

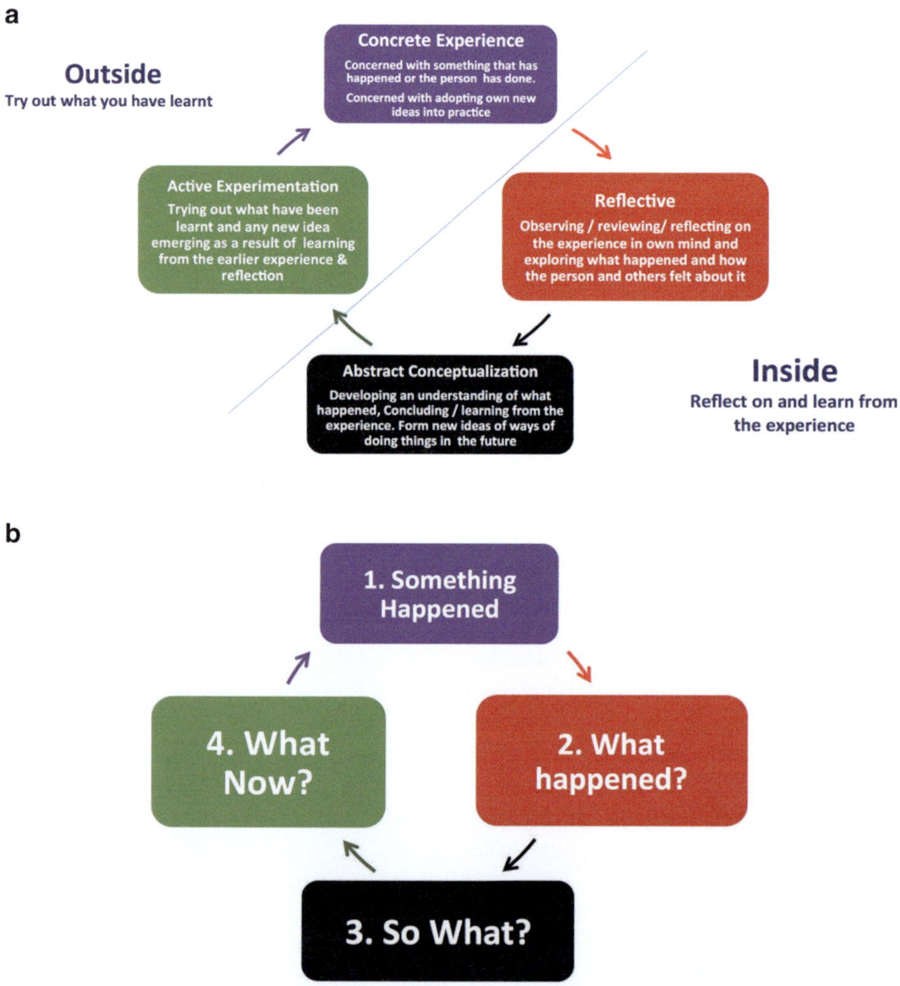

Fig. 12.1 Kolb cycle. (**a**) Following the cycle in a clockwise direction with the student, after having had an experience, the candidate should reflect on what has been experienced or done, by reviewing the whole situation in own mind. This can be assisted by looking at it, discussing it with others, thinking abstractly about the event for a while and seeking advice or further information. Eventually the scholar will possibly come up with ideas or suggestions for approaching the situation differently next time. The student will then try out these ideas to see whether they are effective. The learner will thus complete the learning cycle and start over again with a view to refining own actions. This is an ongoing process, so we will never achieve perfection. Always there will be other ways of doing things based on our learning from previous experiences. To make Kolb's model (**a**) more understandable, Pedler et al. [13] simplify the terminology (**b**)

In his proposal, Kolb [12] highlights an important point. Individuals tend to have a preference for carrying out one part of the learning cycle over the others, for example, theorizing in the "abstract conceptualization" or the "so what" in Pedler's model [13]. In many cases this is not problematic, so long as a level of skill is maintained in the other areas. However, if an individual develops a very strong preference for one part of the cycle, then they may neglect and become deskilled in the other areas. This can cause the subsequent learning to become skewed and unbalanced. Therefore, maintaining a level of competence in all parts of the learning cycle is essential to ensure comprehensive learning. The "experiential learning" model published by Kolb [14] is based directly on Kolb's experiential learning cycle where active experimentation leads to a transfer of learning from current cycle to a new cycle. There are four main components to the cycle, and the individual can enter the model at any one of these points (Fig. 12.2). Table 12.1 summarizes the four components of the cycle.

In 1988, Professor Graham Gibbs proposed reflective cycle (Fig. 12.3) which appears in learning by doing [15, 16]. Gibbs' model is developed from the earlier theoretical Kolb's four-stage experiential learning model. Whereas Kolb's model is sometimes referred to as an experiential learning model (which simply means learning through experience), Gibbs' model is sometimes referred to as an iterative model (which simply means learning through repetition). The version of Gibbs' model given to students may be slightly adapted, such as the one that appears in Bulman and Schultz [17].

Gibbs' model is composed of six stages (Table 12.2); these include:

1. Description. In this section, the person needs to explain what he/she is reflecting on to the reader. This should include background information, such as what it is being reflected upon, and who was involved. The information provided should be relevant and to the point. Waffle on about unrequired details should be avoided.

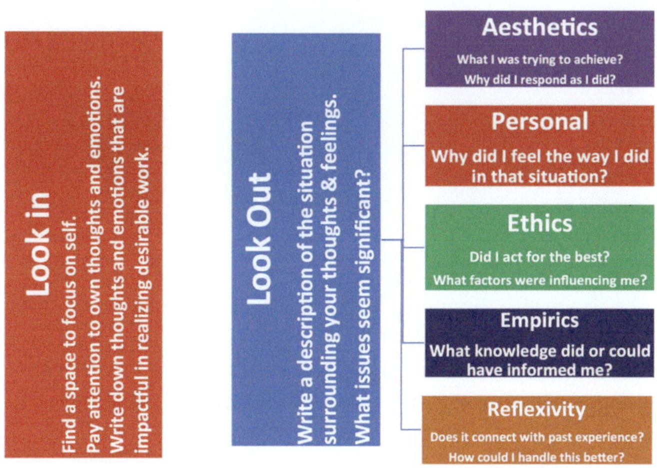

Fig. 12.2 Maughan and Webb structure for production of reflective writing

Table 12.1 The four components of Kolb's reflective cycle

Concrete experience	Reflective observation	Abstract conceptualization	Active experimentation
This relates to the incident or event prompting the reflection and involves the physical act of being involved in or having hands-on experience. Although in theory you can enter the model at any stage, this tends to be the main point of entry	After the event comes the initial reflection. This entails stepping back and viewing the event or incident from an objective perspective. This should provide some insight into what you did and why you did it	These initial reflections are then explored in greater detail. Conceptualization involves interpreting events and actions, looking for connections between these and the process of applying some theoretical premise to make understand events	Once this deeper understanding has been established, the individual translates it into predictions about what is likely to happen next or what actions should be taken to refine the way similar events may be handled in the future

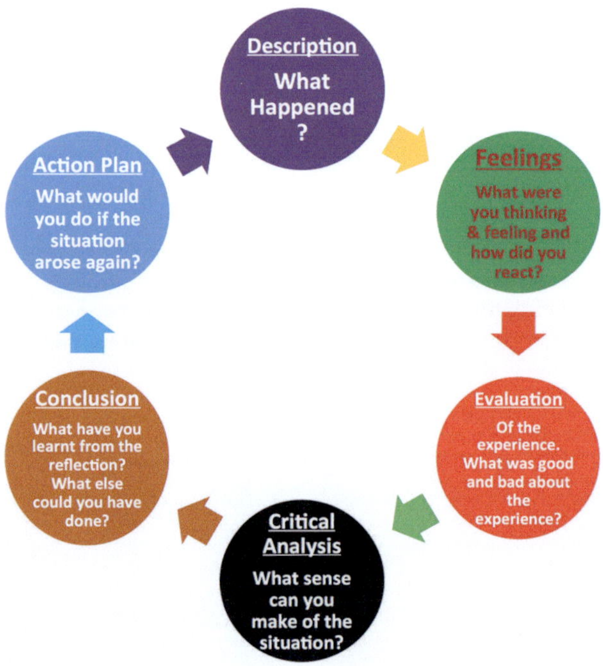

Fig. 12.3 Gibbs reflective model (1998)

2. Feelings. Feelings and thoughts about the experience should be discussed at this stage. This involves how the person felt at that time, what did he/she think of at the time and what was the feeling and thoughts about the incident afterwards. Emotions can be discussed honestly, but within the academic frame, hence, chatty texts should be avoided.
3. Evaluation. This includes how well things went, what was the reaction to the situation, how did other people react, what was good and what was bad regarding

Table 12.2 Gibb's cycle

Description	Feelings	Evaluation	Analysis	Conclusion and action plan
When and where did the situation take place?	What were your feelings before this situation?	What went well/ was positive? Why?	What assumptions are you making?	What will you do differently?
Why were you there?	What were your feelings at the time?	What did not go so well/was less positive? Why?	What insights are now available to you?	What skills do you need to develop to achieve this?
Who else was there?	What were your feelings afterwards?	What was your contribution?		Who and what will support your development in this area?
What happened?	What do you think the others in the situation were feeling?	What was the contribution of others?		
What did you do?				
What you didn't do?				
What did they do?				
What they didn't do?				
What happened?				

the experience, how did other people react, was the situation resolved afterwards and why/why not. It is important to include references in reflective writing.

4. Analysis. This should include analysis of what might have helped or hindered the event. There is a good opportunity to compare the current experience with similar experiences reported in the literature. This section is very important, particularly for higher-level writing. Many students receive poor marks for reflective assignments for not bringing the theory and experience together.
5. Conclusion. In this section it is important to acknowledge whether anything else could have been done, what was learnt from the experience and was it possible to respond in a different way. If a positive experience is being discussed, would the person do the same again to ensure a positive outcome, or would changing anything might help to improve things even further? If the incident was negative, how could it have been avoided and how to avoid it from recurring?
6. Action plan. This should sum up anything needed to be known and done to improve for next time. Perhaps learning about something or attending some training could be of help. Could some advice be sought from the tutor or supervisor? How to cope with similar events in the future? [18]

In theory, Gibb's reflective process follows the six steps of the model so that each step informs the next. In practice, students often confuse the evaluation, analysis and conclusion stages. These parts seem to ask similar questions and as a result, there can be a lot of repetition. Analytical writing is only required in the analysis stage. The other five steps are made up of statements of description, statements of value (whether something was good or bad), statements of summation or statements of justification (why something was done).

The aims of using Gibbs' reflective cycle include (1) to challenge your assumptions, (2) to explore different/new ideas and approaches towards doing or thinking about things, (3) to promote self-improvement (by identifying strengths and weaknesses and taking action to address them) and (4) to link practice and theory (by combining doing or observing with thinking or applying knowledge).

A model for structured reflection was proposed in the year 2000 by Johns [19]. This model focuses on uncovering and making explicit the knowledge that is used in the standard teaching practice. It can be used as a guide for analysis of a critical incident or general reflection on experience or more complex decision-making. In the model, the author suggests that in addition to guided reflection, students should use a reflective diary since noting, reflecting on and sharing such experiences can lead to greater understanding than by reflection as a lone exercise. The model involves "looking in on the situation", which includes focusing on the person, targeting the person's thoughts and emotions. It then advises "looking out of the situation" and writing a description of the situation based on five sources of knowledge, each of which has a number of cues (Fig. 12.2).

Reflective writing is an evidence of reflective thinking. In an academic context, reflective thinking usually involves (1) looking back at something (often an event, i.e. something that happened, but could also be an idea or object), (2) analysing the event or idea (thinking in depth and from different perspectives, and trying to explain, often with reference to a model or theory from your subject) and (3) thinking carefully about what the event or idea means for you and your ongoing progress as a learner and/or practising professional. Therefore, reflective writing is more personal than other kinds of academic writing. It also involves writing in the first person rather than the traditional third person associated with academic writing, which can initially be a challenge. Although we may engage in basic reflection on a daily basis, reflective writing requires the individual to go deeper and to analyse the rationale and consequences of their actions and to learn from the experience.

In 2001, a new reflective model for reflective writing has been proposed by Rolfe [20], which is based upon three simple questions: What? So what? Now what? (Fig. 12.4). Table 12.3 shows a list of questions that you may choose to answer in response to the three elements. The model starts by introducing the problem meant to be reflected upon, before making any observations about the issue, and finally concluding by telling the reader what they would change next time. Therefore, "What?" should include a briefing of the specific tasks shared out either individually or among the team members (the tasks may not be seen as equally difficult by all team members); "So what?" entails reflection on what this experience tells the person and the personal views about it; "Now what?" deals with the suggestions for the next steps to maintain the development or improve the outcomes.

Another structure for reflective writing was suggested by Maughan and Webb in 2001 [21], in which they state that while reflective thinking and writing can be an unstructured process, the individual is commonly required to demonstrate some editorial skills in the presentation and structure of the final diary/journal. As a result, they propose a three-part structure to produce reflective writing: description, interpretation and outcome (Fig. 12.5).

More recently, a new model of reflection in clinical practice has been developed by Nick Butcher and Andy Whysall through their work as trainers in their company Sherwood Training [22]. The "REFLECT model" (Fig. 12.6) is composed of seven

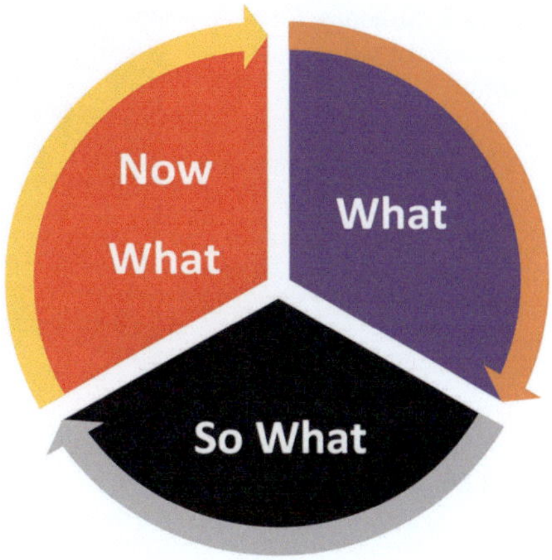

Fig. 12.4 Rolfe et al.'s [20] reflective model

Table 12.3 Rolfe et al., model of critical reflection

What	So what	Now what
Is the problem/difficulty/reason for being stuck/reason for feeling bad/reason we don't get on?	Does this tell me/teach me/imply/mean about me/my class/others/our relationship/my patient's care/the model of care I am using/my attitudes/my patient's attitudes?	Do I need to do in order to make things better/stop being stuck/improve my teaching/resolve the situation/feel better/get on better/etc., etc.?
Was my role in the situation?	Was going through my mind as I acted?	Broader issues need to be considered if this action is to be successful?
Was I trying to achieve?	Did I base my actions on?	Might be the consequences of this action?
Actions did I take?	Other knowledge can I bring to the situation?	
Was the response of others?	Could/should I have done to make it better?	
Were the consequences for the student? Myself? Others?	Is my new understanding of the situation?	
Feelings did it evoke in the student? Myself? Others?	Broader issues arise from the situation?	
Was good/bad about the experience?		

stages and aims at ensuring that a thorough reflective learning cycle takes place, while the mnemonic makes it extremely easy to understand and remember. The main concept is that the model can be used from memory, making it more useful in the practice setting than those requiring textbooks (Table 12.4).

In conclusion, while using a reflecting model can help users focus on learning and self-awareness after an incident and avoid simply retelling the events, there are several reflection models available. The challenge is that many of these models consist of similar stages. Choosing which model to use often is based on personal preferences. However, some of these reflection models are oversimplified and do not address all the relevant issues (they allow users to approach the process in a

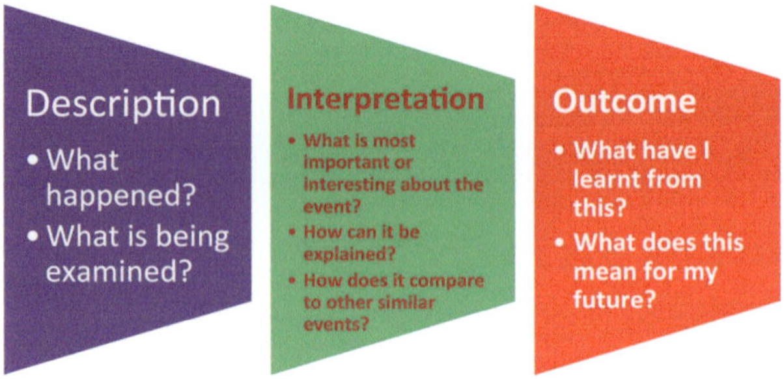

Fig. 12.5 Structure for production of reflective writing

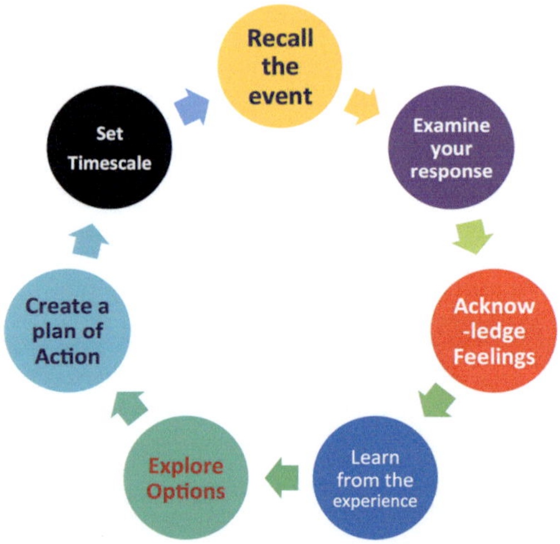

Fig. 12.6 REFLECT

Table 12.4 The seven stages of the REFLECT model

R	E	F	L	E	C	T
Recall the event	Examine your responses	Acknowledge feelings	Learn from the experience	Explore options	Create a plan of action	Set timescale
Stage 1:	Stage 2	Stage 3	Stage 4	Stage 5	Stage 6	Stage 7
Give a brief overview of the situation upon which you are reflecting. This should consist of the facts – a description of what happened	Discuss your thoughts and actions at the time of the incident upon which you are reflecting	Highlight any feelings you experienced at the time of the situation upon which you are reflecting	Highlight what you have learned from the situation	Discuss options for the future if you were to encounter a similar situation	Create a plan for the future – this can be for future theoretical learning or action	Set a time by which the plan outlined in stage 6 will be complete

superficial way), while others are overly complex, more structured and prescriptive and difficult to remember without a textbook in hand [23]. In general, in standard practice, it is advisable to use models that are easy to remember and do not require the use of a textbook to implement. Furthermore, while reflection is by definition about looking back, a forward-looking step is fundamental to make its use worthwhile to encourage learning.

Characters of Reflective Learning

Types of Reflection

Earlier studies identified two main types of reflection, namely, dialogic and critical reflection. Hatton and Smith [24] distinguish between both types and the engagement level associated with each one of them. "Dialogic reflection" refers to a less intensive approach that involves "discourse with the self" to explore a given event or incident. It involves considering the decisions and judgements made and possible reasons for these. An example of dialogic reflection is the basic model proposed by Brockbank and McGill [25] (Fig. 12.7). The individual thinks about what they are going to learn in their lecture, about the information they would like to convey, the methods they intend to use, the level of engagement and so on, in advance of the

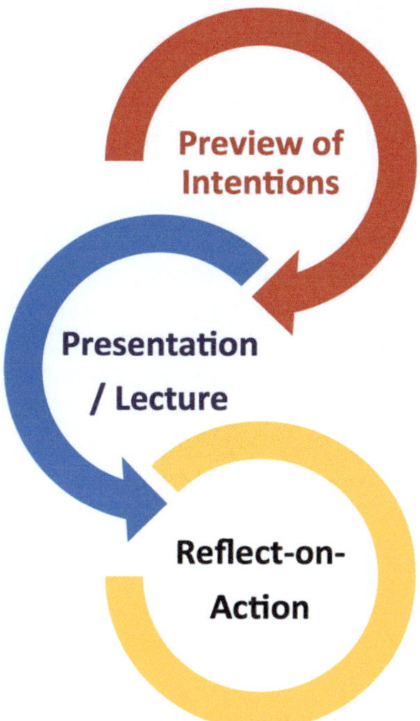

Fig. 12.7 Dialogic reflection: the individual thinks about what they are going to learn in their lecture, about the information they would like to convey, the methods they intend to use, the level of engagement and so on, in advance of the delivery of the class. Afterwards they then consider how well they achieved their intended goals and which aspects require further attention

delivery of the class. Afterwards they then consider how well they achieved their intended goals and which aspects require further attention. As with all forms of reflection, this approach is couched in constructivism and requires the individual to re-evaluate their own personal view of education, teaching and learning. While this is an important first step and may lead to increased confidence or sense of pride, awareness alone doesn't necessarily result in an improvement of the situation [26].

"Critical reflection" refers to efforts to accounting for the broader historic, cultural and political values in framing practical problems to arrive at a solution [22]. This process has been described as Boyd and Fales [27] as "... the core difference between whether a person repeats the same experience several times becoming highly proficient at one behaviour or learns from experience in such a way that he or she is cognitively or affectively changed". Critical reflection facilitates transformational learning that can happen either gradually or from a sudden or critical incident and alter the way people see themselves and their world [28].

Methods of Reflection

Action Research

Reflective practice can be more formally encouraged and directed as action research [28]. Action research involves systematically changing your teaching using "on the ground" evidence that suggests the changes you make are in the right direction and enhancing student learning. The target of action research is the teacher, not the change that's being implemented.

Transformative Reflection

In action research the term "reflection" has been considered as misleading. Brockbank and McGill [25] suggest that teaching is being altered as a result of the reflection and is deemed more accurate (Fig. 12.8). Engaging in action research to improve teaching practice, however, involves a more explicit theory of teaching [29]. While many teachers have an implicit theory of teaching, there is a need for a more consciously worked-out theory that generates answers to teaching problems. This helps to rephrase the unhelpful and not very useful "there is something wrong with my teaching" to the more manageable and approachable "students are only regurgitating what I gave to them in class". The latter also brings it back to the teaching, not the students, and allows the problem to be framed in a way that can be addressed by the teacher [25, 28, 30].

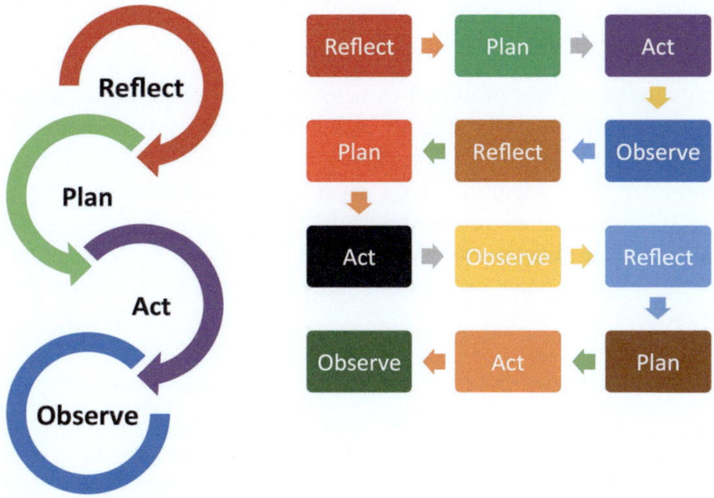

Fig. 12.8 Action reflection: is an approach to improve your own teaching practice. It starts with identifying a problem in the teaching practice (e.g. students do not spend enough effort in reviewing course materials; or difficulty in learning a particular topic in the course). Faced with the problem, the action researcher will go through a series of phases (reflect, plan, action, observe) called the action research cycle to systematically tackle the problem. In practice, things rarely go perfectly according to plan first time round. Usually new ways can be identified to improve the action plan in light of the teacher's experience and feedback from the students. One cycle of planning, acting, observing and reflecting therefore usually leads to another, in which you incorporate improvements suggested by the initial cycle. In such transformative reflection, projects often do not fit neatly into a cycle of planning, action, observation and reflection. It is perfectly legitimate to follow a somewhat disjointed process whenever appropriate or necessary

Guided Reflection

To help progress reflection from dialogic to critical, Johns [19] developed the concept of guided reflection. This involves engaging with a series of questions that help you to explore and reconsider your motivation or rationale for your actions. These can be designed by a third party or by the individual themselves and serve as a guide through the reflection process. Questions can include: What was I trying to achieve?, Why did I do [activity] as I did?, What were the consequences of [activity]?, etc. This can be designed to form a reflective diary, with one side of the page consisting of the descriptive material and the other consisting of the reflection and exploration [25] (Table 12.5).

Frameworks

Several models have been proposed to help promote reflection on teaching; they were discussed earlier in this chapter under the science of reflection. Each tool advocates using some questions to reflect on a situation. Table 12.6 shows a summary of the main items identified in the most famous reflection models. In the first level, they all start with the individual reflecting on the situation. This is followed by different approaches to the establishment of an action plan (reflect-on-action). It is up to the reader to use whichever model he/she feels happy to use for reflection in standard practice.

Table 12.5 The main characteristics of the performance and development review

Aims	Benefits for the person	Benefits for the organization
Review the past year, identifying successes and problems	A formal opportunity to review progress and plan for future activity and development	Improved communications between the professional service and the individual
Plan for the future, taking into consideration the objectives of the professional service or organization	An exchange of experience and feedback at both personal and professional levels	Identification and pursuit of common goals and alignment of individual career goals to the professional service and university strategies
Identify learning and development opportunities	Clarification of roles and responsibilities	
Have ongoing, continuous conversations	Opportunity to suggest improvements and changes	Better planning for learning and development for the individual, as well as professional service
Understand how individual person can contribute to the place of work objectives	A formal record of experience and learning over time	

Table 12.6 Examples of guided reflection

Incident	Reflect on a critical incident in your teaching – a situation in which you thought that your teaching or assessment had not gone quite how you would have liked it to have gone	
Questions	a. What is the most important/interesting/useful/ relevant about the object, event or idea?	a. What was the problem? What went wrong? What was the evidence for the problem?
	b. How can it be explained (e.g. with theory?)	b. What was (were) the cause (s) of the problem?
	c. How is it similar to and different from other issues events?	c. How did you deal with the problem then?
	d. What have I learned from this?	d. How did your solution to the problem relate to your theory of teaching and learning?
	e. What does this mean for my future situations?	
Author	Maughan and Webb [18]	Biggs and Tang [27]

Reflecting on Your Practice: How to Identify Your Learning and Development Needs

The key point is that reflection involves thinking about personal practice to identify learning and development needs. This is applicable to both the employee as well as employer. Everyone should be aware of how to reflect on the quality of the person's own practice in order to identify the learning and development needs. Similarly, employers may also need to understand the learning and development needs of their own employees as this may help them deliver their service and meet the objectives. While it is important to devote sometime that is appropriate for reflection, it is also essential for every person to record the identified learning and development needs.

What Do We Mean by Reflection on Practice?

Perhaps this is the first question that needs to be clear in the person's mind before starting the reflection process. Reflection means creating opportunities to step back from oneself practice considering (1) how the person thinks he/she is performing, (2) what has been learnt from the experience and (3) what can be done differently in the future.

Reflection can be done either at a "transactional" level (i.e. reflecting on the work that is being currently done or has recently been completed) or at a more general level (e.g. considering the work generally or a particular type of job being done often). Reflection includes both things identified happening or happened during work which the person considers as have been done well (and which demonstrates the person's ongoing competence as a healthcare professional or any other profession) and things which could have been done better and which, upon reflection, the matter can be done better next time or you may not be sure and need some external help about how to handle better next time.

This approach is applicable to all types of skills whether technical, soft or knowledge. As healthcare professionals, to help thinking about own practice, the person should think about own profession, asking the following questions: (1) What are my strengths and weaknesses?; (2) Could I have done that better? If so, what? (And how?); (3) Does it have to do with knowledge, technical skills or "soft" skills/behaviours? If so, what knowledge, skills or behaviours are lacking?; and (4) In relation to that knowledge or those skills or behaviours, how would I describe where I am now compared to where I need to be? And what do I need to do to get to where I need to be?

When to Reflect?

Based on the fact that reflection is a tool that is used extensively in health and social care, for both education as well as standard practice, it should adopt a malleable course when it comes to the question of "when to reflect?". Reflection can be used as part of portfolio development, evidence of practice-based learning, or as part of continuous medical education. It has also been recognized as a beneficial tool for use after critical incidents have occurred, to help practitioners and students reflect on experiences and generate new knowledge. Reflective writing is a valued tool for teaching students and for documentation, support as well as knowledge generation. As reflection is considered a self-awareness framework and a main domain of a broader healthcare perception [22], it does not require specific schedule and can be done at any time in relation to the assessed matter. Every individual is expected to regularly dedicate time to reflect on own practice. Identified learning and development needs can be captured in a development record.

Healthcare professionals can reflect by looking at their performance at scheduled intervals (e.g. every 3 months, 6 months and 12 months). As appraisal became mandatory for healthcare professionals in the modern medical service, organizations such as the Royal College of Physicians and General Medical Council, UK, have included reflection as essential part of their annual feedback given by the healthcare professionals. For every continuity professional development entry, the healthcare professionals are asked to give their feedback as well as for the whole year in general. After setting the development targets, the healthcare professional should look back over the last period trying to answer: Where do I think I am at against my development objectives; and am I continuing to provide a proper standard of service? Looking forward over the next 12 months, what do I think I need to do to achieve and/or maintain my development objectives and ensure I continue to provide a proper standard of service? By doing this regular scheduled reflection, the healthcare professionals imply they are reviewing both their development plan as well as development record.

More recently, the General Medical Council (GMC), UK, has released a new guidance (March 2018) [31] and has requested the healthcare professional reflection for each of the four domains: knowledge, skills, performance as well as safety and quality. This has become a prerequisite for the healthcare professional to maintain their licence and get revalidated.

Challenges here include time, both the time required to develop the necessary skills and the time needed to record everything thoroughly, as well as the candidate having the cognitive abilities necessary to be able to reflect [22].

Practical Approaches to Identifying Learning and Development Needs

In healthcare service as well as other professional or business facilities, identifying learning and developmental needs involves the evaluation of the person's capabilities alongside an understanding of current or anticipated gaps in knowledge or skills. This analysis can be conducted at the individual, team or organizational level. In any case, the outcomes are expected to enable the identification of the appropriate learning provisions required to demonstrate that the person's work is in line with the expected principles and values. There are a number of ways to identify the person's learning and development needs (Fig. 12.7).

Personal Approach

Healthcare professionals or other employees may find it helpful to talk with a colleague, manager, client or someone external to their organization who knows the person and the nature of his/her work and can help the person obtain an objective view on any learning and/or development needs and identify if any is required.

Performance Appraisal

Healthcare professionals should be given the chance to sit down with an appraiser who could be a clinical manager, supervisor or a trained colleague, at least once a year and have a performance appraisal. This is an opportunity to look together at (1) how the healthcare professional has developed over the last year, particularly around any specific objectives agreed previously; (2) whether the person is still producing the necessary level of performance in relation to the competencies set out for his/her role – if the healthcare professional is employed by the NHS England, for example, this will almost certainly mean looking at how the person is doing over the six core dimensions of the Knowledge and Skills Framework (these include communication, personal and people development, health, safety and security, service improvement, quality, equality and diversity) [31] – (3) what education and training opportunities are required over the coming year; (4) producing a personal development plan; and (5) setting specific objectives to achieve over the coming year.

The agreed objectives should be what is called SMART, that is, **S**pecific (the objective is clearly and easily understood), **M**easurable (both the appraisee and the appraiser should be able to look back in a year's time and actually be able to see whether the objectives have been achieved or not), **A**greed and achievable (the appraisee should be happy with the objectives and they should not be so challenging that he/she could never achieve them), **R**ealistic and relevant (the objectives should reflect the person's skills, experience and grade and should relate directly to the work being done) and **T**ime-related (both parties should set realistic timescales over which the objectives are expected to be achieved) [32].

It has to be emphasized that the performance appraisal is not about trying to find weaknesses in the persons' practice or punishing for them. Rather, it is about the appraiser and appraisee having the opportunity to look at the person's performance in the round, highlight where he/she is clearly achieving the necessary performance and identify what kind of support is needed to help reaching even higher levels. Therefore, it is about supporting the person to make the best possible contribution to the team's work and develop own knowledge and skills into the bargain.

Performance and Development Reviews

All healthcare professionals are required to participate in an annual appraisal for their "performance and development review". The performance and development review complements the more regular reviews and one-to-one conversations that are usually held with line managers and aims at assessment of the person's performance, professional as well as personal development and identification of any learning or developmental needs required (Table 12.5 shows the main characteristics of the performance and development review) [33, 34].

Some hospitals or health authorities started to issue "Healthcare Evaluation Data" reports for each of their employed healthcare professionals. The system allows healthcare organizations to utilize analytics which harness Hospital Episode Statistics, national inpatient and outpatient information as well as Office for National Statistics mortality datasets. The report usually contains information on various parameters including (1) performance indicators (a data grid containing indicators based around performance, including average length of stay, day case rates and number of elective spells where no procedure was performed); (2) inpatient workload volumes (presented as a data grid containing a breakdown of the finished consultant episodes for the healthcare professional, e.g. consultant), along with trust and national average; (3) outpatient workload indicators (performance indicators for outpatient attendances, presented in comparison to the trust and national values); (4) outpatient procedure indicators (showing indicators for outpatient procedures, broken down by procedure); and (5) governance indicators – details on the consultant's mortality rates, including the nonstandardized value along with the hospital standardized mortality ratio (HSMR) and Summary Hospital-level Mortality Indicator (SHMI) score and the trust and national scores. The data can also be displayed in a bar chart [35].

Monitoring Changes in Practice

Learning and development needs can be identified by monitoring developments in the healthcare service regulations, changes in practice, and guidelines. Changes are released in various forms including online guidelines update message, briefings, electronic alerts and journals. Auditing would be the best approach to monitor the service development and identifying any pitfalls or learning requirement. In healthcare audit is a process used by health professionals to assess, evaluate and improve care of patients in a systematic way. Audit measures current practice against a defined (desired) gold standard. It forms part of clinical governance, which aims to safeguard a high quality of clinical care for patients. In the meantime, it evaluates the current service provided by the healthcare professional(s).

Reviewing Feedback

Reviewing feedback, satisfaction surveys, incident reports or complaints from patients and colleagues can help the healthcare professionals identify their learning and development needs. Most of the healthcare organizations have arranged for such process. A 360-degree feedback (also known as multi-rater feedback, multisource feedback or multisource assessment) is a process through which feedback from an employee's subordinates, colleagues and supervisor(s), as well as a self-evaluation by the employee themselves, is gathered. Such feedback can also include, when relevant, feedback from external sources who interact with the employee, such as customers and suppliers or other interested stakeholders. 360-degree feedback is so named because it solicits feedback regarding an employee's behaviour from a variety of points of view (subordinate, lateral and supervisory).

Peer Reviewing

It is vitally important for doctors to regulate themselves and this represents a major component of clinical governance. Peer review is a clinical governance tool whose primary aim is ensure that departments meet minimum standards and facilitate improvement in quality of clinical services. Several medical specialties have developed peer review programmes, notably the British Thoracic Society with the support of the Royal College of Physicians. More recently NHS England through the National Peer Review Programme has supported specialist areas such as cancer, paediatric diabetes and trauma service. A typical peer review programme comprises of an ordered series of individual specialist unit visits by teams of health professionals randomly selected from other units in the programme.

Peer reviewing is a positive, formative process aiming for service improvements and individual development. It has been suggested that medical departments should participate in peer review on a 5-yearly basis as a means to facilitate improvement in clinical services and to ensure basic core standards are met. The benefits of peer review are multifactorial and can be both at an organizational level (e.g. in line with care quality commissioning (CQC), supporting specialist commissioning, etc.) and at an individual level through providing evidence for CPD and revalidation purposes. In regions where peer review is active, the process is seen as mutually beneficial and educational for reviewers and those reviewed. The outcome of visits commonly addresses staffing needs and results in expansion of nursing, medical, secretarial or associated healthcare professional jobs [36].

The Art of Reflective Teaching

Both good students and good teachers recognize the value of reflection. Reflection takes an experience and turns it into a learning event; hence the reflection concept may expand to become a standard of life with positive impact on the individual's personality. Earlier, Aldous Huxley describes experience as "Experience is not what happens to a person; it is what a person does with what happened." [37]. While reflection might look like a quiet session of daydreaming, it is actually an active process during which the person enriches his/her own life and encourage personal growth by reviewing parts or period of own day or life. Richert [38] describes reflection as "the ability to think about what one does and why – assessing past actions, current situations, and intended outcomes – is vital to intelligent practice, practice that is reflective rather than routine. As the time in the teaching process when teachers stop to think about their work and make sense of it, reflection influences how one grows as a professional by influencing how successfully one is able to learn from one's experiences". Therefore, reflecting on how the person is doing can help him/her take ownership of own career as well as learning and identify areas for improvement.

The Importance of Purpose in Education

With all the pedagogical and andragogical theories handling in depth the role of dialogue in learning, the skill of making the students able to understand and discover a sense of purpose in their learning remains the cornerstone in the whole education process. In their learning path, students should get a metacognitive boost by pausing to think back on how and why they performed learning tasks. Teachers should mindfully craft authentic learning reflections along the way for their students. This may come through questions that lead them to think about their interests. Furthermore, the insights gained from reflective questions can be used by students and teachers to develop links between various subjects and spark interests in multiple curricular areas. The transfer of key understandings and the information that applies to multiple concepts can provide inspiration and clarity to the confused and disaffected learner.

Frameworks for Reflection

While reflection is an analysis of the performance, it aids in deeper learning and supports better performance in the future because it boosts the individual's sense of self-efficacy. However, if reflection was left open without a framework, it either gets very superficial or gets diversified and in both scenarios will lose its impact and targets. It all starts with questions, which should form the basic frame for the reflection process. In the learning process, where, traditionally, units build on each other, this approach comes in handy at the end of a unit, acting as a bridge to the next. It's also a very useful informal assessment for the teacher.

To enhance the framework concept for reflection, Anna Durfee [39] suggested using shapes to help guide reflection. The teacher draws a triangle, a square and a circle on the board. The question for the triangle is, "What three concepts am I taking away from this experience/lesson?" For the square, "What about the lesson squares with my beliefs?" And for the circle, "What questions are still circling my mind?". This shapes protocol was found to be useful at the end of the teaching activity in which new concepts were introduced or expounded on.

Keeping Students Tuned

Maintaining the learners' interest and attention throughout the whole teaching session is a challenge. This interaction in teaching and learning is highly needed and requires the lecturer to be motivated and enjoy his/her job. Some lecturers just do not have such an important skill. Reflection ensures the students stay tuned and attentive. This can be on individual bases or in groups. Group work is an activity that benefits learners, not only because it is a more dynamic and entertaining way of learning but also because they acquire more knowledge and skills, and their learning process becomes more useful. Examples of how a cooperative reflection/learning process could be organized include interactive peer group teaching methods. The interactive groups style [40] is an approach where groups of four or five students are formed and work on an activity for 20 min, mentored by a person of the educational community. This person is in charge of assuring that students follow the activity with the help of their peers and promoting the interactions between them. The interactive groups teaching style achieves two goals. The first one is related to being and learning together, because students of different cultures, gender and academic levels learn to help each other, and this is a way to promote solidarity and open dialogue. The second one is related to instrumental skills. Thanks to interactive groups approach, the learning process strengthens as well as improves the students' learning and enables them acquire more knowledge. Peer group supervision or reflective practice group has been used in the management of personality disorders which involves setting ambitious targets to deliver a more integrated, multidisciplinary service which is more psychologically minded and responsive to patients' needs. Group supervision creates more sight lines and more opportunity to spot parallel process. By sharing the load, the group is able to put words to the experience in more detail [41].

Role of Reflection in Learning

Critical and Reflective Thinking

Both critical thinking and reflective thinking terms are often used synonymously. Halpern [42] describes critical thinking as "… the use of those cognitive skills or strategies that increase the probability of a desirable outcome…thinking that is purposeful, reasoned and goal directed – the kind of thinking involved in solving problems, formulating inferences, calculating likelihoods, and making decisions when the thinker is using skills that are thoughtful and effective for the particular context and type of thinking task. Critical thinking is sometimes called directed thinking because it focuses on a desired outcome".

On the other hand, reflective thinking is a part of the critical thinking process referring specifically to the processes of analysing and making judgements about what has happened. Dewey [8] suggests that reflective thinking is an active, persistent and careful consideration of a belief or supposed form of knowledge and of the grounds which support that knowledge and the further conclusions to which that knowledge leads. Learners are aware of and control their learning by actively participating in reflective thinking – assessing what they know, what they need to know and how they bridge that gap – during learning situations.

In summary, critical thinking involves a wide range of thinking skills leading towards desirable outcomes, whereas reflective thinking focuses on the process of making judgements about what has happened. However, reflective thinking is most important in prompting learning during complex problem-solving situations because it provides students with an opportunity to step back and think about how they actually solve problems and how a particular set of problem-solving strategies is appropriated for achieving their goal.

As modern medical curricula got more complex, this has reflected on the teaching approaches prompting learners to constantly rethink, switch directions and change problem-solving strategies. Thus, it is increasingly important to prompt reflective thinking during learning to help students develop strategies to apply new knowledge to the complex situations in their day-to-day activities. Reflective thinking helps learners develop higher-order thinking skills by prompting learners to (1) relate new knowledge to prior understanding, (2) think in both abstract and conceptual terms, (3) apply specific strategies in novel tasks and (4) understand their own thinking and learning strategies.

When students are faced with a perplexing problem, reflective thinking helps them to become more aware of their learning progress, choose appropriate strategies to explore a problem and identify the ways to build the knowledge they need to solve the problem. The KaAMS model of problem- based learning [43] incorporates various components to prompt students' reflective thinking during the learning process (Fig. 12.9).

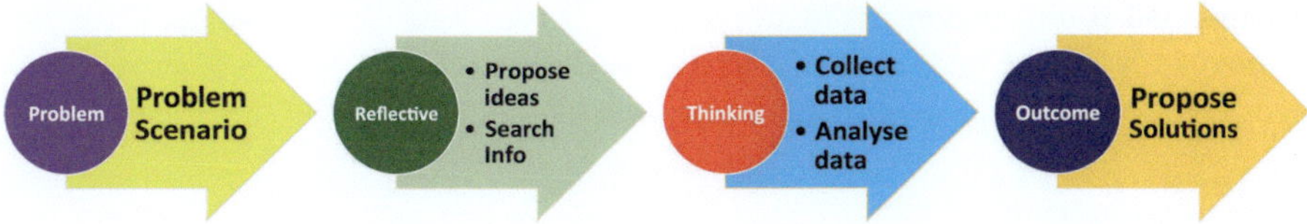

Fig. 12.9 KaAMS model of problem-based learning and its relationship to reflective thinking

Becoming a Reflective Learner

Reflective learning is a way of allowing students to step back from their learning experience, have a look at what happened and develop this skill of critical thinking skills and consequently improve on future performance by analysing their experience. However, it can be a challenge to learn the reflection habit or to instil this approach among learners. Thanks to technology, the Internet and a global obsession with efficiency, adults and children alike are always trying to press forward and move onto the next step or action. Furthermore, such low enthusiasm in reflection might be attributed to the false concept of reflection being a research tool. Reflection is not only important for academic work; but it is beneficial also for everyone in the standard daily lives both at home and at work. Reflection forms part of a learning cycle in which we look over the things that went well or badly in a task, refine and tweak our processes to carry forward to the next attempt. If you remove reflection, the cycle stops – it simply becomes repetition, and from experience this rarely has positive results (Fig. 12.6).

A learner can become more reflective by going over work he/she doesn't feel confident about. For example, it could be an exercise done in a topic that proved difficult for the learner. From there, the learner could ask questions such as how do I improve? How can I move from this point to that one? Student can also seek the help of their teacher and ask them these questions. The learner needs to see the reflection as a way to progress in a given subject. If the person started to implement such approach to several challenges or difficulties that might face him/her, soon the individual will realize that it can be effective in the long haul, and it should become a habit in the learner's life.

While it may be easy to see why reflecting is so important, it remains unexplainable why people do not dedicate more time to it, even the adults. Most of us would love to move forwards with things quickly; this can be enhanced by looking at ways to bring more reflection into my life. Approaches to do so include:

Allocate a Specific Time for It

Whether as you finish your work or after checking your mobile/emails, make sure you allot sometime to think over what happened recently, what you would like to repeat and how would you avoid things you do not. Assign the same time every day for this and it will become a matter of habit before long. Just make sure it is not immediately before bed, as it will impact negatively on your sleep. Nobody manages a good night's sleep with a racing mind!

Summarize Each Day in a Sentence

Summarize each day in a single sentence, and then bring that into your reflection routine by the end of the year. Electronic diaries can help in simple recording of the events on daily basis, and you can record the reflection in the same diary. Not only will it be fascinating, but you could refresh ideas that you had long forgotten.

Involve Others in Reflection

Reflection can be a group activity rather than a lonely process. You can talk about incidents or through the day with colleagues or friends, or if it is more comfortable for the person, it can be through prayers or meditation.

Ask the Right Questions

For reflection to be useful, the right questions need to be asked. While "What did I do today?" is a good place to start, the important questions always begin with "How". "How can I get that done faster next time?" or "How did that affect others?" are always better than "Why was I so slow?" or "Why were they unhappy?". While the journey to be a reflective learner is not an easy one in this fast-paced life, refining a process is surely better than rushing to finish it and start another.

How Can I Become a Reflective Practitioner?

Reflective practice is a term strongly associated with learning in professional contexts such as teaching, medical, nursing or social work and can be thought of in a number of ways. In fact, reflection in teaching and healthcare career is essential. It can be described as a learning tool, something that is going to help professionals to synthesize, explain, make sense of and ultimately develop meaningful outcomes, from their own experiences.

Learning from your experience in workplace is central to the individual professional development. During work or educational courses, practical skills and knowledge will start to develop and provide the professionals with opportunities to demonstrate their learning. To help understanding how to learn effectively, there are some challenges and tips that could help the person to become a reflective practitioner, and these include the following.

Complexities of Workplace Learning

Working in any specific professional context is likely to highlight differences of opinion. These may be the result of differences between (1) members of staff about what strategies they employ or the beliefs they hold, (2) the andragogy of different educators, (3) variety of concepts and knowledge attained from reading journals or books as well as personal experience in the working place and (4) person's own beliefs, views and assumptions and those of other people.

These differences in perspectives are a normal occurrence in any workplace-based learning. How to deal with these situations is important, as they can be a stimulus for learning if some questions were asked such as: (1) Why such discrepancy of the views occurred? (2) How far is the impact of the personalities of the people involved and their beliefs and values? (3) Is there a possibility of contraindications that might have happened? (4) How far the person's own assumptions, beliefs and values are linked to this?

Reflective practice requires the person to think of these perspectives, make links between them and make informed, reasoned decisions about what to take forward into your own practice and what not to.

Professional Judgement and Practice Wisdom

Professional judgement means the application of relevant training, knowledge and experience, within the context provided by auditing, accounting and ethical standards, in making informed decisions about the courses of action that are appropriate in the circumstances of the audit engagement. The divide between practice/experience and theory has existed since the profession emerged, and practice wisdom is the bridge to this gap (Fig. 12.10). Therefore, practice wisdom is the foundation for effective practice and encompasses both the art and science of social work [44]. What often lies behind professional judgements or practice wisdom is years of experimenting with different approaches, incorporating different ideas from research, theory and practice and constant critical reflection [45, 46].

Critical analysis and reflection is a key tool in helping learners as well as tutors learn from the encountered contradictions and complexities. Critical reflection facilitates the synthesis of different perspectives (whether from other people or literature) to help explain, justify or challenge the encountered own or other people's practice. It may be that theory or literature which gives an alternative perspective that the person should consider, it may provide evidence to support own views or practices or it may explicitly challenge them. Critical reflection also facilitates the analysis of what has been learned and how it was taught. This enables the individual to take control of own development. It is in light of these two functions that a great deal of importance is placed on critical reflection in the professional development.

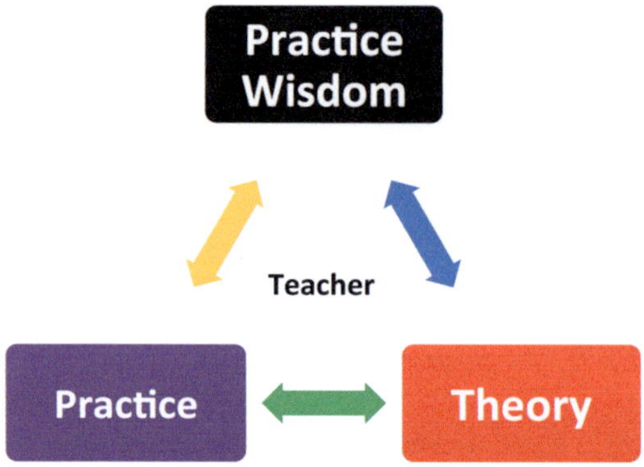

Fig. 12.10 The triangular relationship between practice wisdom, theory and practice/experience. Practice wisdom is the foundation for effective practice and encompasses both the art and science of social work. The divide between practice and theory has existed since the profession emerged and practice wisdom is the bridge to this gap

Which Type of Reflection to Adopt

Reflection has two aspects: reflection-in-action and reflection-on-action [9]. Reflection-in-action refers to the quick thinking and reaction that occur as things are being done (e.g. while teaching a topic, the tutor may notice difficulty in conducting the message to his students). The reflection-in-action allows the teacher to see this, consider why it is happening and respond by doing it differently. This could involve reframing the tutor explanation or approaching the topic from a different perspective. Reflection-on-action is what occurs outside the teaching session, when the tutor is able to reconsider the whole situation, deep thinking about why the learners did not understand, what caused the situation, what were the available options, why that particular option was chosen and not another. The responses will depend on the tutor's existing level of knowledge, experience, values as well as extent of understanding of theories.

Features of Reflection

Reflective practice is widely considered to be an important activity for professional development. There is a huge amount of literature exploring and debating reflection and reflective practice; however, there are some widely accepted key features of reflection:

– Reflection results in learning – through changing ideas and understanding of the situation.
– Reflection is an active learning process – it is more than thinking or thoughtful action.

- Reflection involves problematizing teaching by recognizing that practice is not without dilemmas and issues.
- Reflection is not a linear process, but a cyclical one where reflection leads to the development of new ideas which are then used to plan the next stages of learning.
- Reflection encourages looking at issues from different perspectives, which enables considering the issue and analysing own values, assumptions and perspective.

Therefore, when the term "critical reflection" is used, it refers to a combination of the analytical, questioning (or critical thinking) and reflective approaches. It is this combination that would characterize a critically reflective conversation.

Critical Reflection in Reading and Writing

As part of the education process or professional development, a written report might be requested demonstrating critical reflection. Maughan and Webb [21] state that while reflective thinking and writing can be an unstructured process, the individual is commonly required to demonstrate some editorial skills in the presentation and structure of the final report. As a result, they propose a three-part structure to produce reflective writing: description, interpretation and outcome. Based on the structure above, Maughan and Webb provide some suggestions for words and phrases for reflective writing. While using any of these words and phrases will not automatically result in "good reflection", they do help with the vocabulary required in this style of writing. Table 12.7 shows the main features of critical reflection in reading and writing.

Ensuring Reflection Leads to Learning

The main target of reflection is to ensure that reflective practice leads to learning (Fig. 12.11). Both Finlay [47] and Ixer's [48] criticisms of reflective practice hint at a discrepancy between surface-level reflection (routinized, bland and unthinking) and a deeper-level reflection (conscious control, self-analysis, metacognition). LaBoskey identified three types of reflective thinkers: (1) common sense thinkers, (2) alert novices and (3) the pedagogical thinker [49]. Cartwright [50] reported that LaBoskey makes a distinction between "common sense thinkers" and those who are "pedagogical thinkers". This distinction gets to the heart of how to ensure reflection is an effective learning tool. LaBoskey defines "common sense thinkers" as those who reflect in an unconscious way, suggesting they are happy to use a "trial-and-error" approach to learning to address short-term issues that are context specific. "Pedagogical thinkers" are more conscious of their actions asking the questions

Table 12.7 Main features of critical reflection in reading and writing

Reading for critical analysis and reflection involves	Writing in a critically reflective and analytical style involves
Making judgements about the way arguments are made in the text	Applying these ideas to facilitate arguments development
Are they convincing? Are they based on reliable evidence?	Use evidence and demonstrate the link between theoretical perspectives and experiences in practice
Considering the arguments from a detached position which allows you to carefully scrutinize what is being said	Description:
What is missing or doesn't relate to own understanding of the issues?	If describing an idea, for example, a theory or model, it is usually best to use the present tense, e.g. "Social interdependence theory recognises…" (not "recognised")
Reading target is to understand different ways of thinking about a subject rather than just collecting information or quotes	Events, of course, are nearly always described using the past tense
Considering how the literature relates to personal own practical experiences. Does it support, challenge or even undermine person's experiences?	Interpretation:
	For me, the [most]
	Significant aspect(s) was
	Important element(s) were
	Relevant experience(s)
	Useful issue(s)/idea(s)
	Learning arose from…/happened when…/resulted from…
	Previously, though (did not think)
	At the time, felt (did not feel)
	At first, noticed (did not notice)
	Initially, questioned (did not question)
	Subsequently, realized (did not realize)
	Later,
	Outcome:
	Having……. read………… I now….. think
	Experienced ……feel
	Applied ……realise
	Discussed …….wonder
	Analysed ……. questioned
	Learned ……. Know
	Additionally, I have learnt that…..
	Furthermore,
	Most importantly,
	I have significantly developed my skills in……..
	I have slightly improved my understanding of…I have ………………………… my ability to
	However, I have not sufficiently ……………
	This means that ……..

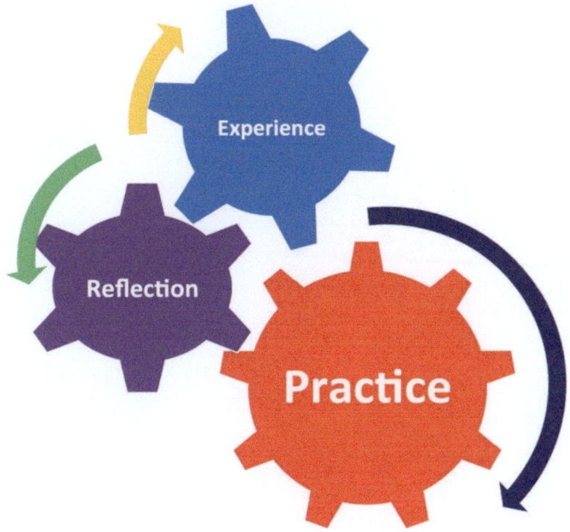

Fig. 12.11 Reflective practice

"What is my intuitive response to this, and why am I feeling or acting this way?" Labosky suggests that it is by taking conscious control that pedagogical thinkers "take a long-term view of how to solve problems… remain open to learning… recognise there are no simple answers and the conclusions they reach are likely to be tentative" [49, 50].

Tools for Reflection

Several approaches are available for reflection. These include learning journals (via blogs or offline formats), webfolios, written assessment tasks, lesson evaluations as well as tutorials or meetings with the mentor or tutor. Whatever the format, these tools provide an opportunity to demonstrate deep-level reflection but are all susceptible to the kind of surface-level reflection that Finlay, Ixer and LaBoskey warn against [9, 47, 48]. Understanding the basic concepts of the reflection models (Table 12.8) will help to evaluate whether these tools are being used effectively.

Transformational Learning

Mezirow [51] argues that reflection only leads to learning if it leads to transformation. Merizow suggests that transformation occurs where the original starting point causes a dilemma that needs to be addressed and then suggests that there are a series

Table 12.8 Summary of the most common models used for reflection on teaching

	The experiential learning cycle	Gibbs' reflective cycle	Johns' model for structured reflection	Rolfe et al.'s reflective model	Reflective writing	REFLECT
	1. Concrete experience (a new experience or situation is encountered or a reinterpretation of existing experience)	1. Description: what happened?	Looking in:	1. What?	1. Description:	– RECALL the events (stage 1) – Give a brief overview of the situation upon which you are reflecting. This should consist of the facts – a description of what happened
		2. Feelings: what were you thinking or feeling?	Find a space to focus on self	… is the problem/ difficulty/ reason for being stuck/reason for feeling bad/reason we don't get on?	What happened?	
		3. Evaluation: what was good/ bad about the situation?	Pay attention to your thoughts and emotions		What is being examined?	
	2. Reflective observation of the new experience (of particular importance are any inconsistencies between experience and understanding)	4. Analysis: what sense can you make of situation?	Write down these thoughts and emotions	2. So what?	2. Interpretation:	
		5. Conclusion: what else could you have done?	Looking out:	… does this tell me/teach me/imply/mean about me/my class/others/our relationship/my patient's care/the model of care I am using/my attitudes/ my patient's attitudes?	What is most important/interesting/ useful/relevant about the object, event or idea?	E – EXAMINE your responses (stage 2) – Discuss your thoughts and actions at the time of the incident upon which you are reflecting
			Write a description of the situation		How can it be explained e.g. with theory?	
	3. Abstract conceptualization (reflection gives rise to a new idea or a modification of an existing abstract concept)	6. Action plan: if situation arose again, what would you do?	What issues seem significant	3. Now what?	How is it similar to and different from others?	
			Aesthetics	… do I need to do in order to make things better/stop being stuck/ improve my teaching/ resolve the situation/ feel better/get on better/ etc., etc.?	3. Outcome	

	4. Active experimentation (the learner applies them to the world around them to see what results)		What was I trying to achieve? Why did I respond as I did? What were the consequences for myself and others? How were others feeling? How did I know this? Personal Why did I feel the way I did within this situation? Ethics Did I act for the best? What factors were influencing me? Reflexivity How does this situation relate to previous experiences? How could I have handled this better? What would have been the consequences of alternative actions? How do I feel now about the experience? How can I support myself and others better in the future?		What have I learned from this? What does this mean for my future?	F – Acknowledge FEELINGS (stage 3) – Highlight any feelings you experienced at the time of the situation upon which you are reflecting L – LEARN from the experience (stage 4) – Highlight what you have learned from the situation E – EXPLORE options (stage 5) – Discuss options for the future if you were to encounter a similar situation C – CREATE a plan of action (stage 6) – Create a plan for the future; this can be for future theoretical learning or action T – Set TIMESCALE (stage 7) – set a time by which the plan outlined in stage 6 will be complete
Author	Kolb [12]	Gibbs [15]	Johns [19]	Rolfe et al. [20]	Maughan and Webb [21]	Butcher and Whysall [22]

Table 12.9 Phases of transformational learning as suggested by Mezirow [51]

Phases of transformational learning
A disorienting dilemma – loss of job, divorce, marriage, back to school or moving to a new culture
Self-examination with feelings of fear, anger, guilt or shame
A critical assessment of assumptions
Recognition that one's discontent and the process of transformation are shared
Exploration of options for new roles, relationships and actions
Planning a course of action
Acquiring knowledge and skills for implementing one's plans
Provisional testing of new roles
Building competence and self-confidence in new roles and relationships
A reintegration into one's life on the basis of conditions dictated by one's new perspective

of possible phases which may be gone through (Table 12.9). In his report, Merizow emphasizes the role of conscious, self-managed learning. However, it has to be noted that the learning is not a mere direct result of the experience, it happens when the individual takes charge of their critical reflection and explicitly plans and carries out steps to learn from it. This level of personal responsibility for learning is crucial during professional development.

The Next Step

Reflective practice is a career-long learning. Therefore, it is important the individual keep on updating their understanding of critical reflection, as well as the reflective practice. MacGregor and Cartwright [52] report that deep and extended reflection begins to develop into "reflexivity". Reflexivity is the process of reflecting on yourself "the researcher", to provide more effective and impartial analysis. It involves examining and consciously acknowledging the assumptions and preconceptions you bring into the research and that therefore shape the outcome. Bordieu and Wacquant [53] have derived the meaning of reflexivity from its Latin definition, "to turn back on oneself". Thus, to be reflexive means to think about one's own concepts, values and what they bring to any situation. In concordance, MacGregor and Cartwright [51] report that reflexivity is about self-awareness and how we, as teachers, impact on situations and our pupils. This can in turn lead to experimentation, developing research questions that the person wants to explore further and ultimately can lead to them becoming researchers.

In conclusion, teaching is a very demanding work. It requires a lot of energy, stamina and fortitude. Learning new techniques for teaching is like the fish that provides a meal today; reflective practice is the net that provides meals for the rest of your life [25]. Reflection can be defined broadly as the deliberate, purposeful, metacognitive thinking and/or action in which educators engage in order to improve their professional practice. Reflection is viewed as a process of becoming aware of one's context and of the influence of societal and ideological constraints on previously taken-for-granted practices and gaining control over the direction of these influences. Different theories, models and levels of reflection have been published to facilitate the reflection process in standard practice.

References

1. Effective pedagogy, The New Zealand Curriculum. 2014. p. 34. http://nzcurriculum.tki.org.nz/The-New-Zealand-Curriculum#effective_pedagogy. Accessed on 6 Apr 2018.
2. Boud D, Keogh R, Walker D. Reflection: turning experience into learning. London: Kogan Page; 1985.
3. Johns C, Freshwater D. Transforming nursing through reflective practice. London: Blackwell Science; 1998.
4. Reid B. 'But we're doing it already!' Exploring a response to the concept of reflective practice in order to improve its facilitation. Nurse Educ Today. 1993;13:305–9.
5. Jarvis P. Reflective practice and nursing. Nurse Educ Today. 1992;12:174–81.
6. Kahneman D. Thinking, fast and slow. New York: Farrar, Straus and Giroux; 2013.
7. Johnson M. The forgotten 'R': using reflection to speed student learning. 2017. https://matthewmjohnson.com/2017/11/30/why-your-students-should-probably-be-doing-more-reflections/. Accessed on 8th Apr 2018.
8. Dewey J. How we think. Boston: D.C. Heath; 1910. p. 6.
9. Schon D. The reflective practitioner: how professionals think in action. London: Temple Smith; 1983.
10. Schon D. Educating the reflective practitioner. San Francisco: Jossey-Bass; 1987.
11. Kolb DA, Fry R. Toward an applied theory of experiential learning. In: Cooper C, editor. Theories of group process. London: Wiley; 1975.
12. Kolb DA. Experiential learning: experience as the source of learning and development. New Jersey: Prentice Hall; 1984.
13. Pedlar M, Burgoyne J, Boydell T. A manager's guide to self-development. 4th ed. Maidenhead: McGraw-Hill; 2001.
14. Kolb DA, Boyatzis RE. Experiential learning theory: previous research and new directions. In: Sternberg RJ, Zhang LF, editors. Perspectives on cognitive learning and thinking styles. New Jersey: Lawrence Erlbaum; 2000.
15. Gibbs G. Learning in doing: a guide to teaching and learning methods. London: Oxford Centre for Staff and Learning Development, Oxford Polytechic; 1988.
16. Gibbs G. Learning by doing: a guide to teaching and learning. London: Brookes Oxford University; 1998.
17. Bulman, Schultz. In: Bulman C, Schutz S, editors. Reflective practice in nursing. 4th ed. Hoboken: Wiley-Blackwell; 2013.
18. Gibbs' reflective cycle. Academic Services & Retention Team, University of Cumbria; 2016. https://my.cumbria.ac.uk/media/MyCumbria/Documents/ReflectiveCycleGibbs.pdf. Accessed on 8th Apr 2018.
19. Johns C. Becoming a reflective practitioner. Oxford: Blackwell Science; 2000.
20. Rolfe G, Freshwater D, Jasper M. Critical reflection in nursing and the helping professions: a user's guide. Basingstoke: Palgrave Macmillan; 2001.

21. Maughan C, Webb J. Small group learning and assessment. 2001. Retrieved 11 Apr 2018, from the Higher Education Academy Web site: http://www.ukcle.ac.uk/resources/temp/assessment.html.
22. Barksby J, et al. A new model of reflection for clinical practice. Nurs Times. 2015;111(34/35):21–3.
23. Forrest MES. Learning and teaching in action. Health Inf Libr J. 2008;25:229–32.
24. Hatton N, Smith D. Reflection in teacher education-towards definition and implementation. Teach Teach Educ. 1995;11(1):33–49.
25. Brockbank A, McGill I. Facilitating reflective learning in higher education. 2nd ed. Berkshire: Open University Press; 2007.
26. Surgenor P. Reflective practice: a practical guide. UCD teaching and learning. 2011. https://www.ucd.ie/t4cms/Reflective%20Practice.pdf.
27. Boyd E, Fales A. Learning: the key to learning from experience. J Humanist Psychol. 1983;23(2):99–117.
28. Kember D, Kelly M. Improving teaching through action research, HERDSA Green Guide no. 14. Sydney: HERDSA; 1993.
29. Baumgartner LM. An update on transformational learning. New Dir Adult Contin Educ. 2001;2001:15–24. https://doi.org/10.1002/ace.4.
30. Biggs J, Tang C. Teaching for quality learning. Berkshire: SRHE & Open University Press; 2007.
31. www.gmc-uk.org/guidance/good_medical_practice.asp.
32. Craft M. Reflective writing and nursing education. J Nurs Educ. 2005;44(2):53–7.
33. Burrows DE. The nurse teacher's role in the promotion of reflective practice. Nurse Educ Today. 1995;15(5):346–50.
34. The NHS Knowledge and Skills Framework (NHS KSF) and the development review process, Department of Health, October 2004. Available from www.nhsemployers.org/agendaforchange.
35. Healthcare evaluation data system (HED). https://www.hed.nhs.uk/info/hed-system.htm.
36. The British Society for Rheumatology. Peer Review Guidance. https://www.rheumatology.org.uk/Portals/0/Policy/Peer%20review/Peer%20Review%20Guidance.pdf.
37. Huxley A. Texts & pretexts: an anthology with commentaries. https://www.goodreads.com/quotes/92753-experience-is-not-what-happens-to-a-man-it-is.
38. Richert AE. Teaching teachers to reflect: a consideration of program structure. J Curric Stud. 1990;22(6):309–527.
39. Durfee A. Frameworks for Reflection. Eutopia. 2018. https://www.edutopia.org/article/frameworks-reflection. Accessed on 14th Apr 2018.
40. Elboj C, Puigdellívol I, Soler M, Valls R. Comunidades d Aprendizaje. Transformar la educación. Barcelona: Graó; 2002.
41. Edmunds H. A model for reflective practice and peer supervision groups. 2012. http://www.brightontherapycentre.org.uk/wp-content/uploads/2011/11/Edmunds-H-2012-Model-for-Reflective-Practice-and-Peer-Supervision-in-Mental-Health-Services.pdf. Accessed on 14th Apr 2018.
42. Halpern DF. Thought and knowledge: an Introduction to critical thinking. 5th ed. New York: Psychology Press; 2014.
43. Loszalka T. Learning and Instruction Section (NY) KaAMS: a PBL environment facilitating reflective thinking. 2001.
44. Lunenberg M, Korthagen F. Experience, theory and practice wisdom in teaching and teacher education. Teach Teach. 2009;15(2):225–40.
45. Hobson A. Student teachers perceptions of school-based mentoring in initial teacher training (ITT). Mentoring Tutoring Partnership Learn. 2002;10(1):5–20.
46. Jones M, Straker K. What informs mentors practice when working with trainees and newly qualified teachers? An investigation into mentors' professional knowledge base. J Educ Teach. 2006;32(2):165–84.

47. Finlay L. Reflecting on reflective practice. PBPL CETL, Open University. [Online]. 2008. Available at http://www.open.ac.uk/opencetl/resources/pbpl-resources/finlay-l-2008-reflecting-reflective-practice-pbpl-paper-52. Accessed 15 Apr 2018.
48. Ixer G. There's no such thing as reflection. Br J Soc Work. 1999;29(4):513–27.
49. LaBoskey VK. Development of reflective practice. A study of preservice teachers. New York: Teachers College Press; 1994.
50. Cartwright L. How consciously reflective are you? In: McGregor D, Cartwright L, editors. Developing reflective practice: a guide for beginning teachers. Berkshire: Open University Press; 2011.
51. Mezirow J. Learning to think like an adult: core concepts of transformation theory. In: Mezirow J, et al., editors. Learning as transformation. San Francisco: Jossey-Bass; 2000. p. 3–34.
52. McGregor D, Cartwright L. Developing reflective practice: a guide for beginning teachers. Berkshire: Open University Press; 2011.
53. Bordieu P, Wacquant L. An invitation to reflexive sociology. 1st ed. Chicago: University of Chicago Press; 1992.

Chapter 13
e-Learning, Adaptive Learning and Mobile Learning

Introduction

The significant developments in how healthcare is delivered as well as the advances in the medical care protocols and treatment guidelines resulted in constrains on today's medical educators who have been facing the challenge of keeping up to date with the new developments in their specialities. This, consequently, led to a reduction in the time available for teaching, than has previously been the case [1]. In concordance, the shift in healthcare delivery sites, from acute care institutions to community-based settings for chronic care, has mandated further adaptations in educational approach [2]. Finding time to teach "new" fields such as gerontology, genomics, palliative care and complementary medicine is difficult while medical schools' curricula are already challenged to cover conventional materials. On the other hand, the traditional teacher-centred learning model is yielding to a student-centred approach which puts the students in control of their own learning. A recent shift towards competency-based curricula emphasizes the learning outcome, not the process, of education [3]. These advances in medical education content required similar advances in medical education strategies. These new strategies aim at facilitating the access to the learnt content, better understanding of the learning process, increasing the learners' retention by improving the educational experience, as well as making learning affordable. One of these new approaches is "e-learning" that refers to "electronic learning", in which instruction is delivered through a wide range of electronic means including computer- and Internet-enabled learning. e-Learning has expanded and is not only reflects the use of technology to deliver a broad array of solutions that enhance knowledge and performance but also the social dynamics of networking [4, 5].

Technologies on their own will not alter the fundamental fact that learning medicine, always, requires considerable effort from both the student as well as

Y. El Miedany, *Rheumatology Teaching*,
https://doi.org/10.1007/978-3-319-98213-7_13

the teacher. However, there is growing evidence that technology can enhance teaching and learning when used thoughtfully and appropriately [6]. e-Learning can be viewed as computer-assisted learning and as pedagogy for student-centred and collaborative learning. Different definitions have been proposed (Table 13.1) which reflect the different aspects of the concept. e-Learning can be used by medical educators to improve the efficiency and effectiveness of educational interventions in the face of the social, scientific and pedagogical challenges. Such electronic pedagogical approach aims to encourage interaction (teacher–teacher, teacher–student, student–student), collaboration and communication. It has gained popularity in the past decade; however, its use is highly variable among medical schools and appears to be more common in basic science courses than in clinical clerkships [7–9]. Examples of e-learning are independent learning using available online learning modules; access to online medical information and learning resources; web-based synchronous presentation by a teacher to a group of students; online group of students learning in real time, facilitated by a tutor; asynchronous discussion forums or chat rooms/bulletin boards; social networks such as Facebook, Twitter, and WhatsApp; interactive multimedia activities including games and stimulations whether online or on DVD; virtual patient who interacts with the learner; and video or audio recordings of lectures distributed via online streaming and podcasts using mobile devices. This chapter will review the current state of e-learning in medical education outlining the reasons for introducing e-learning, educational features and the role of the teacher, the components of e-learning, the evidence for its effectiveness, faculty development needs for implementing e-learning, evaluation strategies for e-learning and its technology, and the potential for e-learning to be considered evidence of academic scholarship.

Table 13.1 Definitions of e-learning. How compelling is the evidence for the effectiveness of e-learning in the post-16 sector?

e-Learning in education	e-Learning in medical education	e-Learning in the commercial/training sector
Learning with the aid of information and communications technology tools	The use of Internet technologies to deliver a broad array of solutions that enhance knowledge and performance	e-Learning is the effective learning process created by combining digitally delivered content with (learning) support and services
Examples: the Internet, intranets, computer-based technology or interactive television. Also, the use of e-technology to support traditional methods of learning, e.g. using electronic whiteboards or video conferencing	e-Learning incorporates (1) formal knowledge and learning resources; (2) learning networks; (3) contact, administration and assessment; (4) information management skills	Work based e-learning: the delivery and administration of learning opportunities and support via computer, networked and web-based technology to help individual performance and development, undertaken in or linked to the workplace

e-Learning, e-Teaching, and e-Training

There has been significant development on comparing the past versus the current forms of online learning. Years ago was the earlier type called computer-based instruction or training which focused on the interaction between the student and computer drills, tutorials or simulations. This has developed now to be computer-mediated communication, where the primary form of interaction between students and instructors, is mediated by the computer. While, the computer-based instruction is usually individualized (self-study) learning, the computer-mediated communication involves teacher/tutor facilitation.

Essential When It Comes to Educating Healthcare Professionals
While many people use the terms e-learning and e-training interchangeably, there are actually some important differences distinguishing "learning" and "training". Understanding what makes each of these concepts unique is essential when it comes to educating healthcare professionals, as both are required in order to develop a competent staff. In e-training, the raining focuses on helping healthcare professional trainees develop the skills they need to perform specific tasks. E-training does this in an online environment. Speeches, demonstrations, videos, text documents and other materials can all be useful instruction methods for e-training. On the other hand, learning is the process of acquiring knowledge and applying that information in potentially unanticipated ways. Therefore, while training teaches medical protocol for specific situations, learning enables training doctors to overcome non-specific issues that suddenly arise on their own. In essence, training may make healthcare professional ready for expected situations, whereas learning prepares them for the unexpected (e-learning, obviously, does this in an online setting).

Although there are huge opportunities to enhance clinical teaching through e-learning, a number of challenges exist in addition to determining pedagogical aspects. Teachers will need to be familiar with the range of innovations available so that they can select appropriate means of developing content, facilitating the process of learning and enabling communication. Other challenges include becoming familiar with new systems, processes and online environments, making time to filter through and select appropriate materials, having time to support learners as they use e-learning and keeping materials and activities up to date.

Reasons for Introducing e-Learning

As medicine incorporated its part of the electronic revolution, the traditional static concept of medical education has changed into a dynamic pattern. The style of the passive doctor who is to be compelled to education has been replaced by a creative doctor interested and trained on problem-solving in practice (self-directed). The vast diversity and extensive rapid developments of biomedical science have persuaded doctors to search for recent updates and techniques to enhance their career; otherwise they will be on the wrong doing side. In fact, today, each doctor or senior medical student became a role model in his/her work and, in the meantime, an educator. This may expand to include younger colleagues, nurses, patients, relatives and students.

Endorsing the student-centred approach, e-learning got famous for being "individualized learning", with "just-for-you" teaching approach as well as "just-the-right-place" education. In contrast to the traditional way of education, e-learning introduced several new terms in the education process, the first one is "learning flexibility". The students have the control over the content, learning sequence, pace of learning, time and often media which allows them to tailor their experience to meet personal learning objectives. This gives the students the opportunity to learn how to work independently and contact their supervisor or colleagues [10, 11]. "Learning delivery" is another term that is considered one of the most often cited privileges of e-learning. This includes increased accessibility to information, ease in updating content, personalized instruction, ease of distribution, standardization of content, and accountability [4, 12]. Another term is "learning accessibility" which refers to the user's ability to find what is needed, when it is needed. Improved access to educational materials is crucial, as learning is often an unplanned experience [13]. "Learning novelty" is another term where regular updating of the online information becomes a standard in our day-to-day practice. This got the momentum particularly as updating electronic content has got much easier than updating printed material. Therefore, e-learning technologies have enabled the educators to revise their resources and update their knowledge simply and quickly [14].

e-Learning goes beyond being an educational tool, to be an educational style and living approach. In the virtual environment era, there is no meaning for information without a context. Living in the age of information, the attained data expand the person's senses, and experience occurs in the context of the virtual environment. The target also changes from just obtaining information or data to the quality of the data attained. The ability of having access to variable educational resources from different institutions where some superior quality of the knowledge can be gained gives the achieved target a 3D form. Furthermore, e-learning not only is a cost-effective approach that can be adapted to the education needs and financial resources but also increases the capacity of the educational institution. It also facilitates a uniform distribution of the information.

e-Learning and the Science of Adult Learning

e-Learning technologies offer educators a new educational paradigm based on adult learning theory, which states that adults learn by relating new learning to past knowledges, by linking learning to specific needs and by practically applying learning, resulting in more effective and efficient learning experiences [15]. Learning enhancement permits better learner interactivity and promotes learners' efficiency, motivation, cognitive effectiveness and flexibility of learning style. Learning is a deeply personal experience: The people learn because they want to learn. By enabling learners to be more active participants, a well-designed e-learning experience can motivate them to become more engaged with the content. Interactive learning shifts the focus from a passive, teacher-centred model to one that is active and learner centred, offering a stronger learning stimulus. Interactivity helps to maintain the learner's interest and provides a means for individual practice and reinforcement. Evidence suggests that e-learning is more efficient because learners gain knowledge, skills and attitudes faster than through traditional instructor-led methods. This efficiency is likely to translate into improved motivation and performance. e-Learners have demonstrated increased retention rates and better utilization of content, resulting in better achievement of knowledge, skills and attitudes. Multimedia e-learning offers learners the flexibility to select from a large menu of media options to accommodate their diverse learning styles [16].

e-Learning has introduced a new paradigm shift in medical education. It has been suggested that, like a Trojan horse, e-learning can be introduced not only for the attributes it brings with it but also for the hidden curricular changes included. e-Learning meets the criteria specified in the CRISI framework for effective continuing education. This includes:

- Convenience: flexibility in the time and place where the trainee can learn.
- Relevance: linking theory to practice. The use of virtual patients expands the learners' clinical experience.
- Individualization: e-learning can be tailored to the individual student's needs.
- Self-assessment: students can evaluate their own performance through questions incorporated in the e-learning activity.
- Interest: the dynamic nature of e-learning, being user-friendly and able to engage the learner enhance the student's learning academic knowledge and clinical experience.
- Systematic: the e-learning programme can systematically cover a topic identified in the medical education curriculum.

As the Internet has provided opportunities for correspondence among the medical universities and share the educational materials, medical universities started to work on grounds to integrate e-learning and medical education. The key factors of success which are vital in e-learning have been determined through several research studies. The main three items identified to ensure the e-learning place in the adult learning process include the learner, the educational body/organization and the technical resources (Fig. 13.1). As for the learner factor, having the motivation to obtain the learning materials, communication with colleagues and social and financial factors and having regular access to Internet and experience in using computers are the bridges linking the learners, the institute and other participants to as well as establishing emails among the learners and safeguard the e-learning process at its baseline. The educational authority preparedness plays also a dynamic role in the success of the e-learning process. Setting up the learning process and environment, communication (whether unidirectional or bidirectional), well-trained and professional academic staff, curricula design and content, financial reward as well

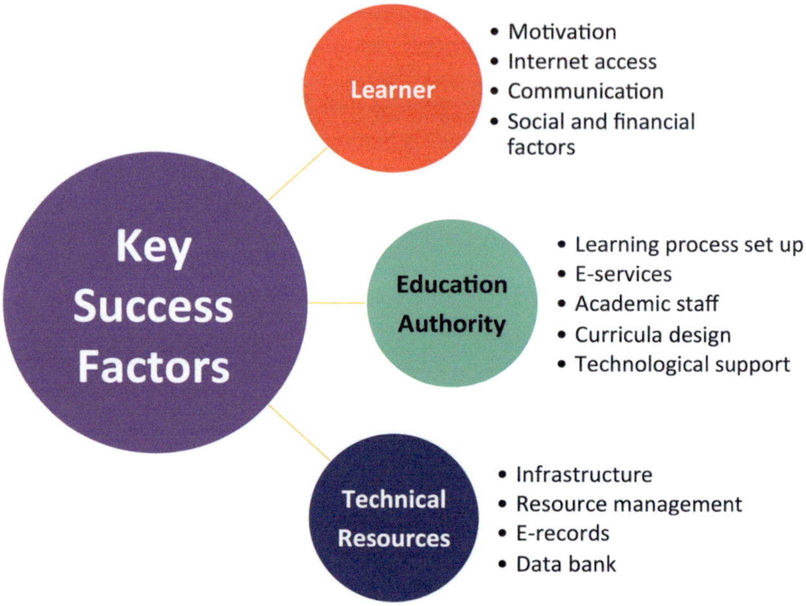

Fig. 13.1 The main three items identified to ensure the e-learning place in the adult learning process are: the learner, the educational body/organization and the technical resources

as technological support and e-services represents the main mediators for the e-learning success [17]. The infrastructure provided by the technical resources represents the third main pillar for success. These include resource management, availability of software and hardware, accessibility to the online saved data and easy download process, e-records and databank regular updates. Briefly, the key factors of success of e-learning rely mainly on the preparedness and inter-connectivity of the three critical factors recognized.

Components of e-Learning

A digital learning object is defined as any grouping of digital materials structured in a meaningful way and tied to an educational objective [18]. Creating an e-learning material goes in several phases, which are linked to the curriculum and tailored to meet the education targets. The main components of e-learning include developing the content, which should be then managed, delivered and then standardized. The content is developed comprising all instructional information, which range in complexity from individual items to larger instructional modules identified to meet the learning objectives. Learning objects represent distinct, self-reliant units of instructional material gathered and reassembled around explicit learning outcomes, which are used to build larger educational materials such as lessons, modules or complete courses to meet the requirements of a specified curriculum [19]. Examples include tutorials, case-based learning, multimedia, simulations and game-based learning modules. Content creators use instructional design and andragogical principles to produce learning objects and instructional materials.

The second component “content management” includes all the administrative functions (e.g. e-storing, e-indexing) required to make e-learning content accessible by learners. Examples include portals, repositories, digital libraries, learning-management systems, search engines and e-portfolios. A learning-management system is an Internet-based software which facilitates the delivery and tracking of e-learning across the organization [20]. A learning-management system can serve several functions beyond delivering e-learning content. It can simplify and automate administrative and supervisory tasks, track learners’ competencies and achievement of the targeted outcomes and operate as a foundation for instructional resources that is available 24 h a day [21]. Examples of learning-management systems familiar to medical educators include 360Learning, Absorb, Cornerstone, Docebo, iSpring Learn and Latitude Learning. In general, there are more than 200 commercially available systems, a number that is growing rapidly.

The third component “content delivery” may be either synchronous or asynchronous. [5] Synchronous delivery refers to real-time, instructor-led e-learning, where all learners receive information simultaneously and communicate directly with other learners. Examples include teleconferencing (audio, video or both), Internet chat forums and instant messaging. With asynchronous delivery, the transmission and receipt of information do not occur simultaneously. The learners are responsible for pacing their own self-instruction and learning. The instructor and learners communicate using email or feedback technologies, but not in real time. A variety of methods can be used for asynchronous delivery, including email, online bulletin boards, Listservs, newsgroups and Weblogs [12].

In addition to establishing, managing and delivering content, a fourth component is part of the e-learning equation, that is, standardization. It is becoming increasingly clear that standards are needed for the creation of new e-learning material. Such standards promote and ensure compatibility and usability of products across many computer systems, facilitating the widespread use of e-learning materials.

Several organizations have been engaged in creating broad e-learning standards. [17] Although not specifically designed for medical education, these standards offer medical educators important advantages. The most well-known set of standards is the Advanced Distributed Learning: Sharable Content Object Reference Model (SCORM). SCORM is a group of specifications developed through a collaborative effort of e-learning organizations funded by the US Department of Defense [22]. SCORM is a set of technical standards for e-learning software products. SCORM tells programmers how to write their code so that it can “play well” with other e-learning software. It is the de facto industry standard for e-learning interoperability. Specifically, SCORM governs how online learning content and learning-management systems communicate with each other. SCORM does not speak to instructional design or any other pedagogical concern – it is purely a technical standard. The interaction of the learning-management system allows for the prescription of the learning experience and tracking of learner performance. In medical education, the MedBiquitous Consortium (MedBiquitous) is the American National Standards Institute (ANSI)-accredited developer of information technology standards for healthcare education and quality improvement. Recently, MedBiquitous has announced the launch of a new standard designed to unify competency and achievement data to draw a complete and accurate picture of how a learner progresses throughout his or her career [23]. The educational achievement standard, an American National Standard, also streamlines the process of documenting decisions about learner entrustment.

The new standard allows systems to exchange competency data and follow a learner through his or her entire career, from medical or nursing school to training, fellowship and eventually practice. The standard enables integrated processes for documenting learner progress and milestones at transition points along the educational continuum. Such processes could streamline certification procedures for clinicians, as certifying boards may rely on entrustment information to make decisions in the future.

The Role of the Teacher in e-Learning

The teacher's role in e-learning is dynamic and definitely, not redundant. Good collaboration between content experts, educationists and technologists is vital and mandatory for the e-learning process. In this new approach of education, the teacher maintains all the known roles; however, it may be carried out in a different style to meet the e-learning techniques and objectives [24]. Figure 13.2 shows the main teacher roles in e-learning which include:

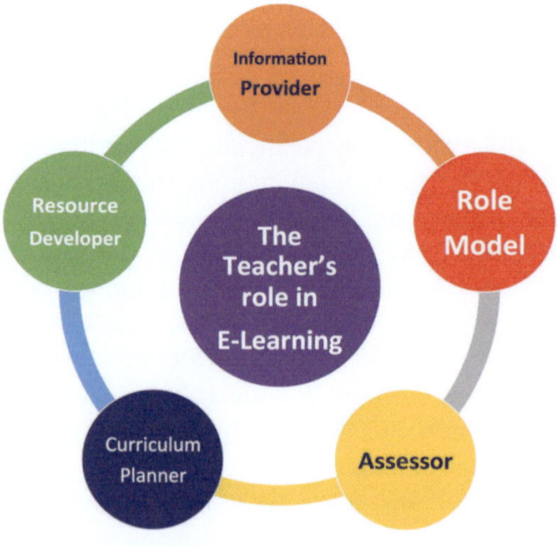

Fig. 13.2 The teacher's role in e-learning

Information Provider

Traditionally a face-to-face lecture is the standard approach the teacher would provide the students with the planned information. In e-learning, this lecture can be reformatted and recorded to include a higher level of students' interaction. The lecture can be uploaded on the system to be available for the students. Video clips presenting a topic or showing how to do a procedure can be also made available. Students worldwide can also view the presentations using web-based platforms.

Role Model

Teachers will remain to be the role model whether they lectured the students in the classroom or online. The teachers' performance and how they present and handle the challenges play an important part in shaping their students' attitude and professionalism.

Facilitator

In concordance with the modern teaching styles, in e-learning the teacher's role shifts significantly from providing the student with information to one of giving them the key and supporting them to open the door to the vastly growing amount of information. This can be done in different ways, e.g. playing the role of e-tutor or e-mentor; working with the students online, answering their queries and supervising their e-portfolio; and helping the students to be able to find out information for themselves and assess the quality of information sources. Being a facilitator endorses the student-centred teaching approach.

Assessor

Digital technology has enabled the incorporation of the "assessment component" into the learning resources. This paved the way for a significant change in the assessment concept, where assessment is no longer viewed as "assessment of learning" but "assessment for learning". This support the learners with a richer learning experience. This, in turn, encouraged the learners to assess their achievement of the targeted learning outcomes and if necessary adjust their pace or learning path. This approach has led to improvement of the effectiveness and efficiency of the learning process. Results of earlier study revealed that progress has been made about online assessment for both formative and summative purposes [25].

Curriculum Planner

Planning for the curriculum is the essential role of successful teaching and the teachers are the planners. In fact, the quality of teacher education is maintained by curriculum of teacher education. Before anything else, the teacher must develop a "flight plan". Like any good flight plan, it must lay out a destination and the path to that destination. The curriculum development should follow a dynamic path to accommodate challenges or recent developments and give room for the use of digital technology in standard education.

Resource Developer

The development of online resources that combine the technology with the standard andragogy education is not an easy mission. In view of the fact that specialized skills are required for this task and that few teachers possess such skills, a team approach has been endorsed. The team includes content expert, instructional designer, educationist and a technologist. Teachers play an important role in identifying the learning resources and learning objectives; consequently, the information about resources with attached annotations can be incorporated in the students' study guide.

Evaluating e-Learning Processes and Outcomes

Before launching or after completion of an e-learning course, it is important to identify whether there are still changes that need to be made or can better results be achieved next time. This is the value of evaluating the e-learning activity. In fact evaluation should be an ongoing process; and constant evaluation of the e-learning course is important in order to keep improving it and making regular changes and updates. This way, the learners will appreciate their teachers' efforts by experiencing the e-learning course offered to them to the fullest.

How to conduct e-learning course evaluation? In concordance with other educational approaches and policies, there are two major methods to evaluate the e-learning approach: the process and the outcomes.

Evaluation of the e-learning process examines the e-learning programme's strengths and weaknesses and how its results are produced, often providing information that will allow others to replicate it. Peer review is one type of process evaluation. Traditional peer review for journal articles can be adopted to verify the quality of content. Collecting feedback from the learners by running focus groups from a sample audience, in order to evaluate the e-learning experience that the course has offered. In general, the evaluation process should consider seven aspects:

- *e-Learning objectives:* The first step is to identify the e-learning objectives and the expected outcomes the students should achieve. After identifying the objectives, it has to be determined if the e-learning content and the learning material chosen can serve these objectives.
- *Level of interactivity:* Interactivity is essential for an e-learning course, because it boosts your learners' engagement and knowledge retention, both of which lead to a more effective e-learning experience. It is important to assess whether the e-learning course has succeeded in integrating enough interactive elements. It is expected that the more interactive elements included, the more time and maybe money is invested; however, the better e-learning preferences are offered to the learners.
- *Visual impact:* Attractive visual impact engages the learners and vice versa. Therefore, it is important to examine the e-learning course and determine whether the images and graphics chosen are aesthetically appealing, expressive as well as suitable to the content. Unnecessary elements are expected to distract the learners from the course content.
- *Language:* Language is a key element of the e-learning course. The learners should be able to completely comprehend what they are reading or listening. Questions to be answered include: Is the content well written and does it stimulates critical thinking? If the targeted audience is a large group, is the jargon used clear for all the learners? Are the examples given or scenarios relevant to the topic as well as the learners or can some be excluded? Finally, if a humour is used to make a point, is it appropriate or are there some groups in the audience who may find it offensive? These points should be answered satisfactorily in order to ensure that the language used in *the e-learning course is* comprehensible, respectful and to the point.
- *Technical functions:* The technological aspect of the e-learning course is also important to be evaluated throughout. It is expected that the learners should use the e-learning course comfortably as well as intuitively. Points to be evaluated include: are interface and navigation effective? What about the content's display and sound? Do all the buttons work and the text and images look as they should? Are multimedia elements used effectively? Can the learners easily access the Internet while taking the e-learning course if they need to? Do all the links work? It is important to be quite meticulous while examining the technology facet of the e-learning course.
- *Time:* Another factor that needs to be checked in order to successfully evaluate the e-learning course is the critical factor of seat time. There are several opinions on how lengthy an e-learning course should be. However, in average, an effective length of time per topic should range between 15 and 30 min.
- *Cost:* Cost-effectiveness is an important issue to tackle when an e-learning course is evaluated. Even if all the aforementioned criteria have been met, if the

e-learning course is too costly, this represents a real challenge. Cost factor should be stratified into (a) the cost of designing and developing the e-learning course (instructional design, working time, purchasing cost, etc.), (b) the cost of running the course (licenses and so on) and then (c) the cost per learner. Cost estimation may also include other factors such as reusability and scale of use.

Evaluation of the e-learning outcomes can be assessed by judging the changes in the learners' knowledge, skills or attitudes. This, in turn, allows the e-learning developers to gauge programme effectiveness. The evaluation framework outlined by Kirkpatrick in the 1950s and later adapted to healthcare education can be used to evaluate e-learning interventions. The Kirkpatrick model (Fig. 13.3) defines four levels of evaluation based on outcome: satisfaction, learning, change in learner behaviour and organizational change/patient outcome [26].

Satisfaction measures: The most popular way to evaluate an e-learning course after it has been created is by conducting surveys: direct questioning of the learners regarding the e-learning course design, relevance and timing; was it easy or hard to use, fun or boring; if their skills/knowledge/work performance has been improved by using what they were taught in the e-learning course; and their reactions to the material. But satisfaction measures alone do not measure learning. For example, excellent content that learners find difficult to use may be rated as poor. Likewise, a module that is highly entertaining in its use of multimedia but superficial in its content may be rated as excellent.

Tracking and monitoring learners' knowledge, attitudes and skills via a learning-management system can greatly simplify the process of evaluating the gains made through e-learning. An approach that combines assessment of skills and attitudes using e-learning technology with facilitator-mediated observation would allow a more in-depth evaluation of skills and behaviour. In contrast, evaluating the direct result of an education programme by measuring changes in learners' behaviours,

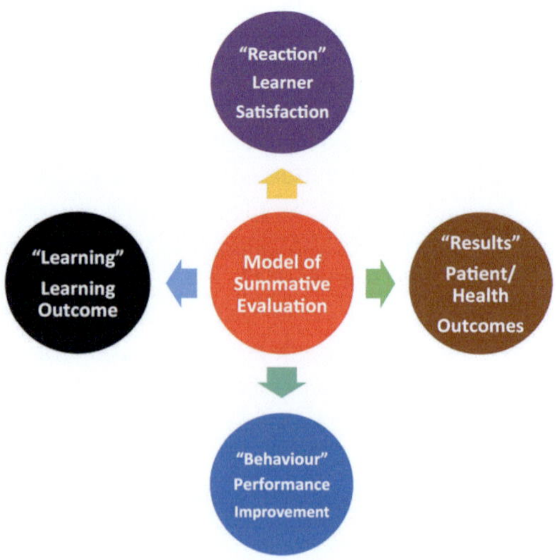

Fig. 13.3 Kirkpatrick s model of summative evaluation

institutional changes, and better patient care is often complex, time-consuming, and costly. e-Learning assessments can be one valuable component in such overall evaluation of medical school curricula.

e-Learning and Virtual Patients

Medical education is most successful when learning occurs in context. One way of achieving this online is by using virtual patients for whom a student may take different roles – junior doctor, consultant, nurse or even as patient himself. By definition, virtual patients are "interactive computer simulations of real-life clinical scenarios for the purpose of medical training, education, or assessment" [27]. The first virtual patient systems emerged in the early 1970s [28] and since then have evolved significantly, taking advantage of new possibilities offered by the Internet and multimedia technologies. Research has shown that such systems enable students to learn clinical problem-solving more efficiently [29]. Increasingly, more and more medical schools are utilizing virtual patients and indeed embedding them into their curricula.

Most virtual patients are entirely computer based and should not be confused with standardized patients – i.e. human actors playing the role of patients [30] – nor with high-fidelity computer simulators connected to realistic robot mannequins [31]. However, some learning scenarios use a combination of these techniques. In these roles, they are presented with a digital scenario describing the patient and the details of the case. The doctor may need to simulate taking a history, carrying out an examination, ordering tests, interpreting test data or images or making a diagnosis and prescribing treatment.

Virtual patients offer a wide variety of (anonymous) patient-related data including medical history, physical and technical examinations, as well as laboratory tests. In most cases, the goal of the student is to find the right diagnosis and propose a correct medical treatment based on the data presented. Virtual patients provide a training opportunity in a risk-free environment before students are allowed to take part in bedside teaching. They may also be used to document the fact that all students have been exposed to all diseases defined by curricular objectives.

Adaptive Learning in Medical Education

In spite of the significantly positive role of technology in several facets of medical education, one of the prime apprehensions from a learning point of view is its current lack of recognition of the learner's needs. Currently technology-enhanced learning is delivered in a standard style to a large cohort of learners irrespective of individual understanding, knowledge or skills. This represents a challenge as it is a common sense that learners during training have variable degrees of understanding and subsequent knowledge gaps. While competency might be achieved by some learners relatively quickly, others may struggle to do so. Disparity in rates of competency attainment is well recognized but is not easily resolved when teaching is delivered on a big scale. From a teacher perspective, during large-scale lectures and seminars, engaging with learners one on one and recognizing each individual's strengths and weaknesses are simply not possible. This has been attributed to time constraints, personal factors (such as learner's embarrassment of asking or getting involved in open discussion) and the fact that the information is delivered in a passive fashion [32]. Perhaps that is the reason why education researchers had high hopes for technology-enhanced learning and its potential to transform the learning process and enhance faculty–learner interactions, as well as learner–content interactions [33]. By ensuring that content is learner specific, a personalized and adaptive learning environment can help individuals better meet their competency requirements.

At its primary level, adaptive learning is a process that provides an individualized learning experience with technologies designed to determine a learner's strengths and weaknesses [34]. Once an individual's strengths are identified, the computer-based technology can adapt the learning material to focus on the individual's limitations. One example comes from the University of New South Wales, which offered a massive open online course, "Learning to Teach Online". In this course, there were thousands of learners with just two core teachers and hence educational support on an individual basis was impossible. This situation was handled by engaging the learners with assessment and reflective activities that generated personalized learning content based on their responses and self-reflection information. From an exam and course participation perspective, research by the Educational Growth Advisors on the use of adaptive learning has demonstrated an 18% increase in pass rates and 47% decrease in withdrawal from educational courses [35].

Adaptation is however not just confined to the content for learners based on their particular learning requirements. Other forms of adaptation include an adaptive system interface where learner preferences are met with respect to navigation and structure of the course content and the discovery and assembly of content from multiple sources – such as learning sources available on the web and discussion forums to connect peers and faculty with each other, based on a specific understanding of each individual learner and their requirements [36].

In the medical field, there has been little in the way of formal research into adaptive learning uses; yet this is likely to change as time passes. Elsevier currently utilizes an adaptive learning platform powered by Cerego to assist health science users. Performance is predicted per user to determine what they already know and what they need to know, helping to ensure an understanding of higher level tasks [37]. More recently, the NEJM launched an adaptive learning process, in recognition of the fact that frequent updates in the medical field conflict with clinicians' limited time. The resource focuses on clinical scenarios which aim to mirror real-life occurrences with the knowledge and learning system designed to aid preparation for internal medicine exams [38].

Another example in relation to adaptive learning in medical education is the repeat delivery of specific knowledge items or categories if mistakes are made which was assessed in the work done by Kellman [39]. There is also use of "interleaving", where information is delivered in an alternating or mixed fashion to better ensure learning gains, while "mastery criteria" ensure specific learning objectives are reached before a learner can be deemed competent [34]. These techniques have been trialled during delivery of the dermatology histopathology curriculum at UCLA with significant improvements in pre and post-test scoring ($P < 0.0001$) [40]. In the future, there is also hope for the utilization of adaptive learning in relation to more procedural and high-fidelity simulation-based tasks [34]. Table 13.2 gives two examples of adaptive learning.

Perceptual and Adaptive Learning Modules

In recent years, there has been an explosion of research in perceptual learning as an expression of the brain plasticity. Perceptual learning is defined as the process by which the ability of sensory systems to respond to stimuli is improved through experience. Perceptual learning occurs through sensory interaction with the environment as well as through practice in performing specific sensory tasks. The new technology of perceptual learning has proven effective in accelerating the development of expert information extraction skills in several domains such as flight training, surgery, mathematics, mammography and areas of military field medicine [41–45]. These developments indicated that perceptual learning can be systematically advanced by particular kinds of interactive learning experiences. Complementing this emerging technology of perceptual learning is the use of adaptive learning techniques in which learner's accuracy and speed in interactive learning is used to guide the spacing and sequencing of learning events, leading to be more efficient

Table 13.2 Examples of adaptive learning in musculoskeletal medicine

	Problem-solving learning	Examination learning
Case	Acute gouty arthritis	Case: rheumatoid arthritis
Module	On management of acute conditions as part of continuing professional development (CPD)	On assessment of rheumatoid arthritis case
Adaptive learning system	Recognizes optimum knowledge of the features of acute arthritis but poor knowledge of pain and inflammation management in acute gouty arthritis	Recognizes optimum knowledge of clinical manifestations of rheumatoid arthritis but poor knowledge of treatment guidelines and medication escalation
Action	Computerized delivery of information on prescribing anti-inflammatory therapy for acute inflammatory arthritis to ensure an understanding of this poorly learnt aspect	Computerized delivery of treatment guidelines and escalation of therapy to ensure an understanding of this poorly learnt aspect

and durable learning, as well as implementation of objective and comprehensive mastery criteria [46].

Perceptual and adaptive learning modules present an alternative route for training. These modules are intelligent, online tools created to enhance the development of pattern recognition [45]. Pattern recognition relies on perceptual learning which, in turn, underlies enhancement of information extraction from the environment as a result of deliberate practice. Perceptual learning is characterized by a discovery process (distinguishing relevant features from irrelevant variation) and the development of fluency (or "automaticity") in recognition [47, 48]. The principles underlying perceptual learning apply to high-level complex tasks, such as those involved in medical pattern recognition [46].

With perceptual and adaptive learning modules, learners sequentially observe a series of unique items (e.g. images, video clips) and classify them into appropriate groups (e.g. diagnoses), each group consisting of a large number of unique, but related, items. An algorithm uses response accuracy and delay to sequence and space exemplars from each category with learners receiving feedback after each trial. Perceptual learning represents an important element of diagnostic reasoning, and training approaches directed at perceptual learning have been shown to improve several clinical interpretation skills [41–43]. Recent studies have demonstrated the effectiveness of perceptual and adaptive learning modules in training recognition of histopathologic processes [44] and dermatologic lesions [40, 45].

Blended Learning

Blended learning, a fairly new term in education, is an approach that combines e-learning technology with traditional instructor-based education. Blended learning is a system of education that turns teaching on its head. It's a hybrid teaching methodology, making technology and e-learning a more integral part of the classroom experience. It's more than having computers in classrooms; it's about combining e-learning, traditional teaching methods and independent study to create an entirely new learning environment for students.

While, the term blended learning may be new, the concept is familiar to most educators. While, on one hand, faculty, administrators and learners find that multimedia and e-learning are able to enhance both teaching and learning, on the other hand, there has been a general educational trend in favour of employing both e-learning and traditional face-to-face classroom teaching. This approach enables medical educators to design programmes that implement the most appropriate learning modalities and technologies to stimulate and promote an effective learning process [49]. Examples includes a lecture supplemented with an online tutorial, a group assignment showing surgical procedures (e.g. laparoscopy) via video streaming or the use of virtual online patients and robot technology [50].

Interestingly, students do not see e-learning as replacing traditional instructor-led training but as a complement to it, forming part of a blended learning strategy. Many universities are now developing full suites of undergraduate and postgraduate programmes in blended curricula that can, in part, be run online through asynchronous teaching (using discussion boards and text-based assignments) and synchronous teaching (using instant messaging, real-time audio tutorials and teleconferencing). Such programmes also involve face-to-face and practical sessions, deemed essential for subjects like medicine, which require learning complex practical, clinical and communication skills underpinned by an extensive knowledge base [49].

In general, supporters of the methodology, whether educators or learners, have a strong feeling that blended learning is the future and that it's the way to make the most of class time while making sure that students get all the background material they need to support their classroom learning. Flexibility and personalisation are two of the main benefits the methodology offers. The combination of real-time teaching with online work at times to suit each individual student means that the student is able to tailor their learning to meet his/her learning needs.

How Does Blended Learning Work?

Blended learning differs slightly from classroom to classroom, depending on how the facilitator feels it works best with their course material, but it has three main components.

1. In-person classroom activities led by the facilitator: One of the biggest advantages of blended learning is that it frees up class time to focus on interactive activities, making the classroom experience more dynamic and allowing students to use their all-important class time to work on projects with peers to make the most of face-to-face time with the facilitator. Taking silent study out of the classroom changes the learning environment hugely and moves the role of teacher disseminating the information to that of facilitator helping the student access and digest information switches up the roles of teacher and student.
2. Online learning materials and study resources: Materials that the students can study online can include prerecorded lectures – often by the same facilitator leading the classes. They're always accessible, so the student can control the time, place and pace of study.
3. Structured independent study time with material from the lectures and using the skills the student has developed in the classroom. Having students access resources on their own time and outside of the classroom puts them at the centre of their own education, encourages them to take responsibility for their own learning and empowers them to take an active role in their education process. It also allows them to develop their skills that they have developed in the classroom, with guidance and support from the facilitator [51].

m-Learning "Apps and Adds"

Mobile learning (m-learning) refers to learning via a mobile device such as a tablet or smartphone. Such devices are ubiquitous among doctors [52] and offer an array of potential benefits [53]. Downloadable applications (apps) give access to an assortment of materials to support workplace learning and decision-making for practitioners [54, 55]. Examples include key medical textbooks configured for use on small devices [56], medical calculators to assist in drug calculations, guidelines (both national and local) and checklists and score systems for diagnosis. In their systematic review of healthcare apps, Mosa et al. [54] reported that apps for disease diagnosis, medical calculators and drug reference were thought to be most useful. Similar findings were reported by Franko and Tirrell [57] where the most common apps were drug guides and medical calculators. A systematic review [58] of handheld computers in clinical practice concluded that, by providing access to information at the point of care, their use could improve healthcare professionals' clinical decision-making. Smartphones with point-of-care tools have also been shown to be valuable in resource-limited settings [59].

In addition to apps, there are also "adds" (or plug-ins) which are hardware extras that are attached to mobile devices. These include thermometers, blood pressure and heart rate monitors, breathalyzers, stethoscopes and ECG monitors and are being used by clinicians and patients [52, 60, 61].

On another front, medical applications (apps) have been suggested to support clinical decision-making, improve communication between hospital staff and improve patient management [62–64]. Studies have indicated frequent use of apps as reference and information management tools in clinical practice, with a trend towards increasing app use among medical practitioners with less training [65–67]. Resident physicians have reported increasing usage of apps in their clinical practice, most commonly drug guides, medical calculators, coding and billing apps and pregnancy wheels [67]. While previous literature has examined the utility of apps for physicians in various medical specialties, less is known about the popularity, reliability and usage of medical apps by medical students [68, 69].

Smartphone app has also been developed and used to collect day-to-day feedback from doctors-in-training and their trainers [70]. The app provides feedback about the training doctors clinical training and supervision and, for trainers, provides feedback about the trainees' performance. This app would be simple to use and very quick to access, meaning that synergistic feedback between doctors-in-training and their trainers could easily be collected on a day-to-day basis after every clinical session. This would overcome the problems of placement feedback being collected infrequently, often at the end of the placement. This feedback could then be used to identify patterns of concern or good practice and areas for development, on a much more regular basis, improving on the current annual review process and providing a much more accurate assessment of training. Ultimately, the aim of this project is to improve patient care and promote excellent healthcare for all through better medical training [71].

Integrating e-Learning into Medical Education

Perhaps the first step should be incorporating e-learning in the medical curriculum. However, the integration of e-learning into existing medical curricula should be the outcome of a well-designed assessment which starts with evaluation of the needs and accomplishes with the decision to use e-learning [72]. Although some institutions have tried to use e-learning as a stand-alone solution to updating or expanding their curricula, the majority preferred starting with an integrated strategy that considers the benefits and burdens of blended learning before revising the curriculum. In undergraduate medical education, e-learning offers learners materials for self-instruction and collaborative learning. In graduate medical education, the Accreditation Council for Graduate Medical Education has established six core competencies towards which e-learning can be applied. e-Learning materials suited for each of these competencies can be integrated into the education of residents and fellows, replacing lectures and other synchronous methods of instruction. Asynchronous e-learning can be effectively used during demanding clinical care rotations, especially when duty hours are limited yet curriculum requirements remain high. In continuing medical education, physicians with daily clinical obligations can attend medical "e-conferences" using e-learning. The complexity and breadth of medical education content, together with the scarcity of experts and resources in e-learning, make the creation of centres of excellence in e-learning a reasonable proposition. The Federal Interagency Working Group on Information Technology Research and Development has recommended the establishment of centres to explore "new delivery modes for educating medical practitioners and providing continuing medical education" [73]; e-learning clearly fits that description. Such centres could offer a wide range of services, including system deployment and administration, training of faculty and administrators, assistance in content development, the design of learning pathways and programmes, marketing and support, supervision, maintenance, research and consultation. The Internet2 is a US-based, collaborative, university-led project started in 1996 to develop additional infrastructure for the Internet backbone capable of superhigh bandwidth [74]. The Internet2's vision of extremely fast-speed, complex real-time multimedia capabilities and quality of service would provide educators enormous potential to enhance the learning experience [12]. Larger bandwidth offers the promise of sophisticated immersive simulations and the use of full-motion video in real time, in both asynchronous and synchronous modes of instruction, delivered to any desktop computer [75]. Many medical schools and healthcare organizations are already producing high-fidelity e-learning materials, such as virtual patient simulations, which could soon be within the reach of any educator and learner [75–77].

The Future of e-Learning in Medical Education

The direction of the future of e-learning in medical education is heavily influenced by three major trends: (1) the rapid adoption of emerging communication, simulation and information technology in undergraduate, graduate and continuing medical education; (2) a national call for competency-based, patient outcome-oriented training across the continuum of education; and (3) the rapidly changing healthcare environment including advances in the biomedical sciences as well as in the diagnoses and management of diseases, organization, financing and delivery of healthcare services and changes in the societal expectations [78].

Developments in e-learning and technologies are creating the groundwork for a revolution in education, allowing learning to be individualized (adaptive learning), enhancing learners' interactions with each other (collaborative learning) and transforming the role of the teacher (from disseminator to facilitator). To complement the traditional teaching, interactive tutorials are developed on a teaching website or what is called a virtual learning environment. The virtual learning environment can contain, for example, clinical cases which are in a problem-based learning format that closely resemble real-life medical scenarios. Cases mainly cover the common cardiac, respiratory or rheumatologic scenarios; they may also include other common emergencies. Links should be also available to useful educational sites, and current clinical guidelines are provided with each case via national or international organizations. Adaptive learning uses technology to assess learners' knowledge, skills and attitudes at the beginning of online training in order to deliver educational materials at the level most appropriate for each learner [15]. Adaptive learning is the ultimate learner-centred experience because it individualizes a unique learning path for each learner that is likely to target his or her specific learning needs and aptitudes. Perceptual learning is a process by which the ability of sensory systems to respond to stimuli is improved through experience. Perceptual learning occurs through sensory interaction with the environment as well as through practice in performing specific sensory tasks.

One of the major challenges to be tackled in e-learning technologies is the potential for collaborative learning to break the isolation of the e-learners. Advances in synchronous distance education and collaborative technologies like Weblogs, message boards, chats, email and teleconferencing are making such collaborative learning more readily available. Quantitative and qualitative studies of collaborative learning in medicine have shown higher levels of learner satisfaction, improvements in knowledge, self-awareness, understanding of concepts, achievement of course objectives and changes in practice [79, 80].

An evolving emphasis within medical education on lifelong learning and competency-based education has forced educators to re-evaluate their traditional roles. In this changing paradigm, educators no longer serve as the sole distributors of content but are becoming facilitators of learning and assessors of competency. e-Learning offers the opportunity for educators to evolve into this new role by providing them with a set of online resources to facilitate the learning process [11].

In conclusion, e-learning can be defined as the act of learning through the use of electronic means to enhance understanding, to improve skills or to gain experience. e-Learning provides potential benefits and vast opportunities for both learners and clinical teachers, enabling access to a massive amount of resources and facilitating communication when face-to-face learning is difficult. However, it is vital to maintain the main focus on improving teaching and learning while acknowledging that new technologies can enhance and facilitate teaching and learning.

References

1. Ozuah PO. Undergraduate medical education: thoughts on future challenges. BMC Med Educ. 2002;2:8–10.
2. Nair BR, Finucane PM. Reforming medical education to enhance the management of chronic disease. Med J Aust. 2003;179:257–9.
3. Leung WC. Competency based medical training: review. BMJ. 2002;325:693–6.
4. Rosenberg M. E-Learning: strategies for delivering knowledge in the digital age. New York: McGraw-Hill; 2001.
5. Wentling T, Waight C, Gallaher J, La Fleur J, Wang C, Kanfer A. E-Learning: a review of literature 2000. http://learning.ncsa.uiuc.edu/papers/elearnlit.pdf. Accessed 14th Feb 2018. 2005. Urbana: University of Illinois National Center for Supercomputer Applications; 2000.
6. Rice S, McKendree J. In: Swanwick T, editor. Understanding medical education: evidence, theory and practice. 2nd ed. Oxford, UK: Wiley; 2014. p. 161–73. Chapter 12.
7. Moberg TF, Whitcomb ME. Educational technology to facilitate medical students' learning: background paper 2 of the medical school objectives project. Acad Med. 1999;74:1146–50.
8. Ward JP, Gordon J, Field MJ, Lehmann HP. Communication and information in medical education. Lancet. 2001;357:792–6.
9. Ellaway R, Masters KAMEE. Guide 32: e-learning in medical education. Part 1: learning, teaching and assessment. Med Teach. 2008;30:455–73.
10. Masic I. E-learning as new method of medical education. Acta Inf Med. 2008;16(2):102–17.
11. Chodorow S. Educators must take the electronic revolution seriously. Acad Med. 1996;71:221–6.
12. Ruiz J, Mintzer M, Leipzig R. The impact of E-learning in medical education. Acad Med. 2006;81(3):207–12.
13. Ward JP, Gordon J, Field MJ, Lehmann HP. Communication and information technology in medical education. Lancet. 2001;357:792–6.
14. Chu LF, Chan BK. Evolution of web site design: implications for medical education on the Internet. Comput Biol Med. 1998;28:459–72.
15. Gibbons A, Fairweather P. Computer-based instruction. In: Tobias S, Fletcher J, editors. Training & retraining: a handbook for business, industry, government, and the military. New York: Macmillan Reference USA; 2000. p. 410–42.
16. Clark D. Psychological myths in e-learning. Med Teach. 2002;24:598–604.
17. Emami H, Najafi L. Key success factors in E-learning in medical education. Aust J Basic Appl Sci. 2011;5(10):1359–64.

18. Smith R. Guidelines for authors of learning objects. http://www.nmc.org/guidelines/NMC/20LO/20Guidelines.pdf. Accessed 22 Mar 2018. Austin: The New Media Consortium; 2004.
19. Littlejohn A. Issues in reusing online resources. In: Littlejohn A, editor. Reusing online resources: a sustainable approach to eLearning. London: Creative Print and Design; 2003. p. 1–6.
20. Johnson CE, Hurtubise LC, Castrop J, et al. Learning management systems: technology to measure the medical knowledge competency of the ACGME. Med Educ. 2004;38:599–608.
21. Phelps C, Michea YF. Learning management systems' evaluation focuses on technology not learning. AMIA Annu Symp Proc. 2003:969.
22. Fallon C, Brown S. E-learning standards: a guide to purchasing and deploying standards-conformant E-learning. Boca Raton: St Lucie Press; 2003.
23. The MedBiquitous Consortium: new educational achievement standard unveiled to track learner progress and milestones. 2017. https://www.medbiq.org/new_educational_achievement_standard_unveiled_to_track_learner_progress_and_milestones. Accessed on 25 Mar 2018.
24. Harden R, Laidlaw J. E-Learning. In: Essential skills for a medical teacher. Churchill: Elsevier; 2012. p. 165–70.
25. Dennick R, Wilkinson S, Purcell N. Online assessment. AMEE guide No 39. Med Teach. 2009;31:192–206.
26. Kirkpatrick DL. Evaluating training programs: the four levels. San Francisco: Berrett-Koehler; 1994.
27. Ellaway R, Poulton T, Fors U, McGee J, Albright S. Building a virtual patient commons. Med Teach. 2008;30:170–4.
28. Harless WG, Drennon GG, Marxer JJ, Root JA, Miller GE. CASE: a computer-aided simulation of the clinical encounter. J Med Educ 1971. 1971;46(5):443–8.
29. Kononowicz A, Hege I. Virtual patients as a practical realisation of the e-learning idea in medicine. In: Soomro S, editor. E-learning experiences and future. InTech. ISBN: 978-953-307-092-6. Available from: http://www.intechopen.com/books/e-learning-experiences-and-future/virtual-patients-as-apractical-realisation-of-the-e-learning-idea-in-medicine.
30. Barrows HS. An overview of the uses of standardized patients for teaching and evaluating clinical skills. AAMC Acad Med. 1993;68(6):443–51. discussion 451–3
31. Bradley P. The history of simulation in medical education and possible future directions. Med Educ. 2006;40:254–62.
32. Zemsky R, Massy WF. Thwarted innovation – what happened to e-learning and why? A final report for the weather station project of the learning alliance at the University of Pennsylvania in cooperation with the Thomson corporation. Pennsylvania: The University of Pennsylvania; 2004. p. 1–76.
33. Miayzoe T, Anderson T. Interaction equivalency in an OER, MOOCS and informal learning era. J Interact Media Educ. 2013;2:Art 9. Available online from: http://jime.open.ac.uk/articles/10.5334/2013-09/. Last accessed Mar 2018
34. Itself, Sharma N, Doherty I, Dong C. Adaptive learning in medical education: the final piece of technology enhanced learning? Ulster Med J. 2017;86(3):198–200.
35. Zimmer T. Rethinking higher Ed: a case for adaptive learning. Forbes. 2014. Available online from: http://www.forbes.com/sites/ccap/2014/10/22/rethinking-higher-ed-a-case-for-adaptive learning/#65a9f1126293. Last accessed Nov 2016.
36. Paramythis A, Loidl-Reisinger S. Adaptive learning environments and eLearning standards. Electron J e-Learning. 2004;2:181–94.
37. Plass, J. (2014). Elsevier adaptive learning. [Internet]. Available online from: http://www.elsevieradvantage.com/article.jsp?pageid=12132. Last accessed Mar 2018.
38. McMahon GT, Drazen JM. Introducing NEJM knowledge+ and its adaptive personalized learning. New Engl J Med. 2014;370(17):1648–9.

39. Kellman PJ. Adaptive and perceptual learning technologies in medical education and training. Mil Med. 2013;178(10 Suppl):98–106.
40. Krasne S, Hillman J, Kellman P, Drake T. Applying perceptual and adaptive learning techniques for teaching introductory histopathology. J Pathol Inf. 2013;4:34.
41. Kellman PJ, Kaiser MK. Perceptual learning modules in flight training. Proceedings of the 38th annual meeting of the human factors and ergonomics society, vol. 18. Santa Monica: Sage Publications; 1994. p. 1183–7.
42. Guerlain S, La Follette M, Mersch TC, Mitchell BA, Poole GR, Calland JF, et al. Improving surgical pattern recognition through repetitive viewing of video clips. IEEE Trans Syst Man Cybern A Syst Hum. 2004;34:699–707.
43. Kellman PJ, Massey CM, Son JY. Perceptual learning modules in mathematics: enhancing students' pattern recognition, structure extraction, and fluency. Top Cogn Sci. 2010;2:285–305.
44. Sowden PT, Davies IR, Roling P. Perceptual learning of the detection of features in X-ray images: a functional role for improvements in adults' visual sensitivity? J Exp Psychol Hum Percept Perform. 2000;26:379–90.
45. Kellman PJ. Adaptive and perceptual learning technologies in medical education and training. Mil Med. 2013;178:98–106.
46. Mettler E, Massey C, Kellman P. Improving adaptive learning technology through the use of response times. In: Carlson L, Holscher C, Shipley T, editors. Proceedings of the 33rd Annual Conference of the Cognitive Science Society. Boston: Cognitive Science Society; 2011. p. 2532–7.
47. Nodine CF, Kundel HL, Mello TC, Weinstein SP, Orel SG, Sullivan DC, et al. How experience and training influence mammography expertise. Acad Radiol. 1999;6:575–85.
48. Speelman C, Martin K, Flower S, Simpson T. Skill acquisition in skin cancer detection. Percept Mot Skills. 2010;110:277–97.
49. Albarrak A. E-learning in medical education and blended learning approach. In: Mendez-Vilas A, editor. Education in a technological world: communicating current and emerging research and technological efforts. Badajoz: Formatex; 2011. p. 147–53.
50. Hayashi T, Tominaga H, Yamasaki T. Blended learning contents for university education. In: The 7th International conference on information technology based higher education and training. Piscataway: IEEE; 2006. p. 499–502.
51. Oakman H. Blended learning – the new normal. Education technology. 2016. https://edtechnology.co.uk/Article/blended-learning-the-new-normal. Accessed on 26 Mar 2018.
52. Gagliani SM, Topol EJ. iMedEd: the role of mobile health technologies in medical education. Acad Med. 2014;89:1207–9. https://doi.org/10.1097/ACM.0000000000000361.
53. Payne KB, Wharrad H, Watts K. Smartphone and medical related app use among medical students and junior doctors in the United Kingdom (UK): a regional survey. BMC Med Inform Decis Mak. 2012;12:121. https://doi.org/10.1186/1472-6947-12-121.
54. Mosa AS, Yoo I, Sheets LA. A systematic review of healthcare applications for smartphones. BMC Med Inform Decis Mak. 2012;12:67. https://doi.org/10.1186/1472-6947-12-67.
55. Bullock A, Fox F, Barnes R, et al. Transitions in medicine: trainee doctor stress and support mechanisms. J Workplace Learn. 2013;25:368–82. https://doi.org/10.1108/JWL-Jul-2012-0052.
56. Hardyman W, Bullock A, Brown A, et al. Mobile technology supporting trainee doctors' workplace learning and patient care: an evaluation. BMC Med Educ. 2013;13:6. https://doi.org/10.1186/1472-6920-13-6.
57. Franko OI, Tirrell TF. Smartphone app use among medical providers in ACGME training programs. J Med Syst. 2012;36:3135–9. https://doi.org/10.1007/s10916-011-9798-7.
58. Mickan S, Atherton H, Roberts NW, et al. Use of handheld computers in clinical practice: a systematic review. BMC Med Inform Decis Mak. 2014;14:56. https://doi.org/10.1186/1472-6947-14-56.

59. Chang AY, Ghose S, Littman-Quinn R, et al. Use of mobile learning by resident physicians in Botswana. Telemed J E Health. 2012;18:11–3. https://doi.org/10.1089/tmj.2011.0050.
60. Lippman H. How apps are changing family medicine. J Fam Pract. 2013;62:362–7.
61. Bullock A, Webb K Technology in postgraduate medical education: a dynamic influence on learning? In: Postgraduate Medical Journal Published Online First. 2015. https://doi.org/10.1136/postgradmedj-2014-132809.
62. Dala-Ali BM, Lloyd MA, Al-Abed Y. The uses of the iPhone for surgeons. Surgeon. 2011;9(1):44–8.
63. Ozdalga E, Ozdalga A, Ahuja N. The smartphone in medicine: a review of current and potential use among physicians and students. J Med Internet Res. 2012;14(5):e128.
64. Prgomet M, Georgiou A, Westbrook JI. The impact of mobile handheld technology on hospital physicians' work practices and patient care: a systematic review. J Am Med Inform Assoc. 2009;16(6):792–801.
65. Boruff JT, Storie D. Mobile devices in medicine: a survey of howmedical students, residents, and faculty use smartphones and other mobile devices to find information. J Med Libr Assoc. 2014;102(1):22–30.
66. Ventola CL. Mobile devices and apps for health care professionals: uses and benefits. Pharm Ther. 2014;39(5):356–64.
67. Franko OI, Tirrell TF. Smartphone app use among medical providers in ACGME training programs. J Med Syst. 2012;36(5):3135–9.
68. Oehler RL, Smith K, Toney JF. Infectious diseases resources for the iPhone. Clin Infect Dis. 2010;50(9):1268–74.
69. Aungst TD. Medical applications for pharmacists using mobile devices. Ann Pharmacother. 2013;47(7–8):1088–95.
70. Gray TG, Hood G, Farrell T. BMJ Innov. 2015;1:25–32. https://doi.org/10.1136/bmjinnov-2014-000011.
71. UK Department of Health. High quality care for all. 2008. http://webarchive.nationalarchives.gov.uk/+/www.dh.gov.uk/en/healthcare/highqualitycareforall/index.htm. Accessed 27 Mar 2018.
72. Kern D, Thomas P, Howard D, Bass E. Curriculum development for medical education. Baltimore: Johns Hopkins University Press; 1998.
73. Reddy R, Wladawsky-Berger I. President's information technology advisory committee. Transforming health care through information technology. Arlington: National Coordination Office for Information Technology Research & Development; 2001.
74. Internet 2 Web page http://www.internet2.edu. Accessed 22 Nov 2005. Ann Arbor: Internet 2 Consortium. 2005.
75. Walker R, Dieter M, Panko W, Valenta A. What it will take to create new Internet initiatives in health care. J Med Syst. 2003;27:95–103.
76. Tidmarsh PJ, Cummings J, Hersh WR, Freidman CP. Distributed medical informatics education using Internet2. Proc AMIA Symp. 2002:787–91.
77. Vincent DS, Berg BW, Hudson DA, Chitpatima ST. International medical education between Hawaii and Thailand over Internet2. J Telemed Telecare. 2003;9(2 suppl):S71–2.
78. Kim S. The future of e-learning in medical education: current trend and future opportunity. J Educ Eval Health Prof. 2006;3:3. https://doi.org/10.3352/jeehp.2006.3.3.
79. Wiecha J, Barrie N. Collaborative online learning: a new approach to distance CME. Acad Med. 2002;77:928–9.
80. Wiecha JM, Gramling R, Joachim P, Vanderschmidt H. Collaborative e-learning using streaming video and asynchronous discussion boards to teach the cognitive foundation of medical interviewing: a case study. J Med Internet Res. 2003;5:e13.

Chapter 14
Simulation in Medical Education

Introduction

Simulation has been defined as "the technique of imitating the behaviour of some situation or process" (whether economic, military, mechanical, medical, etc.) by means of suitably analogous situation or apparatus, especially for the purpose of study or personal training [1].

In medical training, simulation has a long history. The start was the use of very basic models to enable learners to practice skills and techniques (such as in obstetrics). In spite of such early start, medical simulation did not attain any fame or widespread use over the past decades. This was attributed to reluctance to implement new teaching methods, characters of the educators (educators mostly represent generation X), lack of technological facilities or cost. With advances in knowledge, educational theories and computer sciences, a wide range of modalities have been developed such as virtual reality, high-fidelity manikins and perceptual learning. These science and technology advances, together with increased awareness of patient safety, increased pressure on educators both in time and number as well as the characters of the new generation, the Millennials, who has always been treated as special and important, able to work under pressure and tech savvy, have promoted simulation as an option to traditional clinical skills teaching (Fig. 14.1). Although a wide range of simulation activities has been developed and is available, these are still linked with specific medical specialities rather than centrally managed or resourced.

There is widespread agreement, supported by robust research, systematic reviews and meta-analysis, on what makes effective simulation. Simulation-based learning has been implemented in undergraduate, as well as postgraduate, education, in both general and speciality-based curricula, as well as clinical and nonclinical contexts. Simulation endorses the acquisition of procedural skills through repetition, deliberate practice with feedback. It also supports the acquisition of nontechnical skills such as communication, teamworking and leadership.

Y. El Miedany, *Rheumatology Teaching*,
https://doi.org/10.1007/978-3-319-98213-7_14

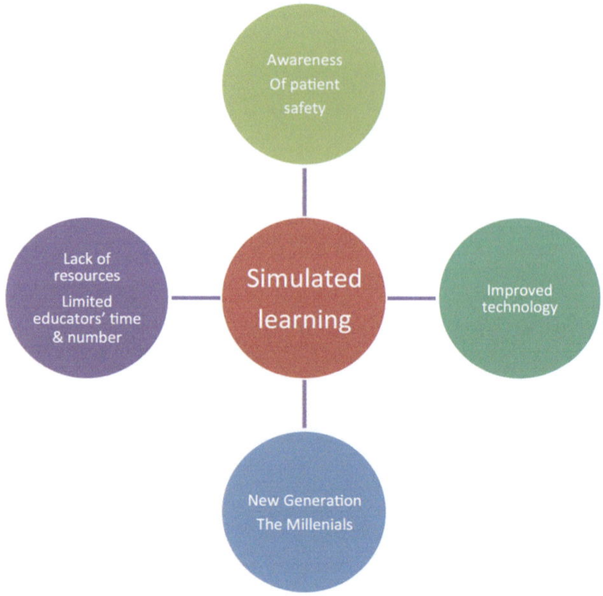

Fig. 14.1 Promoting factors for developing simulated learning

Providing high-quality educational experiences is vital if learners are to engage in simulation with all its challenges; however, assessment drives much of the learning, and stimulation has a huge role to play in ensuring that health professionals are fit, safe and competent to practice. Simulation can be implemented in preparation for both formative (developmental) and summative (contributing to grade or score) assessments. Well-designed simulation provides excellent opportunities for learners to receive timely and specific feedback from the educators as well as real, virtual and simulated patients which in turn is expected to endorse the trainee's clinical and communication skills.

This chapter will discuss the art and science of simulated learning, the simulation fidelity continuum (low to high, multimode) and how it can be tailored to the learner's needs. It will also discuss using simulation for assessment, how to design an effective simulation-based medical education activity as well as approach to evaluation of a simulation learning activity. It will expand to include curriculum integration and simulated learning in rheumatology and then will conclude with future directions of simulation-based education.

The Science of Simulation-Based Learning

Simulation plays a central role in the student-directed learning model [2, 3]. It enhances the concept of "need to know", as it mimics real-life situations and gives students the chance to perform and practice procedures, both with a safe controlled environment and the possibility to determine in advance the nature of the cases to be assessed. Thus, it becomes feasible to cover in an ordered manner the most important and relevant disorders whether acute that require immediate intervention or chronic that require assessment of the disease activity/severity and its associated comorbidities. It also helps in overcoming the expected variability of real scenarios in the hospital setting.

In simulation-based learning, the training is mainly focused on skills learning which in the healthcare education setting reflects a variety of tasks including perceptual, cognitive, motor, technical, problem-solving, decision-making and social interaction. Clinical skills learning in simulation context often involves a composite of several of these aspects in addition to a biomedical knowledge base and some coordinated physical, cognitive and/or social activities [4]. On another front, a critical aspect of simulation is constant feedback [5]. This task is mainly done through debriefing, which must be seen as a unique opportunity to reinforce the core assumptions of adult learning as well as provide external motivation and stimulate guided reflection. Understanding how the experience affects future practice is a crucial step to improve performance [6].

In spite of the diversity of contexts and numerous targets, the outcomes of simulation-based learning are similar. In fact, various objectives can be accomplished by adopting simulation, but in all cases it can be tailored to meet the adult learning assumptions. Dreyfus and Dreyfus [7] reported that this approach helps learners progress from apprentice to skilled and from stepwise task executer performing a rule-based action or ticking box to instinctive and situationally fluent actions. The purpose of the educational use of simulation is to provide learning opportunities for the participants. The "as-if" during simulation is a "cognitive tool" for learning not the goal [8]. According to this line of thinking, some as-if processes help people to learn, orient oneself in the world and construct relevant meaning.

On the facilitators' side, the different phases of the simulation setting imply different roles for them. During the introduction to the simulation, facilitators might instruct, whereas, during the scenario, it might be necessary for the instructor to leave the educational role and become a protector, if the participants engaged in dangerous activities (e.g. unsafe handling of the defibrillator). During the debriefing, the facilitator might have a floating role, sometimes facilitate, and other times can be coach or devil's advocate. However, in all scenarios, the effective facilitator should have the skills to move seamlessly into different appropriate roles and to develop meaningful learning relationships with the learners [4, 9].

The social nature of simulation-based learning implies that the interaction between those involved impacts on learning, and learners need to feel motivated, engaged in the fiction contract and open to learning [5]; feeling like being tricked and exposed during simulation inhibits learners engagement [10]. One the other hand, one of the advantages of simulation settings is that they offer possibilities for augmented feedback. Feedback can be an in-built part of the simulation (e.g. vital signs that change, providing feedback about treatment options) or via comments from role players. It can also specifically be part of an augmentation of simulation, where special monitors or displays provide the additional information or where role players are introduced in their augmented role. Strategies to stop and restart the scenario or leave the framework of the simulation completely (having time out) can help participants develop specific abilities.

Simulation Fidelity Continuum (Low to High, Multimode)

The degree of practicality or authenticity ranges along a scale from completely artificial to an actual real-life situation. A stem of a patient scenario or a clinical vignette that involves the learner to make a clinical decision is a simulation at the low end of the fidelity continuum. Assessments using simulated patients are at the high end of the fidelity continuum, giving a more realistic context for measuring clinical skills and competencies [11, 12].

In their report, Norcini and McKinley [13] noted that test designers may try to reconstruct actual life circumstances or elaborate tasks in a simulation that will result in a long test with narrow sampling. Due to practical limitations, a long test will contain few problems, which limits the generalizability of scores to the domain of interest. They recommend balancing fidelity and breadth of sampling as these will affect reliability, validity, educational impact, feasibility and acceptability of the assessment method.

Multimode simulation is the combination of inanimate models with standardized patient to provide a convincing learning environment. Standardized patient takes part in realistic quasi-clinical scenarios, where procedures can be practiced on models attached to the standardized patient [14–16]. Kneebone et al. suggested the integration of technical clinical skills with effective communication skills. A study was carried out to explore the feasibility and benefits of a conceptual model for integrated skills teaching [14]. The feasibility of a simulated activity was assessed where clinical skills including suturing a wound and urinary catheter insertion are taught and evaluated coincidentally with attention to doctor–patient interaction, patient comfort and patient privacy. Results revealed that the integrated model was feasible and valuable. Benefits included the opportunity to integrate, within a safe environment, and skills which are often taught separately. It was suggested that promoting reflective practice may also enable the successful transfer of these integrated skills to other procedures. Therefore the multimode simulation offered the advantage of merging the best features of inanimate simulation with animate standardized patients to present realistic clinical challenges for education and evaluation [16].

Simulation Fidelity Tailored to the Learner's Level

Though the value of simulations has been assessed in several studies and reported to be valuable, few articles have compared the educational outcomes between high- and low-fidelity simulations. While Matsumoto et al. [17], Lee et al. [18] and de Giovanni et al. [19] did not find any significant differences in performance on comparing subjects trained on a low- to those on high-fidelity simulator, based on assessment of the learnt skills, Scerbo et al. [20] reported better performance in the low-fidelity simulator-trained group. In contrast, Crofts et al. [21], Grady et al. [22] and Rodgers et al. [23] reported better performance in favour of higher-fidelity simulator training. However, the outcomes of these three studies [21–23] which reported superior performance in the cohorts trained by a high-fidelity simulator were highly criticized. The criticism was based on the finding that the outcome performance of both low- and high-fidelity simulator trained groups was evaluated using the high-fidelity simulator. This was considered as a bias as the training was carried out on the lower-fidelity simulator, while the high-fidelity simulator was used for performance evaluation [24].

In two studies, performance was evaluated based on a neutral task where the optimal goal was transfer of knowledge/skills to a real patient. In the de Giovanni et al. study, diagnostic accuracy and communication skills were equivalent regardless of the degree of simulator fidelity [19]. In another study carried by Scerbo et al. [20], transfer of phlebotomy training to a real patient was better with the low-fidelity trained group. This was attributed to what Smallman and St. John described as "naive realism" (naive realism describes people's tendency to believe that they perceive the social world "as it is"—as objective reality—rather than as a subjective construction and interpretation of reality). This term describes the desire among users for higher fidelity despite contrary to its efficacy evidence [25]. Simulators are meant to support learning objectives. A study which reviewed 109 articles for conditions of high-fidelity simulations that lead to effective learning [26] reported that the 3 conditions linked to effective learning (which were most cited in 25–47% of the articles) were provision of feedback, repetitive practice and curriculum integration. These are features of learning and are not characteristics of simulation fidelity.

In view of these findings, a question was raised regarding which parameters should be considered when selecting the appropriate simulation-based learning approach. Earlier studies reported that different levels of fidelity may be needed for different objectives and levels of trainees [21, 27]. This agreed with another work which reported that the level of fidelity should be appropriate to the type of task and training stage [28]. To facilitate learning and improve user performance of simulations, Smallman and St. John [24] suggested that training systems should be developed from a minimalist perspective, presenting only the essential material needed for a given level of performance. Therefore, a novice can achieve similar or higher skills transfer with a simple simulator, for example, a clinical vignette, than with a complex training aid such as a simulated environment [12, 29]. At more advanced levels of training, the level of fidelity should support higher levels of speed and practice of a task (Fig. 14.2). In laparoscopy training, the low-cost and low-fidelity training box for assessment of skills was found to be superior to high-cost and high-fidelity virtual reality laparoscopy training [28]. This has also been confirmed in a randomized crossover study [30]. Similar findings were noted in the learning outcomes for a neonatal resuscitation programme (NRP). In a randomized controlled study, use of the low- and high-fidelity mannequin simulators resulted in similar levels of objectively measured neonatal resuscitation programme (NRP) outcomes for integrated skills station and teamwork performance [31]. On the other hand, high fidelity was more advantageous than low fidelity in shoulder dystocia training and nursing learning [21, 32]. These variations in findings are merely due to the approach of evaluating a simulation-based learning programme and the design of the studies. Therefore, it can be concluded that a simulator is best utilized if used in alignment

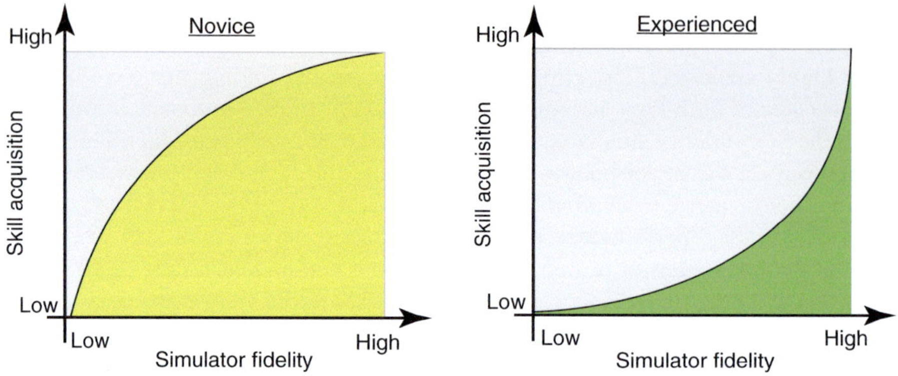

Fig. 14.2 Simulation fidelity tailored to the learner's level: low-fidelity vs high-fidelity simulators. A novice can achieve higher skills with a simple low-fidelity simulator than with a complex training aid. At more advanced levels of training, the level of fidelity should support higher levels of speed and practice of a task; hence, high-fidelity simulator is advised

with educational goals that underpin its use within a programme and that one of the arts of simulation is tailoring educational objectives according to available resources, a process in which innovation and student participation may play a central role.

The Art of Simulation: The Teamwork

Failures of the teamwork have been highlighted as a chief contributor to poor patients' outcomes. The growing complexity of the healthcare delivery mandated a similar growing need for healthcare service to be provided as a teamwork to be able to serve the patients' best interests. Simulation-based learning is a good example of such team cooperation. Simulation-based team training can also be used to improve communication and performance within the healthcare system. Though when talking about simulated learning, the use of advanced tools, gadgets and facilities dominates the discussion, effective simulated learning methodology is based also on two other pillars: the educators and the simulated patients. Here comes the art of the simulation-based learning where the translation of learning between different complexity settings and grades is a vital insight to develop in learners, especially if trying to support the course of learning to develop from the stage of achieving competency to that of proficiency, mastery and even expert performance. The educator plays a critical role in exercising this mental model and reinforcing the need for learners to reflect "on practice", "in practice" and "for practice" in order to improve individual performance. The important role of the simulated patients is also getting more acknowledged and professionalized to maintain their high level of contribution and ensure regular assessment of the simulated patients' capabilities and skills. Therefore, ensuring the harmony, cooperation and training among the team members is essential for the success of the simulation learning process. The spectrum of ways in which simulation is applied to healthcare and determines the appropriate relation between the educator and participants has been suggested in a review article about the future vision of simulation in healthcare [33]. The author provided a comprehensive framework for understanding the diversity of applications of simulation in healthcare, as categorized by 11 different dimensions (Fig. 14.3), to provide a vision of how fully integrating simulation into the structures and processes of healthcare can be used to revolutionize patient care and patient safety and to provide an overview of the driving forces and implementation mechanisms by which different entities may, or may not, disseminate simulation.

Simulation-Based Faculty

"Faculty" is a term that has got variable interpretations among healthcare educational and clinical practice communities. The term "faculty" is often used interchangeably to describe simulation-based educators, healthcare simulation educator, clinical educator, teacher or other individuals who facilitate learning. The purpose and nature of the educational activity would have an impact on how the educator and learner would interact. It may also mandate the adoption of variable interaction approaches between the faculty educator and the learners. Approaches of interaction between the faculty and the learners during simulation-based activities include: (1) Instructor

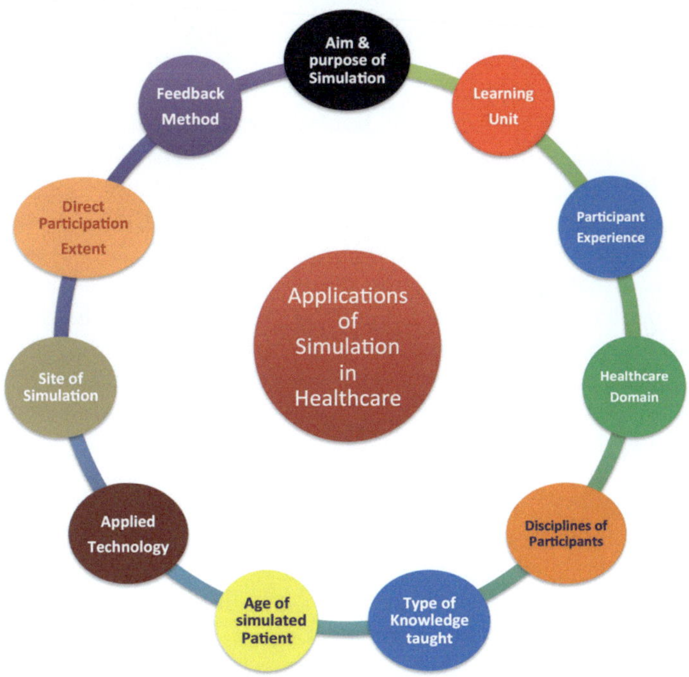
Aim & purpose of Simulation
Learning Unit
Participant Experience
Healthcare Domain
Disciplines of Participants
Type of Knowledge taught
Age of simulated Patient
Applied Technology
Site of Simulation
Direct Participation Extent
Feedback Method
Applications of Simulation in Healthcare

Fig. 14.3 Spectrum of applications of simulation in healthcare. (Adapted from Gaba [45], with permission)

or expert: Likely to be analytical, such as in learning new skills like cannulation or basic life support skills where the educator will adopt a directive instructional style whether during the learners' performance or in the feedback. (2) Coach: Likely to be didactic tuition, where the coach demonstrates the procedure or behaviour and provides more direct feedback with clear guidance about improving performance. (3) Mentor: Likely to be supervision or facilitation, where the educator encourages the learners to critically question their own reasoning and assess their decision-making actions as well as behaviour. Feedback is given through open questioning giving the learners the chance to reflect on their performance and how this can be improved and how to achieve this. (4) Examiner: Likely to be assessor or researcher, where the examiner interacts with the learner in a way to actively and objectively optimize observation of key actions with little immediate feedback regarding analysis of performance. (5) Quality improvement lead: Likely to be dealing with quality improvement, patient safety, governance or leading a clinical service. The nature of the interaction between the educator and those participating in the simulated practice activity is determined by its purpose [34–36].

Simulated Patients

The term "simulated patient" is often used interchangeably with standardized patient, role player, medical actor, simulator, clinical teaching associate, patient educator (instructor) or patient expert. Simulated patients were first used in the 1960s, with their use in medical undergraduate and postgraduate education expanding rapidly since the 1980s [37].

Simulated patient is someone who has been trained to play actively a specific patient when given a history of a case incorporating relevant symptoms, signs, emotions and behaviour, whereas standardized patient incorporates simulated patients as well as real patients who have been coached to present their own illness in a standardized way.

Training is essential to making simulated encounters as real and as standardized as possible, particularly in high-stakes summative assessments. There is wide international experience of using simulated patients in most clinical specialties, although children, the very elderly and some mental health problems are difficult to simulate in this medium and are therefore perhaps underrepresented in assessment and training. Alternatives such as videoing clinical encounters for teaching and assessment are being implemented.

Ker and Bradley [38] summarized the potential applications of such simulation as follows: (1) Routine learning and rehearsal of clinical and communication skills at all levels (2) Routine basic training of individuals and teams (3) Practice of complex clinical situations (4) Training of teams in crisis resource management (5) Rehearsal of serious and/or rare events (6) Rehearsal of planned, novel or infrequent interventions (7) Induction into new clinical environments and use of equipment (8) Design and testing of new clinical equipment (9) Performance assessment of staff at all levels (10) Refresher training of staff at all levels.

Using Simulation for Assessment

Simulation provides a wide range of opportunities to assess learners. A critical review of simulation-based medical education research published by McGaghie et al. [34], defined the importance of quality assessment when simulation is used as a training modality. The comprehensive review identified 12 characteristics and best practices, which every simulation teacher should recognize, to achieve maximum education benefit using medical simulation. The review highlighted that assessment is integral to at least seven of the best practice elements: (1) Secure that chances for feedback (both formative and summative) are used appropriately. (2) Offer facilities for deliberate rehearsal involving focused repetitive practice and assessment. (3) Confirm curriculum integration so that simulation is incorporated into the wider curriculum to complement clinical education. (4) Outline outcome measurements for educational interventions to establish reliability and validity of those interventions. (5) Provide opportunities/programs for mastery learning (deliberate practice with clearly defined learning objectives with set minimal standards required before progression to further stages). (6) Establish use for high-stakes testing procedures including undergraduate/postgraduate examinations and licensing of professionals. (7) Ensure simulation training is used in the correct educational and professional context.

Schuwirth and van der Vleuten categorized simulation-based assessment methods using Miller's pyramid model of medical competence [39]. Written and computer-based simulations are aimed at measuring the "knows how" layer, observation-based techniques such as standardized patient-based examinations, and objective structured clinical examinations target the "shows how" layer, and performance practice measures assess performance at the "does" layer (Fig. 14.4). Examples of these methods include the patient management problem, clinical vignettes, followed by multiple-choice questions or short answers, extended matching questions and script concordance tests. The patient management problem (PMP), a device increasingly used for assessment of medical competence, responds to the concern that more traditional techniques for objective evaluation, such as use of the multiple-choice question (MCQ), are often restricted in their content or scope. Though they can reliably test what is known about various aspects of health and illness, they commonly fail to evaluate realistically the process of healthcare. The patient management problem attempts to put the student or physician (the "test-taker") figuratively into a setting recognizable as belonging to real life, and within that setting (where specified resources are available) presents a clinical problem for solution or management. Given a clearly stated problem in a defined setting, the test-taker is asked to choose among a variety of alternatives for action, some of which may be appropriate, others either not appropriate or even contraindicated. In contrast to the MCQ, which would simply have the choices scored as correct or incorrect, the patient management problem not only records such scores but, in addition, gives the test-taker the results of the actions selected, usually through development of a latent image embodied in invisible ink. For example, if a blood test is selected as appropriate, the test taker who follows instructions to develop a latent image placed opposite the choice will see the

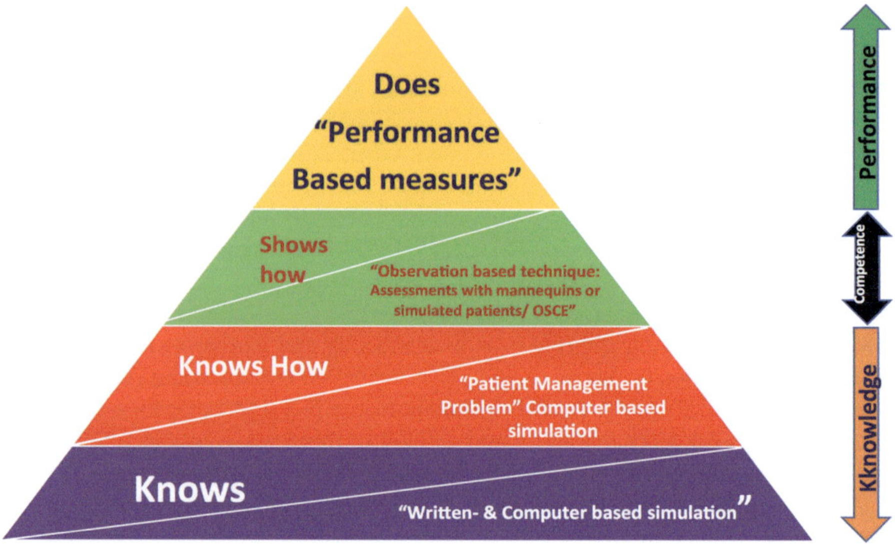

Fig. 14.4 Categorized simulation-based assessment methods using Miller's pyramid model of medical competence. Written and computer-based simulations are aimed at measuring the "knows how" layer, observation-based techniques such as standardized patient-based examinations and objective structured clinical examinations target the "shows how" layer and performance practice measures assess performance at the "does" layer

results of the test appear [40]. Assessments with mannequins or simulated patients test at the shows how level. Performance in actual healthcare practice tests at the level of does. No single simulation-based assessment method will assess the entire range of medical competencies [41]. A suitable combination is needed to cover all layers of Miller's pyramid.

A high-stakes test is any test used to make important decisions about students, educators, schools or districts, most commonly for the purpose of accountability, i.e., the attempt by federal, state or local government agencies and school administrators to ensure that students are enrolled in effective schools and being taught by effective teachers. In general, "high stakes" means that test scores are used to determine punishments (such as sanctions, penalties, funding reductions, negative publicity), accolades (awards, public celebration, positive publicity), advancement (grade promotion or graduation for students) or compensation (salary increases or bonuses for administrators and teachers). A "low-stakes test" would be used to measure academic achievement, identify learning problems or inform instructional adjustments, among other purposes [42].

Simulation-based educational programmes may require relatively heavy resources in terms of faculty: participant ratio as well as the programme capital costs to set up. However, simulation provides excellent chances to create authentic scenarios and observe skills which may be difficult to assess using other assessment tools [43]. In high-fidelity simulation, formative assessment commonly takes the form of the post-scenario debrief and covers both technical and nontechnical aspects of the performance. The importance of the debriefing has been widely highlighted by educationalists as a powerful tool where reflective practice can increase the value of the educational experience. A formative assessment, accompanied by comprehensive feedback, can inform learners about their current levels of performance, highlight their individual strengths and weaknesses and point the way towards future learning and development. The educational impact of such an assessment can be positive and strong. On the other hand, a summative assessment that reports no more than a simple pass/fail decision for each examinee gives those who fail little idea how they might pass next time and therefore has little effect on learning. Therefore, the use of immediate feedback performed in simulated learning has been reported to be very beneficial [44].

The potential advantages of simulation include the highly reproducible nature of activities and scenarios plus the ability to observe how actually individuals perform. In this way, simulation can reveal competence of a doctor who "shows how" rather than just "knows how" in Miller's clinical assessment hierarchy [45]. Furthermore, in response to fresh attempts to identify what professionalism is and how to evaluate it, behaviours and attitudes can be assessed which can elicit aspects of the participant's professionalism [46]. Simulation, including the use of clinical skills assessment, simulated patient, objective structured clinical examinations (OSCE) and immersive simulation, can be used alongside workplace-based assessment methods to assess a trainee's ability at the performance levels of "shows how" and "does". Simulation may also have an increasing part to play in performance-based assessment which is usually used to assess clinical skills and behaviour [47].

Lastly, using simulation to assess the trainees' performance and competence may facilitate the standardization of assessments with key index cases and the ability to use the same assessors for some specific cases. The potential to use simulation for standardizing the assessment of procedural skills has been highlighted in the medical education literature in parallel with the need for development of appropriate, reliable and valid metrics [48].

Criticisms remain regarding the use of simulation for high-stakes assessment including limited realism of medical simulators, inability to control for simulator related behaviours such as hypervigilance (increased state of vigilance and awareness which may result in over reaction) and cavalier attitudes (behaviour induced by the knowledge that this is not a real patient, which may hamper how well the simulated setting mirrors the way the participant would respond to real life), plus the use of complicated scoring methods [49]. Further work is required to address these criticisms including scoring refinement methods and the development of feasible assessment models that implement suitable numbers of scenarios and assessors to establish acceptable reliability for high-stakes assessment. These models should be appraised in high-stakes setting with criterion-related measures embedded, so that comparisons can be made with current standards of assessment in such circumstances.

How to Design an Effective Simulation-Based Medical Education Activity

Defining Goals and Modality

The effectiveness of medical simulation depends on the appropriate application of its methodology and on the knowledge of its different modalities. The simulation modalities can be classified into five major groups (Fig. 14.5) [50, 51]:

1. Low technology: relatively low-cost models or mannequins used to teach basic knowledge or particular psychomotor skills
2. Screen-based computer simulators: software for training and assessment of clinical knowledge and decision-making
3. Simulated/standardized patients: actors trained to play patients, which enables training and assessment of history taking, physical examination, communication skills and professionalism

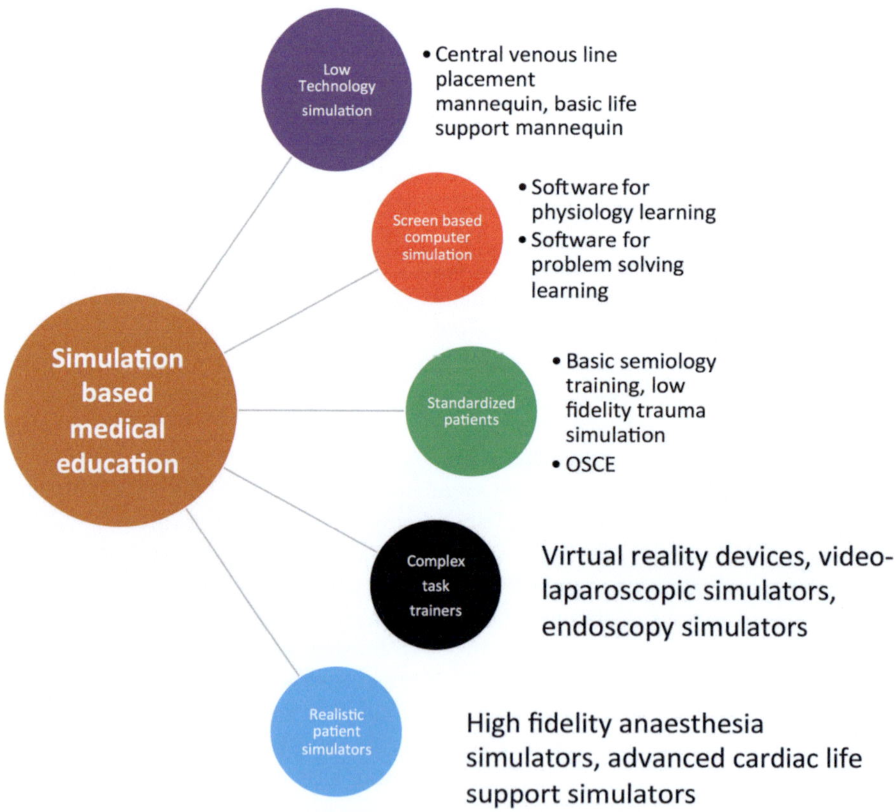

Fig. 14.5 Simulation modalities and examples of applications of simulation-based medical education that can be applied for each modality

4. Complex task trainers: computer-based simulators used for high-fidelity training of procedures
5. Realistic patient simulators: computer-based mannequins used for high-fidelity replication of complex and high-risk clinical conditions in lifelike settings

Despite there are different simulation methodologies with wide applicability, there is no right or wrong template for a simulation exercise. Several combinations of techniques are possible depending on who the target population, previous background and the specific educational goals of the activity.

How the Medical Simulation Session Works

According to Pazin et al. [52], a simulation session is characterized by the presence of four core components (Fig. 14.6). The first component is termed "exposure", which consists of the trainees' introduction to the problem ahead, and it is also referred as "briefing". The second element is "sequence", defined by a progressively escalating complexity during the session, which helps the trainees to build upon consolidated knowledge and allows them to have a better performance throughout the exercise. The third core component is named "feedback", and it refers to the continuous exchange of information between trainer and trainee. This process takes place during and/or after the simulation session, and the instructor must be observant of the trainees' abilities and performance in order to guide the learning process. Finally, the last component is "repetition", which provides improved retaining of

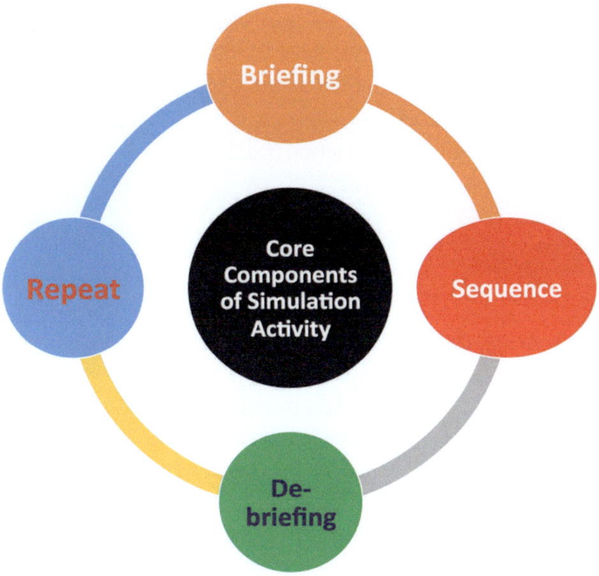

Fig. 14.6 Core components of simulation activity

knowledge learned during a session. The methodology of simulation-based medical education was reviewed in an article published by Jones et al. [53]. The medical simulation activity should include:

Preparation

The preparation of a simulation session involves the creation of a welcoming and positive learning environment. Trainees should be presented to all materials and resources that may be used during simulation, as well as become familiarized with terms and singular aspects of simulation—such as which decisions should be explicitly mentioned, what aspects of physical examination will be measured or told by the trainer and others. Such systematic approach avoids unexpected breaks in the virtual reality pact, an agreement with all involved personnel that commits them to the scenario and provides the concentration and emotional binding that are essential to educational success [52].

Conduction

Dealing with the trainee during simulation is a dynamic and complex task. There are different ways to approach this task, and there is no single best method. The decision on how to perform an intervention, whether or not to help with clues, how flexible to be with various types of conduct deviations and when to stop, allowing, forbidding or forcing a "patient" to die are all key aspects that should be addressed when defining how the trainer will guide the scenario. These decisions should be taken according to learning objectives and trainee preparation [53].

When using sophisticated manikins, it is usually necessary to sketch a flowchart with all possible pre-set scenarios. This may be useful also for training standardized patients and for less experienced trainers.

Debriefing

Debriefing, also referred to as guided reflection, is a planned session after the simulation and is led by the instructor, who provides students with the time to assess their decisions, actions, communication and ability to deal with the unexpected. The goals of a debriefing session are to give the opportunity to the trainees to conceptualize the learning goals set by the trainers and gain insight towards a better understanding of the event and its application on future experiences [54].

Although there are several models of debriefing techniques [54–57], there is no gold standard approach to the debriefing session. However, debriefing is generally considered to be a time for the participant to reflect on the event, discuss it with others, learn and modify behaviour as a result. During the briefing session, it is recognized that the trainer must act as a facilitator, and his or her ability to assess the trainees' skill is fundamental for the learning process. In addition, facilitators must create a nonthreatening environment that promotes active participation of trainees through the use of open-ended questions and positive reinforcement [56]. The use of audio-visual tools helps trainees to analyse, synthesize and evaluate the experience in order to be able to apply the lessons in future events.

Debriefing provides learners an opportunity to learn from their mistakes, and therefore is the one of the ways in which many of the advantages of simulation occur, as previously discussed. It is also applied following real clinical settings, and it has been successfully implemented in obstetrics [58], resuscitation [59] and critical care [60].

Approach to Evaluation of a Simulation Learning Activity

Norman and his colleagues defined five characteristics for simulations: fidelity, reliability, validity, learning and feasibility (Fig. 14.7) [61]. First, fidelity is the extent to which the appearance and behaviour of the simulation match the appearance and behaviour of the simulated system [12]. In 1954, Miller made an important distinction in simulations between the engineering or physical fidelity and the psychological or functional fidelity. Engineering fidelity is the extent to which the simulation replicates the physical characteristics of the actual task. This involves the environment and simulation device or tool. Psychological fidelity is the extent to which the skills of the real task are captured by the simulated task [62]. Matthews and Yachemetz described four levels of simulation fidelity. The aim was to develop a common language in clinical simulation terminology [63]. Level 1 (SF1) is state-of-the-art fidelity, in which a computer-aided mannequin interacts with the trainees. Level 2 (SF2) is high fidelity, which includes a complex scenario that may involve multiple mannequins. Level 3 (SF3) is intermediate fidelity, which involves a series of procedures put together to resemble a simple scenario found in a clinical setting. Level 4 (SF4) is low fidelity, which is meant to demonstrate a simple skill, for example, airway management on an intubation head.

As far as the second character "reliability" is concerned, Ebel and Frisbie operationally defined reliability as the following: "The reliability coefficient for a set of scores from a group of examinees is the coefficient of correlation between that set of scores and another set of scores on an equivalent test obtained independently from the members of the same group". The definition has three main points that should be highlighted. First, reliability is a measure of the measurement tool when applied to a specific group of participants. The better the fit between the exam difficulty and participant ability, the higher the reliability. Second, the definition states that a correlation coefficient is used as a measure of reliability. A property of the correlation coefficient is that it is a relative not an absolute measure. This implies that if the differences between the scores for the same candidate are small relative to the differences between the scores for different candidates, the test will yield high

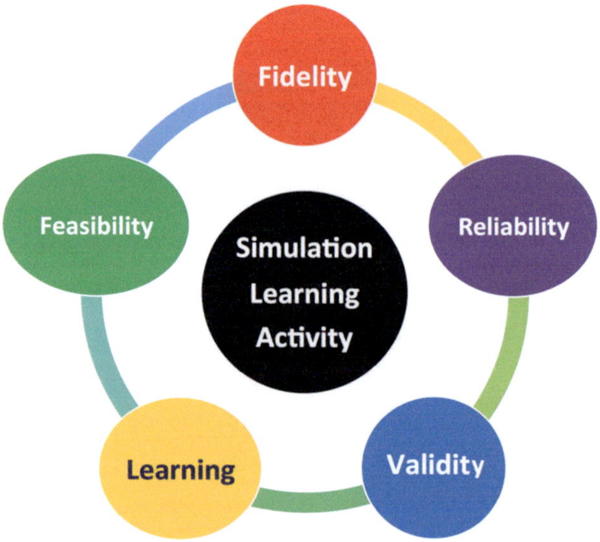

Fig. 14.7 Evaluation of a simulation learning activity: the five characteristics for simulation learning activity assessment

reliability [64]. The definition emphasizes two or more independent measures obtained from equivalent tests of the same construct for each candidate within the group being assessed. This mandates the foundation of the various types of reliability such as test-retest, equivalent forms and split-halves.

The third character "validity" is defined as the extent to which a measurement tool measures the intended outcome. Palter and Grantcharov categorized the tools for assessing technical skills in clinical simulations into high and moderate validity [65]. High-validity tools include global rating scales and virtual reality simulators. The global rating scale relies on the assessment of an expert observer using predefined criteria to assess ability. Virtual reality simulators provide immediate feedback on performance by recording performance metrics such as time. Moderate-validity tools include checklist scales, analysis of dexterity and procedure-specific checklists. Checklist scales and procedure-specific checklists are observational tools that rely on an expert assessor. Analysis of dexterity measures performance by the speed and number of a surgeon's hand movements. The evidence for validity of all of the high- and moderate-validity measurement tools were outlined based on observational studies [24].

Fourth, the "learning" impact of simulation studies can be categorized by Kirkpatrick's four levels of training evaluation: reaction, learning, behaviour and results [66]. The first level includes the assessment of participants' reactions to the use of simulation. The second level involves a quantitative indicator to measure the increase in knowledge or improvement of skills due to the learning experience. The third level is the assessment of the behavioural change or knowledge application in improving performance in a clinical setting. In other words, the third level assesses the transfer of skills learned through simulations to actual clinical encounters. Level 4 involves a broader impact of simulation training on the organization.

Last, “feasibility” describes the degree to which the simulation is affordable and feasible to implement. The two criteria to judge feasibility are required cost and value to be attained [61].

Curriculum Integration

Simulation-based medical education is one of many educational approaches that is used most powerfully and effectively to achieve learning objectives in concert with other educational methods. It complements clinical education but cannot substitute for training grounded inpatient care in real clinical settings [67, 68].

When a simulation programme is implemented, it usually complements an existing curriculum. Simulation is one of several teaching strategies available to healthcare educators. Others include lectures; problem-based learning; hospital, ambulatory and community-based clinical experience, peer-assisted learning; and multimedia computer-based learning. Incorporating simulation into the curriculum by first determining where it will best be used leads to a more effective use of the modality. The simulation experience must be planned, scheduled, implemented and evaluated in the context of a broader medical curriculum. Integration of simulation can occur at the course level or on a larger scale across an entire curriculum. The general concepts and principles are the same for both approaches. Importance of curriculum integration in simulation-based healthcare education simulation exercises is most successful when they become part of the standard curriculum and not an extraordinary, additional component [34, 69]. Determining which components of a curriculum are enhanced using simulation-based education, and incorporating the exercises into the existing model, results in a more goal-directed and sustained use of the tool. This approach has the added benefit of helping determine what personnel, equipment, space and economic resources will be needed to carry out the training. Also, for an existing curriculum, it allows for a critical review of how the curriculum is being administered and how learning objectives are best met using the different teaching modalities available to the healthcare educator. Developing a comprehensive plan before implementation will save time and valuable resources [70].

Simulated Learning in Rheumatology

The inadequacy of the medical curriculum to address musculoskeletal disorders and diseases has long been recognized and has received increased attention in the last decade. One of the major challenges for curriculum developers in the health professions is that the musculoskeletal system has multiple varying conditions, injuries and pathology [71].

In concordance with healthcare training, teaching musculoskeletal medicine has traditionally depended on patient contact. However, changes in healthcare delivery and the availability of real patients, coupled with concerns about lack of standardization of clinical examinations, led to the introduction of the simulation-based learning. This was supported by experience attained over the past 20 years, where there has been increasing interest in simulation as a tool to develop student and trainee procedural skills in a realistic but safe environment. Simulation can vary from part-task trainers (e.g. joint injection manikins), through integrated simulators (e.g. SimMan), simulated patients (trained actors) and simulated environments (e.g. hospital wards). These approaches meet the criteria required for adult learning, that is, problem-orientated experiential learning. Furthermore, they facilitate the development of a community of practice, particularly if such programmes provide longitudinal experience within the same group. Inter-professional training sessions using integrated simulators have been shown to improve the subsequent teamworking climate, with improved ability to communicate disagreement between professional groups. Results of an earlier study [72] documented the growing evidence that simulated learning environments such as simulated wards can be used to develop the musculoskeletal nontechnical skills. However, more recently rheumatology practice has moved progressively away from inpatient care, and ward-based simulation may therefore no longer be the ideal setting for such educational interventions. Studies were carried out to assess simulated educational approaches to management of rheumatology patients in outpatient or community settings. A pilot simulation course was run for rheumatology trainees to provide education in the identification and management of rheumatology emergencies and aid development of nontechnical skills. Five scenarios were used including scleroderma renal crisis, methotrexate pneumonitis, acute lupus myocarditis, catastrophic antiphospholipid syndrome and ANCA-positive vasculitis presenting with pulmonary haemorrhage. The running of the scenarios lasted 20 min, with debriefing taking between 30 and 40 min. Post-course questionnaires assessing confidence scores, session rating as well as general feedback were used to assess the course. Results revealed overall improved trainee confidence in identifying and managing these rheumatology emergencies. It also highlighted nontechnical skills and was felt to be a satisfactory teaching method by all the participants and trainers. Other studies were carried out simulating gouty arthritis [73], rheumatoid arthritis and psoriatic skin severity affection (PASI scoring) [74]. Other simulation courses were also carried out for biologic therapy and its cost-effectiveness [75–79]. Using simulated activities for postgraduate teaching showed also significant impact. In an earlier study carried out to assess Simulated Teaching in Rheumatology and the value of an Interactive E-Learning Postgraduate Rheumatology Teaching Module, results revealed that simulated teaching approach was a valid tool to increase the exposure of postgraduate trainees to interactive diagnostic and treatment procedures that mimic real-world scenarios but with fewer resource implications [80].

Overall, there is a wide room for simulated teaching in rheumatology. The higher-fidelity approaches have certainly face validity, and investment in simulated musculoskeletal teaching (at both undergraduate and postgraduate level) should be part of the curriculum, notwithstanding the need for further research to help define the optimum length and evaluation of such experiences that focus on learners' outcomes in the short and longer terms.

Future Directions of Simulation-Based Education

Over the past decade, there has been significant change in the healthcare educational paradigm. Initially, it has become increasingly clear that exposure to patients in a clinical environment with ad hoc educational sessions is not sufficient to create competent healthcare practitioners [81–85]. Furthermore, it has become evident that there is a need for curriculum standardization, deliberate skills practice, structured exercises and outcomes-based evaluation with feedback. Training without these components leaves competency largely up to chance. Given the high-risk nature of medical practice, and that the outcomes directly impact patients' health and livelihoods, this is less than acceptable. The growing and sustained focus on medical error reduction and patient safety, and the need to provide safe, learner-centred and ethical training, leads us to a model that incorporates simulation-based health education. The future direction of simulation in healthcare education was reviewed in a "Guide" authored by Motola et al. [70] in which it was noted that simulation-based healthcare education has great potential for use throughout the healthcare education continuum, from undergraduate to continuing education. It can also be used to train a variety of healthcare providers in different disciplines from novices to experts.

Considering the new model of healthcare education, simulation should be incorporated as a complement to clinical exposure, in a framework that incorporates mastery learning and ample opportunities for deliberate practice to achieve the expected competencies. Evidence increasingly shows that simulation-based healthcare education with deliberate practice led to improved and lasting results compared with traditional clinical education [86]. Simulation may also substitute for clinical experience to ensure the needed exposure to a range of clinical cases. This is a necessity, due to increasing limitations for clinical training opportunities. Simulation-based education is also part of the solution in the context of medical error reduction and patient safety. Simulations used to address miscommunication and other sources of error, especially in the context of team training and systems-based practice, are a crucial component in improving patient outcomes [87–89]. Simulations will increasingly be used to supplant animal and live-tissue models as pressures mount to curtail their use and as the fidelity of the replicated tissue models increases. Simulation is also being increasingly considered as an enabling technology to facilitate implementation and translational sciences [90].

Although hesitant at first, over the past decade, there has been a steady progress towards simulated learning. The Society for Medical Simulation (SMS) in the United States and the Society in Europe for Simulation Applied to Medicine (SESAM) provided technical and political leadership for the simulation community. Individual schools, training programmes and hospitals adopted systematic simulation training for certain domains and disciplines. Typical targets were students and trainees, although continuing education for experienced personnel caught on, and hospitals began to train specific work units. A variety of professional organizations around the world took an early lead in promulgating simulation training, encouraging other professional societies to follow. An important driver was the public raising growing concern about patients' safety. By 2010, owing to the continued occurrence of highly publicized cases of death or brain damage linked to significant errors by clinicians and organizations, the public became fully aware of how haphazard is the training and assessment of clinical personnel. This trend was seized upon by malpractice attorneys who developed novel theories of negligence based on the inability of healthcare institutions to ensure the safety of patients from error chains of accident evolution or even to systematically assure the competence of personnel. Healthcare institutions turned to simulation as a means to respond to this challenge, and the liability insurers in turn provided incentives (discounts on premiums) to adopt simulation and later disincentives (refusal of coverage) for those who did not adopt it. Ultimately, governmental regulators and non-governmental accrediting agencies (e.g. the Joint Commission for the Accreditation of Healthcare Organizations – JCAHO – for hospitals in the United States) institutionalized these changes. Again, they first offered incentives for conducting simulation training but eventually required such training as a standard. Medical device regulators, such as the Food and Drug Administration in the United States, first encouraged and then required the submission of data from simulations as part of the approval process for devices. This was particularly relevant for testing the usability of equipment and especially on the user interfaces of diagnostic and therapeutic equipment [45].

In addition to traditional methods, simulation has booked its place in healthcare professional certification and continuous education. Simulation has been used as a tool for accreditation for licensure and maintenance of certification [91–94]. Simulation-based training and assessment have also been incorporated in some specialties in a variety of countries for high-stakes examinations, and certification bodies are increasingly examining ways to incorporate simulation into requirements for initial certification, continuing education and ongoing certification [95, 96].

This interest in simulation has opened the floor for further research in this field. Research questions were categorized into three main themes: instructional design, outcomes measurement and translational research [97]. As far as instructional design, questions still remain about how best to structure simulation interventions and the best frequency and timing for effective learning acquisition and skill retention. Deliberate practice has been shown to be an effective method for skill acquisition, but research is needed to determine the required intensity, duration and feedback characteristics [98]. Regarding outcome measures, as outcomes-based education is increasingly adopted, assessment tools that yield reliable data should be developed and refined. Rigorous measures will allow for valid judgments about competence and are required for adequately evaluating progress and determining areas for improvement. Future studies are needed to set appropriate mastery standards for procedures and clinical skills, as are studies into the way in which simulations with a range of difficulty can best be used to achieve improved patient care practices that are retained over time. Concerning translational science, similar to the biomedical translational science model that aims to transfer the results from laboratory research to the patient bedside, McGaghie et al. [90, 99] reported that simulation-based health education translational science "demonstrates that results achieved in the educational laboratory (T1) transfer to improved downstream patient care practices (T2) and improved patient and public health (T3)". Much of simulation research, until recently, has focused on showing improved educational outcomes. Of late, some studies have shown that what healthcare trainees and practitioners learn using simulations transfers to behaviours in the clinical setting and can lead to improved patient outcomes and decreased errors and complications. Additional research is needed that substantiates the skills learned using simulation-based health education translate to improved patient outcomes and, ultimately, population health.

In conclusion, simulation takes many different shapes, all of which may be appropriate for assessment in a variety of contexts. An important focus for future progress is to identify those forms of simulations that have high utility proven in specific contexts. Simulation providers have an important role to play in incorporating simulation within the principle assessment programmes and helping to evaluate the future role of simulation for assessment.

References

1. Oxford English Dictionary. www.oed.com. Accessed 29 Mar 2018.
2. Datta R, Upadhyay K, Jaideep C. Simulation and its role in medical education. Med J Armed Forces India. 2012;68(2):167–72.
3. Akaike M, Fukutomi M, Nagamune M, Fujimoto A, Tsuji A, Ishida K, et al. Simulation-based medical education in clinical skills laboratory. J Med Investig JMI. 2012;59(1–2):28–35.
4. Dieckmann P, Ringsed C. Pedagogy in simulation-based training in healthcare. Chapter (4). In: Forrest K, Mckimm J, Edgar S, editors. Essential simulation in clinical education. Wiley; 2013. pp. 43–58.
5. Abela JC. Adult learning theories and medical education: a review. Malta Med J. 2009;21(1):11–8.
6. Kaufman DM. Applying educational theory in practice. BMJ Br Med J. 2003;326(7382):213–6.
7. Dreyfus H, Dreyfus S. Mind over machine: the power of human intuition and expertise in the era of the computer. Oxford: Basil Blackwell; 1986.
8. Vaihinger H. The philosophy of AS if. Abingdon: Routledge; 2000.
9. Dieckman P. Simulation settings for learning in acute medical care. In: Dieckman P, editor. Using simulations for education, training and research. Lengerich: Pabst. p. 40–138.
10. Diekman P, Manser T, Wehner T, Rall M. Reality and fiction cues in medical patient simulation, an interview study with anesthesiologists. J Cogn Eng Decis Making. 2007;1:148–68.
11. Tekian A, McGuire C, McGaghie W. Innovative simulations for assessing professional competence: from paper-and-pencil to virtual reality. University of Illinois at Chicago, Department of Medical Education; 1999.
12. Maran NJ, Glavin RJ. Low- to high-fidelity simulation – a continuum of medical education? Med Educ. 2003;37(Suppl. 1):22–8.
13. Norcini JJ, McKinley DW. Assessment methods in medical education. Teach Teach Educ. 2007;23(3):239–50.

14. Kneebonee R, Kidd J, Nestel D, Asvall S, Paraskeva P, Darzi A. (2002)An innovative model for teaching and learning clinical procedures. Med Educ. 2002;36:628–34.
15. Kneebone RL, Kidd J, Nestel D, Barnet A, Lo B, King R, Yang GZ, Brown R. Blurring the boundaries: scenario-based simulation in a clinical setting. Med Educ. 2005;39:580–7.
16. Kneebone R. Simulation and transformational change: the paradox of expertise. Acad Med. 2009;84:954–7.
17. Matsumoto ED, Hamstra SJ, Radomski SB, Cusimano MD. The effect of bench model fidelity on endourological skills: a randomized controlled study. J Urol. 2002;167(3):1243–7.
18. Lee KHK, Grantham H, Boyd R. Comparison of high- and low-fidelity mannequins for clinical performance assessment. Emerg Med Australas. 2008;20(6):508–14.
19. De Giovanni D, Roberts T, Norman G. Relative effectiveness of high- versus low-fidelity simulation in learning heart sounds. Med Educ. 2009;43(7):661–8.
20. Scerbo MWP, Schmidt EAM, Bliss JPP. Comparison of a virtual reality simulator and simulated limbs for phlebotomy training. J Infus Nurs. 2006;29(4):214–24.
21. Crofts JF, Bartlett C, Ellis D, Hunt LP, Fox R, Draycott TJ. Training for shoulder dystocia: a trial of simulation using low-fidelity and high-fidelity mannequins. Obstet Gynecol. 2006;108(6):1477–85.
22. Grady J, Kehrer R, Trusty C, Entin E, Entin E, Brunye T. Learning nursing procedures: the influence of simulator fidelity and student gender on teaching effectiveness. J Nurs Educ. 2008;47(9):403–8.
23. Rodgers DLE, Securro SJE, Pauley RDE. The effect of high-fidelity simulation on educational outcomes in an advanced cardiovascular life support course. Simul Healthc E J Soc Simul Healthc Winter. 2009;4(4):200–6.
24. Munshi F, Lababidi H, Alyousef S. Low- versus high-fidelity simulations in teaching and assessing clinical skills. J Taibah Univ Med Sci. 2015;10(1):12–5.
25. Smallman HS, John MS. Naive realism: misplaced faith in realistic displays. Ergon Des Q Hum Factors Appl. 2005;13(3):6–13.
26. Issenberg B, Mcgaghie WC, Petrusa ER, Lee Gordon D, Scalese RJ. Features and uses of high-fidelity medical simulations that lead to effective learning: a BEME systematic review. Med Teach. 2005;27(1):10e28.
27. Rudolph JWP, Simon RE, Raemer DBP. Which reality matters? Questions on the path to high engagement in healthcare simulation. Simul Healthc E J Soc Simul Healthc Fall. 2007;2(3):161e163.
28. Aggarwal R, Mytton OT, Derbrew M, Hananel D, Heydenburg M, Issenberg B, MacAulay C, Mancini ME. Training and simulation for patient safety. Qual Saf Health Care. 2010;19(Suppl 2):i34–43.
29. Grober ED, Hamstra SJ, Wanzel KR, Reznick RK, Matsumoto ED, Sidhu RS, et al. The educational impact of bench model fidelity on the acquisition of technical skill: the use of clinically relevant outcome measures. Ann Surg. 2004;240(2):374–81.
30. Steigerwald SN, Park J, Hardy KM, Gillman LM, Vergis AS. Does laparoscopic simulation predict intraoperative performance? A comparison between the fundamentals of laparoscopic surgery and LapVR evaluation metrics. Am J Surg. 2014; https://doi.org/10.1016/j.amjsurg.2014.08.031. pii: S0002-9610(14)00526-1
31. Tan SC, Marlow N, Field J, Altree M, Babidge W, Hewett P, Maddern GJ. A randomized crossover trial examining lowversus high-fidelity simulation in basic laparoscopic skills training. Surg Endosc. 2012;26(11):3207e3214. https://doi.org/10.1007/s00464-012-2326-0.
32. Curran V, Fleet L, White S, Bessell C, Deshpandey A, Drover A, Hayward M, Valcour J. A randomized controlled study of manikin simulator fidelity on neonatal resuscitation program learning outcomes. Adv Health Sci Educ Theory Pract. 2015;20(1):205–18.
33. Merchant DC. Does high-fidelity simulation improve clinical outcomes? J Nurses Staff Dev. 2012;28(1):E1–8. [quiz E9–10]
34. McGaghie WC, Issenberg SB, Petrusa ER, Scalese RJ. A critical review of simulation based medical education research: 2003–2009. Med Educ. 2010;44:50–63.

35. Vaughan V III. The patient management problem as an evaluative instrument. Pediatr Rev. 1979;1(3):67–76.
36. Epstein RM, Hundert EM. Defining and assessing professional competence. J Am Med Assoc. 2002;287(2):226–35.
37. High-stakes test. Education reform. https://www.edglossary.org/high-stakes-testing/. Accessed on 30th Mar 2018.
38. Gale T, Roberts M. Assessment. Chapter 5. In: Forrest K, Mckimm J, Edgar S, editors. Essential simulation in clinical education. Willey; 2013. pp. 43–58.
39. Schuwirth LW, van der Vleuten CP. The use of clinical simulations in assessment. Med Educ. 2003;37(Suppl. 1):65–71.
40. Miller GE. The assessment of clinical skills/competence/performance. Acad Med. 1990;65:S63–7.
41. Ker J, Bradley P. Simulation in medical education. Edinburgh: Association for the Study of Medical Education; 2007.
42. Smith AF, Greaves JD. Beyond competence: defining and promoting excellence in anaesthesia. Anaesthesia. 2010;65:184–91.
43. Postgraduate Medical education and training board. Developing and maintain an assessment system – a PMETB guide to good practice. London: PMETB; 2007.
44. Epstein RM. Assessment in medical education. NEJM. 2007;356:387–96.
45. Gaba D. The future vision of simulation in health care. Qual Saf Health Care. 2004;13(Suppl 1):i2–i10.
46. Weller JM, Bloch M, Young S. Evaluation of high fidelity patient simulator in assessment of performance of anaesthetics. Br J Anaesthesia. 2003;90:43–7.
47. Johnson KB, Syroid ND, Drews FA. Part task and variable priority training in first-year anaesthesia resident education: a combined didactic and simulation-based approach to improve management of adverse airway and respiratory events. Anesthesiology. 2008;108:831–40.
48. Baxendale B, Coffey F, Buttery A. The roles of faculty and simulated patients in simulation. Chapter 6. In: Forrest K, Mckimm J, Edgar S, editors. Essential simulation in clinical education. Willey; 2013. pp. 87–110.
49. Barrows H. An overview of the uses of standardized patients for teaching and evaluating clinical skill. Acad Med. 1993;68:443–53.
50. Ziv A, Small SD, Wolpe PR. Patient safety and simulation-based medical education. Med Teach. 2000;22(5):489–95.
51. Ziv A, Wolpe PR, Small SD, Glick S. Simulation-based medical education: an ethical imperative. Acad Med. 2003;78:783–8.
52. Pazin Filho A, Romano MMD. Simulacao: aspectos conceituais. Rev Fac Med Ribeirao Preto. 2007;40(2):167–70.
53. Jones F, Passos-Neto CE, Braghiroli OF. Simulation in medical education: brief history and methodology. Princ Pract Clin Res. 2015;2(1):56–63.
54. Decker S. Integrating guided reflection into simulated learning experiences. In: Jeffries PR, editor. Simulation in nursing: from conceptualization to evolution. New York: National League for Nursing; 2007. p. 73–85.
55. Dismukes RK, Gaba DM, Howard SK. So many roads: facilitated debriefing in healthcare. Simul Healthc. 2006;1(1):23–5.
56. Fanning R, Gaba D. The role of debriefing in simulation-based learning. Soc Simul Healthc. 2007;2(2):115–25.
57. Rudolph JW, Simon R, Dufresne RL, Raemer DB. There's no such thing as "non-judgmental" debriefing: a theory and method for debriefing with good judgment. Simul Healthc. 2006;I(I):49–55.
58. Cho SJ. Debriefing in pediatrics. Korean J Pediatr. 2015;58(2):47–51.
59. Couper K, Perkins GD. Debriefing after resuscitation. Curr Opin Crit Care [Internet]. 2013;19(3):188–94.

60. Clay AS, Que L, Petrusa ER, Sebastian M, Govert J. Debriefing in the intensive care unit: a feedback tool to facilitate bedside teaching. Crit Care Med. 2007;35(3):738–54.
61. Norman G, Muzzin L, Williams R, Swanson D. Simulation in health sciences education. J Instr Dev. 1985;8(1):11–7.
62. Miller R. Psychological considerations in the design of training equipment. Report no. WADC-TR-54-563, AD 71202. Wright Patterson Air Force BAse, OH; Wright Air Development Center. Wright-Patterson Air Force Base; 1954.
63. Yachemetz T, Matthews LR. Clinical simulation terminology within the context of respiratory therapy education: a discussion paper. Can J Respir Ther. 2008;44(4):29.
64. Ebel R, Frisbie D. Essentials of educational measurement. 5th ed. Englewood: Prentice Hall College Div; 1991.
65. Teodor PG, Vanessa NP. Simulation in surgical education. Can Med Assoc J. 2010;182(11):1191.
66. Bates R. A critical analysis of evaluation practice: the Kirkpatrick model and the principle of beneficence. Eval Program Plann. 2004;27(3):341–7.
67. Kyle RR, Murray WB. Clinical simulation: operations, engineering, and management. Burlington: Academic; 2008.
68. Issenberg SB. The scope of simulation-based health care education. Simul Healthc. 2006;1:203–8.
69. Issenberg SB, Mcgaghie WC, Petrusa ER, Gordon DJ, Scalese RJ. Features and uses of high-fidelity medical simulations that lead to effective learning: a BEME systematic review. Med Teach. 2005;27:10–28.
70. Motola I, Devine LA, Chung HS, Sullivan JE, Barry Issenberg S. Simulation in healthcare education: a best evidence practical guide. AMEE Guide No. 82. Med Teach. 2013;35(10):e1511–30.
71. Monrad SU, Zeller JL, Craig CL, DiPonio LA. Musculoskeletal education in US medical schools: lessons from the past and suggestions for the future. Curr Rev Musculoskelet Med. 2011;4:91–8.
72. Sabanathan A, Fent G, Purva M. OP0279 developing and running a rheumatology emergency simulation course. Ann Rheum Dis. 2016;75:163–4.
73. Sabanathan A, Purva M, Helliwell P, Thurairajah T, Fernando X, Prakash A. Can you simulate gout teaching? Rheumatology. 2015;54(suppl 1):i147.
74. El Miedany Y, El Gaafary M, Youssef S, Almedany S, Palmer D. Using simulation in clinical education: psoriasis area and severity index (PASI) score assessment. Curr Rheumatol Rev. 2016;12(3):195–201.
75. Russell A, Beresniak A, Bessette L, et al. Cost-effectiveness modeling of abatacept versus other biologic agents in dmards and anti-tnf inadequate responders for the management of moderate to severe rheumatoid arthritis. Clin Rheumatol. 2009;28:403–12.
76. Saraux A, Gossec L, Goupille P, et al. Cost-effectiveness modelling of biological treatment sequences in moderate to severe rheumatoid arthritis in France. Rheumatology (Oxford). 2010;49:733–40.
77. Cimmino MA, Leardini G, Salaffi F, et al. Assessing the cost-effectiveness of biologic agents for the management of moderate-to-severe rheumatoid arthritis in anti-TNF inadequate responders in Italy: a modelling approach. Clin Exp Rheumatol. 2011;29:633–41.
78. Beresniak A, Ariza-Ariza R, Garciallorente JF, Ramirez-Arellano A, Dupont D. Modelling cost-effectiveness of biologic treatments based on disease activity scores for the management of rheumatoid arthritis in Spain. Int J Inflamm. 2011;2011:727634.
79. Puolakka K, Blåfield H, Kauppi M, et al. Cost-effectiveness modelling of sequential biologic strategies for the treatment of moderate to severe rheumatoid arthritis in Finland. Open Rheumatol J. 2012;6:38–43.
80. El Miedany Y, El Gaafary M, Youssef S, et al. OP0312 simulated teaching in rheumatology: assessment of an interactive e-learning postgraduate rheumatology teaching module. Ann Rheum Dis. 2015;74:191.
81. Joorabchi B, Devries JM. Evaluation of clinical competence: the gap between expectation and performance. Pediatrics. 1996;97:179–84.

82. Mangione S, Nieman LZ. Cardiac auscultatory skills of internal medicine and family practice trainees. A comparison of diagnostic proficiency. JAMA. 1997;278:717–22.
83. Lypson ML, Frohna JG, Gruppen LD, Woolliscroft JO. Assessing residents' competencies at baseline: identifying the gaps. Acad Med. 2004;79:564–70.
84. Friedman Z, Siddiqui N, Katznelson R, Devito I, Davies S. Experience is not enough: repeated breaches in epidural anesthesia aseptic technique by novice operators despite improved skill. Anesthesiology. 2008;108:914–20.
85. Bell RH Jr, Biester TW, Tabuenca A, Rhodes RS, Cofer JB, Britt LD, Lewis FR. Operative experience of residents in US general surgery programs: a gap between expectation and experience. Ann Surg. 2009;249:719–24.
86. McGaghie WC, Issenberg SB, Cohen ER, Barsuk JH, Wayne DB. Does simulation-based medical education with deliberate practice yield better results than traditional clinical education? A meta-analytic comparative review of the evidence. Acad Med. 2011;86:706–11.
87. Birnbach DJ, Salas E. Can medical simulation and team training reduce errors in labor and delivery? Anesthesiol Clin. 2008;26:159–68.
88. Kuehster CR, Hall CD. Simulation: learning from mistakes while building communication and teamwork. J Nurses Staff Dev. 2010;26:123–7.
89. Salas E, Diazgranados D, Weaver SJ, King H. Does team training work? Principles for health care. Acad Emerg Med. 2008;15:1002–9.
90. McGaghie WC, Draycott TJ, Dunn WF, Lopez CM, Stefanidis D. Evaluating the impact of simulation on translational patient outcomes. Simul Healthc. 2011a;6:S42–7.
91. Ziv A, Rubin O, Sidi A, Berkenstadt H. Credentialing and certifying with simulation. Anesthesiol Clin. 2007;25:261–9.
92. Steadman RH, Huang YM. Simulation for quality assurance in training, credentialing and maintenance of certification. Best Pract Res Clin Anaesthesiol. 2012;26:3–15.
93. Holmboe E, Rizzolo MA, Sachdeva AK, Rosenberg M, Ziv A. Simulation-based assessment and the regulation of healthcare professionals. Simul Healthc. 2011;6:S58–62.
94. Buyske J. The role of simulation in certification. Surg Clin N Am. 2010;90:619–21.
95. Ben-Menachem E, Ezri T, Ziv A, Sidi A, Brill S, Berkenstadt H. Objective structured clinical examination-based assessment of regional anesthesia skills: the Israeli National Board examination in anesthesiology experience. Anesth Analg. 2011;112:242–5.
96. Levine AI, Schwartz AD, Bryson EO, Demaria S Jr. Role of simulation in U.S. physician licensure and certification. Mt Sinai J Med. 2012;79:140–53.
97. Issenberg SB, Chung HS, Devine LA. Patient safety training simulations based on competency criteria of the Accreditation Council for Graduate Medical Education. Mt Sinai J Med. 2011a;78:842–53.
98. McGaghie WC. Research opportunities in simulation-based medical education using deliberate practice. Acad Emerg Med. 2008;15:995–1001.
99. McGaghie WC. Medical education research as translational science. Sci Transl Med. 2010b;2:19cm8.1–3.

Chapter 15
Flipped Learning

Introduction

Flipped learning is a pedagogical teaching approach in which the conventional notion of classroom-based learning is inverted, so that students are introduced to the learning material before class, with classroom time then being used to deepen understanding through discussion with peers and problem-solving activities facilitated by teachers [1]. The same concept was applied later in the andragogical learning.

In the early mid-2000s, in the shadow of Colorado's Pikes Peak, veteran Woodland Park High School chemistry teachers Jonathan Bergmann and Aaron Sams stumbled onto an idea. Struggling to find the time to reteach lessons for absent students, they plunked down $50, bought software that allowed them to record and annotate lessons and posted them online. Absent students appreciated the opportunity to see what they missed. But, surprisingly, so did students who hadn't missed class. They, too, used the online material, mostly to review and reinforce classroom lessons. And, soon, Bergmann and Sams realized they had the opportunity to radically rethink how they used class time. Chemistry teachers Jon Bergman and Aaron Sams [2] and the founder of the Khan Academy, Salman Khan [3], were the first to popularize the phrase "flipped learning" into general use.

The concept of flipped learning, however, goes back much earlier than this. In the 1990s, a model of "peer instruction" was developed by Harvard Professor Eric Mazur, in which he provided material for students to prepare and reflect on before class. The class time was then used to encourage deeper cognitive thinking via peer interaction and instructor challenge. He called this "just in time teaching" [4]. This model was later expanded to include technological elements. At the International Conference on College Teaching and Learning in 2000, a presentation was delivered on "The Classroom Flip: Using Web Course Management Tools to Become a Guide by the Side" [5]. It was the first time the "flip" concept was introduced with emphasis on the learning management systems' role in delivering materials to

Y. El Miedany, *Rheumatology Teaching*,
https://doi.org/10.1007/978-3-319-98213-7_15

students before class. Significantly, the role of the teacher was amended and called facilitator and coach or "guide on the side". Subsequent research focused on the notion of "inverting the classroom" as a means of providing an inclusive learning environment in which personalized coaching and mentoring were the norm [6].

Fast forward to the current and the dramatic growth of online content which provided practitioners with an access to ample toolkits as well as resources for delivering flipped learning. Video creation (e.g. Screenr and Webinaria) and distribution tools (e.g. YouTube and Vimeo) provide the opportunity to create flipped content with ease [7]. Alternatively, there is a wealth of pre-existing media available for reuse (e.g. iTunes, Khan Academy and Open Yale Courses). While technology is not a prerequisite (flipped text-based content is just as valuable as video content), there is no doubt that the intersection of web 2.0 technology and learning theory has enabled flipped learning to become a valuable addition to the spectrum of blended learning. This chapter will discuss how the flipped learning model can be used to bring medical education into the twenty-first century. It will start with presenting the science of flipped learning, followed by "What should we know before flipping?", subsequently, flipped learning models will be summarized then the art of flipping. The chapter will conclude with discussing flipped learning in medical education and rheumatology and lastly challenges to flipped learning.

The Science of Flipped Learning

According to the constructivist, inquiry-based, learning cycle model [8–10], teaching consists of two phases (Fig. 15.1): a phase in which students are gaining conceptual understanding (hereafter referred to as the content attainment phase) and a phase in which students learn to apply and/or evaluate those concepts in novel situations in order to broaden their conceptual understanding beyond the context in

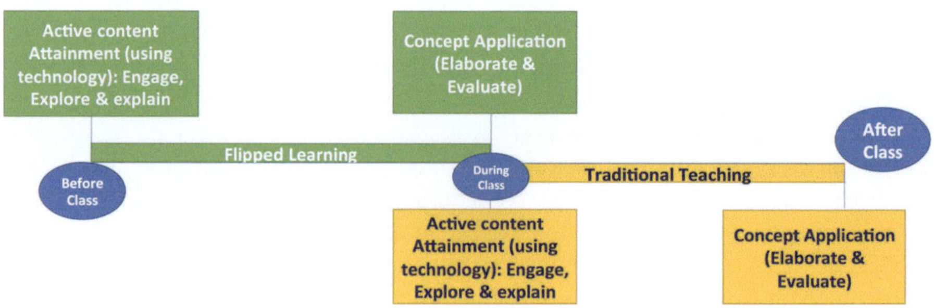

Fig. 15.1 Teaching phases: comparison between flipped and traditional learning. Teaching consists of two phases: (1) content attainment (a phase in which students are gaining conceptual understanding) and (2) concept application phase (a phase in which students learn to apply and/or evaluate those concepts in novel situations in order to broaden their conceptual understanding beyond the context in which they learned it)

which they learned it (hereafter referred to as the concept application phase). In a traditional teaching model, the instructor facilitates content attainment through various means in a classroom setting. Students are then given the responsibility of applying the concepts, generally in the form of homework assignments. In a flipped model, the roles are reversed, with students being responsible for attaining the content before coming to class, at which time the instructor facilitates the application process. It appears that the main difference between these models is the role of the instructor: to facilitate content attainment or concept application. Does it matter where you place instructor and student responsibilities?

While often defined simplistically as "school work at home and home work at school", flipped learning is an approach that allows teachers to implement a methodology, or various methodologies, in their classrooms. To counter some of the misconceptions about this term, the governing board and key leaders of the Flipped Learning Network (FLN) have composed a formal definition of flipped learning: "Flipped Learning is a pedagogical approach in which direct instruction moves from the group learning space to the individual learning space, and the resulting group space is transformed into a dynamic, interactive learning environment where the educator guides students as they apply concepts and engage creatively in the subject matter" [8]. Defining the term helped also to distinguish between a flipped classroom and flipped learning. These terms are not interchangeable. Flipping a class can, but does not necessarily, lead to flipped learning. Many teachers may already flip their classes by having students read text outside of class, watch supplemental videos or solve additional problems; but to engage in flipped learning, there are four pillars which teachers should incorporate into their practice (Fig. 15.2).

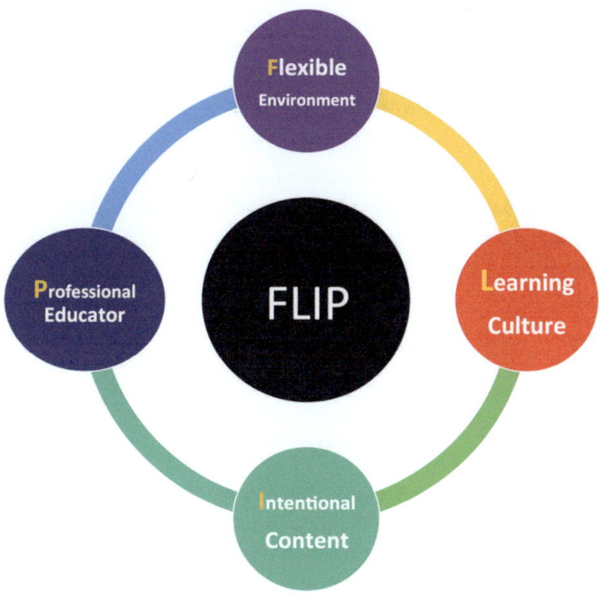

Fig. 15.2 The four pillars of flipped learning: flexible environment, learning culture, intentional content and professional educator

Flexible Environment

In contrast to the traditional learning style, flipped learning allows for implementation of a variety of learning modes. Physical rearrangement of the learning spaces is required to support either group work or independent study or accommodate a lesson or unit. Educators may require also to create flexible spaces in which students are able to choose when and where they learn. Furthermore, educators who flip their classes should be flexible in their expectations of student timelines for learning and in their assessments of student learning.

Learning Culture

In contrast to the traditional teacher-centred model, where the teacher is the primary source of information, in the flipped learning model, there is a fundamental shift of the educational model to a learner-centred approach, where in-class time is dedicated to exploring topics in greater depth and creating rich learning opportunities. Consequently, students are actively involved in knowledge construction as they participate in and evaluate their learning in a manner that is personally meaningful. As the year progresses, the educators should be able to see their students asking better questions and thinking more deeply about the content.

Intentional Content

Flipped classroom teachers almost universally agree that it's not the instructional videos on their own but how they are integrated into an overall approach that makes the difference. Flipped learning educators should constantly revise and consider how they can implement the flipped learning model. During class time flipped learning model can be implemented in standard teaching practice to help students develop conceptual understanding, as well as procedural fluency. They determine what materials students should explore on their own and what they need to teach. Students cannot just "watch the video and be done with it". Educators should use intentional content to maximize classroom time in order to adopt methods of student-centred, active learning strategies, depending on the subject matter and grade level.

Professional Educator

In contrast to the standard teaching style, in flipped classroom, the role of a professional educator is even more important and often more demanding. As it usually takes a little while for students to get used to the system, educators are expected to continually observe their students, providing them with feedback relevant in the moment, supervising and assessing their work. Professional educators are reflective in their practice, accept constructive criticism, connect with each other to improve their instruction and tolerate controlled chaos in their classrooms. All aspects of instruction should be rethought to best maximize the scarcest learning resource. While professional educators take on less visibly prominent roles in a flipped classroom, they remain the essential ingredient that enables flipped learning to occur [11].

The main advantage of flipped teaching model is that it enables the educator to work individually with students. Classically, in the traditional classroom, the most outgoing and engaged students ask questions, while struggling students may act out. The flipped learning allows the educator to spend more time with struggling students, who may require help through challenging problems in the class. Advanced students have more freedom to learn independently. And, while students may occasionally lapse on their homework assignments, the new arrangement endorses better relationships between the educator and the student with greater student engagement and higher levels of motivation.

Concerning the video presentation which lies in the core of the out-of-class learning component (content attainment), cognitive theory of multimedia learning should be used to guide the video production process [12]. It is important to keep the students engaged while watching these instructional videos. Mayer [13] proposed 12 design principles to enhance the multimedia instructions. For example, segmenting principle stresses that a long presentation should be divided into a series of short videos. Specifically, empirical findings suggested that students' median engagement time of watching instructional videos was 6 min [14]. Thus, the desirable length of each video should be within 6 min. Also, personalization principle suggests that the presentation in videos should be spoken in a conversational style. Teachers should use an informal conversation with students (e.g. "I" and "you"), instead of a non-personalized style speaking in a third-person formal monologue. In addition, signaling principle states that learning is enhanced when essential materials are highlighted. Teachers may consider using PowerPoint-embedded presentation such as screencasts [15–17]. It can offer a step-by-step instruction to guide students' video watching [15] and assist students in note-taking [17].

What Should We Know Before Flipping?

Flipped learning can be an excitement for both educators and students alike. Enthusiasm for flipped learning is not limited to a certain education level or age. With the concept gaining more mainstream attention, a growing number of education faculty started implementing flipped learning. Lectures that were once held live in large halls are now recorded, searchable and viewable from anywhere and anytime, opening up new ways to interact, learn and share during the "in-class" time [18].

Proper implementation of flipped learning has been reported to be associated with several benefits [19]. It can lead to increased and better interaction between teachers and students and reduced student stress concomitant with higher student achievement scores. In addition, it can facilitate individualized teaching tailored to the student's requirements. Moreover, flipped learning helps teachers personalize lessons and assessments to target students' individual learning styles and abilities. For this reason, it is largely expected that the less clever students are, particularly, expected to benefit from flipped classrooms which offer multiple ways to absorb and learn content.

Simple movement of the course material from the classroom to the home will not improve learning outcomes. A successful flipped classroom is expected to offer a carefully designed learning experience that caters to each learner's own experiences and ideas. The educator can also use powerful analytics to see trends in students' understanding to prepare for class. In addition, teachers who use flipped learning approaches should continue to apply varied teaching strategies and good pedagogy/andragogy as they would with traditional models of learning. Teachers still need to ensure that students are able to transfer their learning to new situations. When starting to use a flipped classroom approach, teachers should start small so that students have time to develop an understanding of the model. Selecting what information to read or the instructional videos to watch at home is also crucial for the flipped learning model. Its content, accuracy and whether it fulfils the required teaching aims play a vital role in the success of the flipped learning experience. As the online tools will continue to multiply, this will offer both the educator and the learner the opportunity to learn and know different views of the same topic.

Flipped Learning Models

While there is no one model, the core idea is to flip the common instructional approach: With the instruction that used to occur "in class" is now accessed at home, in advance of the lesson time in the class. Class becomes the place to work through problems, advance concepts and engage in collaborative learning. At first, the flipped classroom sounds fairly straight forward. Having a closer look, however, it becomes clear that from this basic concept emerge several unique and interesting forms of how a teacher can invert their class. Educators can implement one or more of such flipped concepts which they feel right for their classrooms. Applying such a dynamic strategy of teaching will keep the students attracted and educators excited with the experience. Models of flipped learning include:

- *The standard inverted classroom*: Students are assigned the "homework" of watching video lectures and reading any materials relevant to the next day's class. During class time, students practise what they've learned through traditional schoolwork, with their teachers freed up for additional one-on-one time.

- *The discussion-oriented flipped classroom*: Teachers assign lecture videos, as well as any other video or reading related to the day's subject (e.g. TED Talks, YouTube videos and other resources). Class time is then devoted to discussion and exploration of the subject. This can be an especially useful approach in subjects where context is everything (e.g. history, art or English).
- *The demonstration-focused flipped classroom*: Especially for those subjects that require students to remember and repeat activities exactly (e.g. chemistry, physics and math). It is most helpful to have a video demonstration to be able to rewind and rewatch. In this model, the teacher uses screen recording software to demonstrate the activity in a way that allows students to follow along at their own pace.
- *The faux-flipped classroom*: This is perfect for younger students for whom actual homework might not yet be appropriate. This flipped classroom model instead has those students watch lecture video in class – giving them the opportunity to review materials at their own pace. After watching, the students can start problem-solving either individually or in groups, with the teacher is able to move from student to student to offer whatever individual support each young learner needs.
- *The group-based flipped classroom*: This model adds a new element to help students learn from each other. The class starts the same way others do, with lecture videos and other resources shared before class. The shift happens when students come to class, teaming up to work together on that day's assignment. This format encourages students to learn from one another and helps students to not only learn what the right answers are but also how to actually explain to a peer why those answers are right.
- *The virtual flipped classroom*: For older students and in some courses, the flipped classroom can eliminate the need for classroom time at all. Some college and university professors now share lecture videos for student viewing, assign and collect work via online learning management systems and simply require students to attend office hours or other regularly scheduled time for brief one-on-one instruction based on that individual student's needs.
- *Flipping the teacher*: All the videos created for a flipped learning do not have to begin and end with the teacher. Students too can make use of video to better demonstrate proficiency. Assign students to their record practice role-play activities to show competency or ask each to film themselves presenting a new subject or skill as a means to "teach the teacher" [20].

While it can be a challenge to choose which flipped learning model to use, the facility of using different models gives it a special taste and adds to its excitement. Mark Frydenberg of the Huffington Post noted that "It is not a 'one size fits all' model". He points out that every classroom is different, with different levels of access to technology, different levels of motivation on the part of the students and different technological know-how on the part of the instructors. Additionally, teachers must relearn how to act as the "guide on the side" rather than the "sage on the stage", and that takes time [21].

However, whenever the shift does occur, many experts believe the benefits are well worth the effort. According to ASCD.org, of 453 teachers who flipped their classrooms, 67% reported increased test scores, with particular benefits for students in advanced placement classes and students with special needs; 80% reported improved student attitudes, and 99% said they would flip their classrooms again next year [22].

The Art of Flipped Learning

Ideas and opinions about flipped learning environments vary. Some consider it simply another way of presenting the student-centred learning approach. Others view flipped classrooms as the most cutting-edge approach to learning. Still others see flipping as just another fad that will eventually run its course.

In many definitions and models, flipped learning means students watch a video of pre-recorded lectures before class. Then, when they arrive to class, they work through assignments or activities with their peers and the instructor. However, flipped learning teachers almost universally agree that it is not the instructional videos on their own but how they are integrated into an overall approach that makes the difference. After all, a video of a lecture is still a lecture. Expanding the definition of a flipped learning environment was discussed in an editorial by Barbi Honeycutt and Jennifer Garrett [22].

The essential goals of the flipped classroom are to move beyond the lecture as the primary way to deliver information and structure class time. In this approach the in-class time is "repurposed" for inquiry, application and assessment in order to better meet the needs of individual learners. While a well-developed lecture can be effective in the traditional teaching, the educators rely on it too heavily and often to the exclusion of other more meaningful teaching and learning approaches. Flipped learning enables educators to introduce new strategies of doing things. Yet adding something new generally requires letting go of something old. In the flipped learning, educators need to let go of their reliance on the lecture and focus on other ways to enhance learning by introducing active learning approaches that put students in the centre of the learning experience.

There are other ways to describe the flip. It can be defined as moving from an educator-centred to a student-centred learning environment. It could also be defined as shifting from individual to collaborative strategy. However, it is possible to flip a class using individual activities such as worksheets, quizzes, reflective writing prompts and problem-solving assignments. The key is to complete these activities during class time.

Flipping may or may not include technology. Bergmann and Sams [2] explain, "Ultimately, flipping a classroom involves shifting the energy away from the educator toward the students and then leveraging educational tools to enhance the learning environment". Bearing in mind that educational tools vary and are not confined to technology, the true essence of the flipping is principally to focus on the student.

Therefore, while videos and other technological tools can be effective in a flipped classroom, they are not essential. The true essence of the flipping is principally to focus on the student.

Putting a framework for comparing the lecture-centred style to the flipping approach, the cornerstone will be the "in-class" achievement. In general educators focus on higher-level learning outcomes during class time, whereas lower-level outcomes are expected outside of the class. This means the flipping could be as simple as watching a video before class and then attending class for more in-depth discussions that involve judging, creating and analysing. In contrast to the traditional teaching where the students are not prepared for applying the taught subject, in flipping where students work with the fundamental material before class, they are better prepared to apply the information and engage in higher-level discussions with their peers and the educator.

Another way to think about the flipped classroom is the student role in the process of learning during class. Dr. Honeycutt and Garret put the student in the core of the learning process and referred to the flip as focusing on the learners by incorporating them in the process. This allows students to spend ample time on "in-class" practising with their peers and educator. This adds a new level of complexity to the classroom.

Regardless of the definition or framework used to define flipped learning, the main outcome is a dynamic learning environment. Flipped classrooms are interactive; however, it can sometimes be even "messy", as students, instead of sitting passively listening to the lecture, are working together and solving problems. Flipped learning might also be risky. Educators relinquish a degree of control when the energy in the classroom shifts to the students. Similarly, while some flipped strategies may work, others may not. Educators using any flipping model need to be aware of these challenges when integrating active learning strategies into their classrooms. However, some of these challenges can be mitigated by careful planning. For example, starting with a flipped lesson plan helps determine the appropriate tools and most effective strategies which can help educators maintain control of the flipped classroom and ensure achieving the targeted learning outcomes.

One of the best approaches for educators to start with is by rethinking their role in the teaching room. When considering using new approaches, tools and strategies for teaching, it is expected that the lesson planning process and the assessment process will also change. In several cases, there are mini-lectures that need to be presented, but the majority of class time is spent on active learning. When planning for a flipped lesson, an educator should begin with the question, "what the learning outcomes are and what do the students need to do to achieve them?" This change in perspective will instantly flip the lesson focus since the question highlights the learners' efforts, not the educator. Consequently, the educators plan learning experiences based on what the students need to do and not what the educators are going to talk about. The instructor may give a presentation or a lecture, but any teaching activity must be designed to help students achieve what they need to do with the information or material to accomplish the desired learning outcomes, not just to disseminate information [22].

Flipped Learning in Medical Education

Over the past few years, there has been growing interest in the use of flipped learning in the field of health science education. However, the majority of this work was carried out in pharmacy and nursing [2, 23–34]. O'Flaherty and Phillip [35] published a review of the literature, in 2015, on the use of flipped learning in higher education. Out of 12 studies identified from health science education, only 3 studies were conducted on medical education, none of which used a rigorous design to examine the effect of the flipped learning approach on learning outcomes (i.e. performance indicator or patient care outcomes) [36–38].

Recent review of the literature [39] highlighted four key findings on the current status of research on flipped learning in medical education. First, flipped learning in medical education has gained momentum as there have been a growing number of publication rate in this field over the past few years. Second, the effects of the flipping on learning are inconsistent, with some purported benefits and some reports of negligible improvement over traditional teaching methods. Third, students like the flipped learning teaching approach. Overall, the flipped learning seems a promising teaching strategy in medical education, particularly when the intent is to increase students' motivation, task value and engagement. However, most of the controlled studies focused on learners' perceptions of the intervention and changes in their knowledge and skills, whereas limited outcomes were reported on the higher level of Kirkpatrick's classification (i.e. changes in behaviour, professional practice and patient outcome). The studies published prior to 2015 were largely commentaries, action research, the before and after design without control groups or precourse survey design. In 2016, research on the flipped learning in medical education shifted to more rigorous designs, with almost half of the studies conducted using a controlled design. This suggests that the body of literature on the flipped learning in medical education is not only continuing to grow but is also being conducted using more rigorous research designs. This trajectory must continue in order to develop a strong empirical basis for (or against) the use of the flipped learning in medical education. The majority of work in this area has been carried out in undergraduate medical education. It is unclear if these findings would be generalizable to graduate medical education. This especially holds true for the research carried out in the preclinical years of medical school as this period tends to focus on classroom- and laboratory-based foundational science education. Although the clinical years of medical school are more similar to graduate medical education with regard to clinical learning in the context of a patient care environment, there are still significant differences between the learners (patient responsibilities, hours spent performing clinical work, depth and application of knowledge needed, etc.). Thus, more studies aimed at graduate medical education are needed.

Gain in knowledge and skill sets, when utilizing the flipped learning, was examined in a number of studies, compared with traditional learning methods. Only four studies provided sufficient statistics for effect sizes to be calculated. However, the effects of the flipped learning were generally mixed and inconclusive. One factor that might need to be taken into account in future research in this area is students' compliance with the flipped learning requirements (i.e. did the students complete the assigned preparatory work before the in-class session). This is linked to Heitz et al. note [40] which highlighted that the non-compliant group in their study was quite substantial (31%). Ultimately, students' compliance with flipped learning requirements might drastically affect differential gains in knowledge and skill sets compared with the traditional classroom.

Multiple studies reported positive students' perceptions of and attitudes towards the flipped learning. The students reported benefit were in favour of online modules as a learning resource [41]; and in in-class quizzes as well as follow-up homework as motivation for in-class participation [42]. Students learning through flipped learning methodology also reported greater task value, increased enjoyment and decreased boredom compared with those learning in a traditional classroom. In view of the positive attitudes towards the flipped learning demonstrated by the students, and the data depicting that flipped learning was, at least, as successful as traditional learning methods with regard to knowledge and skill set acquisition, it was concluded that the flipped learning could be considered as a component of medical education.

In order to more firmly support (or refute) the use of the flipped learning in medical education, future studies should be carried out to evaluate the higher levels of Kirkpatrick's framework. The effects of the flipping on learning have been examined across three of Kirkpatrick's classification measures: perception, attitude and change in knowledge and skill sets. Future studies should continue to focus on change in knowledge but should examine potential differential effects of the flipped learning on knowledge requiring different levels of cognitive processes, as highlighted in Morton and Colbert-Getz [43]. Changes in attitudes, as an independent variable and moderator of change in student knowledge, could be worthy of examination. Much of the work on change in knowledge has examined knowledge acquisition. Ultimately, it would be helpful to look at knowledge retention and transfer of this knowledge to professional practice and patient care (the highest two levels of Kirkpatrick's measures).

Flipped Learning in Rheumatology Education

It is important to state that the flipped classroom cannot be the only form of education. Medicine is still a very hands-on practice, and nothing can replace that experience. There must be clinical time in medical school as nothing will replace seeing a patient. Clinical experience and human interaction are too important to the practice of medicine. Thus, the flipped classroom and case-based instruction cannot be the only form of instruction. However, this model represents a potential future as a means for improved instructional efficiency. The flipped classroom enable the students to be better prepared for the clinical experience so they can go further in their training, rather than catching up to where they're supposed to be [44].

Considering rheumatology teaching, earlier studies [45, 46] carried out to assess for educational deficiencies in musculoskeletal medicine revealed that a large majority of recent medical school graduates failed to demonstrate basic competency in musculoskeletal medicine on the clinical skills and examination front. It is therefore reasonable to conclude that medical school preparation in musculoskeletal medicine is inadequate and is in need to fundamental changes. Furthermore, several challenges have been reported, and it is believed that there is room for improvement to enhance the learning curve. Initially, and unfortunately, there is a general perception that the rheumatology curriculum and musculoskeletal learning come in the second place to a number of other specialities [47, 48]. This assertion is made, not only on personal observation, as rheumatology cases are not routinely included in the formal or summative OSCE exams for medical students, but also as an outcome of cross-sectional surveys to assess medical students' knowledge and clinical confidence in musculoskeletal medicine [45]. Furthermore, in contrast with the high prevalence of musculoskeletal conditions in the community, the time devoted to rheumatology teaching within the undergraduate curriculum remains inadequate and relies mainly on the availability of a rheumatologist with special interest in medical education.

Rheumatology can serve as a good model leading the way in changing medical education. Rheumatology is robust in both the basic science as well as clinical applications. This creates an opportunity for rheumatologists to be actively involved in the development of modern teaching approaches and the dissemination of the musculoskeletal knowledge in medical schools. Instead of giving lectures to teach the basic concepts and principles, students learn the basic materials in their own time and then come to class prepared to discuss the clinical applications of that knowledge. This agrees with the findings reported by Dr. Jonas, (Director of the Rheumatology Fellowship Training Program at the University of North Carolina at Chapel Hill School of Medicine), in the ACR conference 2016 [49]. She noted that "New concepts and new technologies are changing what medical school and medical education looks like, and rheumatologists are in the forefront". Considering the unique mix of basic sciences and clinical applications make the rheumatologists some of the best-positioned clinician–educators to guide and lead the shift in medical education.

A recent study was carried out aiming at implementing flipped classroom rheumatology teaching for undergraduate education and to evaluate outcomes of teaching using OSCE assessment and student perceived effectiveness and satisfaction survey [50]. Results of this work revealed that considering both clinical and academic outcomes, there was a compelling evidence to support the claim that students in the flipped learning course were overwhelmingly satisfied and confident. Students indicated high satisfaction levels reflecting that flipped learning was effective and gave them clear ideas of what is expected from them. Also, this approach did enable the students to retain their knowledge (examples, recognition of clinical symptoms and signs of diseases, better ability to perform necessary tasks in a clinical practice). In turn, these knowledge attainment abilities have consequently improved their self-confidence. The result of this study is congruent with other studies done on the use of flipped learning in medical teaching; where results indicated high learners' satisfaction and confidence in their skills with clinical flipped learning [32, 51, 52]. The students' feedback reported in earlier studies comes also in agreement with the outcomes of this work reflecting their satisfaction with this teaching model and its learning outcomes.

Flipped Learning and the Learners' Views

Flipped instruction is gaining popularity in medical schools, but there remain some unanswered questions and items that should be addressed. These include queries regarding the learner beliefs and preferences [53]. Also, the optimum amount of the curriculum to flip and whether flipped sessions should be mandatory.

New media literacy research [54, 55] indicated that the current Internet generation student population is fully engaged in electronic media and audio-visual stimulation. Therefore, it would be logical to use interactive, technology-enhanced instruction as a tool to enhance the students' attention, participation and collaboration, even in small groups' clinical case practice. A study revealed significant improvement of educational outcomes when technology enhanced teaching was implemented [56]. Furthermore, results confirmed that embedding online video clips in the education process enhanced students' interaction and engagement. The tutor and independent observer scores revealed that the students' engagement has improved significantly in three dimensions: flow, interest and relevance, reflecting better understanding and attainment. This agreed with the outcomes of an earlier study which depicted that during a flipped learning setting, students were focused on the task at hand, enthusiastic and willing to finish the assessment task [12].

Demonstrating students how to learn through flipped classroom is vital for the success of the educational approach. Kirvan et al. [57] shared their experience in preparing the students gradually before full implementation of their flipped classroom. Students were asked to view a video lecture during class time. At the same time, they introduced students with some cognitive skills such as making their own notes while watching the video lectures. Providing instructor brief notes to accompany the videos is another useful technique to guide student learning during video lectures [15, 16]. For the in-class activities, students may not be accustomed to the change especially regarding the group learning process [15]. Teachers should provide clear instructions to ensure better communication and efficiency in group activities. For example, Clark [58] would split his students into three groups according to their ability. Each group of students had a clear lesson objective and completed their corresponding learning tasks. The high ability students worked on practice problems in groups without the teacher's assistance, whereas the average students first reviewed the contents with the teacher before doing in-class exercises. As for the underperforming students, they would revisit the instructional videos in groups and gain a better understanding of the materials. In this example, every student in Clark's [58] flipped classroom knew their own learning objective and what to be discussed with their group members.

On another front, the issue of ensuring that the students have watched the video has been raised by Chao et al. [59] who pointed out that "it is difficult to ensure that students had truly previewed the video". In this regard, they designed follow-up quizzes on instructional videos to ensure students had previewed the learning materials. A learning management system (LMS) is therefore required to monitor and record the data of student learning. However, there is still a possibility that students complete the quizzes casually without being well prepared from video lectures. So how can we engage students in learning tasks? Another solution is to create an online discussion forum for students to post their questions and discuss with peers [60]. This will help in extending the learning community outside the classroom.

Outside the contexts of flipped classroom approach, gamification has been recently used in the education field to engage student in learning [61]. Hew et al. [62] found that digital game elements such as points, badges and leaderboard could produce a positive effect on student motivation and engagement. In a gamified environment, they found that students would be more active online (e.g. contribute more on discussion forum) and engage in more difficult tasks. Some learning management systems such as Moodle enable the use of game elements. To motivate student learning, teachers may consider flipping and gamifying their course by using these systems.

Challenges to Flipped Learning

Given education's long history of fascination with new educational approaches which are abandoned later, there's a real challenge that flipping, a seemingly simple idea that is profound in practice, may be reduced into the latest educational fad. And, in today's highly polarized political environment, it also runs the risk of being falsely pigeonholed into one of education's many false dichotomies, such as the age-old pedagogical debate between content knowledge and skills acquisition.

Before flipping the entire course, teachers can start small and proceed at a reasonable pace [15, 17]. Experiment in small ways also enables teachers to gain experiences of using flipped classroom approach. Teachers can cumulate the flipped learning materials by working on two to three topics every year. Grypp and Luebeck [15] further recommended teachers flipping their courses in team. In other words, teachers can share their experiences of implementing flipped classrooms as well as their teaching resources. However, in DeSantis et al.'s [63] experience, the materials created by others may not feature the host teacher. Discussion and agreement on the materials designed are thus necessary if teachers intend to develop a flipped course collaboratively.

While technology plays a big part in a successful flipped learning experience, the challenge remains of getting a fair access to it. It is not just the access but the download speed and the facility to view the educational content. While the majority of elite university students are more likely able to have a smartphone or a laptop with a decent Internet access for at-home lecture listening, this may not be the rule at all universities. This is also highly applicable in public high/secondary schools. This was one of the reasons critics pointed to the digital divide as a strike against flipping. Therefore, supporting the students who have limited access to technology resources is mandatory to the success of the flipped learning strategy. Teachers should consider students' socio-economic status and make IT supports available for them. For example, teachers can extend the use of computer facilities in school to support the implementation of flipped classrooms [16]. Also, teachers can prepare a few additional copies of flipped learning materials in flash drives or DVDs for the students who do not have Internet connection at home [58].

Many students need an incentive to watch videos at home just like they need to be motivated to read their textbooks and do their homework. Students' disengagement in the out-of-class learning is a real challenge to the flipped learning strategy as not all students are motivated to learn on their own. If students are not prepared, it makes it much harder to have a successful in-class experience. It has been suggested, in such cases, that the incentive can be the implementation of a short quiz at the start of class. As mentioned earlier, gamification can also be used in the education field to engage student in learning [61].

On another front, teachers need the knowledge and the time to create or provide targeted informative educational videos. The videos themselves should be focused, clear and relatively short (in average 5 min each). However, it takes time to get such videos right which represent an extra burden for the university/college tutors. Some faculty resort to the available free online videos. On another aspect, some educators need to put their egos aside as they shift from being the "sage on the stage" to becoming the "guide on side". So, instead of the traditional face-to-face time with long lectures, to relay information; interaction with students would be the best approach, as they grapple with course concepts. Furthermore, enriching teachers' knowledge of flipped classroom approach is important to keep the momentum and enthusiasm among the teachers. Institutes can create opportunities for teachers to share their experiences of implementing flipped classrooms as well as to receive feedback from colleagues or other professionals [63]. In Kirvan et al.'s study [57], a student teacher joined the teaching team of their flipped classroom. By enacting the flipped course, the student teacher gained experiences in both video production and lesson design. Kirvan et al. [57] concluded that their intervention could be a critical component of teacher preparation and "may be important for making education theory come alive for new teachers". Therefore, institutes may consider strengthening their teacher training and professional development on flipped classroom approach.

Though thoughtful curriculum or course redesigns may help to improve learning, there is no magic wand to achieve this target. Redesigning the traditional educational approach is a hard job which requires time, effort, support as well as enforcement. It might be quite not realistic to assume that good percentage of the students would love doing homework. However educational strategy redesign presents an opportunity to re-engage students and improve their learning motivation. This is quite achievable with proper use of the technology to set proper expectations and monitoring of their students' performance [12].

The layout of the traditional classrooms is another challenge to flipped learning. Collaboration, communication and creativity are at the heart of this method, but fostering these skills is almost impossible with pupils inactive in rows of desks all day. With a little imagination, savvy teachers can implement a more flexible classroom with the minimum amount of fuss, resource and disruption, boosting student engagement and helping pupils to learn more effectively. Video-conferencing technologies, screen-casting tools and cloud-based platforms that let teachers create and deliver lessons all help to create the flipped classroom. However, with poor-quality, faulty and out-of-date ICT equipment, one of the main reasons for teachers not using technology in the classroom, this can be a barrier to success [21].

There is also another challenge that the flipped classroom could be seen as another front in a false battle between teachers and technology. Bergmann and Sams [2] emphasize that the "only magic bullet is the recruiting, training, and supporting of quality teachers". They reported that instructional videos are powerful tools for teachers to create content, share resources and improve practice. It seems almost certain that instructional videos, interactive simulations and yet-to-be-dreamed-up online tools will continue to multiply. But who will control these tools and whether they will fulfil their potential remains to be seen. Content is vital to creating a successful flipped classroom. However, a new approach often requires fresh resources. With spare time the one thing few teachers have in excess, the thought of designing and creating new content can be enough to turn even the most enthusiastic of teachers off.

Lastly, institutes may consider allocating additional manpower to support the implementation of flipped classrooms. In this way, teachers can develop their flipped learning materials collaboratively [15] and administer the flipped course in team [57, 64]. For example, Kirvan et al. [57] split their students into two groups (reteaching group and exploration group) by referring to their daily assessment results. One teacher provided remedial help for students who need further understanding of the materials (reteaching group), while another teacher helped more capable students explore the materials more deeply (exploration group). Once the re-teaching group was ready to proceed, they would join the exploration group to engage in the advanced learning activities.

In conclusion, flipped learning is a step forward educational approach which incorporates technology in the standard teaching process to enhance the students' learning curve. When compared the learning outcomes with traditional teaching, the previous reviews suggest that flipped classroom approach can improve student performance. However, rather than being viewed as the ultimate solution to improved teaching and learning, flipped classrooms should be used as one of many pedagogical/andragogical educational tools. Flipped learning seems to have great potential but is not the holy grail and needs to evolve beyond a one-size-fits-all solution. Only time will tell whether flipped learning permanently rewrites the classroom script that has been used for thousands of years, but the results to date suggest that flipped classrooms allow us to begin to tackle the biggest barriers preventing learners from succeeding in the classroom.

References

1. Flipped learning. Higher Education Academy. https://www.heacademy.ac.uk/knowledge-hub/flipped-learning-0. Accessed 6 May 2018.
2. Bergmann J, Sams A. Flip your classroom: reach every student in every class every day. Washington, DC: International Society for Technology in Education; 2012.
3. TED. Salman Khan: let's use video to reinvent education. [Internet]. 2011. Available from: https://www.ted.com/talks/salman_khan_let_s_use_video_to_reinvent_education.
4. Crouch CH, Mazur E. Peer instruction: ten years of experience and results. Am J Phys. 2001;69:970–7.
5. Baker JW. The "Classroom Flip": using web course management tools to become the guide on the side. In: The 11th international conference on college teaching and learning. Jacksonville; 2000.
6. Lage MJ, Platt GJ, Treglia M. Inverting the classroom: a gateway to creating an inclusive learning environment. J Econ Educ. 2000;31:30–43.
7. El Miedany Y, El Aroussy N, Youssef S, Almedany S, Palmer D. Teaching the millennials: using youtube for teaching rheumatology in the standard educational setting. Ann Rheum Dis. 2018;77:1782.
8. Heiss ED, Obourn ES, Hoffman CW. Modern science teaching. New York: Macmillan; 1950.
9. Bybee R. An instructional model for science education: developing biological literacy. Colorado Springs: Biological Sciences Curriculum Studies; 1993.
10. Lawson AE. Science teaching and development of thinking. Belmont: Wadsworth/Thompson Learning; 2002.
11. Flipped Learning Network (FLN). The four pillars of F-L-I-P. 2014. https://flippedlearning.org/wp-content/uploads/2016/07/FLIP_handout_FNL_Web.pdf. Accessed 6 May 2018.
12. Lo CK, Hew KF. A critical review of flipped classroom challenges in K-12 education: possible solutions and recommendations for future research. Res Pract Technol Enhanc Learn. 2017;12:4. https://doi.org/10.1186/s41039-016-0044-2.
13. Mayer RE. The Cambridge handbook of multimedia learning. New York: Cambridge University Press; 2014.
14. Guo PJ, Kim J, Rubin R. How video production affects student engagement: an empirical study of MOOC videos. In: Proceedings of the first ACM conference on learning@ scale conference. New York: ACM; 2014. p. 41–50.
15. Grypp L, Luebeck J. Rotating solids and flipping instruction. Math Teach. 2015;109(3):186–93.
16. Schultz D, Duffield S, Rasmussen SC, Wageman J. Effects of the flipped classroom model on student performance for advanced placement high school chemistry students. J Chem Educ. 2014;91(9):1334–9.
17. Snyder C, Paska LM, Besozzi D. Cast from the past: using screencasting in the social studies classroom. Soc Stud. 2014;105(6):310–4.
18. King's Undergraduate Medical Education in the Community (KUMEC). 2016. https://www.kcl.ac.uk/lsm/research/divisions/hscr/study/undergradops/kumec/MBBS-2020.aspx. Accessed 22 Apr 2018.
19. Kurshan B. What you should know before flipping for flipped learning. Forbes: education /#change the world. https://www.forbes.com/sites/barbarakurshan/2017/04/26/what-you-should-know-before-flipping-for-flipped-learning/#1f97e80f23cc. Accessed 6 May 2018.

20. Riddle R. In 7 unique flipped classroom models – which is right for you? https://www.panopto.com/blog/7-unique-flipped-classroom-models-right/.
21. Frydenberg M. The flipped classroom: it's got to be done right. Huffpost. The blog. https://www.huffingtonpost.com/mark-frydenberg/the-flipped-classroom-its_b_2300988.html.
22. Honeycutt B, Garrett J. Expanding the definition of a flipped learning environment. Faculty Focus. 2014. https://www.facultyfocus.com/articles/blended-flipped-learning/expanding-definition-flipped-learning-environment/.
23. Muzyk AJ, Fuller S, Jiroutek MR, Grochowski CO, Butler AC, Byron May D. Implementation of a flipped classroom model to teach psychopharmacotherapy to third-year doctor of pharmacy (PharmD) students. Pharm Educ. 2015;15(1):44–53.
24. Critz CM, Knight D. Using the flipped classroom in graduate nursing education. Nurse Educ. 2013;38(5):210–3.
25. Ferreri SP, O'Connor SK. Redesign of a large lecture course into a small-group learning course. Am J Pharm Educ. 2013;77(1):13.
26. Hawks SJ. The flipped classroom: now or never? AANA J. 2014;82(4):264–9.
27. McGowan BS, Balmer JT, Chappell K. Flipping the classroom: a data-driven model for nursing education. J Contin Educ Nurs. 2014;45(11):477–8.
28. McLaughlin JE, Griffin LM, Esserman DA, Davidson CA, Glatt DM, Roth MT, Gharkholonarehe N, Mumper RJ. Pharmacy student engagement, performance, and perception in a flipped satellite classroom. Am J Pharm Educ. 2013;77(9):196.
29. McLaughlin JE, Roth MT, Glatt DM, Gharkholonarehe N, Davidson CA, Griffin LM, Esserman DA, Mumper RJ. The flipped classroom: a course redesign to foster learning and engagement in a health professions school. Acad Med. 2014;89(2):236–43.
30. McLaughlin JE, Rhoney DH. Comparison of an interactive e-learning preparatory tool and a conventional downloadable handout used within a flipped neurologic pharmacotherapy lecture. Curr Pharm Teach Learn. 2015;7(1):12–9.
31. Simpson V, Richards E. Flipping the classroom to teach population health: increasing the relevance. Nurse Educ Pract. 2015;15(3):162–7.
32. Pierce R, Fox J. Vodcasts and active-learning exercises in a "flipped classroom" model of a renal pharmacotherapy module. Am J Pharm Educ. 2012;76(10):196.
33. Singleton JA, Nissen LM. Teaching pharmacy student show to manage effectively in a highly competitive environment. Pharm Educ. 2014;14(1):21–5.
34. Wong TH, Ip EJ, Lopes I, Rajagopalan V. Pharmacy students' performance and perceptions in a flipped teaching pilot on cardiac arrhythmias. Am J Pharm Educ. 2014;78(10):185.
35. O'Flaherty J, Phillips C. The use of flipped classrooms in higher education: a scoping review. Internet High Educ. 2015;25:85–95.
36. Young TP, Bailey CJ, Guptill M, Thorp AW, Thomas TL. The flipped classroom: a modality for mixed asynchronous and synchronous learning in a residency program. West J Emerg Med. 2014;15(7):938–44.
37. Prober CG, Khan S. Medical education reimagined: a call to action. Acad Med. 2013;88(10):1407–10.
38. Kurup V, Hersey D. The changing landscape of anesthesia education: is flipped classroom the answer? Curr Opin Anaesthesiol. 2013;26(6):726–31.
39. Chen F, Lui A, Martinelli S. A systematic review of the effectiveness of flipped classrooms in medical education. Med Educ. 2017;51:585–97.
40. Heitz C, Prusakowski M, Willis G, Franck C. Does the concept of the flipped classroom extend to the emergency medicine clinical clerkship? West J Emerg Med. 2015;16(6):851–5.
41. Belfi LM, Bartolotta RJ, Giambrone AE, Davi C, Min RJ. "Flipping" the introductory clerkship in radiology: impact on medical student performance and perceptions. Acad Radiol. 2015;22(6):794–801.
42. Tune JD, Sturek M, Basile DP. Flipped classroom model improves graduate student performance in cardiovascular, respiratory, and renal physiology. A J P Adv Physiol Educ. 2013;37(4):316–20.

43. Morton DA, Colbert-Getz JM. Measuring the impact of the flipped anatomy classroom: the importance of categorizing an assessment by Bloom's taxonomy. Anat Sci Educ. 2016. https://doi.org/10.1002/ase.1635..
44. Williams DE. The future of medical education: flipping the classroom and education technology. Ochsner J. 2016;16:14–5.
45. Freedman K, Bernstein J. Educational deficiencies in musculoskeletal medicine. J Bone Joint Surg Am. 2002;84(4):604–8.
46. Truntzer J, Lynch A, Kruse D, Prislin M. Musculoskeletal education: an assessment of the clinical confidence of medical students. Perspect Med Educ. 2014;3:238–44.
47. Goh L, Samanta A, Cavendish S, Heaney D. Rheumatology curriculum: passport to the future successful handling of the musculoskeletal burden? Rheumatology. 2004;43:1468–72.
48. Day C, Yeh A, Franko O, Ramirez M, Krupat E. Musculoskeletal medicine: an assessment of the attitudes and knowledge of medical students at Harvard Medical School. Acad Med. 2007;82(5):452–7.
49. Jonas B. Rheumatology leads the way in changing medical education. ACR conference 2016 daily news. http://www.acrdailynewslive.org/rheumatology-leads-the-way-in-changing-medical-education/.
50. El Miedany Y, El Gaafary M, El Aroussy N, Youssef S. Flipped learning: can rheumatology lead the shift in medical education? Curr Rheumatol Rev. 2018. https://doi.org/10.2174/1573397114666180416170156.
51. de Fátima Wardenski R, de Espíndola MB, Struchiner M, Giannella TR. Blended learning in biochemistry education: analysis of medical students' perceptions. Biochem Mol Biol Educ. 2012;40(4):222–8.
52. Veeramani R, Madhugiri VS, Chand P. Perception of MBBS students to "flipped class room" approach in neuroanatomy module. Anat Cell Biol. 2015;48(2):138–43.
53. Pettit RK, McCoy L, Kinney M. What millennial medical students say about flipped learning. Adv Med Educ Pract. 2017;8:487–97.
54. Johnson L. The sea change before us. Educ Rev. 2006;41:72–3.
55. Oblinger G, Oblinger J, editors. Educating the net generation. Washington, DC: Educause; 2005.
56. Admiraal W, Huizenga J, Akkerman S, Dam G. The concept of flow in collaborative game-based learning. Comput Hum Behav. 2011;27(3):1185–94.
57. Kirvan R, Rakes CR, Zamora R. Flipping an algebra classroom: analyzing, modeling, and solving systems of linear equations. Comput Sch. 2015;32(3–4):201–23.
58. Clark KR. The effects of the flipped model of instruction on student engagement and performance in the secondary mathematics classroom. J Educ Online. 2015;12(1):91–115.
59. Chao CY, Chen YT, Chuang KY. Exploring students' learning attitude and achievement in flipped learning supported computer aided design curriculum: a study in high school engineering education. Comput Appl Eng Educ. 2015;23(4):514–26.
60. Bhagat V, Haque M, Bin Abu Kakar YI, et al. Emotional maturity of medical students impacting their adult learning skills in a newly established public medical school at the east coast of Malaysian Peninsula. Adv Med Educ Pract. 2016;7:575–84.
61. Hamari J, Koivisto J, Sarsa H. Does gamification work? A literature review of empirical studies on gamification. In: 2014 47th Hawaii international conference on system sciences. IEEE; 2014. p. 3025–34.
62. Hew KF, Huang B, Chu KWS, Chiu DK. Engaging Asian students through game mechanics: findings from two experiment studies. Comput Educ. 2016;92:221–36.
63. DeSantis J, Van Curen R, Putsch J, Metzger J. Do students learn more from a flip? An exploration of the efficacy of flipped and traditional lessons. J Interact Learn Res. 2015;26(1):39–63.
64. Mazur AD, Brown B, Jacobsen M. Learning designs using flipped classroom instruction. Can J Learn Technol. 2015;41(2):1–26.

Chapter 16
Social Media and YouTube

Introduction

The twentieth century has seen major advances in biological sciences, as well as information and communication technology in parallel with increasing demands from health services [1–3]. The highly dynamic developmental path of science and technology warranted a similar impactful change in medical education environment. Calls have repeatedly been raised for increasing the learning efficiency and promoting the adoption of evidence-based practice as new standards for medical education [4, 5]. This paved the way for the implementation of online electronic medical resources to be available for learners in the public domain [6–8]. By the beginning of the twenty-first century, these developments reached a mature stage and a new scope of medical learning started to materialize [9]. This was endorsed by the fact that most of the current medical learners belong to a generation that has grown up using modern online information and communication technologies. No wonder, they have been referred to as YouTube and social media generation, Millennials, Generation Y, Generation Next and Net Generation [10–12].

In recent years, Internet-based technologies not only have become part of our standard daily lives but also have dramatically transformed the interaction between undergraduate as well as postgraduate learners, educators and the world of knowledge. At the local level, such big transformation has offered new opportunities but in the meantime created new challenges [13, 14]. On the other hand, adopting the phenomenon of globalization paved the way to proposing a new concept of global health education with key indicators and outcome metrics identified to assess and monitor educational developments [15]. This was paralleled by a new concept of a global profession of medicine that is based on healthcare professionals core competency, regardless of where they have been trained [16, 17].

Y. El Miedany, *Rheumatology Teaching*,
https://doi.org/10.1007/978-3-319-98213-7_16

Use of Technology in Medical Education

Medicine is a unique mix of knowledge, skills, behaviour and attitudes. Different modalities can be used to achieve the targeted learning goals. Standard teaching approaches vary from face-to-face lecturing, bedside teaching, small-group learning, self-study, self-assessment, as well as mentoring. The past few decades have seen a progressive popularity and spread of Internet-based educational technologies particularly in medical education. This in turn has led to a breath-taking metamorphosis of medical curricula. Educational technology tools offer lucrative learning capabilities and provide both the educators and learners with new educational opportunities. These resources can portray basic medical sciences such as anatomy and physiology as well as clinical knowledge and skills whether medical or surgical with notable precision and instructions tailored to the learners' needs, facilitating safe practice, providing standardized instruction and assessment activities and being user-friendly as it is available anywhere, anytime and for everyone.

The spectrum of educational technology is broad. Current educational technologies cover most, if not all, points on the medical education continuum and vary widely in complexity, degree of realism and cost. Such resources include relatively straightforward online multimedia tutorials, high-fidelity virtual patient applications that ask learners to diagnose and manage simulated patients and immersive, team-based simulations designed around lifelike mannequins. Many institutions have purchased commercial products developed for the medical education market, while others have created in-house development teams of educators, illustrators, web designers, programmers and other multimedia specialists, who create excellent products for their own use [18].

Even though the core patient requirements and doctors' expectations remain the same as they have been across the centuries, the current generation of healthcare professionals as well as future doctors must be ready for changing healthcare services delivery with a patient–physician partnership in the decision-making process [19].

The Science of Using Videos and Social Media in Education

Implementing learning theories to develop modern teaching approaches that would keep the students more adherent to the education process, Prober and Heath [20] have suggested that medical education can be improved if the lessons were made more comprehensible and memorable, hence, "stickier" in their minds. Embracing a learning strategy that is self-paced and mastery-based has been endorsed to boost engagement and facilitate creativity. Information technology can meet today's medical students' learning needs by providing multiple curriculum delivery methods [21]. Videos, in particular, have been used effectively in many facets of face-to-face medical education and at a distance [22]. Using videos in medical education settings has been shown to enhance learning outcomes and increase learning retention. Video is proven to be useful in demonstrating patient findings and in teaching physical examination methods, procedural and communication skills [23–25]. Videos can assist learners in understanding complex events and sequences at the cellular and molecular levels [26] and has long been used in surgical education in particular to learn new techniques [27–29]. Studies on the effectiveness of video lectures in medical education have shown an improvement in grades and greater satisfaction with teaching and learning [21, 30].

Earlier studies revealed that students and trainees tend to understand and recall better when they see, hear and do [31]. The level of a learners' understanding of a topic when they see, hear and produce materials during instruction is higher (75%) compared to students who only see during instruction (20%) and see and hear only (40%) [32]. Learning with multimedia elements, such as videos, has been shown to be effective for learning activities, with subsequent improvement in their ability to produce the required behaviours/skills [33]. There is a variety of online media, broadcasting videos which enable these elements to be available. YouTube, TeacherTube and Vimeo are online video repositories in which videos are made available [34]. Users are able to download, view and share video clips on an extensive variety of content which includes film clips, television shows, music and instructional videos, vlogs or videoblogs, as well as amateur video.

Social media were reported to be effective for learning. Learners are able to develop higher-level thinking skills such as decision-making and problem-solving as well as communicate and collaborate using social media [35, 36]. In addition, connections can be made to what they learnt in their classrooms, and learning becomes more engaging [35]. YouTube becomes social media when the videos have been shared and comments and other forms of interaction occurred on the site. Hence, there is a potential for YouTube, as both a video with audio and visual elements and a social media, to be used for instruction.

With over one billion users, almost one-third of all people on the Internet, YouTube has become the most popular video-sharing platform on the Internet. With more than 300 h of video uploaded every minute, each day, Internet users watch a billion hours of video, generating billions of daily views. With this massive number of viewers, YouTube has launched local versions in more than 88 countries, in a total of 76 different languages (covering 95% of the Internet population). These figures paved the way for YouTube to become the podium for all video sectors and a goldmine for socially savvy digital marketers. With this vast growth of watchers and followers of YouTube, a new section dedicated for "education" was launched. This was endorsed by the finding that "YouTube" is an extremely practical teaching tool, with more than half YouTube views coming from mobile devices, not limited by place or time, in contrast to books, lectures and tutorials. YouTube has been implemented in preschool teaching, through to postgraduate level and beyond. Data on YouTube for press [37] revealed that YouTube on mobile alone reaches more 18–34-year-olds as well as 18–49-years-olds than any cable network in the United States. In the United Kingdom, statistical analysis [38] revealed that 46% of YouTube users are 18–24 years old.

YouTube has completely changed how people view content. Videos can have a huge impact on consumer buying decisions and can be very lucrative for education, sharing ideas and selling brands. In education, videos play an important role in supporting the teaching process in the classroom, self-directed learning, revision and continuous medical education. The role of multimedia including videos in medical education has long been documented and has been reported to be more efficient in reducing classroom time and improving examination performance in many instances [39–43]. Earlier studies revealed that students' interest in the subject and their learning process are increased when instruction is integrated with multimedia tools [44, 45].

YouTube users are one of the most important measures of success online. These "Millennials" have attitudes, aptitudes, expectations and learning styles reflecting the environment in which they were brought up [46, 47]. This makes this generation different from that existed when their teaching faculty were raised. Thus, the onus lies with the medical educators who should find lucrative ways of engaging students more critically and creatively. One of these teaching approaches is through the use of social networks like YouTube (YouTube, LLC., San Bruno, CA), Facebook© (Facebook. Palo Alto, CA) and Twitter™ (Twitter, Inc., San Francisco, CA). The use of social networks in an educationally relevant context can change the way students learn and communicate as well as improve interactions between the educators and learners [48, 49]. The growth of these online resources and the advances in Web 2.0 technology have changed the information landscape and have had positive impact on both teaching and learning. Furthermore, earlier studies showed that social networking creates a blended, social constructive learning environment that encourages collaboration, conversation and sharing. Additionally, many social networks offer platforms that can be tailored by the individual learner [50–53].

Basic usage statistics indicating number of views for each video clip, demographics as well as geographics of users, country of origin as well as dates of viewing are available through the YouTube's "creator studio/analytics". This can be used by the educator or researcher, as it will be valuable for updating the teaching content and educational tools.

Health 2.0, Medicine 2.0 and Web 3.0

Over the past two decades, the increased popularity of Internet, which has become an important part of the daily life worldwide [54], paved the way for it to replace the traditional media like television, radio and newspapers [55]. In fact, the opposite happened, as these traditional media tools have joined in and developed web pages or channels to broadcast their content online. The impact of the Internet and other technological developments has not been limited on social or sport activities but has extended to involve healthcare [56, 57]. As a consequence, people started to search the Internet using search engines like Google and Bing for health-related information and advice. In Google, 5% of all searches are health related [58]. Such online activity has developed further to be interactive rather than passive, where patients are able express their feelings and share experiences on weblogs and online forums [56]. Furthermore, patients and professionals can use the Internet to improve communication and the sharing of information on websites such as CureTogether [59] and the Artsennet websites [60] for medical professionals. The use of Internet or web technology in healthcare is called e-Health [54, 61].

In 2004 the term "Web 2.0" was introduced. Since that time, there have been several definitions for the "Web 2.0"; however, most of them have quite a good number of aspects in common. O'Reilly defined Web 2.0 as "a set of economic, social, and technology trends that collectively form the basis for the next generation of the internet, a more mature, distinctive medium characterized by user participation, openness, and network effects" [62]. On the other hand, Hansen defined Web 2.0 as "a term which refers to improved communication and collaboration between people via social networking" [63]. According to both definitions, the main difference between Web 1.0 (the first Internet generation) and Web 2.0 is interaction [64]. Web 1.0 was mostly unidirectional, whereas Web 2.0 allows the user to add information or content to the web, thus creating interaction. This is why the amount of "user-generated content" has increased enormously [65]. Practical examples of user-generated content are online communities where users can participate and share content. Examples are YouTube, Flickr, Facebook and microblogging such as Twitter. Twitter, for example, improves communication and the sharing of information among healthcare professionals [66].

According to some critics, Web 2.0 is not a new generation of the Internet because it is still based on old technologies such as HTML, the predominant markup language. Therefore, the term Web 2.0 simply describes renewal or evolution of these older technologies or of the Internet itself [67, 68]. Nonetheless, the term Web 2.0 seems to be widely used and accepted. The search engine Google reported over 85,000,000 results for the search string "Web 2.0 or Web2.0".

When Web 2.0 technologies are applied in healthcare, the term Health 2.0 may be used [69, 70]. Other authors use the term Medicine 2.0, which combines medicine and Web 2.0 [71]. There are many examples of Health 2.0/Medicine 2.0, such as the websites "PatientsLikeMe" [72] and Hello Health [73]. With the expansion of the medicine 2.0, websites and networks have been organized around specific patient categories [74, 75]. Expected beneficial aspects of these websites include improved quality and efficiency of care [76]. Another concept that appears in the Health 2.0/Medicine 2.0 literature is "patient empowerment 2.0". This has been described as "the active participation of the citizen in his or her health and care pathway with the use of information and communication technologies" [77]. It is assumed that Health 2.0/Medicine 2.0 leads to patient's empowerment, as patients have easier access to health-related information and thereby have better understanding of choices that can be made.

Web 3.0 is slated to be the new paradigm in web interaction and will mark a fundamental change in how developers create websites but, more importantly, how people interact with those websites. Computer scientists and Internet experts believe that this new paradigm in web interaction will further make people's online lives easier and more intuitive as smarter applications such as better search functions give users exactly what they are looking for, since it will be akin to an artificial intelligence which understands context rather than simply comparing keywords, as is currently the case.

Web 3.0 will be a complete reinvention of the web, something that Web 2.0 was not. Web 2.0 was simply an evolution from the original Web which can be compared to a library, as Web 1.0 was essentially an infodump, a place where people just placed walls upon walls of text which people can read but usually not interact with. Web 2.0 changed this by allowing user interaction with dynamic websites that acted more as applications than simply pages of information.

There is no concrete definition for Web 3.0 yet and the technology that will bring us there has not even matured yet. To get a better understanding of Web 3.0, an example might help to clarify the difference. In the current Web 2.0, users can interact with websites that have predetermined behaviours according to the input of users. Users can search for information using various search engines which generally provide satisfactory results if there is enough information regarding the search. However, that search is only for keywords and brings in the most popular information available and does not understand the context of the search. So if a user searches for an insect called a camaro and uses only that one word, then about 90% of the search results are for the Chevy Camaro model of car and not the insect because the car is the most popular search result and has the most prolific information. However, Web 3.0 will be able to get the context from the user and then be able to provide the user with the most useful information about the camaro insect, such as its habitat and even where to find it as a delicacy. Web 3.0 can be likened to an artificial intelligence assistant that understands its user and personalizes everything.

Furthermore, if someone is preparing for a vacation and needs to search for cheap flights and accommodations as well as meals, they must look through a lot of information on the web comparing different selections, and the search might take hours. But Web 3.0 search engines or assistants will be able to scrape all of this information and present it to the user in a very intelligent way, even making highly accurate and favourable suggestions based on the user's profile [78].

Insight into Social Media in Medical Education

In practical terms, Medicine2.0 has become a modern form of educator–learner as well as doctor–patient relationship meant to deliver medical information through up-to-date web technologies and services, with a view to endorsing health education. There are variable patterns for integrating the digital medicine in medical education whether for healthcare professionals or patients' education/management. Examples of such applications of cyber medicine include:

- *Educational/CME*: an increasing number of prestigious medical journals and organizations can be found online (e.g. *British Medical Journal*, World Health Organization, American College of Rheumatology, European League Against Rheumatism [EULAR]), with guidelines for management of different rheumatic diseases and announcements for education events/workshops. Websites like Medscape and UpToDate are also available for continuous medical education and updating the junior as well as senior healthcare professionals.
- *Clinical and research information*: social media has become a very powerful research tool (e.g. studies carried out within the "PatientsLikeMe" online community based on the personal experience of community members, also modern apps and mobile phones have been developed to facilitate the patient recruitment process). Although it is still difficult to replace clinical studies, online recruitment of the patients has a vast research potential, as it is less complicated and less time-consuming.
- *Management tailored to the patient needs*: optimization of the individual patient management based on regular monitoring of the patient's disease activity status using applications or mobile devices (Fig. 16.1) [79, 80] and portable ultrasound systems, as well as the use of games (video, 3D, virtual worlds) in therapy, e.g. for healing acrophobia or claustrophobia.
- *Visual feedback*: consulting charts, statistical data or even personal medical files online. Using such online data in the form of figures or charts endorses the patient education. Earlier study revealed that visual feedback for online recorded patient-reported outcome measures had a disease-modifying impact in the management of patients living with inflammatory arthritic conditions (Fig. 16.2) [81].
- *Online tracking*: social media tools have been used to track health information in real time or assess the cyber behaviour or learning style. The aim is to analyse the available web patterns of information and communication, example is Eysenbach (the epidemiology of information) which frames the online health information tracking process [82].
- *Cyber patient education*: earlier online data analysis (the Pew Internet project) reported that nearly 80% of Internet users have tried online diagnostics, looking for online health information and management. Cyber psychology has also attracted the attention, where research studies focus on the Internet and cyberspace impact on the individuals and groups' psychology, behaviour and interactions.
- *Interactive learning*: through using virtual learning communities on Facebook, Twitter, LinkedIn or WhatsApp, healthcare professionals can build up their network and connect with colleagues in their field. Social media can be a component of interactive learning strategies such as group discussions or case studies. Media could be a film clip, podcast of a lecture or newspaper article. Students can also create their own media. For example, student video projects can be a powerful learning experience.

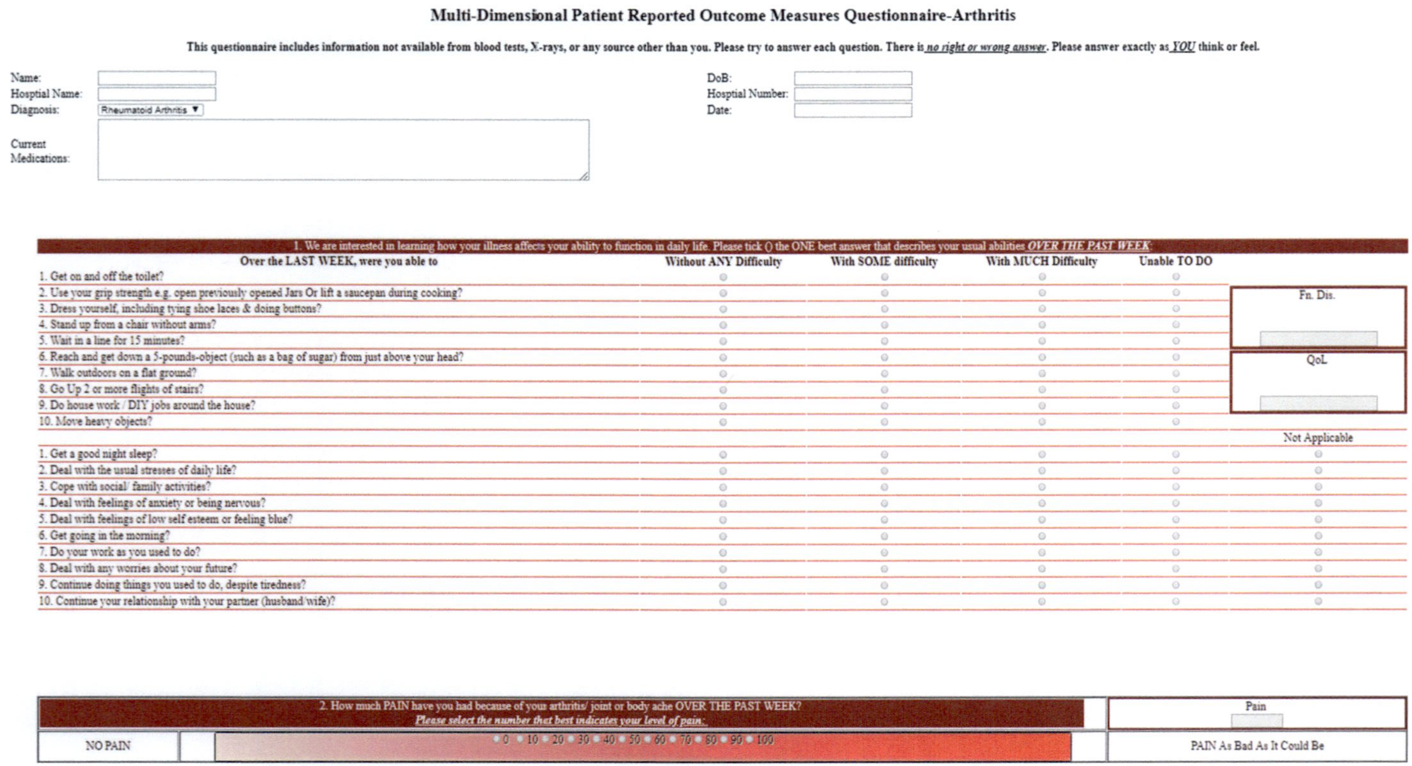

Multi-Dimensional Patient Reported Outcome Measures Questionnaire-Arthritis

This questionnaire includes information not available from blood tests, X-rays, or any source other than you. Please try to answer each question. There is *no right or wrong answer*. Please answer exactly as *YOU* think or feel.

Name:
Hosptial Name:
Diagnosis: Rheumatoid Arthritis ▼
Current Medications:

DoB:
Hosptial Number:
Date:

1. We are interested in learning how your illness affects your ability to function in daily life. Please tick () the ONE best answer that describes your usual abilities *OVER THE PAST WEEK*:

Over the LAST WEEK, were you able to	Without ANY Difficulty	With SOME difficulty	With MUCH Difficulty	Unable TO DO	
1. Get on and off the toilet?	○	○	○	○	
2. Use your grip strength e.g. open previously opened Jars Or lift a saucepan during cooking?	○	○	○	○	Fn. Dis.
3. Dress yourself, including tying shoe laces & doing buttons?	○	○	○	○	
4. Stand up from a chair without arms?	○	○	○	○	
5. Wait in a line for 15 minutes?	○	○	○	○	
6. Reach and get down a 5-pounds-object (such as a bag of sugar) from just above your head?	○	○	○	○	QoL
7. Walk outdoors on a flat ground?	○	○	○	○	
8. Go Up 2 or more flights of stairs?	○	○	○	○	
9. Do house work / DIY jobs around the house?	○	○	○	○	
10. Move heavy objects?	○	○	○	○	
					Not Applicable
1. Get a good night sleep?	○	○	○	○	○
2. Deal with the usual stresses of daily life?	○	○	○	○	○
3. Cope with social/ family activities?	○	○	○	○	○
4. Deal with feelings of anxiety or being nervous?	○	○	○	○	○
5. Deal with feelings of low self esteem or feeling blue?	○	○	○	○	○
6. Get going in the morning?	○	○	○	○	○
7. Do your work as you used to do?	○	○	○	○	○
8. Deal with any worries about your future?	○	○	○	○	○
9. Continue doing things you used to do, despite tiredness?	○	○	○	○	○
10. Continue your relationship with your partner (husband/wife)?	○	○	○	○	○

2. How much PAIN have you had because of your arthritis/ joint or body ache OVER THE PAST WEEK?
Please select the number that best indicates your level of pain:

Pain

NO PAIN 0 10 20 30 40 50 60 70 80 90 100 PAIN As Bad As It Could Be

Fig. 16.1 e-PROMs: electronic patient-reported outcomes online form to be completed by the patient. The patient ticks the box representing what he feels on the assessment day

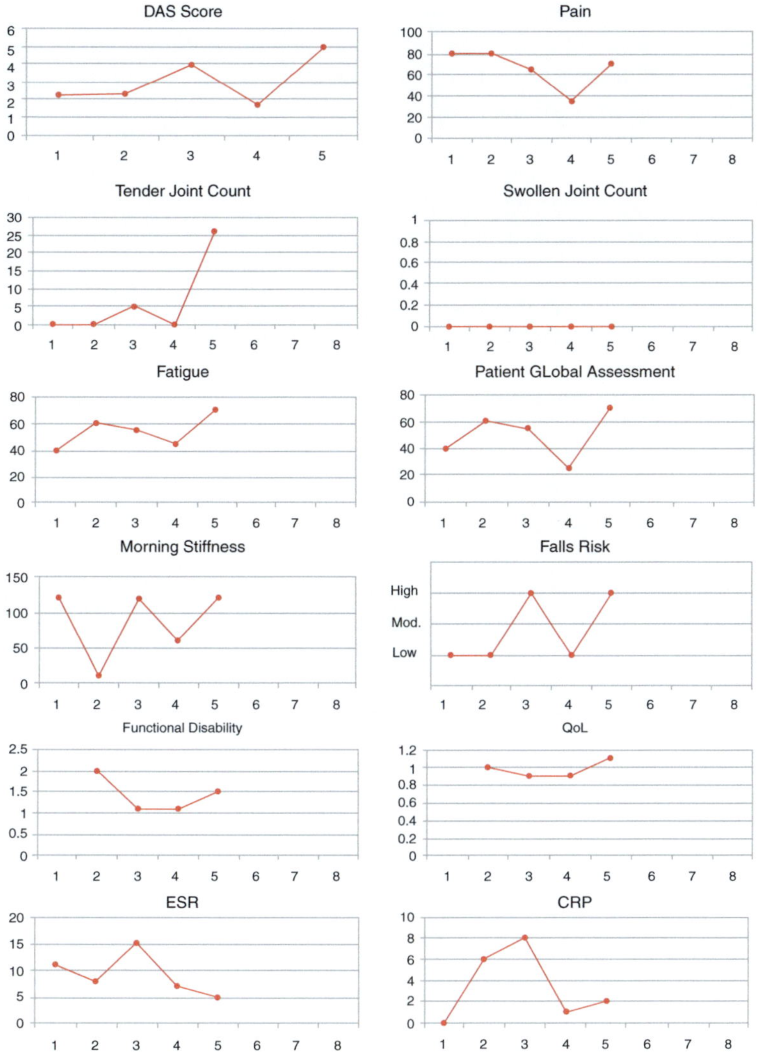

Fig. 16.2 Visual feedback: sharing the patient self-reported outcomes over time has a potential disease-modifying impact on the disease management

Social Media and the Science of Sharing

Over the past years, there has been a significant change in online virtual health environment, which subsequently has transformed the medical practice. For example, sharing stories through social networking, such as Facebook or WhatsApp, can help healthcare professionals learn from each other, improve awareness, educate patients and build trust [83]. Sharing video clips on the social media also can be helpful to both under- and postgraduate learning [84]. Similarly, the use of the creative e-media projects such as audio/video/cartoon content, digital storytelling or interactive motivational clips has been reported to improve competencies such as medical knowledge, practice-based learning, patient care, communication skills as well as professionalism [85]. In concordance, the environment of open e-learning enhanced by Web 2.0 technologies facilitated the spread of open education in terms of open source, free software, open educational resources, open content, open access publication, open teaching as well as open scholarship [86]. Furthermore, the use of mobile applications, smartphones and tablets, QR codes, augmented reality, virtual worlds and gamification play a vital role in creating a virtual learning environment. Therefore, continued social media education can be attained through personal learning networks, learning from experts (e.g. StudentDoctor.net), peer-to-peer learning and mentoring. These innovations in medical education were found suitable particularly for tomorrow's learners [84].

However, social media seemed to be underused by university teachers during their didactic activities. Teachers' negative attitude towards using social media in academic courses reflects their concern of getting out of their usual comfort zone. This has been supported by the concerns regarding ethics in the social media era. Ethical concerns range from digital identity/digital citizenship to proper professional behaviour in the use of social media. These behavioural concerns involve confidentiality, defamation, doctor–patient boundaries [87, 88] as well as following university regulations/the academic social media policy, intellectual property issues, creative commons licence arrangements and concept of information philanthropy [89].

On another front, there have been some concerns regarding the content of the YouTube videos. Clifton and Mann [90] cite unregulated content which can be misleading, inaccurate or even biased. Fernandez et al. [91] and Stohlmann [92] have identified issues such as excess information not relevant to the course or topic of study as well as gaps in the related information which may lead to incomplete or inaccurate understanding. These researchers suggest that it is important for students as well as teachers to sort through the clutter and identify videos that are valuable to advance teaching and learning in the best possible way [91–93].

YouTube and Medical Education

For many years, clinical teachers have been the main sources for teaching their students and helping them learn practical skills [94, 95]. However, with the introduction of problem-based learning and self-directed learning into most medical curricula, more emphasis has been placed on changing the learning and teaching andragogy [96–98]. In these courses, the onus has shifted to lie with the students who should find and use a wide range of learning resources, including review papers, journal articles, textbooks, museum specimens, simulated patients, computer-aided learning programs and multimedia [99–102]. The Internet has become an easily available resource of up-to-date information worldwide [100, 102–106]. This motivated the medical students to start relying on Google and YouTube as the first resources in their research [107–109].

YouTube is the largest Internet video-sharing site and is a useful tool in business, advertising, social communication, news as well as a promising learning resource for students and the general public [107, 108]. YouTube was created as an arena for personal/social communication and for distribution of commercial content. Although similar video-sharing sites are available for public use, YouTube has become the most popular worldwide.

The educational value of YouTube has been epitomized by the launch of YouTube EDU in 2009, which became a home to high-quality educational content from around the world. Its aim is to provide a global platform where anyone can learn or teach anytime and anywhere. In the higher education category, channels from top educational institutions, including colleges and universities around the world, have already subscribed. Several video categories are broadcasted including medical videos [110]. The quality of YouTube educational videos has been evaluated in a number of areas related to medical and patient health information and medical skills [109], including first aid information on thermal burns [111], human papilloma virus vaccinations [112], investigation into the mechanisms of elbow dislocation [113], clinical procedures [114], rheumatoid arthritis [115], as a learning resource for nurses [116], human and surface anatomy [117, 118], cardiopulmonary resuscitation [119], dental education [120], infantile spasms [121] and musculoskeletal conditions (Rheumavideos) [122].

The use of YouTube in education remains a hot topic. A survey in May 2012 on 2nd year MBBS students at the University of Sharjah showed that 98% of students indicated that they use YouTube for acquiring medical knowledge, though with different frequencies [123]. Furthermore, among ten other social networks, YouTube channel ownership (52%) is the second after Facebook account possession (86%) [124]. This results revealed doubling of the YouTube channel owners percentage reported in comparison to the outcomes of a survey carried out 1 year earlier in the same university, where 29% of the students were reported to owe a YouTube channel. In another study [125] done to assess the students' perspective on YouTube video usage as an e-resource in the university classroom, quantitative results showed strong, positive correlations ($p < 0.001$) indicating that, when rightly utilized, YouTube videos can have an overwhelmingly positive educational impact at the university level. Most participants felt that the videos were quite beneficial and valuable to their understanding and clarification of what was taught in the subject.

How to Assess an Educational YouTube Video?

Given the relative easiness of creating channels, producing and uploading videos on the YouTube and its free content, it has become a pool of a huge quantity of educational videos in different specialties uploaded by students and teachers. However, the quality of such uploaded videos has not been scrutinized. In addition the unregulated nature of the information contained within user-generated wiki sites is potentially unsafe to those seeking online information; YouTube is not an exception in this aspect. This mixture of variable content quality videos creates a burden on students who search for an authentic source of information.

The ways social signals are exploited on the search engines and/or Web 2.0 applications are usually not disclosed; however, social features are promising to improve the retrieval performance [126]. Though YouTube is the world's second largest search engine, unlike many professionally oriented databases such as those used for peer-reviewed publications, the search engine utilized by YouTube allows for only a limited degree of search control since it is not best calibrated for searching educational content. Thus, some videos with high-standard educational quality content might not appear on the top of the list [127, 128]. Given the lack of regulation of such videos, it is likely that a proportion of online resources are of poor quality with substantial educational flaws. The student should be observant to quality and not be misled by low-standard educational content videos. Educators can help the student by recommending a short list of relevant videos to the topic under discussion [124].

However, this process, while time-saving to the student, is burdensome to the teacher [123]. Educators should set criteria for rapid selection of a short list of relevant videos by using objective and subjective parameters (Table 16.1). For objectivity, the searching person should look for video information metrics which include the page number on which the video was located in the search results (each page contains 20 videos), duration, date the video was uploaded, number of views, video category and engagement parameters extracted from video statistics including likes, dislikes, comments and favourites. It has been shown that for every "dislike", we get ten "likes" – people like to tell their friends and colleagues about the stuff they watched and liked or disliked [129]. Camm et al. [127] used a "like/dislike" ratio of 0.9 as a cut-off for rating videos. This ratio is calculated by the number of likes divided by the total number of likes/dislikes. The number of comments per se might not be a reliable indicator of a positive feedback as some comments might reflect a negative impact. Other objective information includes those related to the channel on which the video is uploaded and whether the channel is dedicated for educational videos or not. Some channel owners are sporadic producers who have produced the videos once and never added to them. The number of channel views is a collective figure of the views of all videos on the channel. It can be considered as a good reflection of the quality of the channel videos even though the particular video has not by itself attained high-level indicators. The number of channel views is another reliable indicator of the quality of the owner's videos in general. However, in non-dedicated channels, the above-mentioned channel indicators are not reliable in reflecting video or channel quality since the number of channel views or subscribers might have been skyrocketed for the reason of presence of videos of another category like music or social videos [124].

In addition to YouTube metrics, the educators can set their own subjective quality assessment criteria including appropriateness of content to the educational

Table 16.1 Criteria for rapid selection of a short list of relevant YouTube videos by using objective and subjective parameters

Criteria	Reflection
Objective	
The page number on the YouTube search	Indicates the relevance of the video to the search keywords (i.e. those found on the first page are more likely to be seen than those on succeeding pages)
Number of video views	Provides an indication of the popularity of the video
The date the video was uploaded	Gives an idea about the number of views/day (recently uploaded videos will have lower total views than older videos; therefore, this might not serve as a comparative criterion to reflect popularity and usefulness)
The engagement criteria	Indication of the concern of the viewer who might reflect on the video by liking, commenting or adding to his favourites (people like to tell friends and colleagues about the stuff they watched or liked) [19]
Watch time	a sensitive metric of those videos being watched well, rather than got clicked as like or dislike
A brief analysis of the channel to which the video belongs	Provides a better insight on the YouTube channel or video owner
Channel information	Number of subscribers and channel views, number of uploaded videos on the channel and whether the channel is dedicated for educational videos or not
Subjective	
Appropriateness of content to the educational level of the students	The dissociation between usage and community engagement statistics
Authenticity	There are concerns regarding the academic social media policy, intellectual property issues, creative commons licence arrangements and concept of information philanthropy
Fulfilment learning objectives	The introduction of problem-based learning and self-directed learning into most medical curricula has led to a significant change in the learning and teaching andragogy
Communication skills of the presenter	Contract through social networking, such as Facebook or WhatsApp; can improve healthcare professionals communication skills, help them learn from each other, improve awareness, educate patients and build trust
Audio–visual quality of the produced video	Can be considered as a good reflection of the quality of the channel videos

level of their students, authenticity, fulfilment learning objectives, communication skills of the presenter and audio–visual quality of the produced video. This is in view that some authors indicated that YouTube indices of preference (e.g. views, likes, dislikes or search page) are not crucial in determining the value of educational video content [127, 130]. Therefore, teaching institutions or professional societies should endeavour to identify and highlight good online teaching resources.

The Dissociation Between Usage and Community Engagement Statistics

Reports of dissociation of YouTube provided video usage statistics and community engagement statistics with the relevance of the retrieved videos were published before YouTube launched "watch time". Consequently, YouTube updated its suggested videos algorithm in order to focus on "watch time". Thus, the new algorithm for suggesting videos includes prioritizing videos that lead to a longer overall viewing session over those that receive more clicks [131]. By this way it can better surface the videos that viewers actually watch, over those that they click on and then abandon [132]. Previous to this, smart video producers had noticed that YouTube would reward clicks more than actual views. Watch time should thus become an important metric to promote videos on YouTube because it is a sensitive metric of those people who are watching well beyond the first click (Fig. 16.3). However, this new metric has not yet been researched in relation to educational videos [124].

How to Create Your Educational Channel/Video?

YouTube's slogan "Broadcast Yourself" can be easily met by reviewing free self-learning resources. The creator hub on YouTube site (creator studio) provides ample information about how to get started and create a channel or a video. More refined information about creating videos with educational content are provided in YouTube

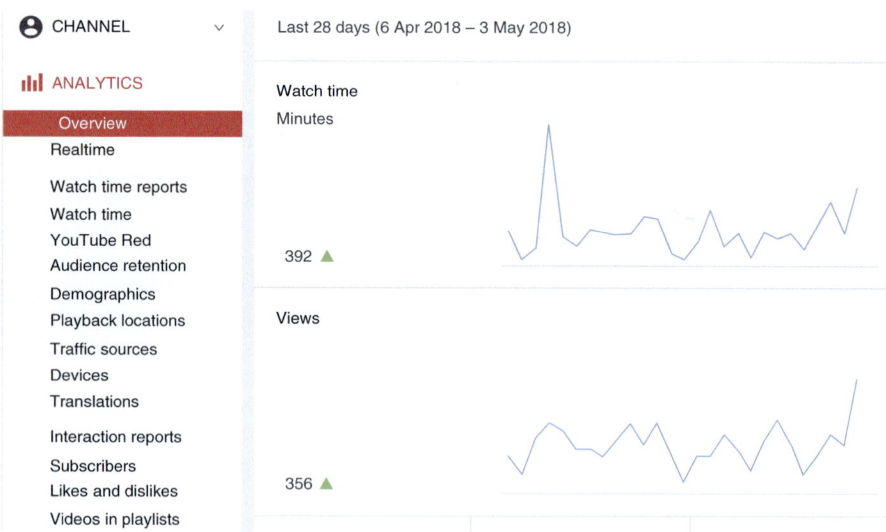

Fig. 16.3 YouTube watch time analytics: YouTube offers detailed watch time analytics which is helpful to monitor who is viewing the channel and the most viewed video clips

EDU Playbook Guide which can be downloaded for free. It also provides information about how to apply for and become part of YouTube EDU [133, 134]. Through the creator studio, YouTube channel offers access to video manager (videos and playlist), live streaming, overview of the channel as well as community (messages, subscribers, credits and community settings).

One of the most important criteria for video capturing and editing methods that are suitable for producing educational videos is to be user-friendly. Educational videos may fail if they go too high-tech and if they go too low-tech. Videos can be captured by video cameras or by using Camtasia Studio software (TechSmith Corporation, Michigan, USA), which is a computer screen capturing programme in which it is also possible to record audio. In this way on-screen PowerPoint presentations can be captured as video. If a drawing pad with a stylus is also used, then writing, drawing illustrations or tracing certain features can be captured at the same time. As for mobile devices, Reflector (Squirrels LLC, USA) can airplay mirror the iPad and iPhone screen on a computer which can then be captured and produced using Camtasia Studio [124].

The captured videos can be edited by using simple software such as Windows Live Movie Maker (Microsoft Corporation, Redmond, WA), Camtasia Studio and the editing tool of YouTube itself. These simple methods of capturing and editing are in many places comparable to those that are used by Khan Academy in producing educational videos [135].

The Art of Using Videos in Education

While science and skill can help in creating a video, there remains the most important task which is "How to optimize your educational video?" In contrast to the traditional classroom setting, where educators are expecting the lecture hall to be full and implementing their educational skills to keep the students attention, in the virtual educational world, there is no visual contact with the learners. Therefore, educators are expected to adopt new methods, different from the traditional face-to-face interaction, to engage the viewers.

Creators of educational videos need to employ certain strategies to optimize their videos to meet several targets including for the educational content, keeping the audience attention and attracting more viewers. The educator can use supplemental or full lessons. The contents can be single or in series. In medical education, as an example, it is advisable to set up a course-based channel in which it is recommended to utilize annotations, metadata and playlists to help the viewer navigate through the videos in a system-oriented or pathology-oriented sequence. In a study carried out to assess the learning potential and educational value of online videos made freely available via a dedicated YouTube channel for undergraduate and postgraduate students studying musculoskeletal medicine, twenty-five videos on joint anatomy and OSCE joint examination were made freely available on a dedicated channel on YouTube (Rheumavideos) [122]. Results revealed that the students reported an increase in knowledge, a positive learning experiences and perceptions of the online teaching model. Student perceived effectiveness and satisfaction was significantly high among the online learning cohort in contrast to the traditional teaching comparative group ($p < 0.05$). Similarly, analysis of the students' assessment scores after the scenario-based learning sessions was higher in the online learning group compared to the students taught by traditional methods ($p < 0.01$).

The metadata (and description in particular) is a great way to communicate and outline the channel content for the viewer. It will help the audience find the right videos as they search. It is also important to give an outline of the objectives of each video session so viewers know what to expect. If the videos are course-based, it should be clear as to how this video session fits into the series or playlist. If such an outline is not provided within the video itself, it can be given in the "about" information tab. Also links should be included to related videos and the sequence they must be watched with both in the "about" information tab and as annotations on the video itself. For the latter purpose, the annotation tab can be used from the edit screen. Hints to the sequence can be included in the video title. These tips can help not only create but also repurpose existing educational materials for YouTube. The use of supplemental subtitles is recommended to engage the viewer. It can also serve to learn difficult medical terminology. Subtitles can be also used to pose questions during the video session which may effectively engage the viewer [124].

Lecture-based videos can often be long. For these videos to become learner-friendly, more consumable as well as accessible, they need to be shortened. If not possible, then an abridged version of the video may guide interested viewers who can then commit to the full-length version. However, viewers often find shorter videos more intelligible. As an example, Stanford University uploaded two versions of the 2005 Steve Jobs commencement speech – a full version included an introduction by the president, and the other video was edited to just feature the speech. The edited version has over 16.5 million views, whereas the full version has 1.5 million [133]. Long videos can be cut into shorter ones each addressing an objective or a group of objectives then the whole series is included in a playlist. Education channels can use the "start and end time" features, allowing the developer to create playlists that feature specific time frames from videos within the playlist. Annotations can be extremely useful to build an interactive, curriculum experience for the viewers and to help them navigate to the previous and next videos in the lesson. Creating an interactive lesson for viewers can be done by annotating to specific time codes of video so that users can jump to a particular section. Annotations can be used for another way of interactivity by posing self-assessment questions for which answers and explanations are provided by hovering the pointer over a highlighted area using the spotlight annotation.

In conclusion, over the past years there has been a growing interest in using social media in all aspects of medical education with rapidly advanced tools and technologies. Social media and YouTube have been reported to have a remarkable potential to help both medical educators and learners, whether undergraduate or postgraduate doctors enter in the Web 2.0 era, enhancing their teaching–learning experiences through customization, personalization and rich opportunities for networking and collaboration. However, medical educators have both opportunities and responsibilities for themselves (supporting their continuing professional development, collaborative research, academic/scholarly communication, publishing and peer review), for their patients (patient education, improve their care and empowers them to have more control over their own health data), for their learners and for the public (gain media coverage, fundraising etc.). Although there are many opportunities offered by Web 2.0 technologies, there is an increased concern regarding the scientific content of some of the published videos. There is also growing need for training in how to use these technologies to enhance teaching and learning to support the medical education process.

References

1. Bleakley A, Bligh J, Browne J. Medical education for the future: identity, power and location. Springer: Dordrecht. isbn: 9789048196913.
2. Masic I, Pandza H, Toromanovic S, Masic F, Sivic S, Zunic L, Masic Z. Information technologies (ITs) in medical education. Acta Informatica Med. 2011;19(3):68–78.
3. Cooke M, Irby DM, Sullivan W, Ludmerer KM. American medical education 100 years after the Flexner report. N Engl J Med. 2006;355:1339–44.
4. Howick J. The philosophy of evidence-based medicine. Chichester: Wiley-Blackwell/BMJ Books; 2011. isbn: 9781405196673
5. Tilson JK, Kaplan SR, Harris JL, Hutchinson A, Ilic D, Niederman R, Potomkova J, Zwolsman SE. Sicily statement on classification and development of evidence-based practice learning assessment tools. BMC Med Educ. 2011;11:78.
6. Taylor P. From patient data to medical knowledge: the principles and practice of health informatics. Malden: Wiley; 2006. isbn: 9780727917731
7. Westwood JD. Medicine meets virtual reality 2001: outer space, inner space, virtual space. Amsterdam: IOS Press; 2001. isbn: 9781586031435
8. Cullen R. Health information on the internet: a study of providers, quality, and users. Westport: Praeger; 2006. isbn: 9780865693227
9. King's Undergraduate Medical Education in the Community (KUMEC). 2016. https://www.kcl.ac.uk/lsm/research/divisions/hscr/study/undergradops/kumec/MBBS-2020.aspx. Accessed on 22 Apr 2018.
10. Borges NJ, Manuel S, Elam CL, Jones BJ. Comparing millennial and generation X medical students at one medical school. Acad Med. 2006;81:571–6.
11. Farnan JM, Paro JA, Higa J, Edelson J, Arora VM. The YouTube generation: implications for medical professionalism. Perspect Biol Med. 2008;51(4):517–24.
12. Miedany E. Flipped learning: can rheumatology lead the shift in medical education? Curr Rheumatol Rev. 2018. [Epub ahead of print].
13. Ruiz JG, Mintzer MJ, Leipzig RM. The impact of E-learning in medical education. Acad Med. 2006;81:207–12.
14. Shamji AI, Law M. The role of technology in medical education: lessons from the University of Toronto. UTMJ. 2011;88(3):150–3.
15. Bozorgmehr K, Saint VA, Tinnemann P. The 'global health' education framework: a conceptual guide for monitoring, evaluation and practice. Glob Health. 2011;7(1):8. https://doi.org/10.1186/1744-8603-7-8.
16. Celletti F, Reynolds TA, Wright A, Stoertz A, Dayrit M. Educating a new generation of doctors to improve the health of populations in low- and middle income countries. PLoS Med. 2011;8(10):e1001108.

17. Schwarz MR. Globalization and medical education. Med Teach. 2001;23(6):533–4.
18. Potomkova J, Mihal V, Schwarz D. In: Kofuji S, editor. Medical education for YouTube generation, e-learning – engineering, on-job training and interactive teaching. isbn: 978-953-51-0283-0. InTech; 2012. Available from: http://www.intechopen.com/books/e-learning-engineering-on-job-training-andinteractive-teaching/medical-education-for-youtube-generation.
19. Palmer D, El Miedany Y. Shared decision making for patients living with inflammatory arthritis. Br J Nurs. 2016;25(1):31–5.
20. Prober CG, Heath C. Lecture halls without lectures – a proposal for medical education. N Engl J Med. 2012;366(18):1657–9.
21. Bridge PD, Jackson M, Robinson L. The effectiveness of streaming video on medical student learning: a case study. Med Educ Online. 2009;14:11.
22. Hurtubise L, Martin B, Gilliland A, Mahan J. To play or not to play: leveraging video in medical education. J Grad Med Educ. 2013;5(1):13–8. https://doi.org/10.4300/JGME-05-01-32.
23. Orientale E Jr, Kosowicz L, Alerte A, et al. Using web-based video to enhance physical examination skills in medical students. Fam Med. 2008;40:471–6.
24. Srivastava G, Roddy M, Langsam D, Agrawal D. An educational video improves technique in performance of pediatric lumbar punctures. Pediatr Emerg Care. 2012;28:12–6.
25. Kalish R, Dawiskiba M, Sung YC, Blanco M. Raising medical student awareness of compassionate care through reflection of annotated videotapes of clinical encounters. Educ Health (Abingdon). 2011;24:490.
26. Azer SA. Mechanisms in cardiovascular diseases: how useful are medical textbooks, eMedicine, and YouTube? Adv Physiol Educ. 2015;38(2):124–34.
27. Koya KD, Bhatia KR, Hsu JTS, Bhatia AC. YouTube and the expanding role of videos in dermatologic surgery education. Semin Cutan Med Surg. 2012;31(3):163–7.
28. Schmidt RS, Shi LL, Sethna A. Use of streaming media (YouTube) as an educational tool for surgeons-a survey of AAFPRS members. JAMA Facial Plast Surg. 2016;18(3):230–1.
29. Rapp AK, Healy MG, Charlton ME, Keith JN, Rosenbaum ME, Kapadia MR. YouTube is the most frequently used educational video source for surgical preparation. J Surg Educ. 2016;73(6):1072–6.
30. Chiu C, Lee GC, Yang J. A comparative study on post-class lecture video viewing. Adv Technol Learn. 2006;3(3):195203. https://doi.org/10.2316/Journal.208.2006.3.208-0886.
31. DeWitt D, Alias N, Siraj S, Yaakub MY, Ayob J, Ishak R. The potential of Youtube for teaching and learning in the performing arts. Procedia Soc Behav Sci. 2013;103:1118–26.
32. Lindstrom R. The business week guide to multimedia presentations: create dynamic presentations that inspire. New York: McGraw-Hill; 1994.
33. Zahn C, Pea R, Hesse FW, Rosen J. Comparing simple and advanced video tools as supports for complex collaborative design processes. J Learn Sci. 2010;19:403–40.
34. Alias N, DeWitt D, Siraj S. Development of science pedagogical module based on learning styles and technology. Kuala Lumpur: Pearson Malaysia Sdn. Bhd; 2013.
35. Bunus P. The Social Network Classroom. Technology enhanced learning: Quality of teaching and educational reform. 2010;73:517–24.
36. Greenhow C, Robelia B. Informal learning and identity formation in online social networks. Learn Media Technol. 2009;34(2):119–40.
37. Youtube.com. Statistics YouTube. 2018. Available from: http://www.youtube.com/yt/press/statistics.html. [cited 22 April 2018].
38. Support.google.com. Demographics report YouTube help. 2018. Available from: https://support.google.com/youtube/answer/1715072?hl=en-GB. [cited 22 April 2018].
39. Leonard W. A comparison of student performance following instruction by interactive videodisc versus conventional laboratory. J Res Sci Teach. 1992;29:93–102.
40. Romanov K, Nevgi A. Do medical students watch video clips in eLearning and do these facilitate learning? Med Teach. 2007;29:490–4.
41. Saxena V, Natarajan P, O'Sullivan PS, et al. Effect of the use of instructional anatomy videos on student performance. Anat Sci Educ. 2008;1:159–65.

42. Bridge PD, Jackson M, Robinson L. The effectiveness of streaming video on medical student learning: a case study. Med Educ Online. 2009;14:11. https://doi.org/10.3885/meo.2009.Res00311. Available from http://www.med-ed-online.org.
43. McNulty JA, Hoyt A, Gruener G, et al. An analysis of lecture video utilization in undergraduate medical education: associations with performance in the courses. BMC Med Educ. 2009;9:6. https://doi.org/10.1186/1472-6920-9-6.
44. Schacter J. The impact of education technology on student achievement: what the most current research has to say. 1st ed. Santa Monika: The Milken Family Foundation; 1999. p. 12. URL: https://bookertdev.ito.lacoe.edu/funding_coordination/docs/impact_of_et.pdf. Accessed 22 Apr 2018.
45. Ruiz JG, Mintzer MJ, Leipzig RM. The impact of e-learning in medical education. Acad Med. 2006;81:207–12.
46. Roberts G. Technology and learning expectations of the net generation. In: Oblinger DG, Oblinger JL, editors. Educating the net generation. 1st ed. Boulder: EDUCAUSE; 2005. p. 3.1–7. Accessed 22 Apr 2018.
47. DiLullo C, McGee P, Kriebel RM. Demystifying the Millennial student: a reassessment in measures of character and engagement in professional education. Anat Sci Educ. 2011;4:214–26.
48. Boulos MN, Maramba I, Wheeler S. Wikis, blogs and podcasts: a new generation of web-based tools for virtual collaborative clinical practice and education. BMC Med Educ. 2006;6:41–8.
49. Wilen-Daugenti T. Twenty-first century trends for higher education. 1st ed. San Jose: Cisco Systems; 2007. p. 12. URL: http://ftp.ucv.ve/Documentos/Evento_Cisco/Top_trends_in_Education_White_Paper.pdf. Accessed 22 Apr 2018.
50. Stanciu A, Mihai F, Aleca O. Social networking as an alternative environment for education. Acc Manag Inf Syst. 2012;11:56–75.
51. Lei C, Krilavicius T, Zhang N, et al. Using Web 2.0 tools to enhance learning in higher education. A case study in technological education. In: Proceedings of the international multi-conference of engineers and computer scientists (IMECS). vol. II. 2012. URL: http://www.iaeng.org/publication/IMECS2012/IMECS2012_pp1153-1156.pdf. Accessed 22 Apr 2018.
52. Nicole A. Buzzetto-more social networking in undergraduate education. Special section on social networking, teaching, and learning. Interdiscip J Inform Knowl Manag. 2012;7:63–90.
53. Forgie S, Duff J, Ross S. Twelve tips for using Twitter as a learning tool in medical education. Med Teach. 2013;35:8–14.
54. Hans O, Carlos R, Murray E, Alejandro J. What is eHealth (3): a systematic review of published definitions. J Med Internet Res. 2005;7(1):e1. https://doi.org/10.2196/jmir.7.1.e1. http://www.jmir.org/2005/1/e1/v7e1.
55. Centraal Bureau voor de Statistiek. Webcite: Statline. http://statline.cbs.nl/StatWeb/publication/?DM=SLNL&PA=71098ned&D1=33-133&D2=0-2&D3=a&VW=T.
56. Ebrahim R. Exploring technology impacts of healthcare 2.0 initiatives. Telemed J E Health. 2009;15(3):255–60.
57. voor de Volksgezondheid R. Webcite: Health 2.0: plan van aanpak. 2010. http://www.rvz.net/data/download/4372-09_plan_van_aanpak_definitief.doc.
58. Eysenbach G, Köhler C. Health-related searches on the internet. J Am Med Assoc. 2004;291(24):2946.
59. Cure together. Website: http://www.curetogether.com.
60. Community Artsennet.nl. Website: http://www.artsennet.nl/.
61. Engelen LJLPG. Slideshare. Website: Zorg 2.0 intro Spanje VWS/Nictiz. http://www.slideshare.net/lucienengelen/zorg-20-intro-spanje-vws-nictiz.
62. O'Reilly T. O'Reilly media. Website: What is web 2.0? http://oreilly.com/web2/archive/what-is-web-20.html.
63. Hansen Margaret M. Versatile, immersive, creative and dynamic virtual 3-D healthcare learning environments: a review of the literature. J Med Internet Res. 2008;10(3):e26. http://www.jmir.org/2008/3/e26/v10i3e26.

64. Wikipedia. Website: Web 2.0. http://en.wikipedia.org/wiki/Web_2.0.
65. Organisation for Economic Co-operation and Development. Website: Working party on the information economy. participative web: user-created content. 2007. http://www.oecd.org/dataoecd/57/14/38393115.pdf.
66. Mark T. Twittering healthcare: social media and medicine. Telemed J E Health. 2009;15(6):507–10.
67. Van De Belt T, Engelen L, Schoonhoven L. Definition of Health 2.0 and Medicine 2.0: a systematic review. J Med Internet Res. 2010;12(2):e18.
68. Conn J. Website: Upgrading to Health 2.0. http://findarticles.com/p/articles/mi_hb6375/is_200712/ai_n25529042/.
69. Benjamin H, Indra J, Jonathan W. Health 2.0 and Medicine 2.0: tensions and controversies in the field. J Med Internet Res. 2008;10(3):e23.
70. Scienceroll MB. Webcite: Medicine 2.0. http://scienceroll.com/medicine-20/.
71. Gunther E. Medicine 2.0: social networking, collaboration, participation, apomediation, and openness. J Med Internet Res. 2008;10(3):e22.
72. Patients Like Me. Website: http://www.patientslikeme.com/.
73. Hello Health. Website: http://hellohealth.com/.
74. Kremer J. De digitale IVF poli. Website: http://www.patientenepd.nl/wpc/wp-content/uploads/2007/09/apeldoorn-kremer-2007.ppt.
75. Slideshare BB. Website: Parkinson net. http://www.slideshare.net/lucienengelen/bloem-zorg.
76. De Rijksoverheid KA. Voor Nederland. Website: Behandeling Parkinson voorbeeld van patient centraal. http://www.rijksoverheid.nl/documenten-en-publicaties/toespraken/2008/12/01/behandeling-parkinson-voorbeeld-van-patient-centraal.html.
77. Bos L, Marsh A, Carroll D, Gupta S, Rees M. icmcc.org. Website: Patient 2.0 empowerment. http://www.icmcc.org/pdf/ICMCCSWWS08.pdf.
78. Web 3.0. Techopedia. https://www.techopedia.com/definition/4923/web-30. Accessed on 5 May 2018.
79. El Miedany Y, El Gaafary M, Youssef S, Bahlas S, Almedany S, Ahmed I, Palmer D. Toward electronic health recording: evaluation of electronic patient-reported outcome measures system for remote monitoring of early rheumatoid arthritis. J Rheumatol. 2016;43(12):2106–12.
80. El Miedany Y, El Gaafary M, El Aroussy N, Bahlas S, Hegazi M, Palmer D, Youssef S. Toward electronic health recording: evaluation of electronic patient reported outcome measures (e-PROMs) system for remote monitoring of early systemic lupus patients. Clin Rheumatol. 2017;36(11):2461–9.
81. El Miedany Y, El Gaafary M, Palmer D. Assessment of the utility of visual feedback in the treatment of early rheumatoid arthritis patients: a pilot study. Rheumatol Int. 2012;32(10):3061–8.
82. Popoiua MC, Grosseck G, Holotescu C. What do we know about the use of social media in medical education? Procedia Soc Behav Sci. 2012;46:2262–6.
83. Kim K, Yoo-Lee E, Joanna Sin S. Social media as information source: undergraduates' use and evaluation behavior. Proc Am Soc Info Sci Tech. 2011;48:1–3.
84. El Miedany Y, El Gaafary M, El Aroussy N, Youssef S. Flipped learning: can rheumatology lead the shift in medical education? Curr Rheumatol Rev. 2018. https://doi.org/10.2174/1573397114666180416170156.
85. Madanick RD. Social media in medical education: embracing a new medium. Paper given at the University of North Carolina School of Medicine on October 27, 2011, as part of the UNC Academy of Educators Lecture Series. 2011. Available at http://www.slideshare.net/ryanmadanickmd/lc11-015so-me-in-meded.
86. Courosa A. Social media, networked learning & identity. 2011. http://www.slideshare.net/courosa/social-media-networked-learning-identity.
87. Chretien KC, Greysen SR, Chretien JP, Kind T. Online posting of unprofessional content by medical students. JAMA. 2009;302(12):1309–15.
88. Jain SH. Practicing medicine in the age of Facebook. N Engl J Med. 2009;361:649–51.

89. Doyle D. E-medical education: an overview. In: Shukla A, Tiwari R, editors. Biomedical engineering and information systems: technologies, tools and applications. Hershey: Medical Information Science Reference; 2011. p. 219–38.
90. Clifton A, Mann C. Can YouTube enhance student nurse learning? Nurse Educ Today. 2011;31(4):311–3.
91. Fernandez V, Simo P, Algaba I, Albareda-Sambola M, Salan N, Amante B, et al. "Low-cost educational videos" for engineering students: a new concept based on video streaming and YouTube channels. Int J Eng Educ. 2011;27(3):518–27.
92. Stohlmann M. YouTube incorporated with Mathematical modelling activities: benefits, concerns, and future research opportunities. Int J Technol Math Educ. 2012;19(3):117–24.
93. Marks R. I learned it from YouTube! (And other challenges of teaching voice). J Sing. 2013;69(5):589–92.
94. Duvivier RJ, van Geel K, van Dalen J, Scherpbier AJ, van der Vleuten CP. Learning physical examination skills outside timetabled training sessions: what happens and why? Adv Health Sci Educ Theory Pract. 2012;17(3):339–55.
95. Bhoopatkar H, Weam A. Medical students describe their patterns of practising clinical examination skills outside time tabled sessions. Med Teach. 2008;30(3):334.
96. Holzinger A, Kickmeier-Rust MD, Wassertheurer S, Hessinger M. Learning performance with interactive simulations in medical education: lessons learned from results of learning complex physiological models with the HAEMOdynamics SIMulator. Comput Educ. 2009;52(2):292–301.
97. Azer SA. Navigating problem-based learning. Marrickville: Elsevier Australia; 2008.
98. Hessinger M, Holzinger A, Leitner D, Wassertheurer S. Hemodynamic models for education in physiology. Math Comput Simul. 2008;79(4):1039–47.
99. Lemley T, Burnham JF. Web 2.0 tools in medical and nursing school curricula. J Med Libr Assoc. 2009;97(1):50–2.
100. Azer SA, Guerrero AP, Walsh A. Enhancing learning approaches: practical tips for students and teachers. Med Teach. 2013;35(6):433–43.
101. Weiner SA, Stephens G, Nour AY. Information-seeking behaviors of first-semester veterinary students: a preliminary report. J Vet Med Educ. 2011;38(1):21–32.
102. Mirando MA, Bewley JM, Blue J, Amaral-Phillips DM, Corriher VA, Whittet KM, Arthur N, Patterson DJ. Extension education symposium: reinventing extension as a resource – what does the future hold? J Anim Sci. 2012;90(10):3677–92.
103. Keene AB, Shiloh AL, Dudaie R, Eisen LA, Savel RH. Online testing from Google Docs™ to enhance teaching of core topics in critical care: a pilot study. Med Teach. 2012;34(12):1075–7.
104. Kingsley K, Galbraith GM, Herring M, Stowers E, Stewart T, Kingsley KV. Why not just Google it? An assessment of information literacy skills in a biomedical science curriculum. BMC Med Educ. 2011;11:17.
105. Boulos MN, Maramba I, Wheeler S. Wikis, blogs and podcasts: a new generation of Web-based tools for virtual collaborative clinical practice and education. BMC Med Educ. 2006;6:41.
106. Baudains C, Metters E, Easton G, Booton P. What educational resources are medical students using for personal study during primary care attachments? Educ Prim Care. 2013;24(5):340–5.
107. Alexa Traffic Rank for YouTube. 2011. Webcite: http://www.alexa.com/search?q=youtube.com%2C&p=&r=.
108. Goodwin D. YouTube now serving 4 billion videos daily. Webcite: Search engine watch. http://searchenginewatch.com/article/2141050/YouTube-Now-Serving-4-Billion-Videos-Daily.
109. Gabarron E, Fernandez-Luque L, Armayones M, Lau AY. Identifying measures used for assessing quality of YouTube videos with patient health information: a review of current literature. Interact J Med Res. 2013;2(1):e6.
110. Azer A, AlGrain H, AlKhelaif R, AlEshaiwi S. Evaluation of the educational value of YouTube videos about physical examination of the cardiovascular and respiratory systems. J Med Internet Res. 2013;15(11):e241–6.

111. Butler DP, Perry F, Shah Z, Leon-Villapalos J. The quality of video information on burn first aid available on YouTube. Burns. 2012;1.
112. Ache KA, Wallace LS. Human papillomavirus vaccination coverage on YouTube. Am J Prev Med. 2008;35(4):389–92.
113. Schreiber JJ, Warren RF, Hotchkiss RN, Daluiski A. An online video investigation into the mechanism of elbow dislocation. J Hand Surg Am. 2013;38(3):488–94.
114. Topps D, Helmer J, Ellaway R. YouTube as a platform for publishing clinical skills training videos. Acad Med. 2013;88(2):192–7.
115. Singh AG, Singh S, Singh PP. YouTube for information on rheumatoid arthritis – a wakeup call? J Rheumatol. 2012;39(5):899–903.
116. Clifton A, Mann C. Can YouTube enhance student nurse learning? Nurse Educ Today. 2011;31(4):311–3.
117. Human Anatomy Education Channel. Akram Abood Jaffar, University of Sharjah, Sharjah, United Arab Emirates. 2011. URL: www.youtube.com/user/akramjfr.
118. Azer SA. Can "YouTube" help students in learning surface anatomy? Surg Radiol Anat. 2012;34(5):465–8.
119. Murugiah K, Vallakati A, Rajput K, Sood A, Challa NR. YouTube as a source of information on cardiopulmonary resuscitation. Resuscitation. 2011;82(3):332–4.
120. Knösel M, Jung K, Bleckmann A. YouTube, dentistry, and dental education. J Dent Educ. 2011;75(12):1558–68. http://www.jdentaled.org/cgi/pmidlookup?view=long&pmid=22184594.
121. Fat MJ, Doja A, Barrowman N, Sell E. YouTube videos as a teaching tool and patient resource for infantile spasms. J Child Neurol. 2011;26(7):804–9.
122. El Miedany Y, El Aroussy N, Youssef S, Almedany S, Palmer D. Teaching the millennials: using YouTube for teaching rheumatology in the standard educational setting. Ann Rheum Dis. 2018;77:1782.
123. Jaffar A. YouTube: an emerging tool in anatomy education. Anat Sci Ed. 2012;5:158–64.
124. Jaffar A. Tips for using YouTube in medical education. Iraqi J Med Sci. 2013;11(2):102–8.
125. Jackman WM, Roberts P. Students' perspectives on YouTube video usage as an e-resource in the university classroom. J Educ Technol Syst. 2014;42(3):273–97.
126. Chelaru SV, Rodriguez C, Altingovde I. Can social features help learning to rank YouTube videos? Web Information Systems Engineering – WISE. 2012. p. 552–66.
127. Camm CF, Sunderlan N, Camm AA. Quality assessment of cardiac auscultation material on YouTube. Clin Cardiol. 2013;36:77–81.
128. Murugiah K, Vallakati A, Rajput K, et al. YouTube as a source of information on cardiopulmonary resuscitation. Resuscitation. 2011;82:332–4.
129. YouTube. About YouTube. San Francisco: YouTube, LLC; 2013.
130. Bruno CA. URL: http://www.youtube.com/t/about_youtube.
131. Tao D, Adsul P, Wray R, et al. Search strategy effectiveness and relevance of YouTube videos. Proc Am Soc Info Sci Tech. 2012;49:1–4.
132. Lardinois F. YouTube changes its search ranking algorithm to focus on engagement, not just clicks. Teckcrunch; 2012. http://techcrunch.com/2012/10/12/youtube-changesits-search-ranking-algorithm-to-focus-on-engagementnot-just-clicks/.
133. YouTube. YouTube support. San Bruno: YouTube, LLC. URL: http://support.google.com/youtube/.
134. YouTube. Playbook guide: education. San Bruno: YouTube, LLC; 2012. URL: http://storage.googleapis.com/support-kmsprod/SNP_2799330_en_v1.
135. Khan Academy. Mountain View: Khan Academy. URL: www.khanacademy.org.

Chapter 17
TED Talks

Introduction

Knowledge is often seen as a rich form of information. Putting "knowledge" in focus, the attention is usually paid to "know-how and know-why"; however, without dissemination and sharing, knowledge would not meet the desired objectives. Over the past decade, the world has changed dramatically with rapid sharing of messages and knowledge and the Internet becoming the most popular and preferred medium of everyday communication. The facility of ideas going viral shows how infectious a concept or news can be shared around the globe in no time. As technological novelties enable swift connection and communication across distances, the landscape of learning has evolved and developed. Lectures can be recorded ahead of time and viewed online, or speakers can use text, voice and video services (e.g. Skype) to present their sessions. Schools of medicine shifted to online teaching and made many of their lectures available for the students online on their websites. Furthermore, some institutions now offer open access to their intellectual property, with a view to increasing accessibility [1].

Technology, Entertainment and Design Talks, commonly known as TED Talks, are an example of how fast great ideas can be disseminated and shared. These, freely available and accessible, online talks, enable people all over the world to watch and listen to thought-provoking speakers talking passionately about their areas of expertise (www.ted.com/talks). The TED community targets sharing "ideas worth spreading" and in doing so potentially educates and informs millions of people. The format of short talks, averaging 10–18 min, given by expert speakers has attracted worldwide interest and attention and has even inspired the launch of local community-organized TEDx events. The TEDx events allow communities to host their own independent TED-like events with a squad of speakers presenting in front of a live audience.

The TED concept continues to evolve in response to its environment, speakers, audiences and users and draws upon TEDx talks from around the world to amass "a

Y. El Miedany, *Rheumatology Teaching*,
https://doi.org/10.1007/978-3-319-98213-7_17

large volume of potentially powerful ideas from which to pick the best". As a result of innovations such as TED Talks, educators now have more opportunity to make use of technology to enhance learning. The impact of exposing learners to thought-provoking speakers who can ignite discussion, debate and reflection, continues long after the speaker's 18 min are over [2]. Therefore, the TED community represents one form of online information sharing which can be used for educational purposes.

This chapter will discuss the science behind TED and try to answer the question "Should TED Talks be teaching us something?". The chapter will discuss also the demographic and academic credentials of presenters and use of TED Talks in education, TED and student/teacher motivation. The chapter will expand to discuss the art of TED Talks and how to design a successful TED Talk and storytelling techniques.

The Science Behind TED Talks

Over the past decade, there has been a major shift from traditional teaching to digital learning. Traditional education, also known as back-to-basics, or conventional education refers to long-established customs that society traditionally used in schools and universities. However, recently, this traditional form of teaching has been challenged to promote the adoption of progressive education practices, a more holistic approach which is student-centred, paying attention to the individual students' requirements and self-control. Social media has played a key role in that shift. In fact, social media has changed how we approach many facets of life in the twenty-first century, one of these aspects is education.

For decades, students only ever expected to see their teachers in a school setting, such as during regular class hours, or perhaps for an extracurricular meeting of some kind. Occasionally teachers would give out their phone numbers to offer assistance with a project or a task which need to be completed within a fixed time frame, but students rarely made calls to their educators after school. However, social media allows students to maintain a direct link to teachers outside of the classroom. This means students will be able to easily ask for help on homework assignments or projects from the comfort of their own homes. Some teachers even report shy students using social media to organize their thoughts and communicate more effectively than when they communicate verbally [3].

Only during the last decade, studies on professional–lay interaction have focused more on mass media, which have become the main channel through which knowledge is shared and popularization is diffused. The media constitute a triangular communication space (Fig. 17.1), a "meeting point" between scientists, the public and mediators (text producers) [4]. The latter are mediators, usually journalists, who master an original technical/scientific language and are able to "translate" a scientific discourse into everyday language. In contrast with the old times where scientific communication used to be conducted through press, radio or television, new online

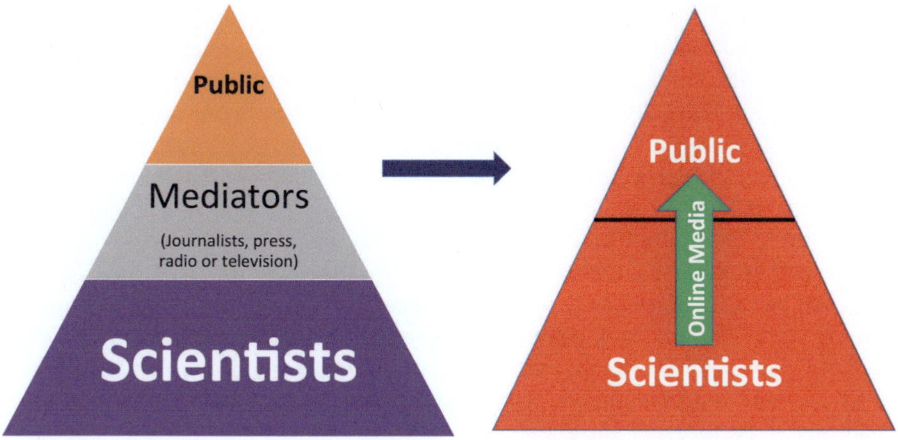

Fig. 17.1 Sharing of knowledge: the triangular communication space and the impact of the online media on this triangle. Online media posed itself as a new tool of popularization that breaches the standard triangularization "scientist–mediator–audience", bringing scientists directly into contact with their audiences

outlets have emerged offering different levels of knowledge sharing. This ranges from mere creation of an online version of previously published in-print materials, to recontextualize the texts adapting them for the web format. This is the case of TED Talks, a non-profit organization devoted to the dissemination of "ideas worth spreading", which constitute an innovation within innovation, as they are a new tool of popularization that breaches the standard triangularization "scientist–mediator–audience", bringing scientists directly into contact with their audiences [5].

In this vein, TED is one of the most effective online producers of popularizing videos. TED's start was in 1984 as a conference dedicated to the dissemination of technology, entertainment and design; however, the real launch was in 2006 when it started hosting videos of the conference talks, eventually becoming a new spoken web-based genre. The videos are provided with a transcription, a translation into a number of languages, a blog and a comment area, giving rise to a phenomenon of style and modality mixture [6]. By breaching the typical triangularization, "TED Talks" brings scientists directly into contact with their audiences. This represent a point of interest, as it enables the facility to analyse the process where a TED talk is presented by its own author, without the use of an external mediator.

In medicine, the goals of education are to support and develop highly responsible, caring and competent physicians with ever expanding roles and responsibilities. While the vast amount of knowledge and skills required to practice are based on principles of best care, this demands adopting the most effective educational approaches possible. Unfortunately, with the current challenges facing the medical service and the constraints of the educators' work schedule, the time available to impart such teaching remains static. Where traditional didactic models might fail to convey the growing complexity of healthcare, innovative educational approaches represent the best available option to ensure that knowledge is disseminated efficiently.

Recently, TED launched its TED-ED site (http://ed.ted.com/), which provides features customized for educators. First, it delivers current content from various talks with added animation for a more visual learning experience. It also affords educators the opportunity to nominate teachers with lessons worth sharing and connects these lessons with gifted animators. The true power of this site, however, lies in its "flipping" function. This function was based on the increasingly popular idea that traditional in-class and homework activities should be flipped, wherein content is introduced outside of class, allowing for deeper and meaningful explorations of the content to occur in class. TED-ED allows educators to "flip" any TED or YouTube video by customizing viewing experience for their students. The educator can adjust the title, add comprehension and higher-level questions and provide additional resources. TED will provide a unique and private uniform resource locator (URL) for students that enables an educator to track who views the video and how each student performs on the questions [7].

As colleges and universities started to endorse online learning and dedicate part of its online webspace for online education and open courseware, it become vital that tutors start to implement such innovative teaching technology to produce meaningful and relevant information that their students can understand and apply. Investing in innovative and dynamic speakers becomes rather a priority now to make use of such incredible worldwide access to the available online educational courses. In-class time can then be spent exploring the content, asking questions, problem-based learning, applying the material to real-life scenarios or developing methods to extend the content.

Should TED Talks Be Teaching Us Something?

TED Talks are an interesting phenomenon for educators to observe and reflect. They are in many ways the antithesis of the traditional way of teaching, i.e. lecturing, which is typically 60–90 min in length and delivered in cavernous halls by faculty members, engaged in everyday academic lives. There are several differences between traditional lecturing and the TED talks (Table 17.1); perhaps the lecture formality is the main superficial difference in contrast with the casual TED Talks [8]. However, TED Talks are not as unstructured as some of the critics may think. Presenters are well trained and advised to follow a specific presentation formula, which maximizes storytelling and highlights passion for the subject. While learning outcomes have not formally been assessed, TED Talks transfer the audience from the passive to the active mode and do seem to accomplish their goals of spreading ideas while sparking curiosity among the learners. The fact that some TED presentations have been viewed more than 16 million times highlights to the effectiveness of the platform in at least reaching learners and stimulating a desire to click, listen and learn. Furthermore, the TED Talks website is the fourth most popular technology website and the single most popular conference and events website in the world [9].

Table 17.1 A comparison between TED talk and traditional academic teaching

Aspect	TED talk	Academic lecture
Concept	Showcase presentation	Traditional academic lecture
Target	Share ideas/engage audience	Educate
Style	Storytelling (good approach delivers the evidence or observation and draws a larger conclusion)	Lecture style – standard/rigid
Composition	New innovative, well-formed ideas, challenge a belief, range from basic great ideas to new or surprising notions	Concept and content follow a specified curriculum. Deliver fundamental principles about established or emerging basic or experiential science
Mode	Digital, async viewing	Mixed (mainly power point)
Venue	Relaxed atmosphere, seating, group interactions	Semester course
Audience	Engaged group of peers	Passive/semi-passive student learners
Speaker	Topic expert, passionate about the idea	Academic, subject matter expert, often dispassionate
Time	18 min	45–90 min
Structure	Explain the idea, make the audience attracted, how the idea can be implemented and affect the audience	Very organized. Starts with introduction, objectives, topics, conclusions
Visuals	Photos and images, graphs, less text	Text bullet points, some images and photos, graphs (usually several points)
Preparation	Script out comments, rehearse	Not scripted, tend to read the slide, usually not rehearsed

Adapted from Romanelli et al. [11] with permission

The TED phenomenon may have both direct and indirect or subliminal messages for academia. However, initially, the main question to consider is whether the TED Talks is a logical educational evolution or a reaction to the Millennial generation and their preference for digital learning which occurs "wherever and whenever" [10]. Cross-sectional analysis of TED fans reveals diversity in background, sex as well as age. This provides an evidence that the digital platform does not solely attract younger generations of learners. In fact, it suggests a shift in adult learning style with adult learners either are more drawn to digital learning than they think they are or than they are likely to admit. The perceived efficacy of TED raises once again the question whether it is time to stop relying on lectures as the primary strategy of learning and consider alternative teaching approaches. However, bearing in mind that the TED Talks do not convey large chunks of information but rather present impressive grander ideas, would TED-like educational modules of 18–20 min be enough to stimulate the students' curiosity across a variety of medical topics, maintain attention span and improve retention, or shall we find a collateral way to include TED education in the standard educational process? Many faculty members who have been recognized as outstanding tutors or lecturers might admit that they already have changed their teaching style and started to teach through a TED-like lens.

Alternatively, TED Talks or TED-formatted learning experiences might be ideal facilitators for incorporation into flipped learning environments where information is gathered and learned at home, while ideas are analysed, debated and assimilated within the classroom [11]. On another front, TED Talks have given scientists, educators as well as researchers a real-time, mass media-driven opportunity to disseminate their research and share their theories, ideas and knowledge that might otherwise have gone unnoticed or presented to a small number of audience. Similar platforms or approaches may be able to provide opportunities for the academy to further transmit research to the general public [10].

Thinking from a different angle, the modern educational approaches and the different style of learners' demand that we all think a bit more productively, more creatively and more rationally, to think from a different angle, with a different set of muscles, as well as a different set of targets and expectations to face the challenges. The debate regarding TED's exact academic role is expected to last for some time while the phenomenon continues to grow and evolve. In the interim, the academy could learn from the TED platform. Romanelli et al. [11] wrote a report raising the question "Should TED Talks be teaching us something?". Even though TED has limitations and is subject to valid criticisms, educators could use the talks as a component of an overall course sequence that helps students connect with material or spark student interest in particular topics that are then explored in greater detail within the curriculum. The TED platform could also be used as an active learning strategy, where students are either asked to critique an existing TED Talk or design their own TED Talk regarding a particular topic of interest or relevance. TED presenters are often selected not only for their expertise on a given topic but also for their ability to effectively and succinctly communicate information to learners. In fact, students familiar with the TED Talk paradigm may hold lecturers to a higher standard given the effectiveness of the platform. In turn, faculty members might be able to improve their own delivery skills by observing TED Talks and adopting techniques used by presenters. Academia as well as administrators in charge of curricula development might familiarize themselves with the platform and its potential implications for future delivery of information in all settings including higher education. Given the vast reach and impact of the platform to date, it would be shortsighted for both individual educators and the academy to ignore what TED phenomenon is able to teach us.

Characteristics and Impact of TED Talk Presenters

Disseminating scientific information and sharing knowledge with the public are not easy; Boulter emphasized that "the public finds much of the detail of science unintelligible" and that academics "need to be aware of their changing status and of the need to respond to the public's demand for more openness" [12]. There is also a challenge in communicating "what science can and cannot do" [12] and making transparent processes such as revisions and retractions [13, 14]. In fact this is not limited to medicine or specific knowledges; certain sections of the population believe that science is not objective but rather used for political or economic purposes [15, 16]. This is particularly problematic when scientific or technical theories become associated with a few outspoken individuals [17]. The situation is further exacerbated in the world of TED Talks [18], where a topic is condensed into 18 min or less of "episodic framing" [19].

For years, visualizations have been the cornerstone in scientific communication, helping both to elucidate and convince [20, 21]; however, in recent years the trend has changed to focus on the audience themselves and how to keep them attracted. A workshop of researchers on science communication concluded that "the greatest challenge to science communication online remains simply reaching audiences" [22]. Therefore, epitomized by the performances of Hans Rosling, called a "master of science communication" [23] and encouraged by the Internet technology and sites such as TED, speakers have increasingly turned to infographics and other visualization methods in order to communicate their ideas to the lay public. A vital component of TED Talks is the entertainment aspect (which is one of the three components of TED's name), which mandates the use of appropriate methods by professional entertainers to package scientific talks as "entertainment". One example that works well for medical teaching is storytelling. Other examples include the use of satire, humour or any other form of comedy to help the public to engage with science [24]. Indeed, "the popularity of scientific claims is inevitably defined by the available technology and preferred aesthetics of contemporary media" [25], and accordingly, it should not be surprising that the visual potentials available on the Internet have been embraced by knowledge disseminators.

Given that TED Talks are an example of popular scientific communication, it is important to identify who would be the best candidate to present at TED, as well as to assess whether these individuals are particularly successful from the perspectives of popular and academic receipt. Information regarding the presenters can provide insights into the credentials of those who are disseminating scientific information on an almost unprecedented scale and the degree to which the viewing public prefers videos presented by academics to those presented by nonacademics (or vice versa).

A study carried out by Sugimoto and colleagues [26] raised three main questions in that aspect: (1) What are the characteristics of academic TED Talk presenters?, (2) What is the relationship (if any) between presenter characteristics and video popularity metrics?, and (3) What impact does giving a TED Talk have on the citation impact of the academic presenters? Bibliometric and webometric techniques were used to gather data on the characteristics of TED presenters and videos and analyse the relationship between these characteristics and the subsequent impact of the videos. The results showed that the presenters were predominately male and nonacademics. Male-authored videos were more popular and more liked when viewed on YouTube. Videos by academic presenters were more commented on than videos by others and were more liked on YouTube, although there was little difference in how frequently they were viewed. The majority of academic presenters were senior faculty, males, from US-based institutions, were visible online and were cited more frequently than average for their field. However, giving a TED presentation appeared to have no impact on the number of citations subsequently received by an academic, suggesting that although TED popularizes research, it may not promote the work of scientists within the academic community. These findings can help to shed light on some theories and beliefs about science popularization. In contrast with earlier reports [27], these outcomes reveal that media can foster positive perceptions of science and technology amongst the public. This can be attributed to the widespread lack of science literacy, which makes the lay people relatively defenceless to the media's influence [27].

Use of TED Talks in Education

TED talks are considered valuable resources in educational settings from two different perspectives: (1) as knowledge resources in their own right containing valuable and accessible content and insights for learners and (2) as educational material, particularly facilitated through the wide range of transcripts [28]. Sir Ken Robinson, one of the most viewed TED speakers, is popular not only for his TED Talk style but also for his message on education reform [29–31]. He argues that the current education process (in the United States as well as most of the schools all over the world) operates as an industrial machine, optimized to achieve outcomes in the form of high grades and performance on standardized tests. In order to facilitate learning, teachers must embrace their profession as a creative one to thereby mentor, stimulate, provoke and engage students as well as pass on learned information. While doing so, his theory has stimulated, provoked and engaged millions of viewers.

Schools were built upon the fundamental premise that teachers and knowledge and information were scarce. This is no longer valid. Now, most of the learners have faster and broader access to the Web, where all of those things are suddenly abundant. Some of the teachers have actually started using educational material available on the web in the standard school teaching. That means that the traditional role of school, to deliver an education, is quickly becoming less and less relevant. If schools continue to be considered as the place where children go to master a narrow list of content, knowledge and skills that were originally defined almost 150 years ago, there is a high risk of putting those kids out into the world with little idea of how to take advantage of the explosion of learning opportunities that now exist. In his TED talk, Sir Ken Robinson outlined "How to escape education's death valley" [31] and how education must change when learning and information become available everywhere. The problem, however, is that most "reform" efforts are aimed almost exclusively in the form of raising test scores. But doing "better" on measures that do not account for this huge shift, both the learners and educators are in the midst of, is the absolute wrong emphasis. This highlight the urgent need for thinking very differently about the experiences, outcomes, skills and literacies expected from students and learners when they go to their schools or universities.

TED talks are valuable resources in educational settings for several reasons, which was reviewed in a review article [32]. First, TED Talks deal with various interesting contents which are related not only to technology, entertainment and design (TED) but also to business, science and all kinds of up-to-date global issues which can draw all kinds of language learners' attention. The total number of tags for all topics of TED Talks is 301. Using this tag function people can find interesting talks easily. TED Talks also can simply be searched on the main webpage according to the ranks of newest releases or popularity (e.g. most viewed, most e-mailed this week, most comments this week, etc.) and by moods of speech (e.g. persuasive, courageous, ingenious, fascinating, etc.).

Second, TED.com has its distinctive "interactive transcript" feature embedded within the script which is different from other online streaming video websites (e.g. YouTube.com). Most TED Talks have a transcript provided in various world languages. Viewers can see the transcript while watching a TED video and can go back and forth when they want to repeat or skip a certain part of the video by just clicking the part of the script. If users wave the mouse cursor over anywhere of the script, the part of script is activated by the phrase. The videos, scripts and transcripts of TED.com can be seen at one site due to its user-friendly arrangement. Consequently, these convenient visual aspects of the webpage create more enjoyable learning experiences to those who are watching TED videos.

Third, TED videos are easy to share with other people by downloading them to a computer hard disk or by using social networking service (SNS), such as Twitter or Facebook. Even when the Internet is not available in the classroom, students can watch a TED video as long as the teacher downloads it from the website in advance. By clicking "download" icon, TED videos can be downloaded simply into MP4 format. Moreover, teachers can directly share the link for TED Talks with students outside the classroom using a class website or social networking service. Therefore, TED Talks can be utilized as materials for in-class activities, group projects or homework assignments by sharing with all participants inside and outside the classroom.

Lastly, TED Talks can be accessed with no bounds on time and place using the latest communications technology. Cha [33] states that this ubiquitous learning enables learners to access to the data anytime and anywhere using mobile devices such as smartphones, tablet or computers. In recent days, smartphones have taken the lead as an ideal tool for satisfying new needs of mobile learning generation with appearance of many kinds of applications (e.g. TED, YouTube, Podcast, iTunes, etc.) providing audio and video clips for authentic learning [34]. Palalas [35] tries to make a set of design principles for effective mobile-assisted listening objects by investigating open access to TED Talk videos including "English as a Second Language" podcasts and vodcasts with flexible retrieval. Kim [36] demonstrated that university students' perceptions and attitudes toward authentic listening materials have been significantly positive.

With these advantages of TED Talks as good authentic materials, instructors can teach and stimulate learner autonomy [37]. By watching TED videos both inside and outside the classroom, learners can get aural and visual input which is useful for their practice, such as the speaker's way of talking and gestures. TED Talks can also increase exposure to world experiences, building up authentic knowledge and various views in diversity of topics interactive and transcript content.

LearnWeb: An Interactive Platform Integrating TED Talks

University teaching requires ever more flexible teaching tools and resources, in order to "incorporate more practice-oriented, media-based assignments to maintain students' interest and to achieve long-term learning outcomes" [38, 39]. LearnWeb is a relatively new tool for an interactive use and management of multimedia resources for pedagogical purposes. Since its creation in 2009, LearnWeb has been used in varied learning scenarios, including language teaching [41], teacher training [38], media education and cooperative learning [40]. To enhance its educational input, LearnWeb has integrated TED Talks an open set of videos with multilingual transcripts that are gaining momentum as multimedia resources for a range of pedagogical purposes, including supporting autonomous language learning [42], increasing student's motivation to study a foreign language [43] or training pre-service perspective teachers [44]. This has added to the educational value of the LearnWeb as TED Talks are valuable resources in educational settings for several reasons [1, 8]. In fact, they offer authentic spoken material, expose language learners to a variety of accents and topics (i.e. vocabulary), are accompanied by transcripts and multilingual translations, are freely available online and are engaging in terms of form, as well as content.

TED and Student/Teacher Motivation

TED talks have been recognized as useful not only for sharing knowledge or improving certain skill such as listening or comprehension [45] but also, more generally, for providing meaningful content that inspires teaching and learning, as well as motivating extended discussion, research and lifelong learning [7, 42, 46]. Motivation is an essential component of learning and has been explored in many educational courses. Many TED Talks address what motivates people, prompting the question of how teachers can inspire students to want to learn. Educators often recognize their goal is to promote "lifelong learning", which is important, given that it is impossible for students to learn everything they need while attending school or university. Unfortunately, how to promote students' motivation is rarely discussed, as the focus in education is often skews toward specific content standards. However, by deliberately asking deeper questions and providing opportunities for students to take responsibility for their learning, this creates the motive to shift that focus to promoting lifelong learning without neglecting the standards [7].

Mihaly Csikszentmihalyi, a leading psychologist and researcher, discussed his most famous contribution to the positive psychology movement: flow. He wanted to understand what makes humans happy, and, after extensive research, he found that it was not money or fame but rather working on a task that is worthwhile and appropriately challenging for one's skill set. Csikszentmihalyi [47] described the conditions needed to facilitate flow, such as a sense of clarity and immediate feedback. If teachers consciously considered how to promote flow among their students, work would become more enjoyable, and students would be more motivated to immerse themselves in their assignments. The essential component of flow is finding tasks that are matched to students' abilities and interests. In content-driven courses, this video could promote examination of pre-assessments and matching assignments to students' skill sets. Further, it could lead to an assignment that encourages students to create a differentiated lesson that begins with pre-assessment and then matches one of multiple assignments to students based on their performance on the pre-assessment.

TED Talks can be used not only to promote student motivation but also to inspire the teachers to introduce us to innovative instructional practices. Teacher educators can create assignments that encourage teachers to explore TED talks or design their own videos. Teachers could then be asked to find a few videos that connect to particular content. These videos could be used as a part of a lesson, an enrichment opportunity or a potential re-teaching tool.

The Art of TED Talks: How to Design a Successful TED Talk

Learning how to breathe life into your slides, instead of draining it out of your audience, is an art before being a science. Every day, audience members are forced to sit through mind-numbing, text-heavy, data-filled presentations that end up doing more damage than good. For a TED talk, presenters are given a maximum slot of 18 min to share their message with the world. Some choose to present without slides. For example, Sir Ken Robinson delivered a very inspiring speech on education without the use of any slides (http://bit.ly/12MPEFx). He felt that his talk didn't require any visual aids, so instead of using slides as a crutch (which is what most mediocre presenters do), he gave his talk without them. Other presenters, however, choose to use slides to help promote the understanding of their message, i.e. use their slides for the audience rather than to help themselves. In another word, they used the slides to amplify the understanding of their message. This section of the chapter will discuss suggestions of how to design a successful TED talk as suggested by Akash Karia [48].

- *Who, why and what?:* Perhaps the first question the speaker should ask him/herself is for "*who*" have the slides been made? Are they to help the audience or to help the speaker? If a slide does not help the audience, then it should not be included in the presentation. Successful and effective presentations are always about the audience, never about the speaker. According to the TEDx speaker guide, which is available for free on the Internet [42], "Slides can be helpful for the audience, but they are by no means necessary or relevant to every talk.

Ask yourself: Would my slides help and clarify information for the audience, or would they distract and confuse them?" Therefore, if a slide helps to clarify the information for the audience, it should be kept. If not, and if it is mainly used as a crutch, then it should be excluded from the presentation. The second question that might raise is: "Why" does the presenter need to spend time making the PowerPoint slides look beautiful? If the audience can get the message, who cares if the slides are crappy?" Actually, nowadays, it's not enough to just display bullet points on the screen. The advice of having six bullet points with six words in each bullet is old and outdated. It results in a boring presentation.

Unfortunately, the audiences judge the speakers and their talks based on the quality of their slides. If the slides are high quality and beautifully designed, the audience will be enthusiastic about listening to the presenter. However, if the slides are badly designed, the audience may think, "If the speaker did not spend much time on designing his/her slides, it is likely that not enough time has been spent in preparing the talk either". In other words, badly designed slides give the audience the impression that the speaker does not care about them. Once they develop a negative perception of the presenter, it will be very difficult keep the audience interested in either the speaker or the message delivered. Is it possible to give a great presentation despite crappy slides? Yes, it's possible. However, a person should be a brilliant speaker in order to overcome the negative perception the slides created. In fact, it is much easier to learn how to create effective and engaging slides instead.

The last question is "what" makes the slides work for the speaker? The presenter should always keep in mind that the target is to create effective slides which promote the understanding of the delivered message. Slides' design is not about making them look pretty and attractive. It is about eliminating clutter, promoting simplicity and enhancing the effectiveness of the delivered message. Implementing these concepts is expected to result in a more visually appealing slide. Whether the slides are prepared for a TED talk or a medical presentation, implementing simple presentation design principles targeting the audience, would make the slides work for the person not against them.

- *The message:* One of the commonest mistakes most presenters make is when they realize they have to deliver a presentation, they immediately start dumping their information onto PowerPoint slides. The result is a lifeless and very dry presentation, filled with too much text and too little inspiration. Instead, the first thing to consider is to identify the "core message" of the talk. The core message refers to the single most important idea the speaker wants to deliver to the audience and to remember from the presentation. What is the one single idea the audience would take away from the presentation?

Nick Morgan, who has coached many TEDx speakers, writes in his blog post on "How to Deliver a 20-Minute TED-Like Talk" (http://bit.ly/18lF6ww): "Begin by choosing one idea. Try to make it an idea that has universal interest, but where your specific expertise can usefully be applied. Then, narrow it down and focus it…". Becky Blanton, who presented at TEDGlobal 2009, emphasized the importance of selecting a core message in an article she wrote for 6 min (http://bit.ly/244tM). In her article titled "How to Deliver the Talk of Your Life", she wrote: "Convey one strong idea. Take time to focus each idea you want to express, then pick the most compelling, the strongest idea".

The presentation core message is of vital importance because it helps the speaker decide what to keep in and what to toss out. Perhaps there is a nice story or example or statistic the speaker may prefer to include in the presentation. Should it be included or tossed out? Simply if it backs up the core message, it should be kept; if not, it should be removed. It may be great, but it does not belong in this presentation. As a result, the final presentation will end up being very clear and laser-focused.

- "I-focused" *vs* "You-focused": The presentation should be kept all the time about the audience, not about the speaker. If the speaker is talking about himself or own business, this is definitely the wrong thing to do. Making the presentations "you-focused" is one of the guidelines included in the TEDx speaker guide [42]: "Don't focus too much on yourself". To elaborate on this guideline, the presentation should include a lot of "you-related words ("you", "your", "you're") than I-related words ("I", "me"). Talk about the audience, not own! As an example is the "you-focused" opening from Simon Sinek's TED talk, "How do you explain when things don't go as we assume? Or better, how do you explain when others are able to achieve things that seem to defy all of the assumptions? For example: Why is Apple so innovative? Year after year, after year, after year, they're more innovative than all their competition" (http://bit.ly/12MP5v9). "Starting with a question "How", ending with "why" and the "you-focused" opening, both immediately grabs the audience's attention. In his presentation, Simon Sinek state: People don't buy what you do; they buy why you do it. Something called the law of diffusion of innovation, and if you don't know the law, you definitely know the terminology. The first two and a half percent of our population are our innovators. The next 13 and a half percent of our population are our early adopters. The next 34% are your early majority, your late majority and your laggards. The only reason these people buy touch tone phones is because you can't buy rotary phones anymore. [Simon Sinek (http://bit.ly/12MP5v9)]
  Though the whole statement could have been done using the "I-focused" approach, Simon used the "you-focused" words, constantly relating his talk to his audience; hence, the focus was on the audience, not on himself.
- *Creating TED meaningful slides storyboarding:* All of us have seen those slides crammed with too much text, with full, grammatically correct sentences, and all the presenter reading the sentences out loud while facing the slide. The reason they fall in this trap is because they dumped the ideas on the slides instead of dumping them on paper. As noted earlier, the first step is to identify the core message(s) and organize them into a logical, easy-to-follow, step-by-step sequence. The best approach to do this is to "storyboard" the presentation.
  Storyboards were first used for movies, but their use has extended to marketing, advertising and presentation design. Why have they been used in presentation

design? Because they free presenters from the self-imposed constraints of using headings and bullet points. By default, presentation software such as PowerPoint pushes presenters into using boring, standard templates, which limits the creativity of the presentations. It's much better for the speakers to free themselves from the software creativity-limiting constraints, step away from the computer and storyboard the presentation using pencil, pen and paper [Nancy Duarte, "The secret structure of great TED talks" (http://bit.ly/yrDGfo), and "What is the best way to start creating a presentation?" (http://bit.ly/SkUByj)].

- *The golden formula*: One of the key factors to create a good presentation for TED talk is to use large, visually stunning images in the presentation. The pictures not only make the presentation attractive but also memorable. John Medina reported that 3 days after a presentation, most people only remember approximately 10% of what they heard. However, if you add a picture, recall shoots up to 65% [49].

  Representing the idea visually is the aid. Images should facilitate delivering the key messages and help the audience understand the presented topic better. The cliché, "An image is worth a thousand words" is true. Usually, a single image will convey an idea better than several paragraphs of text. On creating a presentation, the question should be "Can what I am trying to say be demonstrated visually using a picture?" If it can, then it is advisable to ditch the text and use an image instead. When choosing images for your presentation, choose images that arouse an emotional response in your audience. The best presentations arouse the audience's emotions. How do you know which image is going to arouse your audience's emotions? Here's the guideline: Choose the image that creates the largest emotional response in you. If the image arouses your emotions, it will arouse your audience's.

  Where can a person find visually arresting images able to arouse the audience's emotions? Photos can be bought from stock photography sites such as www.stockphotos.com. Alternatively, the speaker can use www.compfight.com to search for images with a Creative Commons licence. If the speaker is going to use images that have a Creative Commons licence, it is essential to give the author of the image appropriate credit for their work. According to the TED website:

  > You must properly license all images for TED's use in worldwide video and web distribution (we may use the images in TEDTalks, which are distributed globally for free). Don't grab images from the web. Use high-resolution pictures and graphics. Full-quality photos from a digital camera will look better than images pulled off the web. (http://www.TED.com)

  A third alternative is to use the speaker's own photos. If the speaker has taken some high-quality digital images that are aesthetically pleasing and relevant to the point being made, they can be considered for use in the presentation.

  The three-second rule: Lastly, the three-second rule states that the audience should get the slides message within 3 s of seeing it. Therefore, it is advisable to use images that are simple and clearly represent the speaker's point of view. The slide should be like a billboard – it should contain a large image that grabs the audience's attention and understood easily and quickly.

Storytelling Techniques

The art of storytelling is as old as the human race itself. Our earliest forms of communication were deeply visual in nature. Even up today, that hasn't changed. In fact, if anything, having a mastery of visual storytelling techniques has become more important than ever. The success of our marketing, advertising and much of our digital entertainment relies on a solid understanding of such skills.

Academics and marketers alike have found that our brains are hardwired to process and store information in the form of stories. So, when we hear that "once upon a time" there was a certain character in such and such place, our minds are immediately transported to this imaginary scene. Akash Karia, a professional speaker, reported that stories are irresistible to the human mind because they activate our imaginations, and so we have no choice but to follow the mental movies created in our heads. As a result, they are used by many TED presenters who are some of the most inspirational speakers in the world [50]. This is further proven by a study conducted by Chibana [51], on the evolution of long-form multimedia stories published by *The New York Times*. The study revealed that many of the storytelling techniques used thousands of years ago are still applicable today to a wide range of mediums besides the written word.

To start this section appropriately, let us start by telling a story! How many times have you attended a presentation and, within the first 30 s, thought, "Wow, this is going to be good!" Not many? How many speakers have you seen opening their presentations in boring, dull and lifeless ways. The most common (and thus boring) opening is, "Thank you for inviting me. My name is YEM and I want to talk to you about…" This opening literally sucks the excitement out of the room. If the audience members were excited about listening to the speaker, they certainly are not going to be after that opening! So, what is the best way to open a speech? You've probably guessed it: open with a story.

In her great TED talk (http://bit.ly/10gmj3t), titled "The Power of Introverts", Susan Cain masterfully hooked her audience into her speech with the following opening "when I was nine years old, I went off to summer camp for the first time. And my mother packed me a suitcase full of books…". Susan did not bore the audience with an introduction of herself (the introducer/emcee should be the one who introduces you before you get up on stage). She did not bore her audience with gratitude by trying to express how thankful she is that she was invited to speak at TED. Instead, she immediately dives into a story. The best way to thank your audience for the opportunity to speak to them is to deliver a speech that keeps them engaged, interested and involved.

Stories are not only the indispensable tools for novelists; they are useful for presenters, business leaders, marketers and journalists. They can come in all forms, from slide decks and infographics to videos and static images. In her report on storytelling techniques [52], Chibana reviewed the most inspiring TED presentations and highlighted the reasons stories tend to fascinate the audiences. Below are some recommendations which would make a story captivating, along with advice given by leading experts (Fig. 17.2). This may serve a guide to help you make your next presentation a one that your audience will never forget:

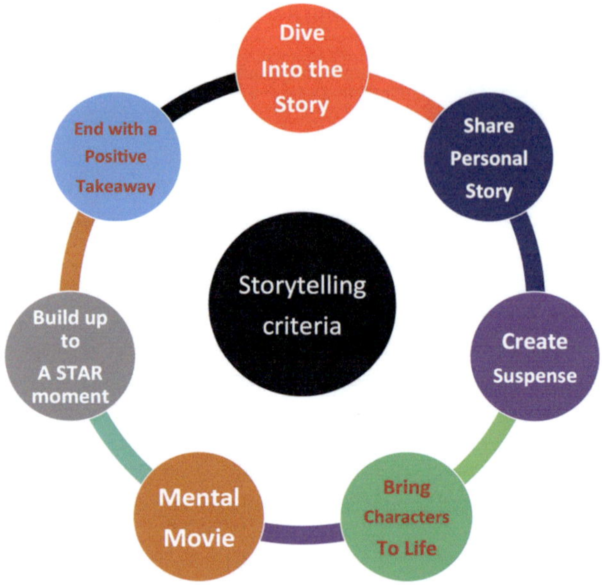
Dive
Into the
Story
Share
Personal
Story
Create
Suspense
Bring
Characters
To Life
Mental
Movie
Build up
to
A STAR
moment
End with a
Positive
Takeaway
Storytelling
criteria

Fig. 17.2 Storytelling techniques: the magic ingredients to create a great memorable presentation

- *Dive into the story and do not forget to immerse your audience in it*: Using basic words and slides with large, graphic images helps to create a clear mental picture of the problem. Another way to immerse the audience in your story is to provide sensory details that will allow them to actually see, hear, feel and smell the different stimuli in your story. Akash Karia [50] noted that this approach will turn the presentation into a mental movie that the audience cannot help but engage in, as is done in TED talks. Therefore, starting with a story, not only is it a beginning of the presentation that is different from how most speakers open their presentations, but it takes the audience along on a journey, mental journey, which is relatable (stories cause people to search their memory banks for similar, relatable experiences). This in turn builds a connection between the speaker and the audience.
- *Share a personal story:* Few things are as captivating as a personal story, especially those of triumph over extreme adversity. In his insightful book *The Seven Basic Plots*, author Christopher Booker [53] reported that there are seven basic story plots that have universal appeal. These include the story of the hero defeating a monster, the rags-to-riches tale, the quest for a treasure and the voyage of a hero who comes back a changed person. These plots are clearly seen in some of the most popular and moving presentations ever given. However, audiences like listening to new things – new ideas, new concepts and new stories. Hearing repeated stories turns audience members off. Therefore, telling a personal story not only gives the audience new material but also improves the presenter's performance, resulting in a more authentic delivery.
- *Create suspense* "makes the story irresistible": Great speeches are not just heard; they're also experienced in the audience's heads. Executive speech coach Patricia Fripp says, "People don't remember what you say as much as

they remember what they see when you say it". If you want your audience to remember and experience your speech, you should paint mental images in their heads.

There are several devices that can increase the level of suspense of your story. One way is to tell a story chronologically and build up to a climactic conclusion, as is done here in this story about a woman who was born without fibula bones and grew up to be an accomplished athlete, actress and model. Another way is to plop the viewer/listener right in the middle of action and then go backwards in time to reveal how all of this occurred. A third way is to begin by telling a predictable story and then surprise the audience by taking a completely different turn from what was expected. For example, this TED talk begins with a presenter who leads his audience to believe he doesn't speak English, only to surprise them in order to make a point about how we construct identity.

- *Bring the characters to life by providing details:* Great speeches are not just heard; they are also experienced in the audience's heads. As characters are at the heart of any story, their fortunes and misfortunes are what make people want to laugh, cry or rejoice. The most successful stories are those which created three-dimensional characters who were easy to identify and, at the same time, had an uncommon characteristic. In order to do this, you must provide enough detail to bring the character to life in the minds of those in the audience.
- *Show and do not tell* "Turn the story into mental movie": Instead of telling your audience about a certain event in a story, try showing them by transporting them to a scene. The reason that the scene affects the audience so much is because it contains a lot of sensory information that brings the scene alive in their minds. As it contains so many vivid details, you can't help but watch the scene playing out in your head. The secret to turning your stories into mental movies for your audience is to make sure your scene is rich in sensory inputs. There are four senses that you need to cover: visual, auditory, kinaesthetic and smell (VAKS) (Craig Valentine: http://www.CraigValentine.com):

  – Visual – what could you see in the story?
  – Auditory – What could you hear?
  – Kinaesthetic – What could you feel?
  – Smell – What could you smell? Smell is a powerful sense for transporting your audience into your scene.

- *Build up to a S.T.A.R. moment:* Similar to a climax, a S.T.A.R. moment is a "Something They'll Always Remember" event that is so dramatic that your audience will be talking about it weeks later. According to presentation expert Nancy Duarte in her book *Resonate* [54], this can come in the form of a dramatization, provocative images or shocking statistics.

  Bill Gates resorted to this technique in a 2009 TED talk when he made the case for increasing investment in eradicating malaria (https://www.ted.com/talks/bill_gates_unplugged). He gave statistics to prove how serious the problem was and then shocked the room by opening a jar full of mosquitos, saying "There's no reason only poor people should have the experience".

- *End with a positive takeaway:* After analysing 200 of the best TED Talks, presentation expert Akash Karia found that the most effective presentations not only had a conflict and a climax but also a positive resolution [47]. On the path to triumph, most characters in these stories received what he calls a "spark", a key piece of wisdom or advice that helped them overcome their obstacles and change for the better. This key takeaway message was then packaged into a short, memorable phrase or sound bite that could easily become viral on social media platforms like Twitter [52].

In conclusion, Technology, Entertainment and Design Talks, commonly known as TED Talks, are an example of our ability to rapidly disseminate great ideas. These online talks, which are freely available and accessible, allow people worldwide to listen to thought-provoking speakers talk passionately about their areas of expertise (www.ted.com/talks). The TED community seeks to share "ideas worth spreading" and in doing so potentially educate and inform millions of people. The format of short talks, averaging 10–18 min, given by expert speakers has garnered worldwide interest and attention and has even sparked community-organized local TEDx events. The TEDx events allow communities to host their own independent TED-like events with a lineup of speakers in front of a live audience. It is expected the TED phenomenon will grow and invade variable aspects of the educational strategies as well as standard practice.

References

1. Nicolle E, Britton E, Janakiram P, Robichaud P, Using TED. Talks to teach social determinants of health maximize the message with a modern medium. Can Fam Physician Méd Famille Can. 2014;60:777–8.
2. Merchant N. When TED lost control of its crowd. Harvard Business Review; 2013. https://hbr.org/2013/04/when-ted-lost-control-of-its-crowd.
3. Hunt T. How social media has changed the traditional classroom. https://www.tintup.com/blog/how-social-media-has-changed-the-traditional-classroom/. Accessed on 31 May 2018.
4. Berruecos V. Las dos caras de la ciencia: Representaciones sociales en el discurso. Rev Iberoam Discurso Soc. 2000;2(2):105–30.
5. Di Carlo G. New trends in knowledge dissemination: TED talks. Acta Sci Lang Cult. 2014. (Maringá;36(2):121–30.
6. Caliendo G. The popularisation of science in web-based genres. In: Caliendo G, Bongo G, editors. The language of popularisation: theoretical and descriptive models. Bern: Peter Lang; 2012a. p. 101–32.
7. DaVia Rubenstein L. Using TED talks to inspire thoughtful practice. Teach Educ. 2012;47:261–7.
8. TED: Our Organization. https://www.ted.com/about/our-organization. Accessed 1 May 2014.
9. Sugimoto CR, Thelwall M, Lariviere V, et al. Scientists popularizing science: characteristics and impact of TED talks. PLoS One. 2013;8(e62403):1–7.
10. Blouin RA, Riffee WH, Robinson ET, et al. Roles of innovation in education delivery. Am J Pharm Educ. 2009;73:154.
11. Romanelli F, Cain J, McNamara PJ. Should TED talks be teaching us something? Am J Pharm Educ. 2014;78(6):113. https://doi.org/10.5688/ajpe786113.
12. Boulter D. Public perception of science and associated general issues for the scientist. Phytochemistry. 1999;50:1–7.

13. Koepsell D. Science ain't an exact science: public perception of science in the wake of the stem-cell fraud. Skept Inq. 2006;30:44–50.
14. Roush S. Fallibility and authority in science. In: Bainbridge WS, editor. Leadership in science and technology: a reference handbook. Los Angeles: SAGE Press; 2012.
15. Luján J, Todt O. Precaution in public: the social perception of the role of science and values in policy making. Public Underst Sci. 2007;16:97–109. https://doi.org/10.1177/0963662506062467.
16. Padlog M. Introductory story: building trust among scientists, authorities and the public. Saf Sci. 2009;47:513–4. https://doi.org/10.1016/j.ssci.2008.07.007.
17. Minkel J. Scientists know better than you–even when they're wrong. Sci Am; 2009. https://www.scientificamerican.com/article/scientists-know-better-than-you/.
18. Heller N. Listen and learn. (Lior Zoref's talk in the Technology, Entertainment and Design conference). New Yorker. 2012;88:69.
19. Iyengar S. Is anyone responsible? How television frames political issues. Chicago: University of Chicago Press; 1991. 206 p
20. Gruber D, Dickerson JA. Persuasive images in popular science: testing judgments of scientific reasoning and credibility. Public Underst Sci. 2012; https://doi.org/10.1177/0963662512454072.
21. Pauwels L. Visual cultures of science: rethinking representational practices in knowledge building and science communication. Lebanon: Dartmouth College Press; 2006. 309 p
22. Bubela T, Nisbet MC, Borchelt R, Brunger F, Critchley C, et al. Science communication reconsidered. Nat Biotechnol. 2009;27:514–8.
23. Müller S. Science marketing and science communication – a breath of fresh air in an ivory tower. n.d. Available: http://www.alumniportal-deutschland.org/en/science-research/article/science-marketing-science-communication.html.
24. Nisbet MC, Scheufele DA. What's next for science communication? Promising directions and lingering distractions. Am J Bot. 2009;96:1767–78.
25. van Dijck J. Picturizing science. The science documentary as multimedia spectacle. Int J Cult Stud. 2006;9:5–24.
26. Sugimoto CR, Thelwall M, Larivière V, Tsou A, Mongeon P, et al. Scientists popularizing science: characteristics and impact of TED talk presenters. PLoS One. 2013;8(4):e62403. https://doi.org/10.1371/journal.pone.0062403.
27. Nisbet MC, Scheufele DA, Shanahan J, Moy P, Brossard D, et al. Knowledge, reservations, or promise? A media effects model for public perceptions of science and technology. Commun Res. 2002;29:584–608.
28. Taibi D, Chawla S, Dietze S, Marenzi I, Fetahu B. Exploring TED talks as linked data for education. Br J Educ Technol. 2015; https://doi.org/10.1111/bjet.12283.
29. Robinson K. Ken Robinson: do schools kill creativity?. 2006. http://www.ted.com/talks/ken_robinson_says_schools_kill_creativity. Accessed 2 June 2018.
30. Robinson K. Ken Robinson: changing education paradigms. 2010. http://www.ted.com/talks/ken_robinson_changing_education_paradigms. Accessed 2 June 2018.
31. Robinson K. Ken Robinson: how to escape education's death valley. 2013. http://www.ted.com/talks/ken_robinson_how_to_escape_education_s_death_valley, Accessed 2 June 2018.
32. Park S-M, Cha K-W. Pre-service teachers' perspectives on a blended listening course using TED talks. Multimed Assist Lang Learn. 2013;16(2):93–116.
33. Cha KW. Teaching English in the age of ubiquitous computing. Multimed Assist Lang Learn. 2006;9(1):167–85.
34. Cho SK. Smartphones used for foreign language learning. Multimed Assist Lang Learn. 2009;12(3):211–28.
35. Palalas A. Mobile-assisted language learning: designing for your students. In: Thouësny S, Bradley L, editors. Second language teaching and learning with technology: view of emergent researchers. Dublin: Research-publishing; 2011. p. 71–94. net.
36. Kim DK. The effects of authentic English listening and reading materials on EFL learners. Multimed Assist Lang Learn. 2008;11(1):61–84.
37. Watkins J, Wilkins M. Using Youtube in the EFL classroom. Lang Educ Asia. 2011;2(1):113–9.

38. Bortoluzzi M, Marenzi I. YELLing for partnership: a social platform for sharing practice and reflection in teacher training for language learning. In: Riem Natale A, Dolce MR, Mercanti S, Colomba C, editors. The tapestry of the creative word in the literatures in English. Udine: Forum; 2013. p. 249–62.
39. Busch-Lauer I-A. A digital revolution in the ESP classroom? The potential of apps, podcasts, e-mags, and social networks revisited. In: Budin G, Lušicky V, editors. Languages for special purposes in a multilingual, transcultural world, Proceedings of the 19th European Symposium on Languages for Special Purposes, 8–10 July 2013, Vienna, Austria. Vienna: University of Vienna; 2014. p. 267–74.
40. Holdack-Janssen E, Marenzi I. Learning about literature on the Web in a German school. In: Vittorini P, Gennari RI, Marenzi I, De La Prieta Pintado F, Corchado Rodriguez JM, editors. Proceedings of the EbTEL workshop, advances in intelligent and soft computing. Berlin: Springer-Verlag GmbH; 2012. p. 57–65.
41. Marenzi I, Kantz D. ESP course design – a multiliteracies approach. In: Proceedings of the 13th IEEE international conference on advanced learning technologies (ICALT 2013). 2013. pp. 221–3. Available at http://www.computer.org/csdl/proceedings/icalt/2013/5009/00/index.html.
42. Takaesu A. TED talks as an extensive listening resource for EAP students. Lang Educ Asia. 2013;4:150–62.
43. Ishinuki F. Learning English with TED talks. Blended learning for learner autonomy. Sophia Linguistica Work Pap Linguist. 2014;62:133–55.
44. Singh J, Zeon TF, Chawla S. LearnWeb-OER: improving accessibility of open educational resources. LinkedUp Vici Challenge, International Semantic Web Conference (ISWC2014). 2014. Available at http://arxiv.org/abs/1509.02739v1.
45. Banker C, Gournelos T. TED talks and the need for a changing education system. Fla Commun J. 2013;41(2):39–56.
46. Csikszentmihalyi M. Mihaly Csikszentmihalyi on flow. [Video file]. 2008. Retrieved from http://www.ted.com/talks/lang/en/Mihaly_csikszentmihalyi_on_flow.html.
47. Karia A. How to design TED-worthy presentation slides. https://www.akashkaria.com/ted-worthy/. Accessed 3 June 2018.
48. TEDx speaker guide. Available on the Internet: http://storage.ted.com/tedx/manuals/tedx_speaker_guide.pdf. Accessed 3 June 2018.
49. Medina J. Brain rules. http://www.brainrules.net/about-brain-rules.
50. Karia A. Storytelling techniques for powerful presentations. https://akashkaria.com/wp-content/uploads/2014/01/TEDTalksStorytellingTechniques.pdf. Accessed on 3 June 2018.
51. Chibana MN. The evolution of online narrative journalism. A content analysis of longform narrative pieces Published on NYTimes.com. https://nchibana.files.wordpress.com/2015/06/the-evolution-of-longform-narrative-journalism.pdf. Accessed on 3 June 2018.
52. Chibana MN. Storytelling techniques used by the most inspiring TED presenters. http://blog.visme.co/7-storytelling-techniques-used-by-the-most-inspiring-ted-presenters/#acEMrBSY8FWLjfO3.99.
53. Booker C. The seven basic plots. https://en.wikipedia.org/wiki/The_Seven_Basic_Plots.
54. Duarte N. Resonate. https://www.duarte.com/resonate/.

Chapter 18
Artificial Intelligence

Introduction

Artificial intelligence (AI) software means computer programmes with the capacity to perform operations analogous to learning and decision-making in humans [1]. Artificial intelligence represents an advancement of computer frameworks able to perform tasks classically requiring human knowledge, for example, basic leadership, visual observation and interpretation between dialects (Fig. 18.1) [1, 2]. In software engineering, perfect knowledge is an adaptable objective where the possibility of achieving a task is amplified. The expression "manmade brainpower" describes a state when a machine imitates "subjective" capacities that people use when dealing with other humans, e.g. "learning" and "critical thinking" [3]. One of the most outstanding AI applications is voice recognition. In contrast to the first models which were awkward and marked by constant defects, they are now capable of responding correctly to all sorts of user requests in the most diverse situations. In the field of image recognition, remarkable advances are also being made, with programmes able to recognize figures – and even cats – in online videos now being adapted for the software to control the autonomous cars set to invade our streets in the coming years [4]. Such advances have persistently pushed back the limits of what was only thought to be achievable by human beings. Along the way, AI research has achieved significant successes: outperforming human beings in complex games (chess, Go) and understanding natural language. It has also played a critical role in the history of mathematics and information technology [5].

Based on the fact that AI, fundamentally, refers to a programme whose ambitious objective is to understand and reproduce human cognition; creating cognitive processes is comparable to those found in human beings. AI research is stratified into subfields that concentrate on particular issues, on particular methodologies, on utilization of specific instrument or towards fulfilling specific applications. Approaches incorporate factual techniques, computational knowledge, delicate processing (e.g. machine learning) and conventional typical AI. Many instruments are utilized as a

Y. El Miedany, *Rheumatology Teaching*,
https://doi.org/10.1007/978-3-319-98213-7_18

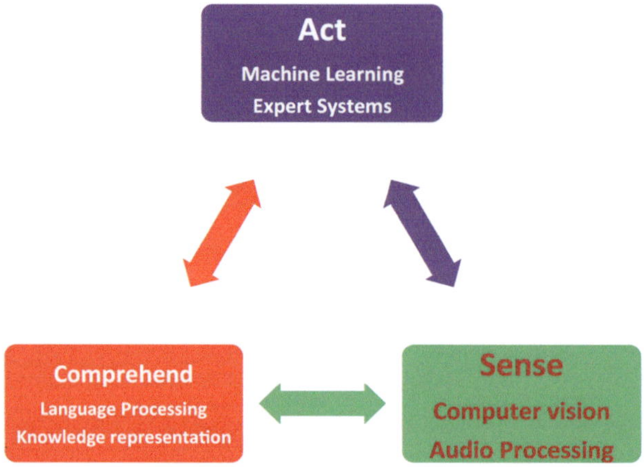

Fig. 18.1 AI refers to multiple technologies that can be combined in different ways to sense, comprehend and act with the ability to learn from experience and adapt over time. In basic terms, AI is a broad area of computer science that makes machines and computer programmes capable of problem-solving and learning, like a human brain. AI includes natural language processing and translation, pattern recognition, visual perception and decision-making. Machine learning, one of the most exciting areas of AI, involves the development of computational approaches to automatically make sense of data

part of AI, including renditions of inquiry and numerical advancement, rationale and techniques in light of likelihood and financial matters [3]. Therefore, a wide scope of specialities is involved in this field, both in terms of the technical procedures that can be employed and the various disciplines that can be called upon, e.g. mathematics, information technology and cognitive sciences. There is a great variety of approaches when it comes to AI; examples are ontological, reinforcement learning, adversarial learning and neural networks. Most of them have been known for decades, and many of the algorithms used today were developed in the 1960s and 1970s [5]. Its visionary nature makes AI one of the most fascinating scientific endeavours of our time; and as such its development has always been accompanied by the wildest, most alarming and far-fetched fantasies that have deeply coloured the general population's ideas about AI and the way researchers themselves relate to their own discipline.

In recent years, artificial intelligence has entered a new era, which gives rise to many hopes. Thanks to complex algorithms, increased computing power and the exponential growth of human and machine-generated data, various applications have been developed; examples include translation, transport (driverless cars), health (cancer detection and disease management) as well as education. Such progress in AI is taking place in a technological context marked by the datafication of the world which affects all sectors of our society and economy, the development robotics and the blockchain (the distributed ledger technology which enables transactions between two, or more, agents without the presence of a trusted third party or institution which most notably underlines cryptocurrencies such as bitcoin). The future of artificial intelligence surely depends on its exposure to these different technological developments [5].

This chapter will discuss the science of AI and explore the importance of big data and AI strategies. It will expand to discuss AI and medicine as well as medical education. It will conclude with discussion of AI and education as well as the future of artificial intelligence.

The Artificial Intelligence Is Changing How We Do Science

In 1992, Patrick Henry Winston [6] defined artificial intelligence as "Artificial Intelligence is the study of the computations that make it possible to perceive, reason, and act". This way, AI differs from most of psychology because of its greater emphasis on computation, and it differs from most of computer science because of its greater emphasis on perception, reasoning and action. One of my points will be that the "reasoning" is particularly essential for higher intelligent functioning. Reasoning involves internal processes that make a subject "think" about what might be the best way of acting before actually moving to act. Cognition about the world and alternate ways of acting in the world add a quality able to differentiate between a smarter and a dumber individual.

The scientific goal of artificial intelligence is to determine which ideas about representing knowledge, using knowledge and assembling systems explain various sorts of intelligence [7]. Artificial intelligence is formed of three main pillars (Fig. 18.2): domain structure, data generation and machine learning. Microsoft has called the full end-to-end AI spectrum "system of intelligence", which is able to ingest human-level knowledge (e.g. via machine reading and computer vision) and use this information to automate and accelerate tasks that were previously only performed by humans. However, it is vital to have a well-defined task structure,

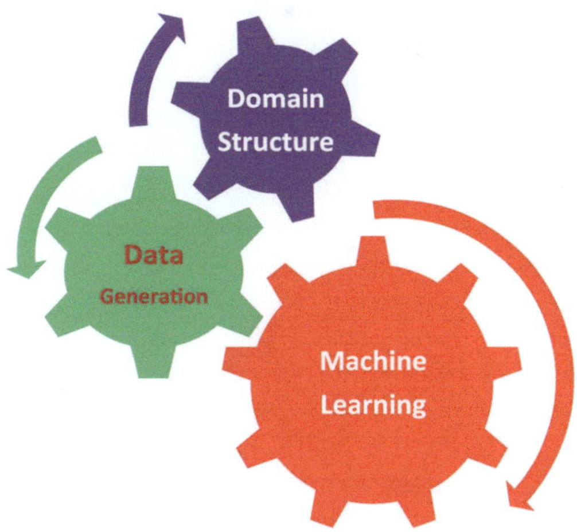

Fig. 18.2 System of intelligence. The three main pillars of artificial intelligence which facilitate the human task automation and acceleration. Domain structure (task structure identified by expertise), data generation (reinforcement learning, big data assets, sensor/video tracking), machine learning (deep neural networks, video/audio/text)

identified and outlined by expertise, to engineer against. A massive bank of data is also essential to get the system up and running, as well as a strategy to continue generating data so that the system can respond and learn. Lastly, machine learning routines able to detect patterns in and make predictions from the unstructured data are also required [8].

Domain structure is the first pillar of AI listed in the system of intelligence. This is the structure which facilitates breaking a complex problem into composite tasks which can be solved with machine learning. The reason that AI firms choose to work with games is that such structure is clear and the rules of the game are codified. This exposes the massive gap between playing games and a system that is able to replace humans in real-world applications. To deal with the real world, the theory should be identified as well as the rules of the relevant game. For example, to develop a system able to communicate with customers, the first step to proceed will be mapping out customer intents and desires in such a way that allows different dialogue-generating machine learning routines for each. Or, for any AI system, in a retail environment, which deals with marketing and prices, it is important to use the structure of an economic demand system to forecast how changing the price on a single item (which might be the job of a single deep neural networks) will affect optimal prices for other products and behaviour of the consumers (who might themselves be modelled with deep neural networks).

Data generation is the second pillar for AI systems. An active strategy of data collection is vital for keeping a steady stream of new and useful information flowing into the composite learning algorithms. In most AI applications, there will be two general classes of data: fixed-size data assets that can be used to train the models for generic tasks and data that is actively generated by the system as it experiments and improves performance. For example, in learning how to play Ms. Pac-Man, the models could be initialized on a bank of data recording how humans have played the game [9] (artificial intelligence first appeared in a digital game in 1979, when the developers of Pac-Man used a technique known as state machine (transitioning between states depending on conditions) to control whether or not a ghost ran towards or away from a player. The AI in most modern digital games builds on this simple approach. As the game-based story unfolds, autonomous non-player characters (agents) take information from both the game and the player and, based on that information, use AI algorithms to determine the most appropriate actions to take). This is the fixed-size data asset. Then this initialized system starts to play the game of Ms. Pac-Man. Recalling that the system is broken into a number of machine learning components, as more games are played, each component is able to experiment with possible moves in different scenarios. Since all of this is automated, the system can iterate through a massive number of games and quickly accumulate a wealth of experience. The general framework of machine learning algorithms actively choosing the data that they consume is referred to as reinforcement learning. This is a hugely important aspect of machine learning-driven AI [10].

Often there is confusion between machine learning and AI. In fact, machine learning is quite distinct from AI; hence, they are different. While machine learning is able to do fantastic tasks, it is principally limited to predicting a future that looks mostly like the past. Machine learning is a tool for pattern recognition. In contrast, an AI system can solve complex problems that have been previously reserved for humans. It does this by breaking these problems into a bunch of simple prediction tasks, each of which can be attacked by a "dumb" machine learning algorithm. AI uses instances of machine learning as components of the larger system (Fig. 18.3). These machine learning instances need to be organized within a structure defined by domain knowledge, and they need to be fed data that helps them complete their allotted prediction tasks. This does not down-weight the machine learning value in AI. In contrast to earlier attempts at AI, the current instance of AI is machine learning driven. Machine learning algorithms are implanted in every aspect of AI, and the evolution of machine learning towards status is described as a general-purpose technology. This evolution is the main driver behind the current rise of AI. Briefly, machine learning algorithms are building blocks of AI within a larger context [8]. Machine learning in its current form has become a general-purpose technology [11]. These tools are going to get cheaper and faster over time, due to innovations in the ML itself and above and below the AI technology stack (e.g. improved software connectors for systems above and improved computing hardware like graphics processing unit (GPUs) below). Machine learning has the potential to become a cloud computing commodity [12].

Machine learning algorithms are often categorized as being supervised or unsupervised. Supervised algorithms require humans to provide both input and desired output, in addition to furnishing feedback about the accuracy of predictions during training. Once training is complete, the algorithm will apply what was learned to new data. Unsupervised algorithms do not need to be trained with desired outcome data. Instead, they use an iterative approach called deep learning to review data and arrive at conclusions. Unsupervised learning algorithms are used for more complex processing tasks than supervised learning systems. The processes involved in

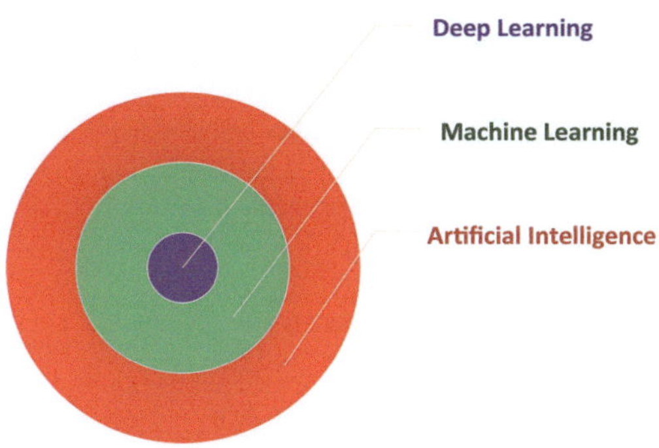

Fig. 18.3 Artificial Intelligence can be described as human intelligence exhibited by machines; whereas, Machine Learning can be described as an approach to achieve Artificial Intelligence. Machine learning is a data driven approach to decision making. At its most basic, Machine Learning is the practice of using algorithms to parse data, learn from it, and then make a determination or prediction about something in the world. Deep Learning is a technique for Implementing Machine Learning. Thanks to Deep Learning, AI has a bright future

machine learning are similar to that of data mining and predictive modelling. Both require searching through data to look for patterns and adjusting programme actions accordingly. Many people are familiar with machine learning from shopping on the Internet and being served ads related to their purchase. This happens because recommendation engines use machine learning to personalize online ad delivery in almost real time. Beyond personalized marketing, other common machine learning use examples include fraud detection, spam filtering, network security threat detection, predictive maintenance and building news feeds. Similarly, Facebook's News Feed, for example, uses machine learning to personalize each member's feed. If a member frequently stops scrolling to read or "like" a particular friend's posts, the News Feed will start to show more of that friend's activity earlier in the feed. Behind the scenes, the software is simply using statistical analysis and predictive analytics to identify patterns in the user's data and use those patterns to populate the News Feed. Should the member no longer stop to read, like or comment on the friend's posts, that new data will be included in the dataset, and the News Feed will adjust accordingly [13].

The pioneering technology within machine learning is the neural network (NN), which is called "deep learning". This mimics (to a very rudimentary level) the pattern recognition abilities of the human brain by processing thousands or even millions of data points. Pattern recognition is pivotal in terms of intelligence. Deep neural networks (deep belief networks) are simple models. Indeed, their simplicity is a strength: basic patterns facilitate fast training and computation. The model has linear combinations of inputs that are passed through non-linear activation functions called nodes (or, in reference to the human brain, neurons). A set of nodes taking different weighted sums of the same inputs is called a "layer", and the output of one layer's nodes becomes input to the next layer. This structure is illustrated in Fig. 18.3. Each circle in the figure is a node. Those in the input (χ on the left) layer typically have a special structure; they are either raw data or data that has been processed through an additional set of layers (e.g. convolutions). The output layer gives your predictions. In a simple regression setting, this output could just be "y" (on the right). Deep neural networks can be used to predict all sorts of high-dimensional objects. As it is for nodes in input layers, output nodes also tend to take application-specific forms [14].

Big Data and Artificial Intelligence Strategies

Nowadays, the Internet is the most common way to collect data electronically using mobile gadgets. In principle, this allows analytics to access a broad range of real-time data. In a report written by Morgan in 2017 [15], it was reported that there are several examples for the value of such data analysis. For instance, online prices of millions of items can be used to assess inflation, the number of customers visiting a store and transacting can give real-time sales estimates, and satellite imaging can assess agricultural yields or activity of oil rigs. Historically, similar data were only available at low frequency (e.g. monthly, weekly rig counts, crop reports, retail sales reports and quarterly earnings, etc.). Given the amount of data that is available, any specialized person can nowadays, in theory, have near real-time macro or centre-/organization-specific data, less likely to be available from the traditional data sources. In practice, useful data are not readily available, and one needs to purchase, organize and analyse alternative datasets in order to extract meaningful signals. Analysis of large or unstructured datasets is often done with the use of machine learning. Successful application of machine learning techniques requires some theoretical knowledge and a lot of practical experience in designing quantitative strategies. This represented in a revolution of how big data can be handled.

Considering the methodology of how datasets can be handled, there are two main approaches: acquiring and understanding the data, as well as using the appropriate technologies and methods to analyse those data. In contrast to the traditional datasets, new datasets are characterized by being often larger in volume, velocity and variability. Another source of datasets include data generated by individuals (social media posts, product reviews, search trends, etc.), data generated by sensors (satellite image data, foot and car traffic, ship locations, etc.) as well as data generated by business processes (company exhaust data, commercial transaction, credit card data, etc.). A level of analysis of these datasets is required, in most cases, before they can be used. This includes analysis of the different data types, evaluation of their relevance for different asset classes as well as their relevance for different styles. Methods to analyse such big datasets can be either the traditional statistics tools or the new techniques such as machine learning. Machine learning techniques include supervised learning (regressions, classifications), unsupervised learning (factor analysis, clustering) as well as novel techniques of deep and reinforcement learning that are often used to analyse unstructured data and show promise in identifying data patterns in structured data.

However, some concerns were raised in relation to the big data analysis as well as the implementation of artificial intelligence. Some key opinion leaders may not have a good understanding of the available data classes and feel uncomfortable about adopting machine learning methods. On a limited basis, many investors have already dealt with alternative datasets and some form of machine learning. For instance, in the 1950s, the founder of Walmart, Sam Walton, used airplanes to fly over and count cars on parking lots to assess real estate investments. The current extensive use of satellite imaging is a more technologically advanced, scalable and broadly available extension of the same idea. Machine learning methods are often simple extensions of well-known statistical analysis methods. Supervised learning methods aim to establish a relationship between two datasets and use one dataset to forecast the other. These methods are often as simple as regression models improved to accommodate changing regimes, data outliers and correlated variables. Unsupervised learning methods aim at understanding the structure of the data and identifying the main drivers behind it. These models are often closely related to well-known statistical methods such as principal component analysis. However, there are significant differences between a simple regression which assess for an outcome variable and one or more risk factors or confounding variables and a big data – machine learning framework. Big data requires new analytical skills and infrastructure in order to derive meaningful signals. Strategies based on machine learning and big data also require understanding of drivers behind data and experience in designing targeted strategies. Therefore, it is expected that the "old" datasets will lose most predictive value and new datasets that capture "big data" will increasingly become standardized. Machine learning techniques will become a standard tool for quantitative investors and perhaps some fundamental investors too. The "big data ecosystem" involves specialized firms that collect, aggregate and sell new datasets and research teams on both the buy side and sell side who evaluate data. As the big data ecosystem evolves, datasets that have high Sharpe ratio signals (viable as a stand-alone funds) will disappear. The bulk of big data signals will not be viable as stand-alone strategies but will still be very valuable in the context of a quantitative portfolio.

The transition to a big data framework will not be without potential pitfalls or setbacks. Certain types of data may lead into blind alleys such as datasets that don't contain alpha and signals that have too little investment capacity, decay quickly or are simply too expensive to purchase. Too much investment might be exerted into unnecessary infrastructure, e.g. build complex models which don't justify marginal performance improvements. Machine learning algorithms cannot entirely replace human intuition. Sophisticated models, if not properly guided, can overfit or uncover spurious relationships and patterns. Talent will present another source of risk – employing data scientists who lack specific professional expertise may not lead to the desired results or lead to clashes of interest. In implementing big data and machine learning in any field, it is more important to understand what is behind data and signals than to be able to develop complex technological solutions. Many big data and AI concepts may sound plausible but will not lead to viable strategies.

A question remains to be answered, what will be the respective roles of humans and machines after the big data/AI "revolution"? Machines are becoming increasingly relevant as they have the facility to quickly analyse news feeds and tweets, process statements, scrape websites and trade on these instantaneously. These strategies are already eroding the option of using fundamental statistical analysis. The current stage of development of artificial intelligence is still in its early phases. Machines will likely not do well in assessing regime changes (market turning points) and forecasts which involve interpreting more complicated human responses such as those of politicians and central bankers, understanding client positioning or anticipating crowding [15].

Artificial Intelligence and Life

Artificial intelligence (AI) is a science and a set of computational technologies that are inspired by – but typically operate quite differently from – the ways people use their nervous systems and bodies to sense, learn, reason and take action. While the rate of progress in AI has been patchy and unpredictable, there have been significant advances since the field's inception 60 years ago. Last year Stanford University published the report "Artificial Intelligence and Life in 2030", exploring the role of AI in various aspects of society, and AI will play a fundamental role in humans' lives [16]. Once a mostly academic area of study, twenty-first-century AI enables a constellation of mainstream technologies that are having a substantial impact on everyday lives. Computer vision and AI planning, for example, drive the video games that are now a bigger entertainment industry than Hollywood. Deep learning, a form of machine learning based on layered representations of variables referred to as neural networks, has made speech-understanding practical on our phones and in our kitchens, and its algorithms can be applied widely to an array of applications that rely on pattern recognition. Natural language processing (NLP) and knowledge representation and reasoning have enabled a machine to beat the Jeopardy champion and are bringing new power to web searches.

While impressive, these technologies are highly tailored to particular tasks. Each application typically requires years of specialized research and careful, unique construction. In similarly targeted applications, substantial increases in the future uses of AI technologies, including more self-driving cars, healthcare diagnostics and targeted treatments and physical assistance for elder care, can be expected. AI and robotics will also be applied across the globe in industries struggling to attract younger workers, such as agriculture, food processing, fulfilment centres and factories. They will facilitate delivery of online purchases through flying drones, self-driving trucks or robots that can get up the stairs to the front door [16].

Artificial Intelligence and Education

Looming as one of the most exciting, yet mysterious, technologies in the coming years, even in schools, artificial intelligence will be able to make the educational experience more efficient and engaging, both for teachers and students [17]. AI is concerned with developing computer systems that can store knowledge and effectively use the knowledge to help solve problems and accomplish tasks. This brief statement sounds a lot like one of the commonly accepted goals in the education of humans. We want students to learn (gain knowledge) and to learn to use this knowledge to help solve problems and accomplish tasks.

Intelligence is a composite from various authors, especially Gardner [18], Perkins [19] and Sternberg [20]. Intelligence is a combination of the abilities to:

1. Learn. This includes all kinds of informal and formal learning via any combination of experience, education and training.
2. Pose problems. This includes recognizing problem situations and transforming them into more clearly defined problems.
3. Solve problems. This includes solving problems, accomplishing tasks and fashioning products.

There is a near universal agreement among researchers that some aspects of our intellectual abilities depend heavily on our experiential histories, and some aspects depend on our genetic makeup. Thus, a person's cognitive abilities are a combination of nature and nurture [21, 22]. Therefore, from a teacher's point of view, it would be ideal to understand that a student's life experiences – which include formal and informal education, as this would reflect on and contribute to the person's intelligence.

As AI is based on computer software which has been programmed to interact with the world in ways normally requiring human intelligence, this means that AI relies on two main pillars: (1) knowledge and (2) algorithms to intelligently process that knowledge. This knowledge is represented in so-called models. Applying this in education, there are three key models at the heart of AI when implemented in education: the pedagogical model, the domain model and the learner model (Fig. 18.4). Integrating these models into the adaptive AI educational software algorithms where the knowledge represented in the models will be processed, leading to the selection of the most appropriate content to be delivered to the learner, according to their individual abilities and requirements (Fig. 18.5). While the content (which can be presented in different ways, e.g. in the form of text, video, animation, sound, game or activity) is delivered to the learner, continuous analysis of the learner's interactions (e.g. the learner's responses and answers, past attainments and current affective state) informs the delivery of feedback (e.g. guidance and/or hints), to help the learner progresses through the content being taught. Deep analysis of the learner's interactions is also used to update the learner model; paving the way to

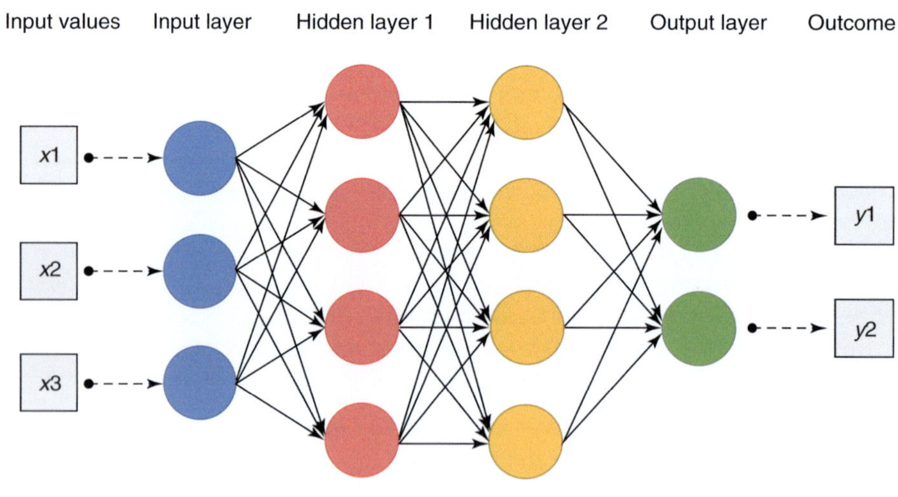

Fig. 18.4 Architectures of deep neural networks. Multilayered feed-forward artificial neural network (a five layer network). (Adapted from Gibson and Patterson [14])

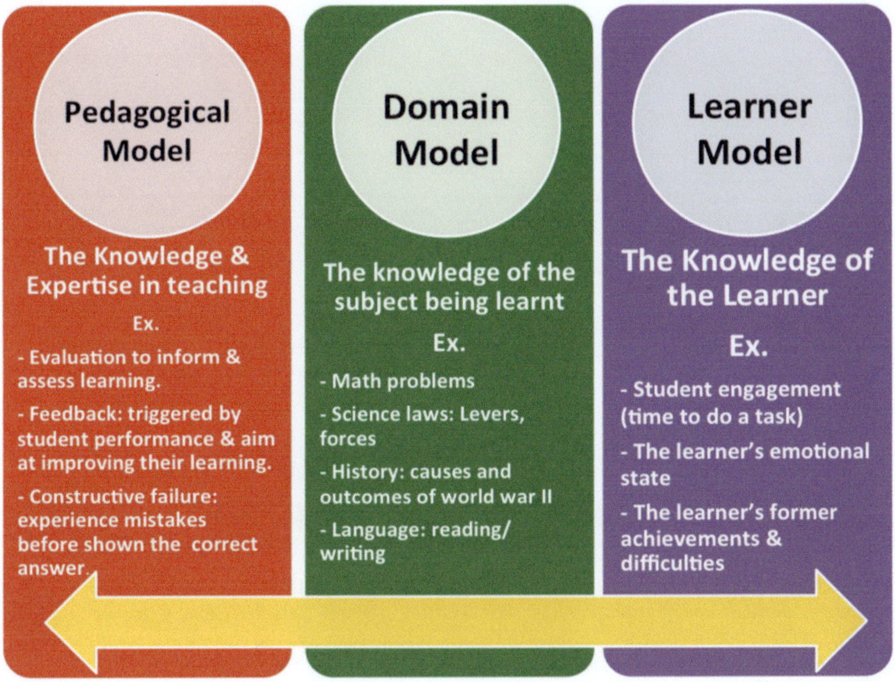

Fig. 18.5 The key models of artificial intelligence in education. The AI system, designed to provide appropriate individualized feedback to a student, should include the knowledge about effective approaches to teaching (the pedagogical model), the subject being learned (the domain model or domain expertise) as well as the student (the learner model)

more precise estimations of the student's present state (e.g. the learner's understanding and motivation) ensures that each learner's learning experience is tailored to their abilities and requirements and efficiently supports their learning.

The "open learner models" are AI systems able to present the analysis outcomes back to both the learners and teachers. The results might comprise important data about the learner's accomplishments, their affective condition or any misconceptions they might hold. This can assist the teachers to recognize their students' approach to learning and facilitate figuring out appropriate future learning experiences. On another front, the "open learner models" can help motivate the learners, by allowing them to track their own progress and encouraging them to reflect on their own learning. One of the advantages of such adaptive educational AI systems is that they typically collect big amounts of data, which can then be computed to dynamically advance the pedagogy and domain models. This process facilitates developing new approaches to provide more efficient, learner-centred support whilst testing and refining our understanding of the teaching processes; enhance learning through guiding teachers as well as motivating learners (Fig. 18.6) [23].

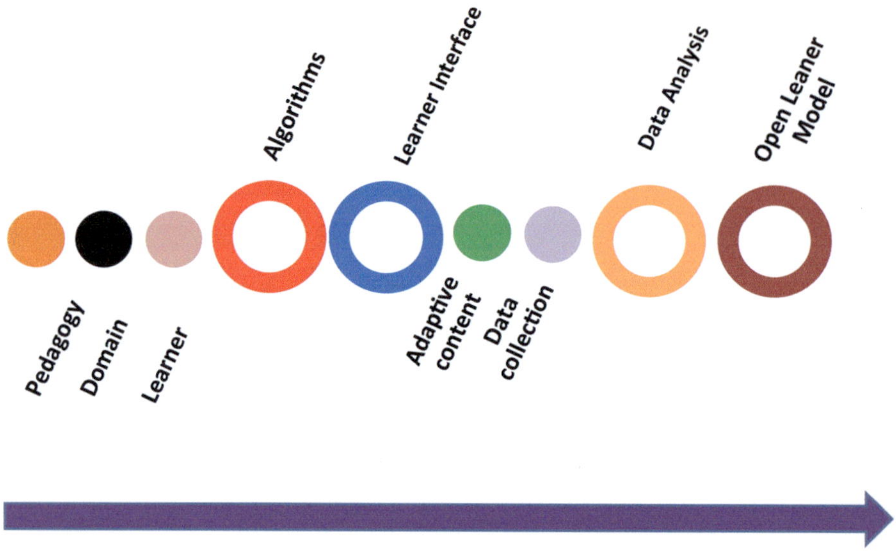

Fig. 18.6 Adaptive AI educational system: algorithms process the knowledge attained from the pedagogy, domain and learner models. The learning content (whether text, video or audio) is adapted to the requirements and abilities of the discrete learner, and the learner's accomplishments, interactions and affections are captured. Analysis of the data is carried out by the AI techniques (e.g. machine learning, deep learning) with feedback to the learner. The stage of open learner model makes the learning overt for both the learners and teachers

What Artificial Intelligence Can Offer Education Now?

At the core of AI, the role in education is the scientific goal to "make computationally precise and explicit forms of educational, psychological and social knowledge which are often left implicit" [22]. Meaning that, in addition to being the engine behind much "smart" educational technology, AI in education is also a powerful tool to open up what is sometimes called the "black box of learning", giving us deeper and more fine-grained understandings of how learning actually happens (e.g. how it is influenced by the learner's socio-economic and physical context or by technology) [23].

Several AI education-driven applications are currently being used in schools and universities. Many incorporate educational data mining (EDM) techniques to "monitor and track" the students' behaviours, e.g. collecting information on class attendance and assignment submission to recognize (and provide support) students at risk of abandoning their studies. Other AI researchers are exploring novel user interfaces, such as natural language processing, speech and gesture recognition, eye tracking and other physiological sensors, which could be used to augment both AI educational and noneducational software. However, there are three categories of educational AI software applications which have been developed to support direct learning. These include personal tutors for individual learners, intelligent support for collaborative learning and intelligent virtual reality.

Intelligent Tutoring Systems

While one-to-one tutoring is practically neither realistic nor practical, AI came as an ideal solution able to facilitate providing an intelligent, personal tutor for every learner. The Intelligent Tutoring Systems implement AI techniques to simulate one-to-one human tutoring, bringing learning activities best matched to the individual learner's cognitive requirements and providing targeted and timely feedback, all without an individual teacher having to be present (Fig. 18.7). Some Intelligent Tutoring Systems enable the learners to be in control of their own learning in order to help students develop self-regulation skills. Others use pedagogical strategies to scaffold learning so that the learner is appropriately challenged and supported [23]. An example of a modern model-based adaptive system is the iTalk2Learn system 16, designed to help young students learn about fractions, used a learner model that included information about the learner's mathematics knowledge, their cognitive needs, their affective (emotional) state, the feedback they had received and their responses to that feedback [24].

Model-based adaptive tutors include a wide range of AI educational tools such as model learners' cognitive and affective states [25] and use dialogue to engage the student in one-to-one learning experiences, which include enquiry and discussion, questioning and answering [26], open learner models to promote reflection and self-awareness [26], metacognitive scaffolding (by providing dynamic help or using a narrative framework) to increase learner motivation and engagement [27] as well as the use of social simulation models (e.g. to enable language learning students to engage more successfully with speakers of their target language by understanding cultural and social norms) [28].

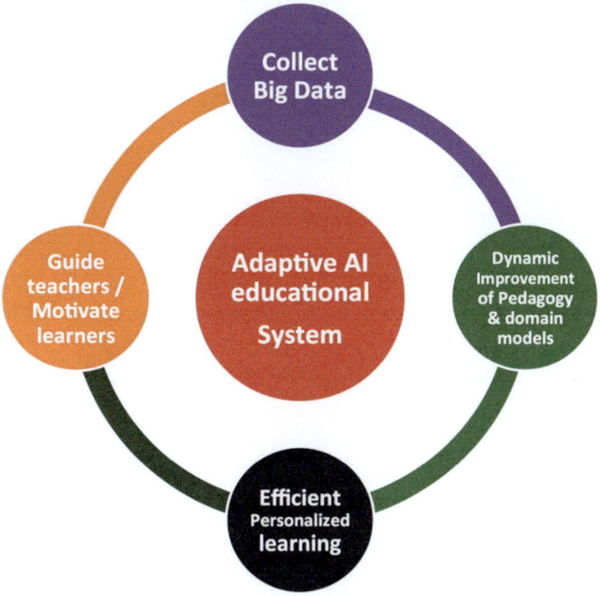

Fig. 18.7 The adaptive educational AI systems is a closed loop starting with big data collection, which then is computed to dynamically advance the pedagogy and domain models. This process facilitates learner-centred educational support while also testing and refining our understanding of the processes of teaching and learning through guiding teachers and motivating learners

Intelligent Support for Collaborative Learning

- Collaboration between students, whether it was between a pair of students undertaking a joined project or a community of students participating in an online course, can foster higher learning performance as well as outcomes than learning solely [29, 30]. Research over decades has suggested that collaborative learning is effective because it encourages participants to articulate and justify their thinking, resolve differences through constructive dialogue, reflect on other explanations and build shared meaning and knowledge. Collaborative learning can also enhance motivation among the students. If students got engaged and cared about the group, they become more committed to the task and achieve better the targeted learning outcomes [31].

  However, on the other hand, an earlier analysis suggested that collaboration between learners does not happen spontaneously [24]. For example, group members might not have the social interaction skills needed to collaborate effectively. This can be especially difficult in the context of online collaborations, where participants rarely meet in person. This is where the AI can play a role in the education process. Several approaches have been investigated in collaborative learning. Table 18.1 shows the most common four approaches, their principles and use. These include adaptive group formation, expert facilitation, virtual agents and intelligent moderation [32].

Intelligent Virtual Reality

- Virtual reality for learning provides immersive authentic experiences (the subjective impression that one is participating in a realistic experience) that simulate some aspect of the real world to which the user would not otherwise have access (such as dangerous environments or somewhere geographically or historically inaccessible, acute medical or surgical condition). Earlier research study reported that giving students the opportunity to explore, interact with and manipulate aspects of a simulated world, perhaps investigating "what if" scenarios (such as "how to manage a person who collapsed, all of a sudden"), enables them to transfer what they have learnt to the real world [33–37].

  Virtual reality becomes "intelligent" when it is augmented with artificial intelligence. AI might be used simply to enhance the virtual world, giving it the ability to interact with and respond to the user's actions in ways that feel more natural. Or, drawing on Intelligent Tutoring Systems, AI might also be integrated to provide ongoing intelligent support and guidance to ensure that the learner engages properly with the intended learning objectives without becoming confused or overwhelmed [23]. Virtual pedagogical agents might also be included, acting as teachers, learning facilitators or student peers in collaborative learning "quests".

Table 18.1 Approaches of how artificial intelligence can provide support for collaborative learning

	Adaptive group formation	Expert facilitation	Intelligent virtual agents	Intelligent moderation
Target	Individual participants	The collaborating students	Intelligent virtual agents	Large student numbers
Principle	AI techniques and knowledge are used in the form of learner models, to form a group best suited for a particular collaborative task	Effective collaboration models, known as "collaboration patterns" – are implemented to provide interactive support to the collaborating students [33]. These patterns are either provided by the system authors or mined from previous collaborations	Involves intelligent virtual agents that are introduced into the collaborative process [35]	When large student numbers work together in multiple collaborative groups, big volume of data is collected, which represent a challenge to a person trying to make sense of such large data volume generated in the participants' discussions
Implementation	To design student groups of similar cognitive level and interests or a group where the participants bring different but complementary knowledge and skills [32]	To train systems identify when students are having trouble understanding the concepts shared among them or provide targeted support of the right form at the right time	Mediate online student interaction, or contribute to the dialogues	Intelligent moderation uses AI techniques such as machine learning and shallow text processing to analyse and summarize the discussions to enable a human tutor to guide the students towards fruitful collaboration

(continued)

Table 18.1 (continued)

	Adaptive group formation	Expert facilitation	Intelligent virtual agents	Intelligent moderation
Examples	Group formation using a set of individual characteristics of group members to form groups that are more likely to have desired group behaviours and that these characteristics can be monitored and updated to dynamically alter group formation	Expert facilitation	An expert participant (a coach or a tutor) A virtual peer (an artificial student at a similar cognitive level to the learner but one who is capable of introducing novel ideas) Someone the participants might themselves teach, e.g. the artificial student might hold deliberate misconceptions or provide alternative points of view to stimulate productive argument or reflection [36]	The system might provide alerts to human tutors to inform them of significant events (such as students going off topic or repeating misconceptions) that may require their intervention or support [37]

These agents might provide alternative perspectives, ask questions and give feedback, all based on a properly specified pedagogical model [38].

Many studies have demonstrated that immersion in intelligent virtual reality can enhance educational outcomes, enabling students to construct their own individual understanding of the world being explored [39]. Some have also been shown to have the potential to release what Chris Dede, a leading learning scientist, calls "trapped intelligence"; that is, they allow low-achieving students to build their self-confidence by shifting their self-image from being a poor academic performer to, for example, a successful virtual scientist [40].

In addition, intelligent synthetic characters in virtual worlds can play roles in settings that are too dangerous or unpleasant for learners. For example, FearNot is a school-based intelligent virtual environment that presents bullying incidents in the form of a virtual drama. Learners, who have been victims of bullying, play the role of an invisible friend to a character in the drama who is bullied. The learner offers the character advice about how to behave between episodes in the drama and, in so doing, explores bullying issues and effective coping strategies

[41]. Intelligent virtual reality can also be used for intelligent team training during which virtual humans are able to reason about individual events, carry out actions and negotiate options, with the aim of guiding human trainees to make similar assessments, e.g. in peacekeeping scenarios [42].

Artificial Intelligence in Medicine

Healthcare is one of the largest and most rapidly growing aspects of AI, driven, predominantly, by innovation in clinical research, robotic personal assistants and big data analytics [43]. Healthcare is poised to accelerate investments in AI over the next 3 years. The influx of healthcare data has resulted in a growing need for AI technology to enhance data mining and computing capabilities. Personalized treatments are being bolstered by growing application of AI in the field of genomics and precision medicine. The emergence of new and promising applications for disease diagnosis and monitoring is anticipated to further drive AI market growth [44].

Recently AI techniques have sent vast waves across healthcare, even fuelling an active discussion of whether AI doctors will eventually replace human physicians in the future. Machines (computers) learn to detect patterns not decipherable using biostatistics by processing massive datasets (big data) through layered mathematical models (algorithms). Correcting algorithm mistakes (training) adds to AI predictive model confidence. AI is being successfully applied for image analysis in radiology, pathology and dermatology, with diagnostic speed exceeding, and accuracy paralleling, medical experts. While diagnostic confidence never reaches 100%, combining machines plus physicians reliably enhances system performance. Cognitive programmes are impacting medical practice by applying natural language processing to read the rapidly expanding scientific literature and collate years of diverse electronic medical records. In this and other ways, AI may optimize the care trajectory of chronic disease patients, suggest precision therapies for complex illnesses, reduce medical errors and improve subject enrolment into clinical trials [45]. Therefore, in the foreseeable future, it is not expected that human physicians will be replaced by machines, but AI can definitely assist physicians to make better clinical decisions or even replace human judgement in certain functional areas of healthcare (e.g. radiology, laboratory or pathology).

Several aspects should be considered when considering the implementation of AI in the healthcare trajectory. These include the span and potential benefits of applying AI in healthcare, big data which can be analysed by AI, tools and devices that enable AI systems to generate clinical meaningful results and disease types that the AI communities are currently tackling systems [46].

The Span and Potential Benefits of AI in Healthcare

The advantages of AI have been extensively discussed in the medical literature [47–49]. AI can use sophisticated algorithms to "learn" features from a large volume of healthcare data and then use the obtained insights to assist clinical practice. It can also be equipped with learning and self-correcting abilities to improve its accuracy based on feedback. An AI system can assist physicians by providing up-to-date medical information from journals, textbooks and clinical practices to inform proper patient care [50]. In addition, an AI system can help to reduce diagnostic and therapeutic errors that are inevitable in the human clinical practice [50–54]. Moreover, an AI system extracts useful information from a large patient population to assist making real-time inferences for health risk alert and health outcome prediction [55].

Healthcare Big Data

Big data represent one of the major assets of medical healthcare. However, before AI systems can be installed for use in healthcare applications, they need to be "trained" through data that are generated from clinical activities, such as screening, diagnosis, treatment pathways as well as outcomes, so that they can learn similar patterns of subjects, associations between subject features and outcomes of interest. These clinical data often exist in the form of, but not limited to, demographics, electronic medical notes, medical devices electronic recordings, physical examinations and laboratory as well as radiologic reports/images [56].

Specifically, at the stage of diagnosis, a substantial proportion of the AI literature analyses data from diagnostic imaging, laboratory results, genetic testing and electrodiagnostic measures and outcomes. In their article, Jha and Topol advised radiologists to adopt AI technologies when analysing diagnostic images that contain vast data information [57]. In another study, Li et al. studied the uses of abnormal genetic expression in long non-coding RNAs to diagnose gastric cancer [58]. In concordance, Shin et al. developed an electrodiagnosis support system for localizing neural injury [59]. On another front, physical examination notes and laboratory results are the other two major data sources. Medical records and physical examination findings could be distinguished from image, laboratory, genetic and electrophysiological (EP) data as they contain large portions of unstructured narrative texts, such as clinical notes, which are not directly analysable. As a consequence, the corresponding AI applications focus on first converting the unstructured text to machine-understandable electronic medical record. For example, Karakülah et al. used AI technologies to extract phenotypic features from case reports to enhance the diagnosis accuracy of the congenital anomalies [60].

Tools and Artificial Intelligence Devices

Artificial mechanisms involved in healthcare can be stratified into two major categories. The first one is the machine learning techniques which analyse structured data such as imaging, laboratory, genetic and electrophysiologic data. In the medical applications, the machine learning procedures attempt to cluster patients' traits or infer the probability of the disease outcomes [61]. The second category includes natural language processing (NLP) methods which work on turning texts to machine-readable structured data, which can then be analysed by ML techniques [62]. In addition, the natural language processing procedures extract information from unstructured data such as clinical notes/medical journals to supplement and enrich structured medical data.

For better presentation, the flow chart in Fig. 18.8 depicts the road map from clinical data generation, through natural language processing procedures data enrichment and electronic medical recording. This big data then feed into machine learning data analysis, leading to the outcome of clinical decision-making. This in turn will feed into clinical activities which subsequently will feed into the big clinical data. As powerful as AI techniques can be, they have to be motivated by clinical problems and be applied to assist clinical practice in the end.

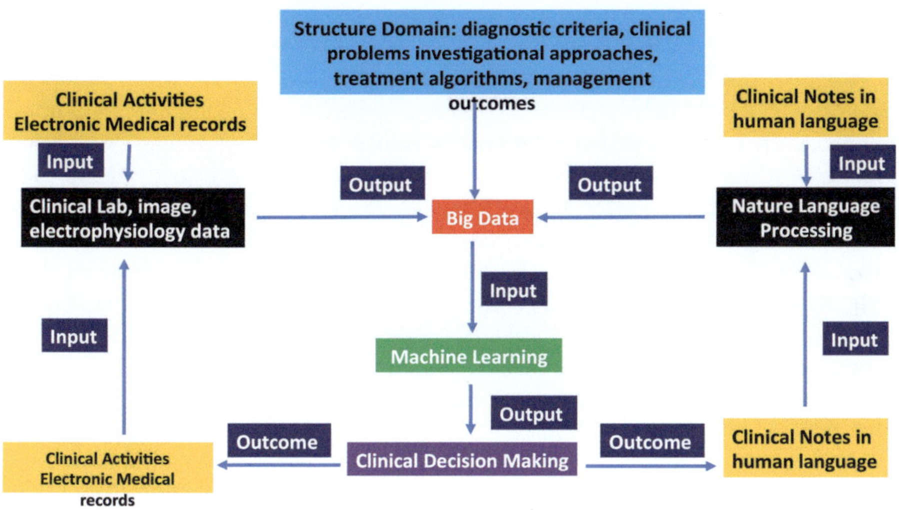

Fig. 18.8 Artificial intelligence in medicine road map: starting with the structure based on the agreed diagnostic and management criteria, then big clinical data generation supported by natural language processing data enrichment and electronic medical recording, to machine learning data analysis, leading to the outcome of clinical decision-making. As powerful as AI techniques can be, they have to be motivated by clinical problems and be applied to assist clinical practice in the end

Disease Specific Use

The increasingly rich AI literature in healthcare has motivated studying the use of AI in different diseases; examples are presented below.

Cancer

Earlier published double-blinded validation study [63] demonstrated that the IBM Watson for oncology would be a reliable AI system for assisting the diagnosis of cancer. In another study, Esteva et al. [64] studied the potential of deep convolutional neural networks (CNNs) [65, 66], trained end-to-end from images directly, using only pixels and disease labels as inputs for classification and identification of skin cancer subtypes. The convolutional neural networks achieved performance on par with all tested experts for the identification of the most common cancers, as well as the deadliest skin cancer across both tasks. This demonstrates that AI is capable of classifying skin cancer with a level of competence comparable to dermatologists. Outfitted with deep neural networks, mobile devices can potentially extend the reach of dermatologists outside of the clinic. It is projected that 6.3 billion smartphone subscriptions will exist by the year 2021 [67] and can therefore potentially provide low-cost universal access to vital diagnostic care [64].

Neurology

Bouton et al. developed an AI system, through applied machine learning algorithms to decode the neuronal activity and control activation of the participant's muscles, aiming at restoring the control of movement in patients with quadriplegia [68]. Farina et al. tested the power of an offline man/machine interface that uses the discharge timings of spinal motor neurons to control upper-limb prostheses [69]. A series of motor neuron discharges was mapped into control commands across multiple degrees of freedom via the offline application of direct proportional control, pattern recognition and musculoskeletal modelling. A series of experiments performed on six patients reveal that the man/machine interface has superior offline performance compared with conventional direct electromyographic control applied after targeted muscle innervation.

Cardiology

Dilsizian and Siegel discussed the potential application of the AI system to diagnose the heart disease through cardiac image [47]. Arterys [70] recently received clearance from the US Food and Drug Administration (FDA) to market its Arterys Cardio DL application, which uses AI to provide automated, editable ventricle segmentations based on conventional cardiac MRI images. The medical imaging platform has been approved to be put into use to help doctors diagnose heart problems. It uses a self-teaching artificial neural network which has learned from 1000 cases and will continue to improve its knowledge and understanding of how the heart works with each new case it examines.

Ophthalmology

Long et al. [71] developed an AI system using deep learning and involving convolutional neural networks for diagnostics, risk stratification and treatment suggestions, accurately diagnoses and provides treatment decisions for congenital cataracts, in an in silico test, in a website-based study and in a multihospital clinical trial. The study showed that the AI agent and individual ophthalmologists perform equally well. Moreover, they reported that integrating the AI agent with a cloud-based platform for multihospital collaboration has been helpful to improve disease management for the benefit of patients with rare diseases. In another study, Gulshan et al. [72] used retinal fundus photographs from adults with diabetes, to develop an algorithm based on deep machine learning for detecting referable diabetic retinopathy. The authors concluded that deep learning algorithms had high sensitivity and specificity for detecting diabetic retinopathy and macular edema in retinal fundus photographs.

Rheumatology

Rheumatologic diseases manifest themselves in varying combinations of symptoms and signs, particularly at early stages, and therefore make differential diagnosis a challenge, especially for non-rheumatologists including general practitioners. Since diagnosis at an early stage and adequate treatment improve prognosis, assistance in establishing diagnosis is desirable. Given the substantial progress in computer science in the last years, the idea of computers taking the role of diagnostic support is not far-fetched. Software applications have affected decision processes in clinical routine, for example, in controlling depth of anaesthesia [73] or in detecting drug interactions [74]. Software tools to support physicians in the diagnostic process have been developed in almost every field of medicine. A widely utilized type is the so-called expert system, defined as artificial intelligence programme designed to provide expert-level solutions to complex problems [75].

Pandey and Mishra distinguished between knowledge-based systems and intelligent computing systems [76]. There are three different approaches to knowledge-based systems depending on the form of knowledge representation: rule-based, case-based and model-based. In rule-based reasoning, the knowledge is expressed by rules. The rules can be newly developed or can be extracted from decision tables or decision trees [77]. In case-based reasoning, the inference engine searches the knowledge base for similar cases. Finally, models, that is, biochemical or biophysical, can also form the knowledge [76].

As early as 1983, a knowledge-based computer consultant system in the medical specialty area of rheumatology was described. The system, called AI/RHEUM, uses artificial intelligence techniques to provide non-rheumatologist physicians with diagnostic assistance in this specialty area. AI/RHEUM contains in structured knowledge-based formal criteria for 26 rheumatologic diseases. The system has been retrospectively tested against 384 clinical cases, with an overall correct diagnostic performance of 94% [78]. However, rheumatology may represent a challenge when it comes to implementing AI in clinical rheumatology. This has been attributed to several causes. First, it is not uncommon to find non-specific findings present in multiple rheumatic diseases and consequently complicate the knowledge representation for AI systems. Second, there is a lack of epidemiological data concerning the prevalence and incidence of rheumatic diseases as well as sensitivity and the specificity of single findings in diseases. Third, even if available for a large population, such data vary greatly among ethnic groups and regions becoming an increasing problem in times of global migration. Fourth, for many of the disease-specific findings, there are no internationally established standardized cut-off values. And finally, many rheumatic diseases can coexist with each other in overlap syndromes [79]. Nevertheless, the growing understanding of diseases, development of diagnostic and management guidelines as well as treatment algorithms and unified international disease activity scoring systems are expected to facilitate the representation of medical knowledge and decision processes in the near future.

Artificial Intelligence and Medical Education

Changes to the medical profession mandate similar developments in the medical education which would enable the physicians to effectively implement contemporary practice into their standard daily work. Several proposals for such reforms have been raised. Common themes include renewed emphasis on communication, teamwork, risk management and patient safety. Though these reforms are important, yet they remain insufficient. This was attributed to the recent trend of medicine which is rapidly transitioning from the information age to the age of artificial intelligence. Physicians are expected now to work at the top of their licence, have knowledge spanning the health professions and care continuum, effectively leverage data platforms, focus on analysing outcomes and improving performance and communicate the meaning of the probabilities generated by massive amounts of data to patients given their unique human complexities [80].

In a recent lecture, entitled "Tomorrow's Doctors: Their Future – Our Choice" [81], Dr. Colin Melville, Director of the UK General Medical Council's (GMC) Education and Standards directorate, discussed how changes in medicine will affect the ways in which future doctors are taught. Changes in demographics, advances in technology and treatments, the focus of medical professionals which shifted to the patients' needs rather than diseases as well as growing interest in doctors' communication skills and their approach to patients will all have an impact on how medicine is perceived and taught in the future. The segregation of undergraduate, postgraduate and continuing education into three silos will disappear with a seamless continuum of education in place. In another talk, Wartman advocated a "reboot" of medical education, noting that many of the current reforms that have been identified are necessary but not sufficient for twenty-first century medical education [82]. He also noted that the track record of medical education reform depicts an industry that is slow to adopt meaningful change. The acquisition of twenty-first century skills for medical practice requires, in our opinion, a more radical transformation of medical education. Although the dictum "see one, do one, teach one" may have characterized the way physicians learned clinical skills in the past, it is now clear that, for training to be effective, learners at all levels must have the opportunity to compare their performance to a standard and to continue to practice until competence is achieved.

Pressed by their managers, external stakeholders and a public troubled by lapses in quality of care as well as unsustainable cost increases, healthcare professionals are facing firmer challenges in designing initiatives to link closely the goals of learning with both the delivery of better care and measures of greater responsibility [83]. In view of the new trend of integrating all levels of medical learning, undergraduate, graduate and continuing medical education, physicians are expected to work at the top of their licence in collaboration with other members of the healthcare team; have knowledge that spans the breadth of the health professions and care continuum; leverage data platforms by using smartphones, social media and other electronic devices; and focus on analysing outcomes and improving performance, including customer service [84]. New skills and expertise will be required as we have entered into the artificial intelligence age. These include better use of the findings of cognitive psychology, closer alignment of humans and machines in education and enhanced use of simulations focused on the integration of machines in care delivery and patients as active collaborators in their care [80]. Cognitive psychology has demonstrated that facts and concepts are best recalled and put into service when they are taught, practiced and assessed in the context they will be used for. Several decades of research on clinical expertise have elucidated the thinking of physicians as they evaluate signs and symptoms, select and interpret diagnostic tests and synthesize data to develop clinical assessments and care plans [85].

It was early noted by [86] that "Educational standards need to be refreshed, refined and improved as technology changes and the data fog thickens". There is no disagreement that a fundamental understanding of the biomedical sciences and their interconnectedness with clinical knowledge and expertise in practice should remain central to medical education.

Big Data in Medical Education

Medical education in the twenty-first century is expected to have regular updates in the curriculum to include recent updated strategies and approaches to strengthen the healthcare professionals' ability to practice with more precision in a data-rich environment supported by artificial intelligence. As one example, learners must be exposed to big data in the context of decision-making. They must develop a solid understanding of the four Vs of big data: volume (the amount of data today is vast compared to the amount in the past), variety (data comes from many different sources of varying validity), velocity (data is being generated very fast and momentum is increasing) and veracity (the quality of the data being generated needs to be assessed) [80].

Learners also will need to develop a basic understanding of how data are being aggregated, analysed and ultimately personalized in healthcare delivery through artificial intelligence applications. They will need to be able to think broadly about how to manage the variety of applications, whether embodied in decision support software, robots or more sophisticated social media applications. Yang and Veltri noted earlier that "The most critical challenge is how we can transform the health care data into additional values for precision medicine, preventive medicine, and predictive modelling" [87].

The Next Phase of Artificial Intelligence

The future of AI in education is intimately linked to the future of AI. The increasing consumerisation of AI technologies brings with it an immense increase in the number of specialists working on and developing AI. The pace of innovation and development in general is at its fastest rate ever [88], and the current popularity of AI should mean that innovation in AI will become a target for several industries, e.g. education, healthcare, automotive, financial services, transportation, media, retail and consumer as well as energy.

There is an increasing recognition that the inclusion of AI in standard education will help learners gain twenty-first century skills. These skills are essential for current and future work environments. AI in education has the tools and techniques to facilitate tracking the development of each learner's skills and capabilities as they interact and learn over time. This monitoring of individual learners can then be collated and interpreted as required to provide knowledge about progress at the school, local and national levels. The increasing range of data capture devices – such as biological data, voice recognition and eye tracking – will enable educational AI systems to provide new types of evidence for currently difficult-to-assess skills. For example, a practice-based learning experience that incorporates elements of problem-solving or collaboration might be assessed using a combination of data sources including voice recognition (to identify who is doing and saying what in a team activity) and eye tracking (to explore which learner is focusing on which learning resources at any particular moment in time). Furthermore, the increasing use of educational AI systems will permit the collection of mass data about which teaching and learning practices work best. This data will make it possible to track a learner's progress against different teaching approaches and, in turn, will allow us to develop a dynamic catalogue of the best teaching practices suited to the development of different skills and capabilities, in particular the twenty-first century skills, across a range of environments [23].

Big Data and In-Time Assessments of the Learning Experience

The continued and growing use of technologies in education will permit the collection of increasing data volume about teachers and learners. This so-called big data is already being studied using learning analytics to recognize data patterns of potential educational interest. For example, analytics have been used with high levels of accuracy to predict when a student is likely to fail an assessment or "drop out" from an online course. Soon the sophistication of these learning analytics will be complemented by AI techniques to provide just-in-time information about learner successes, challenges and needs that can then be used to shape the learning experience itself. For example, educational AI systems will enable learning analytics to identify changes in learner confidence and motivation while learning a foreign language, scientific phenomenon or a tricky math equation [89].

Providing New Insights into How Learning Is Progressing

Educational AI will provide new insights into how learning is progressing. In addition to timeliness, the data gathered from digital teaching and learning experiences will give new insights that cannot be ascertained from currently available assessments tools. For example, as well as identifying whether or not a learner gave the correct answer, datasets could be analysed to help teachers understand how the learner arrived at their answer. The data might also help in better understanding of cognitive processes such as remembering and forgetting and the fundamental impact that these have on learning and student outcomes. Educational AI analysis might also identify if and when a student is confused, bored or frustrated, to help teachers understand and enhance a learner's emotional readiness for learning [23].

Moving Beyond "Stop-and-Test"

In their report, Kristen DiCerbo and John Behrens about Impacts of the Digital Ocean on Education, the models and techniques developed by educational AI researchers over the last 25 years have resulted in an ever rising ocean of digital data on learning and teaching, telling us much about the data we need to collect in order to assess students while they learn [90].

With ongoing educational AI analysis of a student's learning activities, there will be no need for the stop-and-test approach that characterizes many current assessments. Instead of traditional assessments that rely upon evaluating small samples of what a student has been taught, AI-driven assessments will be built into meaningful learning activities, perhaps a game or a collaborative project, and will assess all of the learning (and teaching) that takes place, as it happens [91].

AI and educational AI have always been interdisciplinary fields. Moving forward, educational AI will continue to leverage new insights in disciplines such as psychology and educational neuroscience to better understand the learning process and so build more accurate models that are better able to predict – and influence – a learner's progress, motivation and perseverance.

An Example from Education Neuroscience

One example of the way that neuroscience can inform education and the design of educational AI systems can be extracted from the work of Paul Howard-Jones, Professor of Neuroscience and Education at the University of Bristol. His work suggests that learning can be improved when it is linked to uncertain rewards, e.g. in situations where a learner knows that a reward may be given upon their completion of a task, but there is no certainty that the reward will appear on every occasion. This is counter-intuitive to typical education practices where rewards are consistently related to success.

The use of uncertain rewards is commonly used in the world of computer games, hence the current interest in the design of educational games that use the motivational impact of uncertain rewards to engage learners and to enhance their learning. The addition of educational AI techniques to the design of these educational games would enable, for example, the provision of uncertain rewards to be calibrated to a learner's individual reaction to a given level of uncertainty [92].

An Example from Psychology

For several years psychologists have been interested in exploring the role of "mindsets" in learning [93]. They stratified the learners into those who believe that intelligence does not change over time (a "fixed mindset") and those who believe that their abilities can be developed (a "growth mindset"). Learners with a growth mindset see challenges as things to be overcome; they persist and value effort more, which leads to them enjoying more success as learners. There is increasing evidence that a growth mindset can be taught and that changing students' mindsets can have a substantial impact on their grades and achievement test scores [94]. There is already a role for technology when it comes to helping learners to develop a growth mindset; Carol Dweck's team have developed Brainology, a piece of software to provide support and content for promoting a growth mindset [94]. The addition of AI to the technology would bring greater possibilities. For example, with AI the system could adapt to a learner's goal orientation or mindset or scaffold learners towards a growth mindset. More sophisticated learner models would be able to capture learners' mindsets, including how these change over time and adapt teaching accordingly. This might include providing targeted feedback to teachers to enable them to support each learner to develop a growth mindset in the most effective way [95].

Lifelong Learning Partner

Early educational AI research revived the old Chinese story showing that children would learn more effectively with another [96]; hence, new learning companion systems have been developed. These systems provided each learner with a collaborative computer-based learning companion (or companions). It was the role of the companion to use collaboration and competition to stimulate student learning. The companion could also act as a student for the human learner to tutor, and in so doing, the student learns by teaching. The computer-based teacher offered examples and guidance to human and computer student alike and determined the order and content of the topics to be tackled [97].

The next generation of learning companions will offer huge potential for future teaching and learning. There are no technical barriers to the development of learning companions that can accompany and support individual learners throughout their studies – in and beyond school. These lifelong learning companions could be based in the cloud, accessible via a multiplicity of devices, and be operated offline as needed.

Rather than teaching all subject areas, the learning companion might call in specialist educational AI systems or humans with expertise in the particular subject area required by the learner. In addition, the companion could focus on helping learners to become better at learning through developing a growth mindset or an impressive array of twenty-first century skills. And because this type of system can help all learners to access learning resources that are optimal for their needs, it will be suitable for struggling learners as well as those who are high achieving [23].

In conclusion, artificial intelligence has recently surpassed human performance in several standard life domains. In healthcare, there is great hope that AI will create an era of truly personalized medicine and enable better disease surveillance, facilitate early detection, endorse improved diagnosis and uncover novel treatments.

Given the time limitations of a physician, as the time demands for the rote tasks increased and the fact that the number of items to discuss per clinical appointment has vastly outpaced the time allotted per visit, AI is expected to obviate repetitive tasks to clear the way for human-to-human bonding and the application of emotional intelligence and judgement in healthcare. On the other hand, there is profound fear on the part of some that it will overtake jobs and disrupt the physician–patient relationship. The wealth of data now available in the form of clinical and pathological images, continuous biometric data and Internet of things (IoT) devices is ideally suited to power the deep learning computer algorithms which lead to AI-generated analysis and predictions. Consequently, a substantial increase in AI research in medicine is expected over the coming years.

References

1. Tsang L, Kracov DA, Mulryne J, Strom L, Perkins N, Dickinson R, Wallace VM, Jones B. The impact of artificial intelligence on medical innovation in the European Union and United States. J Intellect Prop Technol Law. 2017;29:8. https://www.arnoldporter.com/~/media/files/perspectives/publications/2017/08/the-impact-of-artificial-inteelligence-on-medical-innovation.pdf.
2. Fenton JJ, Taplin SH, Carney PA, et al. Influence of computer-aided detection on performance of screening mammography. N Engl J Med. 2007;356:1399–409.
3. Gawad J, Bonde C. Artificial intelligence: future of medicine and healthcare. Biochem Ind J. 2017;11(2):113.
4. Bentley P, Brundage M, Häggström O, Metzinger T, Gutenberg J. Should we fear artificial intelligence? In-depth analysis. Eur Parliam Res Serv. 2018; https://doi.org/10.2861/412165. Accessed on 13 May 2018
5. Schoenauer M, Bonnet Y, Berthet C, Cornut A-C, Levin F, Rondepierre B. For a meaningful artificial intelligence. 2018. https://www.aiforhumanity.fr/pdfs/MissionVillani_Report_ENG-VF.pdf. Accessed on 13 May 2018.
6. Winston PH. Artificial intelligence. 3rd ed. Reading: Addison-Wesley; 1992. p. 5.
7. Wachsmuth I. The concept of intelligence in artificial intelligence. In: Cruse H, editor. Prerational intelligence: adaptive behavior and intelligent systems without symbols and logic, vol. 1: Springer; 2000. p. 43–55. https://link.springer.com/content/pdf/bfm%3A978-94-010-0870-9%2F1.pdf.
8. Taddy M. Chicago booth and microsoft. The technological elements of artificial intelligence. http://www.nber.org/chapters/c14021.pdf. Accessed on 13 May 2018.
9. van Seijen H, Fatemi M, Romoff J, Laroche R, Barnes T, Tsang J. Hybrid reward architecture for reinforcement learning. 2017. arXiv:1706.04208.
10. Susan A. Beyond prediction: using big data for policy problems. Science. 2017;355:483–5.
11. Timothy B. General purpose technologies. Handb Econ Innov. 2010;2:761–91.
12. Agarwal A, Hsu D, Kale S, Langford J, Li L, Schapire R. Taming the monster: a fast and simple algorithm for contextual bandits. In: Proceedings of the 31 st International Conference on Machine Learning, Beijing, China, 2014. JMLR: W&CP, volume 32. p. 1638–46. http://proceedings.mlr.press/v32/agarwalb14.pdf.
13. Rouse M. Machine learning (ML). 2017. https://searchenterpriseai.techtarget.com/definition/machine-learning-ML. Accessed on 13 May 2018.
14. Gibson A, Patterson J. Major architectures of deep networks. Chapter 4 in deep learning: a practitioner's approach. O'Reilly. 2017. http://opencarts.org/sachlaptrinh/pdf/27976.pdf. Accessed on 13 May 2018.

15. Morgan JP. Big data and AI strategies: machine learning and alternative data approach to investing. 2017. http://valuesimplex.com/articles/JPM.pdf.
16. Artificial Intelligence And Life In 2030. One hundred year study on artificial intelligence. Report Of The 2015 Study Panel. 2016. https://ai100.stanford.edu/sites/default/files/ai_100_report_0831fnl.pdf. Accessed on 15 May 2018.
17. Is artificial intelligence transforming education. Acer education. http://eu-acerforeducation.acer.com/innovative-technologies/is-artificial-intelligence-transforming-education/?gclid=EAIaIQobChMI04Xai9j52gIVTbftCh178wauEAAYAiAAEgI6CfD_BwE. Accessed on 16 May 2018.
18. Gardner H. Multiple intelligences: the theory in practice. New York: Basic Books; 1993.
19. Perkins D. Outsmarting IQ: the emerging science of learnable intelligence. New York: The Free Press; 1995.
20. Sternberg, Robert (1988). The triarchic mind: a new theory of human intelligence. New York: Penguin Books. Information about Sternberg and his writings is available at: http://www.psy.pdx.edu/PsiCafe/KeyTheorists/Sternberg.htm. Accessed 16 May 2018.
21. Moursund D. Brief introduction to educational implications of artificial intelligence. 2006. E:\Teaching Rheumatology\Book chapters\Section IV\Artificial intelligence\educational implications of AI.pdf. Accessed 16 May 2018.
22. Self J. The defining characteristics of intelligent tutoring systems research: ITSs care, precisely. Int J Artif Intell Educ (IJAIEd). 1999;10:350–64.
23. Luckin R, Holmes W, Griffiths M, Forcier LB. Intelligence unleashed. An argument for AI in education. London: Pearson; 2016. https://www.pearson.com/content/dam/corporate/global/pearson-dot-com/files/innovation/Intelligence-Unleashed-Publication.pdf. Accessed on 16th May 2018
24. Italk2learn. http://www.italk2learn.eu.
25. Grawemeyer B, Mavrikis M, Holmes W, Gutiérrez-Santos S. Adapting feedback types according to students' affective states. In: Conati C, Heffernan N, Mitrovic A, Verdejo MF, editors. Artificial intelligence in education 17th international conference, AIEd 2015. Madrid, Spain, June 22-26, 2015 Proceedings, vol. 9112. Madrid: Springer; 2015.
26. Litman D. Language processing in AIEd: successes and challenges. In: Craig SD, Dicheva D, editors. Presented at the panel on the evolution of AIEd @ AIEd09. Brighton; 2009. http://www.questiongeneration.org/AIED2009/.
27. Dimitrova V, Mccalla G, Bull S. Preface: "Open learner models: future research directions". Int J Artif Intell Educ. 2007;17:217–226. IOS Press.
28. Du Boulay B, Rebolledo-Mendez G, Luckin R, Martínez-Mirón E, Harris A. Motivationally intelligent systems: diagnosis and feedback. In: Proceedings of the 31 st International Conference on Machine Learning, Beijing, China, 2014. JMLR: W&CP, volume 32. p. 563–5. http://proceedings.mlr.press/v32/agarwalb14.pdf.
29. Johnson WL, Valente A. Tactical language and culture training systems: using AI to teach foreign languages and cultures. AI Mag. 2009;30(2):72.
30. Dillenbourg P, Baker MJ, Blaye A, O'Malley C. The evolution of research on collaborative learning. In: Reimann P, Spada H, editors. Learning in humans and machine: towards an interdisciplinary learning science. Bingley: Emerald; 1995. p. 189–211.
31. Slavin RE. Co-operative learning: what makes group-work work. In: Hanna D, David I, Francisco B, editors. The nature of learning: using research to inspire practice. Chicago: OECD Publishing; 2010. p. 161–78.
32. Muehlenbrock M. Learning group formation based on learner profile and context. Int J E-Learning. 2006;5(1):19.
33. McLaren BM, Scheuer O, Mikšátko J. Supporting collaborative learning and e-discussions using artificial intelligence techniques. Int J Artif Intell Educ. 2010;20(1):1–46.
34. Upton K, Kay J. Narcissus: group and individual models to support small group work. In: Houben G, McCalla G, Pianesi F, Zancanaro M, editors. User modeling, adaptation, and personalization. Berlin: Springer; 2009. p. 54–65.
35. Vizcaíno A. A simulated student can improve collaborative learning. Int J Artif Intell Educ. 2005;15(1):3–40.

36. One example of this type of virtual agent can be found in Betty's Brain (http://www.teachableagents.org/research/bettysbrain.php), a computer-based learning environment developed at Vanderbilt University.
37. De Laat M, Chamrada M, Wegerif R. Facilitate the facilitator: awareness tools to support the moderator to facilitate online discussions for networked learning. In: Proceedings of the 6th international conference on networked learning. 2008. p. 80–6. http://proceedings.mlr.press/v32/agarwalb14.pdf.
38. Barab SA, Gresalfi M, Ingram-Goble A. Transformational play: using games to position person, content, and context. Educ Res. 2010;39(7):525–36.
39. Hassani K, Nahvi A, Ahmadi A. Design and implementation of an intelligent virtual environment for improving speaking and listening skills. Interact Learn Environ. 2016;24(1):252–71. https://doi.org/10.1080/10494820.2013.846265.
40. Dede C. Immersive interfaces for engagement and learning. Science. 2009;323(5910):66–9.
41. Vannini N, Enz S, Sapouna M, Wolke D, Watson S, Woods S, et al. "FearNot!": a computer-based anti-bullying-programme designed to foster peer intervention. Eur J Psychol Educ. 2011;26(1):21–44.
42. Traum D, Rickel J, Gratch J, Marsella S. Negotiation over tasks in hybrid human-agent teams for simulation-based training. In: AAMAS '03 Proceedings of the second international joint conference on Autonomous agents and multiagent systems. Melbourne: ACM New York; 2003. p. 441–8.
43. Global Market Insights. Healthcare AI market size, competitive market share & forecast, 2024. 2017.
44. The next generation of medicine: artificial intelligence and machine learning. TM Capital. 2017. www.tmcapital.com/healthcare. https://www.tmcapital.com/wp-content/uploads/2017/11/TMCC20AI20Spotlight20-202017.10.2420vF.PDF. Accessed on 20 May 2018.
45. Miller D, Brown E. Artificial intelligence in medical practice: the question to the answer? Am J Med. 2018;131(2):129–33.
46. Jiang F, Jiang Y, Zhi H, Dong Y, Li H, Ma S, Wang Y, Dong Q, Shen H, Wang Y. Artificial intelligence in healthcare: past, present and future. Stroke Vasc Neurol. 2017;0:e000101. https://doi.org/10.1136/svn-2017-000101.
47. Dilsizian SE, Siegel EL. Artificial intelligence in medicine and cardiac imaging: harnessing big data and advanced computing to provide personalized medical diagnosis and treatment. Curr Cardiol Rep. 2014;16:441.
48. Patel VL, Shortliffe EH, Stefanelli M, et al. The coming of age of artificial intelligence in medicine. Artif Intell Med. 2009;46:5–17.
49. Jha S, Topol EJ. Adapting to artificial intelligence: radiologists and pathologists as information specialists. JAMA. 2016;316:2353–4.
50. Pearson T. How to replicate Watson hardware and systems design for your own use in your basement. 2011. https://www.ibm.com/developerworks/community/blogs/InsideSystemStorage/entry/ibm_watson_how_to_build_your_own_watson_jr_in_your_basement7?lang=en. Accessed 20 May 2018.
51. Weingart SN, Wilson RM, Gibberd RW, et al. Epidemiology of medical error. BMJ. 2000;320:774–7.
52. Graber ML, Franklin N, Gordon R. Diagnostic error in internal medicine. Arch Intern Med. 2005;165:1493–9.
53. Winters B, Custer J, Galvagno SM, et al. Diagnostic errors in the intensive care unit: a systematic review of autopsy studies. BMJ Qual Saf. 2012;21:894–902.
54. Lee CS, Nagy PG, Weaver SJ, et al. Cognitive and system factors contributing to diagnostic errors in radiology. AJR Am J Roentgenol. 2013;201:611–7.
55. Neill DB. Using artificial intelligence to improve hospital inpatient care. IEEE Intell Syst. 2013;28:92–5.
56. Administration UFaD. Guidance for industry: electronic source data in clinical investigations. 2013. https://www.fda.gov/downloads/drugs/guidances/ucm328691.pdf. Accessed 1 Jun 2017.

57. Gillies RJ, Kinahan PE, Hricak H, Rj G, Pe K. Radiomics: images are more than pictures, they are data. Radiology. 2016;278:563–77.
58. Li CY, Liang GY, Yao WZ, et al. Integrated analysis of long noncoding RNA competing interactions reveals the potential role in progression of human gastric cancer. Int J Oncol. 2016;48:1965–76.
59. Shin H, Kim KH, Song C, et al. Electrodiagnosis support system for localizing neural injury in an upper limb. J Am Med Inform Assoc. 2010;17:345–7.
60. Karakülah G, Dicle O, Koşaner O, et al. Computer based extraction of phenoptypic features of human congenital anomalies from the digital literature with natural language processing techniques. Stud Health Technol Inform. 2014;205:570–4.
61. Darcy AM, Louie AK, Roberts LW. Machine learning and the profession of medicine. JAMA. 2016;315:551–2.
62. Murff HJ, FitzHenry F, Matheny ME, et al. Automated identification of postoperative complications within an electronic medical record using natural language processing. JAMA. 2011;306:848–55.
63. Somashekhar SP, Kumarc R, Rauthan A, et al. Abstract S6-07: double blinded validation study to assess performance of IBM artificial intelligence platform, Watson for oncology in comparison with manipal multidisciplinary tumour board? First study of 638 breast cancer cases. Cancer Res. 2017;77(4 Suppl):S6–07.
64. Esteva A, Kuprel B, Novoa RA, et al. Dermatologist-level classification of skin cancer with deep neural networks. Nature. 2017;542:115–8.
65. LeCun Y, Bengio Y, Hinton G. Deep learning. Nature. 2015;521:436–44.
66. LeCun Y, Bengio Y. In: Arbib MA, editor. The handbook of brain theory and neural networks., 3361.10. Cambridge: MIT Press; 1995.
67. Cerwall P, Report EM. Ericssons mobility report. 2016. https://www.ericsson.com/res/docs/2016/ericsson-mobility-report-2016.pdf.
68. Bouton CE, Shaikhouni A, Annetta NV, et al. Restoring cortical control of functional movement in a human with quadriplegia. Nature. 2016;533:247–50.
69. Farina D, Vujaklija I, Sartori M, et al. Man/machine interface based on the discharge timings of spinal motor neurons after targeted muscle reinnervation. Nat Biomed Eng. 2017;1:0025.
70. Marr B. First FDA approval for clinical cloud-based deep learning in healthcare. 2017. https://www.forbes.com/sites/bernardmarr/2017/01/20/first-fda-approval-for-clinical-cloud-based-deep-learning-in-healthcare/#41f14f79161c. Accessed on 20 May 2018.
71. Long E, Lin H, Liu Z, Liu Z, Wu X, Wang L, Jiang J, An Y, Lin Z, Li X, Chen J, Li J, Cao Q, et al. An artificial intelligence platform for the multihospital collaborative management of congenital cataracts. Nat Biomed Eng. 2017;1:0024. https://www.researchgate.net/publication/313111785_An_artificial_intelligence_platform_for_the_multihospital_collaborative_management_of_congenital_cataracts.
72. Gulshan V, Peng L, Coram M, et al. Development and validation of a deep learning algorithm for detection of diabetic retinopathy in retinal fundus photographs. JAMA. 2016;316:2402–10.
73. Schmidt GN, M¨uller J, Bischoff P. Measurement of the depth of anaesthesia. Anaesthesist. 2008;57(1):9–30.
74. McKibbon KA, Lokker C, Handler SM, et al. The effectiveness of integrated health information technologies across the phases of medication management: a systematic review of randomized controlled trials. J Am Med Inform Assoc. 2012;19(1):22–30.
75. Buchanan BG. Rule based expert systems: the mycin experiments of the stanford heuristic programming project. Reading: Addison-Wesley Longman; 1984.
76. Pandey B, Mishra RB. Knowledge and intelligent computing system in medicine. Comput Biol Med. 2009;39(3):215–30.
77. Lehmann TM. Handbuch der Medizinischen Informatik. M¨unchen: Hanser; 2002.
78. Kingsland LC, Lindberg DAB, Sharp GC. J Med Syst. 1983;7:221. https://doi.org/10.1007/BF00993283.

79. Alder H, Michel BA, Marx C, Tamborrini G, Langenegger T, Bruehlmann P, Steurer J, Wildi L. Computer-based diagnostic expert systems in rheumatology: where do we stand in 2014? Int J Rheumatol. 2014; https://doi.org/10.1155/2014/672714.
80. Wartman Steven A, Donald CC. Medical education must move from the information age to the age of artificial intelligence. Acad Med. 2017; https://doi.org/10.1097/ACM.0000000000002044.
81. Harden R. Tomorrow's doctors: their future—our choice. A lecture school of medicine. UK: University of Dundee; 2017. http://medicine.dundee.ac.uk/news/ronald-harden-lecture-2017-looks-future-medical-education
82. Wartman SA. Medical education needs a reboot!! 2016 Mansbach lecture. Norfolk: Eastern Virginia Medical School; 2016. http://www.aahcdc.org/Portals/41/PublicationsResources/Presentations/AAHC%20Presentations/Medical-Education-Needs-Reboot.pdf
83. Iglehart JK, Baron RB. Ensuring physicians' competence – is maintenance of certification the answer? N Engl J Med. 2012;367:2543–9.
84. Beck EH. Training AHC graduates for the 21st century workplace. In: A presentation to the 2016 annual meeting of the association of academic health centers. San Diego: Association of Academic Health Centres. p. 2016.
85. Norman G. Research in clinical reasoning: past history and current trends. Med Educ. 2005;39:418–27.
86. American Medical News. Medical education still evolving 100 years after Flexner report. 2010. http://www.amednews.com/article/20101004/profession/310049932/7/. Accessed 3 Apr 2017.
87. Yang CC, Veltri P. Intelligent healthcare informatics in big data era. Artif Intell Med. 2015;65:75–7.
88. Kaminska I. Innovating fast or slow? Gates vs Wolf edition. 2015. Retrieved from http://ftalphaville.ft.com/tag/technology/.
89. Hill P, Barber M. Preparing for a renaissance in assessment. London: Pearson; 2014.
90. Di Cerbo KE, Behrens JT. Impacts of the digital ocean on education. London: Pearson; 2014.
91. Hill, Barber, DiCerbo K. Why an assessment renaissance means fewer tests. 2014. Retrieved from http://researchnetwork.pearson.com/digital-data-analytics-and-adaptivelearning/assessment-renaissance-means-fewertests.
92. Howard-Jones P, Holmes W, Demetriou S, Jones C, Tanimoto E, Morgan O, Davies N. Neuroeducational research in the design and use of a learning technology. Learn Media Technol. 2014;40(2):1–20.
93. Dweck CS, Leggett EL. A social-cognitive approach to motivation and personality. Psychol Rev. 1988;95(2):256–73 or Dweck CS. Mindset: the new psychology of success. New York: Random House; 2006.
94. Dweck CS. Even geniuses work hard. Educ Leadersh. 2010;68(1):16–20. Retrieved from http://www.mindsetworks.com/brainology
95. Harris A, Bonnett V, Luckin R, Yuill N, Avramides K. Scaffolding effective helpseeking behaviour in mastery and performance oriented learners. In: Dimitrova V, Mizoguchi R, Du Boulay B, Graesser AC, editors. AIED 2009, Frontiers in artificial intelligence and applications. IOS Press; 2009. p. 425–32. 200.
96. Cole M. Cultural psychology: a once and future discipline. Cambridge, MA: Harvard University Press; 1996.
97. Chan TW. Integrationkid: a learning companion system. In: Mylopolous J, Reiter R, editors. Proceedings of the 12th international conference on artificial intelligence, vol. 2. Morgan: Kaufmann Publishers; 1991. p. 1094–9.

Chapter 19
Motivation in Education

Introduction

Modern medical education curricula are based on the premise that students have an inherent desire to become physicians and are motivated by internal rather than external factors [1]. The value of motivation in learning behaviour and education has been well researched and established in general education but is much less studied in medical education. Over the past year, the interest of medical educators in motivation has been on the rise. Three major viewpoints [2, 3] paved the way for the issue to come under the focus. White and Gruppen [4] highlight that research relevant to motivation particularly in relation to medical education need to receive more attention. The current motivation paradigm in medical education suggests that components of the learning environment like communication style, curriculum, and assessment methods not only effect how much effort students put forward but the longer-term nature of how they are motivated in their careers. The past few years have seen significant changes in medical education curricula; however, there is high potential of causing significant detriment to the students, if medical schools continue to develop curricula and assessment tools without improving the current concepts of the nature of motivation [5].

Research in medical education can gain a lot from the wealth of knowledge available in general education literature. Earlier educational studies revealed that motivation is a good predictor for learning, academic success, persistence or continuation in a study as well as well-being [6–8]. There are several reasons for endorsing motivation among medical students in comparison to those in the general education. Medical education is characterized by the intertwining of the clinical and academic studies, which is not the standard for higher education. Furthermore, unlike general education, where students have a wide variety of choices to do different things and create unique profiles, medical education works towards one focused and clearly defined profession and career. The environment within which medical teaching and learning occur is highly specific. Also, medical students are considered highly

Y. El Miedany, *Rheumatology Teaching*,
https://doi.org/10.1007/978-3-319-98213-7_19

motivated from the outset having gone through a considerable effort to enter medical school. These proposals highlight the important role of motivation in medical education and inspire the rationale for studying motivation, particularly in medical students.

This chapter will discuss the science of motivation and then will try to answer the important questions: To what extent are medical students intrinsically or extrinsically motivated? Why do we need to know? Which type of motivation is useful in medical education? It will then discuss the science and art of motivation, followed by discussion of motivation and self-regulation. The chapter will discuss also motivation in medical education, teaching, clinical as well as problem-based learning. It will expand to discuss motivation of medical school and medical profession applicants, and then it will conclude with motivation and e-learning.

The Science of Motivation and Engaged Learning

Motivation is relevant particularly to learning as engaging in learning is an active process requiring conscious and deliberate activities. Even the most capable and smart students will not engage in learning if they do not pay attention and exert some effort. Thus, for learners to achieve optimal benefits from their education, teachers need to provide a learning context that encourages students to be motivated and supports them to enthusiastically engage in the learning tasks.

Motivation to Learn

There has been considerable evidence drawn from research on motivation in educational settings for the salience of particular teaching and learning practices for enhancing students' motivation to engage in learning. Looking into the basic foundation of motivation research revealed that there are many different motivation theories in medical education. Brissette and colleagues [5] published a systematic review on motivation in medical education with the intention of providing a framework for educators to consider this important dimension of curriculum development. One of these early motivation theories is that of adult education described by Malcolm Knowles [9]. Knowles proposed that "andragogy" (adult learning) should be distinct from "pedagogy" (child learning), which was attributed to the suggestion that there are fundamental differences between the two groups of learners. The theory has evolved over time and has is based on five fundamental principles, the fifth of which addresses motivation to learn; Knowles proposes that as a person matures, the motivation to learn shifts from external to internal. Reflecting on medical students, as adult learners, they are responsible for their own educational paths and lifelong learning. Adults are autonomous and self-directed; therefore, teaching medical students should focus on learning facilitation, while the students are left free to direct themselves. These principles are applicable in problem-based and self-directed learning.

Misch [3] has raised concerns about the validity and utility of andragogy in medical education. He argues that separating motivation into intrinsic and extrinsic categories may be over-simplistic as they are not dichotomous; rather they are context dependent, not easily distinguishable and interrelate with one another in complex ways. In medicine, it is impossible to create a solely intrinsically motivating environment because many secondary benefits are related to the medical profession, such as respect, admiration, wealth, etc. Misch states that "Rare indeed would be the medical student unaffected by such secondary riches, whose learning was driven solely by the joy of learning and unadulterated altruism" [3]. Medical educators must be careful not to establish the theory of andragogy as fact without critically assessing its limitations.

In 2000, Ryan and Deci [10] present a more complex model of motivation, in keeping with developments in cognitive psychology. Self-determination theory (SDT) is centred on the importance of intrinsic motivation and how it drives human behaviour. Many of the studies on motivation in medical education are based on SDT [10–14]. Engaging in something because it is inherently interesting or enjoyable is deemed intrinsic motivation, while doing something because it leads to a separable outcome is extrinsic motivation. Their approach focuses on three needs: the need for competence, the need for autonomy and the need for relatedness. Self-determination theory recognizes that basic need satisfaction is partly created from engaging in activities that are interesting for the individual. In medical education, providing optimal challenges, positive performance feedback and freedom from demeaning evaluations can facilitate feelings of competence. However, the need for competence must be accompanied by a sense of autonomy, choice and opportunity for self-direction in order for intrinsic motivation to be maintained or enhanced [10]. It is critical to remember that intrinsic motivation will occur only for activities that hold intrinsic interest for an individual. Concerning the material that does not interest the medical student, some suggest making the values or behaviour a part of one's self-identity, internalizing (taking it in) and then integrating it (transforming it into their own). The more the person internalizes the reasons for an action and assimilates them to the self, the more one's extrinsically motivated actions become self-determined. Internalization is achieved by providing a sense of belongingness and connectedness to the medical profession; this is called relatedness and is the third need in "self-determination theory". According to the self-determination theory, intrinsic motivation is enhanced when the three needs are fulfilled [10].

Several studies examined the application of the self-determination theory of motivation [11–14]. A study by Sobral [12] on the importance of autonomy in medical education determined that "autonomy in the learning environment was highly associated with student's perceptions of course quality in terms of the meaningfulness and value of the educational experience". Despite creating a learning environment based on competence and autonomy, it is crucial to realize that extrinsic motivators can undermine intrinsic motivation. Examples of extrinsic motivators are threats, deadlines and competition pressure because people experience these as controllers of their behaviour. The classroom environment, which encompasses goals of the faculty, the attitudes of doctors and lecturers and student assessments, has a direct influence on competence and autonomy and can either enhance or diminish intrinsic motivation.

Koens et al. [11] have developed a dimensional context model, where context is broken down into categories of physical dimension, semantic/cognitive dimension and the commitment/affective dimension. This model attempted to help educators select appropriate contexts in leading medical students from reduced to enriched learning environments, as well as to provide a framework for further research into context. Curry [15] suggests educating medical students about motivation and different learning styles so that students may develop their own learning tactics. Similarity in educational context and learning style contributes to academic success [13]. In essence, context matters.

Further application of self-determination theory emphasizes the importance of autonomy on the outcome of the action. Increasing internal motivation by providing competence feedback, autonomy and relatedness not only creates better educational outcomes but also creates better patient interactions. Williams [14] demonstrated that the values and skills learned in this type of environment created more autonomous students, which then acted in autonomous ways with their patients as they used an autonomy-supportive style to motivate their patients. The patients then became more autonomous with respect to their own care and showed improved adherence to a variety of health relevant behaviours. In theory, "more autonomy-supportive medical education may actually result in more effective health care delivery".

Motivation to Teach

Research has demonstrated that not everyone is motivated to teach but that there are some motivations commonly shared or expressed by those considering a career in teaching. Individual research studies have also investigated the motivations to teach held by different groups of people, including school students, student teachers, new teachers, qualified teachers, principals, school superintendents, teacher educators, women, second-career teachers, minority groups, those with differing levels of academic achievement and those from developing nations.

Research studies have drawn upon different theoretical bases and used a variety of research methods including essays, interviews and questionnaires. While findings differ across individual studies, as a whole, these studies have shown that people are, or would be, attracted to teaching by *calling*, having always wanted to teach [15]; *altruism*, the perceived worth or value of teaching to others, to make a difference in the lives of others, to help other people, to change society or to help a troubled profession [16]; *intellectual stimulation*, including a love of learning, teaching or a particular subject area or the desire to impart knowledge [17]; *the influence of others*, including family members, past teachers or members of the community [18]; *the perceived benefits and/or convenience of teaching,* including work schedules, work hours, vacations, career security and salary [19]; *the nature of teaching work*, especially the opportunities teaching provides for satisfying interpersonal interactions with others [20]; *a desire for a career change*, through dissatisfaction with a previous career, or a stressful life event such as divorce, unemployment or geographic relocation [21]; *the perceived relative ease of entry* into initial teacher education courses, or of the job of teaching itself [22]; and/or, *the status of teaching,* including the opportunities teaching provides for career or social advancement [18].

The Art of Motivation

Dramatic changes in medical education over the years have affected the design and content of curricula, including methods of teaching and learning, assessment and the competencies required of doctors [23–25]. Educational psychology tells us that learning processes can be mapped on three pillars (Fig. 19.1): cognitive (what to learn), affective or motivational (why to learn) and metacognitive regulation (how to learn). The *cognitive* component of learning involves those thinking activities that people use to process content, including selecting, relating, concretizing and applying information [26, 27]. The *affective* component involves coping with the feelings that arise during learning and may affect the progression of a learning process positively, neutrally or negatively [26]. This component includes aspects of motivation. The *metacognitive regulation* component involves orienting, planning, monitoring, testing, diagnosing, adjusting, evaluating and reflecting on the student's learning behaviour and approach [28, 29]. The learning-oriented teaching (LOT) model suggests that in a truly student-centred medical curriculum, all three of these dimensions should guide curriculum developers in constructing learning environments [30].

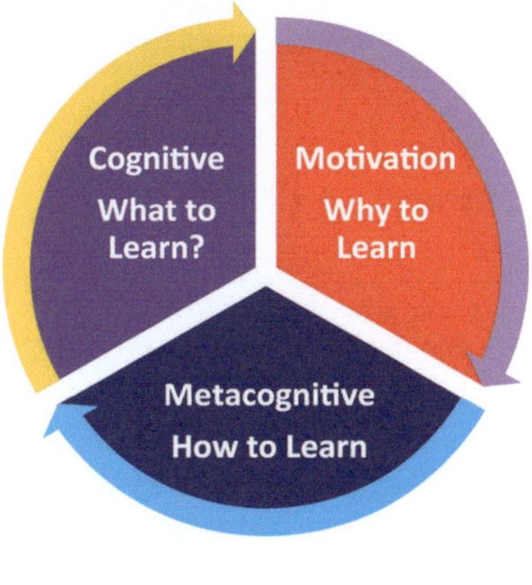

Fig. 19.1 The three pillars of the learning process – educational psychology tells us that learning processes is based on three pillars – cognitive (what to learn), affective or motivational (why to learn) and metacognitive regulation (how to learn)

Though the medical school curriculum should cover the topics and issues in alignment with the intended outcomes, there were concerns raised that the cognitive or "what to learn" dimension has dominated curricular reform for a long time. Examining the concepts described in the different motivation theories shows that motivation theorists have often emphasized the importance of motivation in learning and education [31]. Therefore, it is important to incorporate concepts of student motivation as an integral part of the foundation of medical curricula, particularly the concept of stimulating intrinsic motivation among medical students (i.e. learning for the sake of learning and patients) rather than extrinsic motivation (i.e. learning to be rewarded with good grades, honours, success or money). Intrinsic motivation has been shown to lead to better learning, performance and well-being among medical students [12, 31].

Motivation appears to be characterised by four qualities: *choice*, people tend to choose to do some things rather than others. Why do people prefer to do the things whether academically, socially, and physically? In a very real sense motivation is therefore a personal investment through choice. *Energy*, activities which people are motivated to do are usually characterized by high energy, involvement, enthusiasm, and interest. *Standards*, high personal standards are usually expected in activities in which people are motivated. In most cases, it is not unusual that people do not settle for second best or substandard performance. They try to better their own performance, and, at times, try to beat the performance of others. *Continuing* motivation, when people are motivated, they return to the activity voluntarily, time and again, because they enjoy it and feel rewarded through it. So in the standard learning scene, the students are expected to:

- Choose to do the subject or work rather than to be compelled to do it.
- Invest a lot of energy in their work and to be enthusiastic and interested.
- Set high standards for their work and to try to improve and go beyond the acquisition of basic skills.
- Continue to be motivated by spending voluntary, discretionary time on their work, rather than the minimum time [23].

Such relevance of motivation to the education process has been endorsed by the results of earlier studies which revealed that motivation is a predictor for learning, academic success, persistence or continuation in a study and well-being [7, 8].

Autonomous Motivation in Medical Education

Medical students often study with one target in their minds, which is to be able to exhibit their knowledge in examinations, pursue their desired specialization and handle patients in the right manner. If a student perceives that a topic or subject which needs to be studied does not lead to one of these outcomes, it is sidelined. This is because the activity of studying is dependent on reasons which are external to the student such as "I am expected to learn this" or "My tutor wants me to study this". In concordance, if students study only to get grades in their examinations or enrol for the specialty they want, the reasons for studying are still external. This leads to minimal effort from the student which is sufficient for him to achieve his objective. This also raises the question of "Can this ever lead to deep learning, long-term knowledge, and an attitude of lifelong learning that is expected in the medical profession?" Earlier report [32] revealed that the students' study behaviour is dependent on their motivation. However, this leads to another query "What kind of motivation do we want the medical students and doctors to have?"

Motivation theories provide us guidance in answering these questions. Self-determination theory (SDT), which is one of the well-known motivation theories, is becoming increasingly popular within medical education. Self-determination theory sets store by "autonomous motivation", which means that a student learns out of genuine interest or personal value [33, 34]. On the other hand, "controlled motivation" is the opposite of autonomous motivations, which means that a student learns because of external pressures (such as teachers, parents, examinations) and internal pressures (guilt or shame) or for rewards (such as grades). Autonomous motivation includes the cases in which a student may not feel genuine interest in an activity, but finds this activity personally important or valuable. For example, students may study basic sciences not because they find them genuinely interesting but because they comprehend their relevance to clinical practice. Thus, the students perceive involvement in the activity as their own choice (Fig. 19.2).

Autonomous motivation, in medical education, has been associated with better learning effort and strategies, better academic performance and less exhaustion than controlled motivation [35, 36]. However, the challenge remains regarding "What are the best approaches to keep the students autonomously motivated for medical

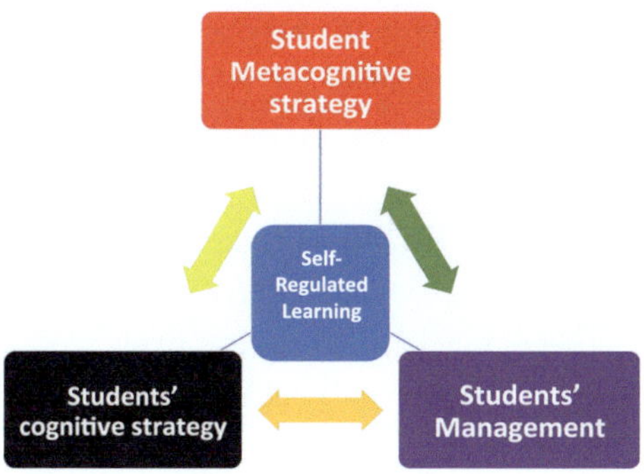

Fig. 19.2 The three components of the self-regulated learning: self-regulated learning includes students' metacognitive strategies for planning, monitoring and modifying their cognition. Students' management and control of their effort on classroom academic tasks has been proposed as another important component. For example, capable students who persist at a difficult task or block out distractors (i.e. noisy classmates) maintain their cognitive engagement in the task, enabling them to perform better. A third important aspect of self-regulated learning that some researchers have included in their conceptualization is the actual cognitive strategies that students use to learn, remember and understand the material

study?" Self-determination theory emphasizes on the fulfilment of three basic psychological needs: autonomy, competence and relatedness [33]. While in several occasions, autonomy has been misinterpreted as independence, that is, working without any help, self-determination theory makes a clear distinction between the two [33]. Human beings have an inherent tendency to grow and develop. Autonomous motivation needs to be nurtured not only by providing an autonomy-supportive environment but also by holding back controlling tendency and behaviour [33]. Autonomy support has been associated with autonomous motivation for medical study and autonomy-supportive medical practice [38]. Autonomy-supportive teaching behaviour has been associated with the students themselves being autonomy-supportive and humanistic in patient care [34]. Medical students have also been shown to choose specialties in which they had autonomy-supportive teachers [37]. The concept of autonomy support is slowly gaining awareness in medical education [38, 39].

There are several strategies of how autonomy support can be exerted in medical education. These include, as examples, small-group teaching, problem-based learning, gradual increase in responsibility of patients (vertically integrated curricula) and opportunities for elective clerkships, to conduct audits or contribute to research to set examples of gold standard or verifying a hypothesis and to get involved in service, educational or professional programmes for higher challenge [38, 40].

The need for autonomy is not restricted to students but applies to teachers as well. For teachers to be autonomy-supportive towards students, it is important that they themselves perceive autonomy in their work. Subsequently, just, as students who have autonomy-supportive teachers become autonomy-supportive towards patients, it is possible that teachers who work in autonomy-supportive institutions are autonomy-supportive towards students. Thus, autonomy support in medical education is not limited to bringing in changes in the medical curriculum for students but encompasses an overall change in the way of thinking and working in medical schools that foster autonomy among those involved in education.

Motivation and Self-Regulation

Self-regulation is the process in which students activate, take control of and evaluate their own learning. Self-regulation of cognition and behaviour is an important aspect of student learning and academic performance in the classroom context [41, 42]. There are a variety of definitions of self-regulated learning, but three components seem especially important for classroom performance (Fig. 19.2). First, self-regulated learning includes students' metacognitive strategies for planning, monitoring and modifying their cognition [43, 44]. Students' management and control of their effort on classroom academic tasks has been proposed as another important component. For example, capable students who persist at a difficult task or block out distractors (i.e. noisy classmates) maintain their cognitive engagement in the task, enabling them to perform better [43]. A third important aspect of self-regulated learning that some researchers have included in their conceptualization is the actual cognitive strategies that students use to learn, remember and understand the material [41, 44]. Different cognitive strategies such as rehearsal, elaboration and organizational strategies have been found to foster active cognitive engagement in learning and result in higher levels of achievement [45].

However, knowledge of cognitive and metacognitive strategies is usually not enough to promote student achievement; students also must be motivated to use the strategies as well as regulate their cognition and effort [46–48]. Although there are classroom situations and tasks that can foster motivation [42, 49], there is also evidence to suggest that students' perceptions of the classroom as well as their individual motivational orientations and beliefs about learning are relevant to cognitive engagement and classroom performance [50, 51]. An earlier work [52] studied the link between the three components of self-regulated learning and the individual differences in student motivation. Results revealed that the students' motivational orientations were linked in important ways to student cognitive engagement and academic performance in the classroom. Self-efficacy was positively related to student cognitive engagement and performance. Students who believed they were capable were more likely to report use of cognitive strategies, to be more self-regulating in terms of reporting more use of metacognitive strategies and to persist more often at difficult or uninteresting academic tasks. These relations were independent of and did not interact with prior achievement levels or intrinsic value and test anxiety. These findings suggest that self-efficacy plays a facilitative role in relation to cognitive engagement as suggested by Schunk [53] but that the cognitive engagement variables are more directly tied to actual performance. This implies that teaching students about different cognitive and self-regulatory strategies may be more important for improving actual performance on classroom academic tasks but that improving students' self-efficacy beliefs may lead to more use of these cognitive strategies [54, 55].

Self-regulation is not the same as motivation. Although motivation and self-regulation share some common elements, there are some critical differences. In motivation, choice (specifically referring to autonomy and control over the situation) does not have to be central to the construct. Self-regulation, however, requires some degree of choice or intentional selection of strategies designed to help the learner achieve a goal or behaviour.

Self-regulated learners are expected to (1) be aware of their strengths and weaknesses; utilize metacognitive strategies, for example, questioning one's learning and monitoring one's learning; to approach academic tasks; and be able to attribute their success or failure to factors within their control.

Therefore, as a process, self-regulation adopts a cyclical course. Students who are motivated to reach a certain goal will engage in self-regulatory activities they feel will help them achieve that goal. The self-regulation promotes learning, which leads to a perception of greater competence, which, in turn, sustains motivation towards the goal and to future goals.

Researchers identified three critical dimensions, or characteristics, of self-regulation (Fig. 19.3): self-observation, self-judgement and self-reaction.

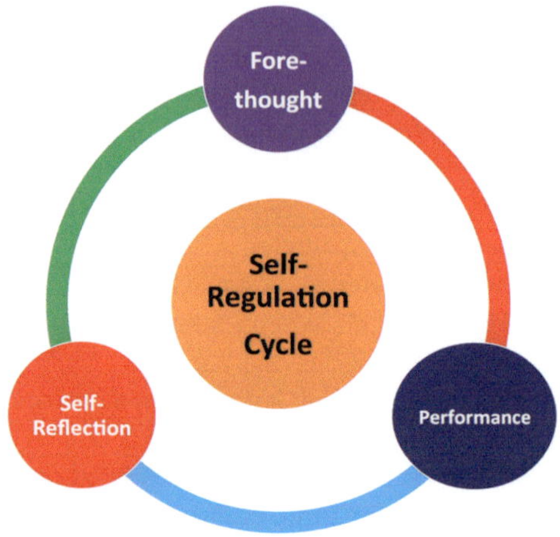

Fig. 19.3 Self-regulation cycle. There are three phases of the self-regulation cycle: forethought, performance (volitional) control and self-reflection

Self-observation refers to the deliberate monitoring of one's activities. Self-observation may take the form of recording frequency, duration or quality of a behaviour. Self-observation is also critical to the regulation of performance and may also lead to higher motivation. For example, if a person realizes his/her study habits were causing the person to perform poorly on certain tests, the way the person study might be adjusted, leading to higher test grades and more motivation to continue to improve the one's study habits.

The second critical dimension of self-regulation is self-judgement. Self-judgement refers to evaluating one's current performance levels compared to the goal level.

The third critical dimension is self-reaction. Self-reaction refers to one's behavioural, cognitive and affective responses to self-judgements. Self-reactions can be motivating if one believes they are making progress towards their goal. Negative self-evaluations are not necessarily demotivating if one believes they can still make changes and progress towards their goal.

The Self-Regulation Cycle

Self-regulation is a cyclical process because during the process of self-evaluation and monitoring, the learner will make alterations to strategies, cognition and behaviours that will alter learning and, ultimately, the end goal. There are three phases of the self-regulation cycle: forethought, performance (volitional) control and self-reflection (Fig. 19.3). Self-regulation begins with the forethought phase. This pre-action phase refers to the processes that set up the learner for action towards their goal. This phase helps the learner to establish a positive outlook, set realistic expectations and address questions such as "When will the work begin? What conditions will help or hinder learning activities towards the goal?" and "How often will tasks be completed towards the goal?" Short-term and long-term goal planning occur in this stage. The next stage is the performance- (or volitional-) control phase. This phase involves processes that occur during learning that affect action and attention. Specific strategies are established during this stage in order to help a learner be successful. Metacognitive strategies are identified; preliminary self-evaluation occurs; and motivational strategies are identified. Questions such as "Am I accomplishing as much as I thought I would? Am I being distracted?" and "What will motivate me to continue working?" are common questions during this phase. Self-reflection is an important skill for learners to develop as it drives the quality of learning insights that comes from feedback. Self-reflection is, in essence, an internal Socratic dialogue, where one asks oneself questions in order to gain a deeper understanding of one's perception, application, outcomes as well as the impact on others [56].

Motivation in Medical Education

Over the past years medical educators have adopted a progressively more complex understanding of the motivation nature as well as its concept. Motivation in medical education was reviewed in a systematic review carried out with the intention of providing a framework for educators to consider this important dimension of curriculum development [5]. The spectrum of motivation started with *Knowles'* assertion that we transit, as we mature from childhood to adulthood, from being externally motivated to internally motivated [9]. This later passed into a more complex view where the person's basic and higher-order needs are driven by multiple motivations that amplify and compete for an action. Furthermore, motivation orientations differ between individuals and within individuals over very short periods of time. More recently, internal motivation is no longer viewed as an absolute result of adulthood, but as the result of a set of conditions, a situation that can be fostered and encouraged by the educational environment.

The current paradigm of motivation in medical education suggests that components of the learning environment like communication skills, curriculum and assessment methods not only affect how much effort students put forward but the longer-term nature of how they are motivated in their careers. If medical schools continued to develop curricula and assessment tools without improving the understanding of the motivation nature, there is a high potential of causing significant detriment to the students. At best, an opportunity may be missing to significantly enrich their lives.

Motivation should be a measure of the quality of medical education. If we truly value the student who engaged, participates and is able to learn deeply, we value a student who is highly motivated. Therefore, the development of a "lifelong learner" is equivalent to a student who is intrinsically motivated. Consequently, the success of an educational programme could be evaluated not only based on knowledge briefly retained or student satisfaction but on the ongoing desire to understand and learn more.

Considering the value of internal motivation, and the suggestion that internal motivation is superior to external motivation (according to self-determination motivational theory), significant consideration must be given when designing curriculum, educational climate and assessment methods. Another study [57] reported that medical students' motivation and self-regulated learning runs a dynamic course as they change over time. The study highlighted the need for change in the medical school's learning environment to facilitate the students' use of cognitive and metacognitive strategies. Supporting student autonomy, sense of competence and need for relatedness lead to increasingly internally motivated students, but the practical implication of these ideas is quite complex and deserve further evaluation.

Motivation in the Clinical Teaching

Health sciences education researchers started to recognize the important role that motivation plays in learning. However, despite the recognition that motivation influences deeper learning and effectiveness of innovations, many health sciences education professionals are unaware of how to influence motivation and how to encourage intrinsic motivation in the clinical teaching environment. Clinical teaching has been suggested as an important factor influencing students' intrinsic motivation and performance [58–61]. A number of studies have found that internalization of students' motivation towards an intrinsic form of clinical medicine learning is associated with increased interest, commitment, effort, learning and satisfaction with education [10, 62, 63]. In contrast, a poor quality of learning occurs when students are not willing to learn [10]. It has been suggested that students in higher education, especially in medical education, have natural tendencies to learn and to know the environment that surrounds them, have a self-concept of being responsible for their own decisions and learn things they need to know for real-life situations [41, 58, 64]. However, these behaviours can be supported or diminished by internal or external factors [41]. Self-determination theory [10] supports the idea of students' innate curiosity and desire to learn. This is achieved by internalizing and integrating psychic components to build an integrated and unified sense of the self [64].

A systematic review article [65] carried out to assess motivation in the clinical teaching environment suggested that clinical teachers should interact with their students in a more "human-centred" teaching style, as these actions predict motivational internalization. Intrinsic motivation and autonomous forms of self-regulation are the desired type of motivation in students, as they have been associated with deep learning, better performance and well-being, in comparison with extrinsic motivation and controlled forms of self-regulation (i.e. under external control) [10, 41, 62]. Teacher behaviours and teaching styles can influence students motivation [64, 66], either in classroom or in clinical environments. Students' own curiosity and interests are potent tools by which teachers can promote their desire to learn.

In contrast, teachers who rely on external factors (e.g. rewards) risk students internal learning aspirations, compromising the quality of the process [64]. An autonomy-supportive teaching style is characterized by providing options and opportunities for self-directed decisions minimizing external pressures [10, 34].

Motivation in Problem-Based Learning

The motivation for learning in problem-based learning (PBL) has been well researched at the level of the tutorial group where students are motivated to learn by interactive discussion of an interesting problem [67]. Problem-based learning has not been implemented only in medicine and dentistry but in various disciplines of education: dentistry, business, engineering as well as law [68]. Problem-based learning improves teaching and learning process focusing mainly on the students' development as self-directed learners in comparison to the traditional lectures which rely on lectures as a spoon-fed teaching approach. Many researchers have shown the effectiveness of problem-based learning in enhancing students' performance in learning [69–71]. Nevertheless, the transition from the conventional teaching method to problem-based learning is a challenging process in most disciplines, as problem-based learning itself will challenge the students' learning behaviour [72].

In the learning environment in which conventional modes remains as the predominant strategy, problem-based learning sounds an attractive mode of teaching particularly for medical education. Problem-based learning is a pedagogical practice employed in many medical schools. While there are numerous variants of the technique, the approach includes the presentation of an applied problem to a small group of students who engage in discussion over several sessions. A facilitator, sometimes called a tutor, provides supportive guidance for the students. The discussions of the problem are structured to enable students to create conceptual models to explain the problem presented in the case. As the students discover the limits of their knowledge, they identify learning issues – essentially questions they cannot answer from their fund of knowledge. Between meetings of the group, learners research their learning issues and share results at the next meeting of the group.

Therefore, motivation plays in important role in ensuring the students learn, achieve the educational targets and attain a new level of performance.

Nevertheless, a question remains "how to motivate students to be mastery-oriented learners, instead of performance approach oriented?" Performance-oriented learners are more likely to compete with their peers to be the best. They will work hard to learn and achieve their personal goal. Grades have value as an external motivator for this group of learners. Unlike performance-oriented learners, mastery-oriented groups attempt to master what they learn, focusing on learning process and making progress rather than being perfect [73, 77].

Biggs and Tang have suggested that the importance of task and students' expectation of success are the two primary factors that can make students learn [70]. Students will immerse in tasks that seem worthwhile for them and promise them the possibility of success. Nobody wants to take a risk if they believe they will fail. This theory is called "*expectancy-value motivation theory*" [74]. Another model of students' motivation from Pintrich [75] also points out the similar views. Three components which could affect motivation were listed as:

- Students' beliefs about the importance and value of the task
- Students' beliefs about the ability to perform the task
- Students' feelings about themselves or their emotional reactions to the task

Motivating Students in Problem-Based Learning

In problem-based learning, there are no given lectures or notes, but students are expected to learn on their own based on the problems. Students will not get information if they do not read, explore or ask for the information. They need to work in a cooperative learning climate, exchange ideas and opinions, proactively argue what others think and be trained to accept failures and mistakes. In addition to that, in problem-based learning, though there is a specific target which is the correct diagnosis and treatment, the students have to find the most appropriate approach. Therefore, there is a room of freedom for them to decide how to work on the problem and which solution they can justify as correct. If possible, students are allowed to surpass their syllabus. These distinctive features of problem-based learning may make students feel uncomfortable and unsecure [68].

Effective facilitation to motivate students is vital for problem-based learning. Having a good structure of the course contents and structured motivating discussion of the case should help the facilitator not only to recover students' strong emotions and enthusiasm but also to maintain their engagement in problem-based learning case studies throughout the course. Several studies have analysed the effective techniques which can be implemented by problem-based learning facilitators to motivate their students. Strategies suggested in the research done in Royal Melbourne Institute of Technology (RMIT) [76] and Center for Teaching and Learning at Stanford University (CTL) [77] are found to be in concordance to that reported earlier by Barbara in her book *Tools for Teaching* [78].

There are six criteria emphasized identified in order to motivate students and stimulate their interest (Fig. 19.4). The cornerstone is the facilitator able to tackle them in the appropriate approach; hence, this will promote better learning and understanding. Usually, traditional instructors in conventional curriculum are only able to deliver the first element of motivation, by highlighting the expected course outcomes at the beginning of the course. They are more likely to neglect other motivation elements. On the other hand, problem-based learning environment requires all six elements to be tackled.

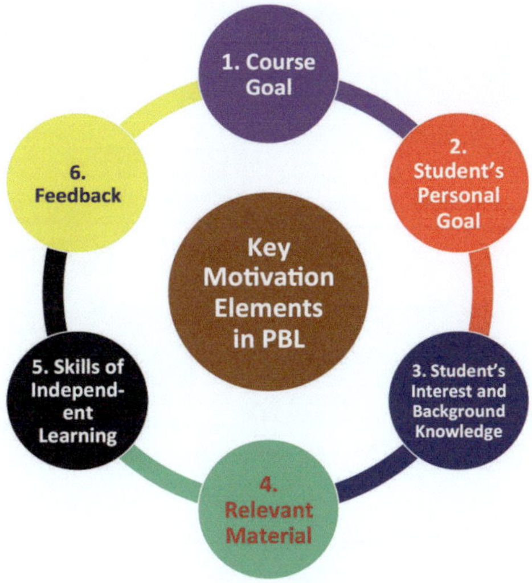
1. Course Goal
2. Student's Personal Goal
3. Student's Interest and Background Knowledge
4. Relevant Material
5. Skills of Independ-ent Learning
6. Feedback
Key Motivation Elements in PBL

Fig. 19.4 Key elements of motivation in problem-based learning (PBL) in educational setting

Motivation of Medical School and Medical Profession Applicants

During selection procedures for medical school, one of the aims is to have an impression of the applicants' motivation [79, 80]. This is assessed based on a description of the applicants' motivation in interviews, multiple mini interviews, personal statements or other approaches [81, 82]. However, while a reliable assessment strategy of motivation is vital for the selection process, it could be difficult to identify the appropriate candidate in high-stake situations such as selection for medical school [83, 84].

By assessing the motivation among medical school and the medical profession applicants, selection committee's main aim is to ensure that the selected students are motivated. Self-determination theory (SDT) [10, 63, 85] stresses that the type of motivation is more important than the quantity of motivation. Motivation is a continuum comprising of different states, namely, a lack of motivation (amotivation), motivation because of internal factors and motivation because of external factors (Fig. 19.5). Autonomous motivation originates from within the individual and represents a sincere interest in (intrinsic motivation), and a positive personal valuation of (identified regulation), the study of medicine. Controlled motivation results from internal pressures, such as feelings of guilt or shame (introjected regulation), and external pressures, such as monetary rewards or parental pressure (external regulation). Autonomous motivation, in contrast with controlled motivation, in students has been found to result in better learning outcomes [12, 36, 86–89]. Moreover, the quality of motivation is a predictor of persistence or dropout [85, 90].

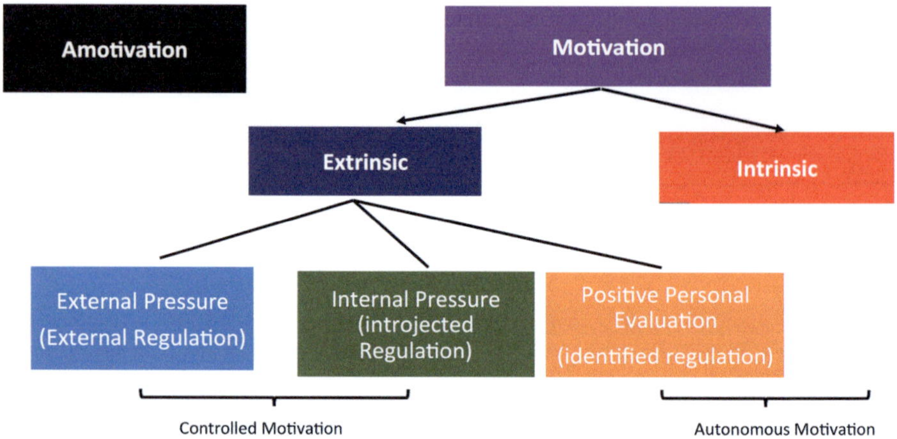

Fig. 19.5 The self-determination continuum of motivation: motivation is a continuum comprising of different states, namely, a lack of motivation (amotivation), motivation because of internal factors and motivation because of external factors. Autonomous motivation originates from within the individual and represents a sincere interest in (intrinsic motivation) and a positive personal valuation of (identified regulation) the study of medicine. Controlled motivation results from internal pressures, such as feelings of guilt or shame (introjected regulation), and external pressures, such as monetary rewards or parental pressure (external regulation). Autonomous motivation, in contrast with controlled motivation, in students has been found to result in better learning outcomes

In many medical schools' selection procedures, applicants are asked to express their motives for the studying medicine in a personal statement. Some studies have found personal statements often evoke heterogeneous responses from the applicants, consequently, complicating the comparison of applicants [3]. Though it is widely used, research on the personal statement's reliability and ability to predict future performance is conflicting [91–98]. In line with this, a more specific writing assignment used in selection procedures (the essay question) has been found to evoke a similar heterogeneity of responses. However, in most of the cases, applicants tend to provide responses that go beyond the scope of the posed question, in order to "show themselves" and "tell their own story", a phenomenon which is expected to occur regardless of the official topic [99]. In some selection procedures a statement on motivation is included. In contrast to personal statements where applicants are expected to write about a variety of issues relevant to their application, a statement on motivation has a particular focus on motivation. An analysis of applicants' motivation statements was carried out earlier [100]. Results revealed that the statements on motivation do not appear to distinguish between applicants in selection for medical school. Both selected and nonselected applicants reported fair degree of motivation (mainly autonomous motivation) for applying and included a lot of additional information, which was beyond the scope of what was asked from them.

Motivation and e-Learning

e-learning has become an increasingly popular approach for medical education and training.

Research on e-learning indicates that, initially, such innovation is expected to fill a niche for those who are not served well or at all by the present system. However, gradually as experience is gained, and the quality of such new teaching model is improved and proved effective, the demand grows over time; consequently, the adoption of e-learning as a teaching approach increases – following a logistic curve, or s-curve [101, 102]. Based on data on the growth of online learning from the North American Council of Online learning and US Department of Education statistics, Christensen et al. [109] predict that 50% of high school courses will be offered online by 2019. In concordance, medical schools have also started to upload several of its teaching courses online. However, in parallel with the e-learning boom, there has been understandable concern about the quality of e-learning. Earlier studies have found that lack of time and lack of motivation are the main factors associated with learner attrition in online courses [103–105].

Fostering motivation to learn is one of the key principles for effective learning. Several research studies have indicated positive correlations between learner motivational levels and academic achievement [106–108]. Student motivation is further important with respect to use of cognitive strategies necessary for effective learning [53]. Perhaps most important, learning experiences which are highly motivating can foster one's propensity for lifelong learning [109]. Furthermore, if students are more motivated to learn, then we would expect them to be less likely to drop out of online courses. This raises the question about how the design of online courses might be improved to increase the students' motivation to learn [110].

Factors Associated with the Learner's Motivation

Analysing earlier published studies for factors that influence learner motivation primarily in computer-based instruction and distance education settings identified three major categories of motivational influences in Web-based instruction; these are internal, external and personal factors [110, 111]. Internal factors are related to the course features itself which can influence the learner's motivation. External factors refer to aspects of the learning environment that can influence the learner's motivation. Personal factors refer to motivational influences caused by the learner. Results of a study [110] carried out to assess what influences motivational change during self-directed online learning revealed that people tend to choose self-directed e-learning when face-to-face classroom instruction is unavailable or not possible due to scheduling conflicts or because of the convenience and flexibility of online training. Learners are more likely to be more motivated when they begin self-directed e-learning if they perceive the learning goals to be more relevant and their competence in use of technology is higher.

Relevance is one of the four factors in Keller's ARCS model of motivation (attention, relevance, confidence and satisfaction) [112–115]. If students are more motivated to learn, then they are more likely to be engaged; and if they are engaged and engaged successfully, they are more likely to achieve the learning objectives [36, 89, 90]. Relevance is also important with respect to First Principles of Instruction [116, 117], in particular the integration principle, which has to do with learner's incorporating what they learn into their own personal lives. Merrill [118] argues that learning is promoted when First Principles of Instruction are used. Students are more likely to be motivated when they solve real-world problems or do authentic tasks (problem-centred principle) and when they are able to incorporate what they have learned into their lives (integration principle).

Competence in using technology is often indicated by the number of different software applications with which one is fluent. Obviously, some degree of technological competence is necessary to use self-directed e-learning. Moreover, automaticity in the use of the technology itself is important to reduce extraneous cognitive load. Extraneous cognitive load can interfere with learning as students are faced with learning how to use the technology when they should be devoting their attention to what it is they are expecting to learn [110]. Maintaining the motivation level during a course (interim level of motivation) and how far has the learner been more motivated after finishing several lessons during a course are good indicator of how successful this educational activity has been. This interim level of motivation is best predicted by the degree of relevance of the course as well as degree of motivation for e-learning at the beginning of a course.

Therefore, learners are more likely to experience increased motivation and satisfaction in self-directed e-learning when they (1) perceive the content to be relevant to their lives, (2) are fluent in technology, (3) are more highly motivated both at the beginning and during the e-learning course and (4) perceive the e-learning experience to be "just right" for them (meaning that the e-learning product embodies first principles of instruction, difficulty level is a good match and they receive institutional support for learning this way). On the other hand, learners for whom e-learning is "not right" for them and who do not want to learn alone are not likely to be motivated either to begin or continue self-directed e-learning or to do so in the future. These learners prefer to work with instructors and peers while they are learning, and thus self-directed e-learning is a poor match for them. These learners tend to be younger and students in university settings, compared with older learners who are not in school and are working professionals [110].

In conclusion, educational psychology indicates that learning processes can be mapped on three main pillars: cognitive (what to learn), affective or motivational (why learn) and metacognitive (how to learn). Motivation is the translation of a person's basic psychological needs and drives, filtered through their view of the world, towards an action with an anticipated result. There is a range of motivational orientations from intrinsically motivated to amotivated; the types of motivation are not dichotomous, and the model itself is not solid, meaning that a person can move between different types of motivation depending on the situation. On the personal level, the individual's motivation is a complex interplay of competing internal and external factors. Educators can foster intrinsic motivation by addressing learner's needs for competence, autonomy and relatedness.

References

1. Mann KV. Motivation in medical education: how theory can inform our practice. Acad Med. 1999;74(3):237–9.
2. Williams GC, Deci EL. The importance of supporting autonomy in medical education. Ann Int Med. 1999;129:303–8.
3. Misch DA. Andragogy and medical education: are medical students internally motivated to learn? Adv Health Sci Educ. 2002;7:153–60.
4. White CB, Gruppen LD. Self-regulated learning in medical education. London: Association for the Study of Medical Education; 2007.
5. Brissette A, Howes D. Motivation in medical education: a systematic review. Webmed Cent Med Educ. 2010;1(12):WMC001261.
6. Vansteenkiste M, Simons J, Lens W, Sheldon KM, Deci EL. Motivating learning, performance, and persistence: the synergistic effects of intrinsic goal contents and autonomy-supportive contexts. J Pers Soc Psychol. 2004;87(2):246–60.
7. Vansteenkiste M, Zhou M, Lens W, Soenens B. Experiences of autonomy and control among Chinese learners: vitalizing or immobilizing? J Educ Psychol. 2005;97(3):468–83.
8. Hustinx PWJ, Kuyper H, van der Werf MPC, Dijkstra P. Achievement motivation revisited: new longitudinal data to demonstrate its predictive power. Educ Psychol. 2009;29(5):561–82.
9. Knowles M. The adult learner: a neglected species. 2nd ed. 1978.The adult learner: A neglected species.(2nd ed).x, 244 Oxford: Gulf Publishing 1978.
10. Ryan RM, Deci EL. Intrinsic and extrinsic motivations: classic definitions and new directions. Contemp Educ Psychol. 2000;25(1):54–67.
11. Koens F, Mann KV, Custers EJFM, OTJ TC. Analysing the concept of context in medical education. MedEduc. 2005;39(12):1243–9.
12. Sobral DT. What kind of motivation drives medical students' learning quests? MedEduc. 2004;38(9):950–7.
13. Curry L. Cognitive and learning styles in medical education. Acad Med. 1999;74(4):409–13.
14. Williams GC, Saizow RB, Ryan RM. The importance of self-determination theory for medical education. Acad Med. 1999;74(9):992–5.
15. Dinham S, Scott C. Moving into the third, outer domain of teacher satisfaction. J Educ Adm. 2000;38(4):379–96.
16. Johnson SM, Birkeland SE. Pursuing a 'sense of success': new teachers explain their career decisions. Project on the next generation of teachers. Am Educ Res J. 2002;40(3):581–617.
17. Gordon JA. Why did you select teaching as a career? Teachers of color [sic] tell their stories, ERIC Document Reproduction Service No. ED383653. East Lansing: National Center for Research on Teacher Learning; 1993.
18. Allard A, Bransgrove E, Cooper M, Duncan J, MacMillan M. 'Teaching is still a good job for a woman': the influence of gender on career and life choices. S Pac J Teach Educ. 1995;23(2):185–94.
19. Yong BCS. The career commitment of primary teachers in Brunei Darussalam: perceptions of teaching as a career. Res Educ. 1999;62:62–70.
20. Crow GM, Levine L, Nager N. No more business as usual: career changers who become teachers. Am J Educ. 1990;98(3):197–223.

21. Hart AW, Murphy MJ. New teachers react to redesigned teacher work. Am J Educ. 1990;98:224–50.
22. Weiner L, Swearingen J, Pagano A, Obi R. Choosing teaching as a career: comparing motivations of Harvard and urban college students, ERIC Document Reproduction Service No. ED357013. East Lansing: National Center for Research on Teacher Learning; 1993.
23. Sinclair C. How can what we know about motivation to teach improve the quality of initial teacher education and its practicum? Chapter 2. In: Towndrow PA, Koh C, Soon TH, editors. Motivation and practice for the classroom. The Netherlands: Sense Publishers; 2008. p. 37–61.
24. Anderson MB, Kanter SL. Medical education in the United States and Canada 2010. Acad Med. 2010;85(9 suppl):S2–S18.
25. Ludmerer KM. Creating the system. In: Time to heal: American medical education from the turn of the century to the era of managed care. New York: Oxford University Press; 1999. p. 3–25.
26. Vermunt JD. Metacognitive, cognitive and affective aspects of learning styles and strategies: a phenomenographic analysis. High Educ. 1996;31:25–50.
27. Greeno JG, Collins AM, Resnick LB. Cognition and learning. In: Berliner D, Calfee R, editors. Handbook of educational psychology. New York: McMillan; 1996. p. 15–46.
28. Schraw G, Moshman D. Metacognitive theories. Educ Psychol Rev. 1995;7:351–71.
29. Bransford JD, Brown AL, Cocking RR. Learning: from speculation to science. In: Bransford JD, Brown AL, Cocking RR, editors. How people learn: brain, mind, experience and school. Expanded ed. Washington, DC: National Academy Press; 2000. p. 3–30.
30. Ten Cate TJ, Snell L, Mann KV, Vermunt J. Orienting teaching toward the learning process. Acad Med. 2004;79:219–28.
31. Kusurkar R, Croiset G, Mann K, Custers E. Have motivation theories guided the development and reform of medical education curricula? A review of the literature. Acad Med. 2012;87:735–43.
32. Kusurkar R, Croiset G. Autonomy support for autonomous motivation in medical education. Med Educ Online. 2015;20(1):27951. https://doi.org/10.3402/meo.v20.27951.
33. Deci EL, Ryan RM. The "What" and "why" of goal pursuits: human needs and the self-determination of behavior. Psychol Inq. 2000;11:227–68.
34. Williams GC, Deci EL. The importance of supporting autonomy in medical education. Ann Intern Med. 1998;129:303–8.
35. Kusurkar RA, Croiset G, Galindo-Garre F, Ten Cate TJ. Motivational profiles of medical students: association with study effort, academic performance and exhaustion. BMC Med Educ. 2013;13:87.
36. Kusurkar RA, Ten Cate TJ, Vos CM, Westers P, Croiset G. How motivation affects academic performance: a structural equation modelling analysis. Adv Health Sci Educ. 2013;18:5769.
37. Williams GC, Wiener MW, Markakis KM, Reeve J, Deci EL. Medical students' motivation for internal medicine. J Gen Intern Med. 1994;9:327–33.
38. Ten Cate TJ, Kusurkar RA, Williams GC. How can self-determination theory assist our understanding of teaching and learning processes in medical education. AMEE Guide 59. Med Teach. 2011;33:961–73.
39. Baldwin CD, Craig MS, Garfunkel LC, Harris JP, Shone LP, Biondi E, et al. Autonomy-supportive medical education: let the force be within you! Acad Med. 2012;87:1468–9.
40. Ten Cate TJ. Entrustability of professional activities and competency-based training. Med Educ. 2005;39:1176–7.
41. Corno L, Mandinach E. The role of cognitive engagement in classroom learning and motivation. Educ Psychol. 1983;18:88–100.
42. Corno L, Rohrkemper M. The intrinsic motivation to learn in classrooms. In: Ames C, Ames R, editors. Research on motivation: vol. 2. The classroom milieu. New York: Academic; 1985. p. 53–90.
43. Brown AL, Bransford JD, Campione JC, Ferrara RA. Learning, remembering and understanding. In: Flavell J, Markman E, editors. Handbook of child psychology: vol. 3. Cognitive development. New York: Wiley; 1983. p. 77–166.

44. Zimmerman B, Pons M. Construct validation of a strategy model of student self-regulated learning. J Educ Psychol. 1988;80:284–90.
45. Weinstein CE, Mayer RE. The teaching of learning strategies. In: Wittrock M, editor. Handbook of research on teaching. New York: Macmillan; 1986. p. 315–27.
46. Paris SG, Lipson MY, Wixson K. Becoming a strategic reader. Contemp Educ Psychol. 1983;8:293–316.
47. Pintrich PR. A process-oriented view of student motivation and cognition. In: Stark JS, Mets L, editors. Improving teaching and learning through research. New directions for institutional research, vol. 57. San Francisco: Jossey-Bass; 1988. p. 55–70.
48. Pintrich PR. The dynamic interplay of student motivation and cognition in the college classroom. In: Ames C, Maehr M, editors. Advances in motivation and achievement: vol. 6. Motivation enhancing environments. Greenwich: JAI Press; 1989. p. 117–60.
49. Malone TW. Toward a theory of intrinsically motivating instruction. Cogn Sci. 1981;4:333–69.
50. Ames C, Archer J. Achievement goals in the classroom: student learning strategies and motivation processes. J Educ Psychol. 1988;80:260–7.
51. Nolen S. Reasons for studying: motivational orientations and study strategies. Cogn Instr. 1988;5:269–87.
52. Pintrich P, De Groot E. Motivational and self-regulated learning components of classroom academic performance. J Educ Psychol. 1990;82(1):33–40.
53. Schunk D. Self-efficacy and school learning. Psychol Sch. 1985;22:208–23.
54. Borkowski J, Weyhing R, Carr M. Effects of attributional retraining on strategy-based reading comprehension in learning disabled students. J Educ Psychol. 1988;80:46–53.
55. Garner R, Alexander P. Metacognition: answered and unanswered questions. Educ Psychol. 1989;24:143–58.
56. The role of motivation in self-regulated learning. https://study.com/academy/lesson/the-role-of-motivation-in-self-regulated-learning.html.
57. Kim K, Jang HW. Changes in medical students' motivation and self-regulated learning: a preliminary study. Int J Med Educ. 2015;6:213–5.
58. Bengtsson M, Ohlsson B. The nursing and medical students motivation to attain knowledge. Nurse Educ Today. 2010;30:150–6. https://doi.org/10.1016/j.nedt.2009.07.005.
59. Kusurkar R, Croiset G, Ten Cate T. Twelve tips to stimulate intrinsic motivation in students through autonomy-supportive classroom teaching derived from self-determination theory. Med Teach. 2011;33:978–82. https://doi.org/10.3109/0142159X.2011.599896.
60. Davies B, Leung A, Dunne S. So how do you see our teaching? Some observations received from past and present students at the Maurice Wohl Dental Centre. Eur J Dent Educ. 2012;16:138–43. https://doi.org/10.1111/j.1600-0579.2012.00733.x.
61. Jahangiri L, McAndrew M, Muzaffar A, Mucciolo TW. Characteristics of effective clinical teachers identified by dental students: a qualitative study. Eur J Dent Educ. 2013;17:10–8. https://doi.org/10.1111/eje.12012.
62. Ryan RM, Deci EL. Self-determination theory and the facilitation of intrinsic motivation, social development, and well-being. Am Psychol. 2000;55:68–78.
63. Vansteenkiste M, Lens W, Deci EL. Intrinsic versus extrinsic goal contents in self-determination theory: another look at the quality of academic motivation. Educ Psychol. 2006;41:19–31.
64. Niemiec CP, Ryan RM. Autonomy, competence, and relatedness in the classroom: applying self-determination theory to educational practice. Theory Res Educ. 2009;7:133–44. https://doi.org/10.1177/1477878509104318.
65. Orsini C, Evans P, Jerez O. How to encourage intrinsic motivation in the clinical teaching environment?: a systematic review from the self-determination theory. J Educ Eval Health Prof. 2015;12:8. https://doi.org/10.3352/jeehp.2015.12.8.
66. Brewer EW, Burgess DN. Professor's role in motivating students to attend class. J Ind Teach Educ. 2005;42:23–47.
67. Dolmans DHJM, Schmidt HG. What do we know about cognitive and motivational effects of small group tutorials in problem-based learning? Adv Health Sci Educ. 2006;11:321–36.

68. Haruna NF, Yusofb KM, Jamaludinc MZ, Hassan SA. Motivation in problem-based learning implementation. Social Behav Sci. 2012;56:233–42.
69. Allen DE, Duch BJ, Groh SE. The power of problem-based learning in teaching introductory science courses. In: Wilkerson L, Gijselaers WH, editors. Bringing problem-based learning to higher education: theory and practice, new directions for teaching and learning, vol. 68. San Francisco: Jossey-Bass; 1996. p. 43–51.
70. Biggs J, Tang C. Teaching for quality learning at university. 3rd ed. New York: McGraw Hill; 2007.
71. Albanese M, Mitchell S. Problem-based learning: a review of literature on its outcomes and implementation issues. In: Lai P, Tang C. Obstacles to the implementation of problem-based learning (PBL) in local universities of Hong Kong. Hong Kong, China; 2000.
72. Stinson JE, Milter RG. Problem-based learning in business education: curriculum design and implementation issues. In: Wilkerson L, Gijselaers WH, editors. Bringing problem-based learning to higher education: theory and practice, new directions for teaching and learning, vol. 68. San Francisco: Jossey-Bass; 1996. p. 3–41.
73. Svinicki MD. Student goal orientation. IDEA Paper. 2005;41:1–5.
74. Feather N. Expectations and actions. In: Biggs J, Tang C, editors. Teaching for quality learning at university. 3rd ed. New York: McGraw Hill; 2007.
75. Pintrich PR. The dynamic interplay of student motivation and cognition in the college classroom. In: Gentry JG. Motivating students: an initial attempt to operationalize the curiosity gap model. Developments in Business Simulation and Experiential Learning, 28. 2001. p. 69–75.
76. Motivating students and stimulating interest: a good teaching tip-sheet. URL: http://mams.rmit.edu.au/p8qsx9780vqxz.pdf. Accessed 26 May 2018.
77. Capturing and directing the motivation to learn. In: Speaking of teaching. Stanford University Newsletter on Teaching. 10 (1); 1998.
78. Barbara G.D.. (1993). Tools for teachingJossey-Bass, San Francisco. URL: http://honolulu.hawaii.edu/intranet/committees/FacDevCom/guidebk/teachtip/motiv.htm. Accessed on 2 May 2010.
79. Turner R, Nicholson S. Reasons selectors give for accepting and rejecting medical applicants before interview. Med Educ. 2011;45:298–307.
80. Breland H, Maxey J, Gernand R, Cumming T, Trapani C. Trends in college admission 2000. A report of a survey of undergraduate admissions policies, practices, and procedures 2002.
81. Albanese MA, Snow MH, Skochelak SE, Huggett KN, Farrell PM. Assessing personal qualities in medical school admissions. Acad Med. 2003;78:313–21.
82. Guyaux J, oude Egbrink MGA, Heeneman S, Houben AJHM, Willekes C, Schuwirth LWT, de Goeij AFPM. Selectie op een combinatie van cognitieve en noncognitieve eigenschappen. Keuzes en ervaringen in de onderzoeksmaster Arts-Klinisch Onderzoeker (A-KO) te Maastricht. Tijdschr Medisch Onderwijs. 2010;29:328–36.
83. O'Neill LD, Korsholm L, Wallstedt B, Eika B, Hartvigsen J. Generalisability of a composite student selection programme. Med Educ. 2009;43:58–65.
84. Kusurkar R, Croiset G, Kruitwagen C, Ten Cate TJ. Validity evidence for the measurement of the strength of motivation for medical school. Adv Health Sci Educ. 2011;16:183–95.
85. Deci EL, Ryan R. Intrinsic motivation and self-determination in human behavior. New York: Plenum; 1985.
86. Kusurkar R, Croiset G, Galindo Garre F, Ten Cate TJ. Motivational profiles of medical students: association with study effort, academic performance and exhaustion. BMC Med Educ. 2013;13:87.
87. Vansteenkiste M, Zhou M, Lens W, Soenens B. Experiences of autonomy and control among Chinese learners: vitalizing or immobilizing? J Educ Psychol. 2005;97:468.
88. Artino AR, La Rochelle JS, Durning SJ. Second-year medical students's motivational beliefs, emotions, and achievement. Med Educ. 2010;44:1203–12.
89. Kusurkar RA, Ten Cate TJ. AM last page: education is not filling a bucket, but lighting a fire: self-determination theory and motivation in medical students. Acad Med. 2013;88:904.

90. Vallerand RJ, Fortier MS, Guay F. Self-determination and persistence in a real-life setting: toward a motivational model of high school dropout. J Pers Soc Psychol. 1997;72:1161.
91. Benbassat J, Baumal R. Uncertainties in the selection of applicants for medical school. Adv Health Sci Educ. 2007;12:509–21.
92. Hanson MD, Dore KL, Reiter HI, Eva KW. Medical school admissions: revisiting the veracity and independence of completion of an autobiographical screening tool. Acad Med. 2007;82:S8–S11.
93. Ferguson E, Sanders A, O'Hehir F, James D. Predictive validity of personal statements and the role of the five-factor model of personality in relation to medical training. J Occup Organ Psychol. 2000;73:321–44.
94. Ferguson E, James D, O'Hehir F, Sanders A, McManus IC. Pilot study of the roles of personality, references, and personal statements in relation to performance over the five years of a medical degree. Commentary: how to derive causes from correlations in educational studies. BMJ. 2003;326:429–32.
95. Dong T, Kay A, Artino AR, Gilliland WR, Waechter DM, Cruess D, DeZee KJ, Durning SJ. Application essays and future performance in medical school: are they related? Teach Learn Med. 2013;25:55–8.
96. Oosterveld P, Ten Cate TJ. Generalizability of a study sample assessment procedure for entrance selection for medical school. Med Teach. 2004;26:635–9.
97. Dore KL, Hanson M, Reiter HI, Blanchard M, Deeth K, Eva KW. Medical school admissions: enhancing the reliability and validity of an autobiographical screening tool. Acad Med. 2006;81:S70–3.
98. Peskun C, Detsky A, Shandling M. Effectiveness of medical school admissions criteria in predicting residency ranking four years later. Med Educ. 2007;41:57–64.
99. White JS, Lemay JF, Brownell K, Lockyer J. "A Chance To Show Yourself" – how do applicants approach medical school admission essays? Med Teach. 2011;33:e541–8.
100. Wouters A, Bakker A, van Wijk I, Croiset G, Kusurkar R. A qualitative analysis of statements on motivation of applicants for medical school. BMC Med Educ. 2014;14:200.
101. Christensen C, Johnson CW, Horn MB. Disrupting class: how disruptive innovation will change the way the world learns. New York: McGraw-Hill; 2008.
102. Rogers EM. Diffusion of innovations. 5th ed. New York: Free Press; 2003.
103. Aragon SR, Johnson ES. Factors influencing completion and noncompletion of community college online courses. Am J Dist Educ. 2008;22(3):146–58.
104. Serwatka JA. Improving retention in distance learning classes. Int J Instr Technol Dist Learn. 2005;2(1):59–64.
105. Visser L, Plomp T, Amirault RJ, Kuiper W. Motivating students at a distance: the case of an international audience. Educ Technol Res Dev. 2002;50(2):94–110.
106. Uguroglu ME, Walberg HJ. Motivation and achievement: a quantitative synthesis. Am Educ Res J. 1979;16(4):375–89.
107. Walberg HJ. Improving the productivity of America's schools. Educ Leadersh. 1984;41(8):19–27.
108. Fyans LJ, Jr, Maehr ML. Sources of student achievement: student motivation, school context and family background. Paper presented at the American Psychological Association, New York. 1987.
109. Wlodkowski RJ. Enhancing adult motivation to learn: a comprehensive guide for teaching all adults. 2nd ed. San Francisco: Jossey-Bass; 1998.
110. Kim KJ, Frick TW. Changes in student motivation during online learning. J Educ Comput Res. 2011;44(1):1–23.
111. Song SH. Research issues of motivation in web-based instruction. Q Rev Dist Educ. 2000;1(3):225–9.
112. Keller JM. Motivational design of instruction. In: Reigeluth CM, editor. Instructional-design theories and models: an overview of their current status. Mahwah: Lawrence Erlbaum Associates; 1983. p. 383–434.

113. Frick TW, Chadha R, Watson C, Zlatkovska E, Green P. Improving course evaluations to improve instruction and complex learning in higher education. Paper presented at the Association for Educational Communications and Technology Summer 2008 Research Symposium, Bloomington. 2008.
114. Kuh G, Kinzie J, Buckley J, Bridges B, Hayek J. Piecing together the student success puzzle: research, propositions, and recommendations. ASHE High Educ Rep. 2007;32(5):1–182.
115. Rangel E, Berliner D. Essential information for education policy: time to learn. Res Points. 2007;5(2):1–4.
116. Merrill DM. First principles of instruction. Educ Technol Res Dev. 2002;50(3):43–59.
117. Merrill DM. What makes e3 (effective, efficient, engaging) instruction? Paper presented at the AECT Research Symposium, Bloomington. 2008.
118. Merrill DM, Barclay M, van Schaak A. Prescriptive principles for instructional design. In: Spector JM, Merrill DM, van Merriënboer JJG, Driscoll MF, editors. Handbook of research on educational communications and technology. 3rd ed. New York: Lawrence Erlbaum Associates; 2008. p. 173–84.

Chapter 20
Virtual Reality and Augmented Reality

Introduction

Virtual reality (VR) is computer-generated simulation of a three-dimensional image or environment that simulates experience through senses and perception. VR consists of a computer-generated, multidimensional environment and interface tools that allow users to (1) immerse themselves in the environment, (2) navigate within the environment and (3) interact with objects and other inhabitants in the environment (Fig. 20.1). Virtual reality may be artificial, such as an animated scene or an actual place that has been photographed and included in a virtual reality app. There are several subtypes of VR (Table 20.1). The immersive environment can be similar to the real world, or it can be fantastical, creating an experience not possible in ordinary physical reality. The experience of entering this environment – this computer-generated virtual world – is compelling. By employing this technology, the user "breaks through" the computer screen and becomes completely immersed in this multidimensional world. Thus immersed, one can walk through a virtual house,

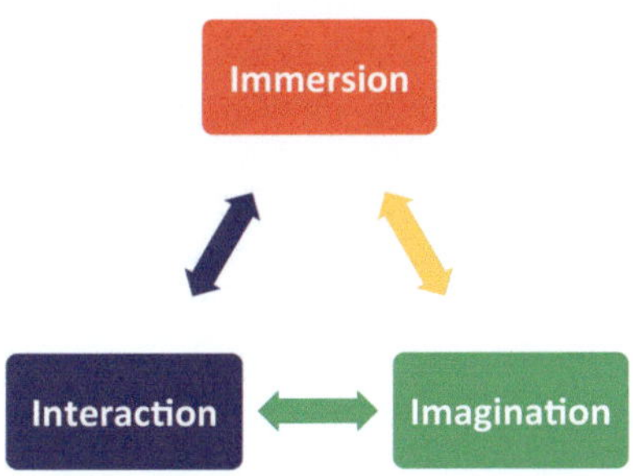

Fig. 20.1 Figure reality triangle. Virtual reality consists of a computer-generated, multidimensional environment and interface tools that allow users to (1) immerse themselves in the environment, (2) navigate within the environment and (3) interact with objects and other inhabitants in the environment

Y. El Miedany, *Rheumatology Teaching*,
https://doi.org/10.1007/978-3-319-98213-7_20

Table 20.1 Types of virtual reality

Virtual reality types
Textual VR (interaction, no immersion)
Desktop VR (interaction, immersion)
Immersive VR (interaction, high immersion)
Augmented VR (interaction, no immersion)

Table 20.2 variable forms of computer-generated simulation

Virtual reality	Virtual reality environment	Immersive virtual reality environment	Augmented reality
A technology that allows the user to explore and manipulate computer-generated 2D or 3D, multimedia sensory environments in real time [1]	Computer-generated representation of a real or artificial environment that can be interacted with by external involvement, allowing for a first-person active learning experience through immersion [2, 3]	Complex technologies that replace real-world sensory information with synthetic stimuli such as 3D visual imagery, spatialized sound and force or tactile feedback [4]	A non-immersive VR and it is based on the idea of taking what is real and adding to in some way so that user obtain more information from their environment [5]
Creates an entire virtual world; difficult to differentiate between what is real and what is not real. Generally achieved by wearing googles or gloves			A mix of the real world and the virtual world; where people interact with both worlds and distinguish between both easily. Generally achieved by holding a smartphone

drive a virtual car or run a marathon in a park still under design. Table 20.2 shows different forms of computer-generated simulation. Recent advances in computer processor speed and graphics make it possible for even desktop computers to create highly realistic environments [1–6].

The field of virtual reality first came to light decades ago; however, recent advances in technology have made it the exciting and emerging field it is today. The practical applications are far reaching. Today, using VR, architects design office buildings; NASA controls robots at remote locations; and physicians plan and practice difficult operations. In medicine, the technology has been implemented for uses such as cognitive rehabilitation post-stroke [7], improving reaction times in children with cerebral palsy [8] and in aiding the diagnosis of psychiatric conditions [9].

Augmented reality (AR) is briefly a non-immersive VR, and it is based on the idea of taking what is real and adding to in some way so that user obtains more information from their environment. AR is defined as "an enhanced version of reality created by the use of technology to add digital information on an image of something". AR is used in apps for smartphones and tablets. AR apps use the phone's camera to show the person a view of the real world in front of him/her and then put a layer of information, including text and/or images, on top of that view [5]. Apps can use AR for fun, such as the game Pokémon GO, or for information,

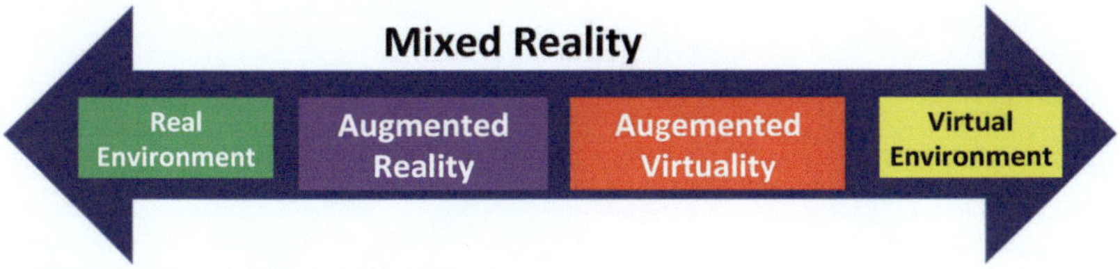

Fig. 20.2 Virtual reality: The basic interaction between the person and virtual world through the interface

such as the app "Layar" (Layar connects our digital lives with the physical world with the Layar Creator, a self-service web application for activating print pages with digital content. Also, the user can upload images of own greeting card, flyer, package or any other item to instantly create a personalized augmented reality (AR) experience) [10].

As shown in Fig. 20.2, according to Milgram [11], virtual reality occupies one extreme of the "virtuality continuum" and is an environment in which the participant observer is totally immersed in, and able to interact with, a completely synthetic world. Augmented reality sits closest to the opposite end of the virtuality continuum and refers to cases in which an otherwise real environment is "augmented" by means of virtual (computer graphic) objects. Mixed reality is a term used to describe the varying types of devices that fall along this continuum [11].

Virtual reality and augmented reality have quickly booked their place and received wide acceptance in the medical community whether researchers, clinicians or educators. Several research studies revealed the significant improvements and outcomes using VR and AR imaging, educating, planning and control techniques. This chapter will discuss the science behind virtual reality technology, the virtual reality environments for health professional education and the use of virtual reality/augmented reality to improve the clinicians' skills. The chapter will expand to discuss designing of realistic virtual patients, advantages and disadvantages of VR and AR for virtual patients as well as virtual reality/augmented reality in medical education. The chapter will conclude with discussion of the use of virtual reality/augmented reality for patient management.

The Science Behind Virtual Reality Technology

The term "virtual reality" describes the experience of interacting with data from within the computer-generated dataset. The computer-generated dataset may be completely synthetic or remotely sensed. Examples are blood dynamics, heart beat regulation, X-ray, MRI or PET images. Interaction with the data is natural and intuitive and occurs from a first-person perspective. The VR technology was reviewed in a report done by Greenleaf [6]. From a system perspective, VR technology can be segmented as shown in Fig. 20.3.

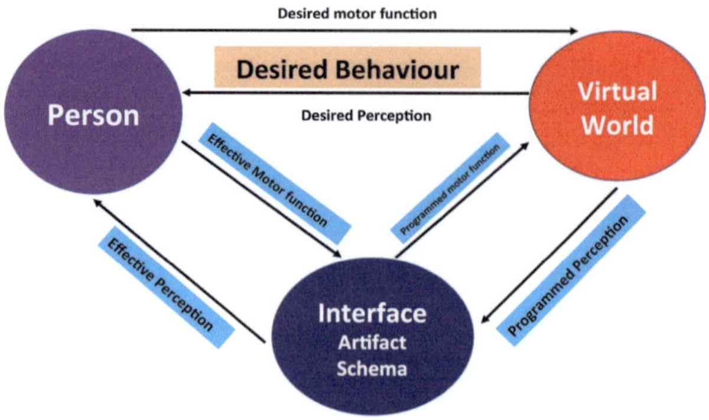

Fig. 20.3 Technology of virtual reality. Virtual reality describes the experience of interacting with data from within the computer-generated dataset

The Computational Tools

The computational tools is the computer-generated environment, or virtual world content, consists of a 3D graphic model, typically implemented as a spatially organized, object-oriented database; each object in the database represents an object in the virtual world.

The Modelling Tools

A separate modelling programme is used to create the individual objects for the virtual world. For greater realism, texture maps are used to create visual surface detail.

Dynamic Generator

The dataset is manipulated using a real-time dynamics generator that allows the object movement within the world according to natural laws such as gravity and inertia or to other variables such as spring rate and flexibility that are specified for each particular experience by application-specific programming. The basic interaction between the person and virtual world through the interface is shown in Fig. 20.4.

Renderers

Powerful renderers are applied to present 3D images and 3D spatialized sound in real time to the observer.

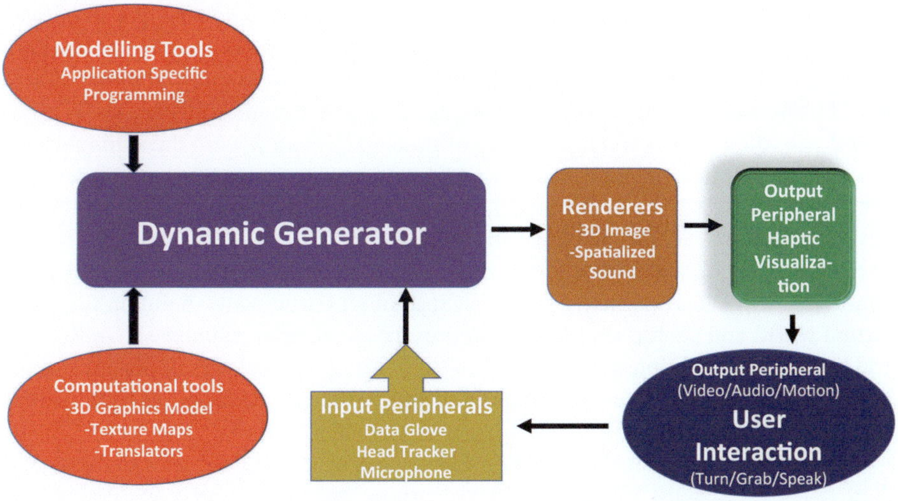

Fig. 20.4 Requirements for designing realistic medical interviews that take advantage of the VR/AR interfaces

Output/Input Interface

The dynamics generator also tracks the position and orientation of the user's head and hand using input peripherals. The interface hardware consists of two components: sensors for controlling the virtual world and effectors for providing feedback to the user. To date, three main computer interface mechanisms, not all of which manifest the ideal sensor/effector duality, have evolved: instrumented clothing, the head-mounted display (HMD) and 3D sound systems. Other VR interface technologies include sense of motion (generated in a VR system by a motion platform, e.g. flight simulators), haptics (haptics is the science of touch) and haptic interface which generates the perception of touch and resistance in VR. Figure 20.3 shows an example of virtual reality technology system.

Virtual Reality Environments for Health Professional Education

Through immersion in a non-real environment that closely mimics the real world, VR provides a good opportunity for enhancing and modifying the learning experience of healthcare professionals [12]. A unique feature of VR environment-based education is that students can experience different situations in the VR environment without physically leaving the classroom setting. This makes the educational experience invaluable. In concordance, VR technology is a good learning tool for students with different needs and learning styles [13, 14]. It also provides opportunities for group work and peer teaching. Students who struggle to be part of a classroom setting can be accepted by their peers thanks to their technology skills [15]. This confidence boost may enable students to learn in a more holistic way. Furthermore, students actively interact with content and role play skills associated with their profession in a VR environment [2]. By allowing the students time to interact with other avatars (animated figures the user may navigate to perform various tasks in a VR environment), it facilitate a safe, simulated environment, with less anxiety and an increase in competency in learning new skills. It also encourages the student to cooperate and collaborate with peers, as well as resolve conflicts. Active learning takes place because other participants, being in the same virtual world and performing tasks to represent ideas, help enhance self-reflection and knowledge [15]. Internet-based 3D VR environment provides opportunities for individuals or groups to engage themselves with the environment, accounting for collective intelligence [16].

A few studies published examining the various aspects of VR environment, and their potential benefits for teaching and learning have collectively yielded a long list of positive capabilities. Mantovani [2] identified VR as an attractive educational tool which can provide a rich, interactive learning environment and an opportunity for experiential learning, which may allow students and trainees to develop a better understanding and learn more thoroughly. The advantage of learning in a VR environment is that it provides new experiences that are not too costly to administer and at the same time provides new experiences in circumstances that might not be feasible to implement in a real-world setting. Jarmon [17] agreed with these suggestions as he reported that "VR tend to provide other instructional benefits, such as allowing for creativity within a rich media environment, providing opportunities for social interaction, facilitating collaboration, increasing a sense of shared presence, dissolving social boundaries, lowering social anxiety, enhancing student motivation and engagement, and accommodating millennial generation learning preferences".

Use of Virtual Reality to Improve the Clinicians' Communication Skills

Communication skills training is one of the main core aspects of medical education, generally introduced early and continued throughout medical school. This is a skill that can be learned, practiced, honed and assessed. Many courses use the Cambridge-Calgary guide to the medical consultation as a useful framework for use in communication skills teaching [18]. It can be broken down and its constituent parts used sequentially during both learning and examining. Medical students can modify the basic model depending on what they have observed in role models and what they feel most comfortable with. In this way, they are able to shape the consultation in the appropriate way to ensure the patient's satisfaction while remaining efficient.

Throughout training and in continuing professional development, medical students and doctors use roleplay with real and simulated patients to practice communication skills. One current training tool involves consultations with a patient actor followed by immediate feedback by experienced staff and the actor. They are often videoed and watched contemporaneously by a group and then kept for personal use to watch in a private space for deeper reflection and understanding. Another tool is to video real patient consultations with consent. This allows for both self-reflection and for an expert to analyse the consultation at a later time.

Communication skills training is also undertaken on the job, for example, in the form of work-based assessments with senior colleagues or as part of a summative assessment for a specialist exit examination. Learning to communicate in complex or emotionally charged situations is challenging: it may occur by reflecting on things that could have gone better or, in worst case scenarios, when having to deal with a complaint, a claim or in court [18].

Often conflicts arise because assumptions about others are made when people come in contact, not least patients. It is important to reflexively consider how culture affects patients' care. Aspects of culture such as race, religion, gender, sexuality, age, experience, background, language and so on undoubtedly have an effect on the views medical professionals hold, and the way in which situations are handled. There are often stereotypes that must be abandoned while working with other professionals to be able to honestly and fruitfully work together. The use of virtual reality, where the appearance of avatars can be easily altered, may allow clinicians to gain a deeper understanding of their own values and how these affect their clinical practice. Fertleman and colleagues discussed the use of virtual reality as a new tool for training healthcare professionals [19].

Virtual reality consultations bring a different perspective to the traditional way of patient communication; it incorporates the patient's (avatar's) interaction and allows the clinicians' responses to be studied, not only by an audience but also by the clinician themselves. It also allows the clinician to recognize the emotions he/she has been through as part of a consultation. In fact, the virtual reality scenario highlights the complex nature of the decision-making process and demonstrates that the clinician has to make the decision based, not just, on clinical evidence but also to consider the latest national or local guidelines. It also exposes the uncomfortable conflict that arises within the doctor's mind during their thought process, knowing that they may cause distress or lose the patient's trust should they fail to meet the patient expectation or answer the patient's queries satisfactorily [20].

The doctor may try one approach in a virtual reality consultation then view their performance and listen to advice on other approaches that could benefit their skills. The doctor can replay the same scenario and see how different approaches, explanations and reactions change the consultation. There are many situations in which virtual reality consultations may be preferable to the use of patient actors. In paediatrics, it is ethically inappropriate to use child actors as victims of abuse for the benefit of teaching. However, practicing child protection scenarios is vital in educating clinicians to notice signs of abuse and react appropriately. Furthermore, consultations with child actors, particularly under the age of five, are particularly challenging due to the unpredictability of child actors. Virtual reality may provide a solution to these respective concerns [7].

Coming across aggressive patients or family members is an unfortunate eventuality in a doctor's career, with conditions such as dementia and mental illness sometimes playing a part. This is another example where virtual reality provides a safe environment to learn and reflect. Virtual reality technology was thought to be particularly useful in such situations in order to protect the doctor's safety. It allows clinicians to take a "trial and error" approach to learn how to respond to these situations, rather than going through this process and putting themselves in danger in real life [5].

Virtual reality may allow the user to work remotely, facilitating distance learning. Clinicians could carry out scenarios at home, providing a novel way to practice communication skills without the need for real actors. On the other hand, there are various downsides and barriers to the use of virtual reality in medical training. In its current form, avatars are not especially realistic, and this may make clinicians less able to immerse themselves in the scenario. Doctors may feel more able to say no to an avatar than a real person. With added funding, the technology could become more sophisticated, with speech recognition and more realistic facial expressions. Creating higher fidelity avatars requires greater funds: another barrier to implementation [19].

Designing Realistic Virtual Patients

Designing more realistic virtual patients requires a framework that comprises (1) a natural user interface aided by natural language processing, (2) appropriate visual and auditory fidelity to represent an emotive virtual patient, (3) the understanding of emotion through both sensing affective state of the user and translating this input into emotive/behavioural states for the patient, and (4) a way to access the training modules asynchronously and without distractions typically associated with computer devices – tedious calibration and setup times, tethered wires, limitations of monitors and other computer peripherals [21].

Recently, there has been an influx of VR/AR technology platforms. VR head-mounted display (HMD) devices range from very inexpensive stereoscopic display devices, such as Google Cardboard, to computer and console systems such as the Oculus Rift, the HTC Vive and PlayStation VR. Some VR devices, like Samsung's Gear VR and Google's Daydream, use the processing capabilities of mobile smartphones. Google also launched an early attempt at a mobile AR with its Google Glass device. Microsoft HoloLens is an example of the evolution of AR head-worn displays. Many others are being developed [22].

Designing realistic medical interviews that take advantage of the growing selection of VR/AR interfaces requires a framework that comprises (1) high-fidelity virtual patients with enhanced, realistic, physical representations, i.e. visual, auditory and behavioural; (2) a cognitive model to govern the virtual patient's emotions, logic and cultural representation; (3) a narrative system for customizable content

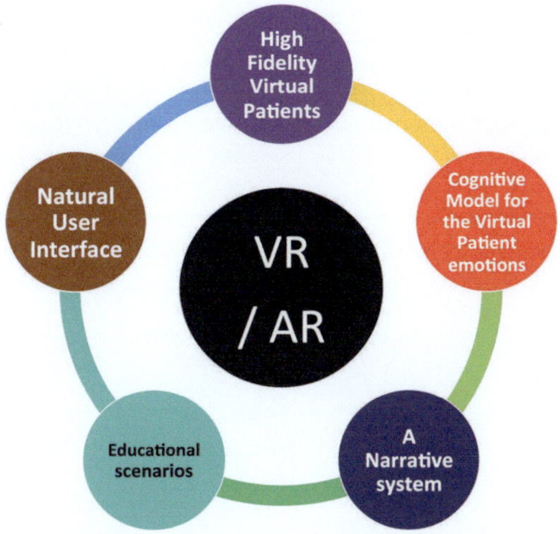

Fig. 20.5 Required characteristics for designing realistic medical interviews that take advantage of the growing selection of virtual reality (VR)/augmented reality (AR) interfaces: (1) high-fidelity virtual patients with enhanced, realistic, physical representations, i.e. visual, auditory and behavioural; (2) a cognitive model to govern the virtual patient's emotions, logic and cultural representation; (3) a narrative system for customizable content presentation through patient stories; (4) educational scenarios with non-linear complexity; and (5) a natural user interface that replaces text with intrinsic human interactions

presentation through patient stories; (4) educational scenarios with non-linear complexity; and (5) a natural user interface that replaces text with intrinsic human interactions – speech and head and body gestures (Fig. 20.5) [23].

VR/AR technologies could allow more realistic interactions with virtual patients by providing both more life-like medical interviews as well as the ability to study how well students verbally and non-verbally demonstrate understanding and empathy. Empathy refers to "an affective response that is more consistent with another person's situation than one's own situation" [7]. Empathy is crucial for the success of social interactions and has been linked to increased patient trust and patient satisfaction [23, 24].

Natural User Interface

A natural user interface (NUI) is a system for human-computer interaction that the user operates through intuitive actions related to natural, everyday human behaviour. Thus, it allows the user to directly interact with a system without a physical controller [25]. A NUI may be operated in a number of different ways, depending on the purpose and user requirements. Some NUIs rely on intermediary devices for interaction, but more advanced NUIs are either invisible to the user or so unobtrusive that they quickly seem invisible. Table 20.3 shows some examples and application of the natural user interfaces. Control over a NUI does not need to be learned

Table 20.3 Examples and applications of natural user interfaces

Touch screen	Gesture recognition	Speech recognition	Gaze tracking	Brain machine interfaces
Interfaces let users interact with controls and applications more intuitively than a cursor-based interface because it is more direct – instead of moving a cursor to select a file and clicking to open it	Systems track user motions and translate those movements to instructions	Allow users to interact with a system through spoken commands. The system identifies spoken words and phrases and converts them to a machine-readable format for interaction	Interfaces allow users to guide a system through eye movements	Read neural signals and use programmes to translate those signals into action
Examples: the user touches a graphic representation of the file to open it. Smartphones and tablets typically enable touch input. Touch is being adapted for non-screen applications as well. For example, Microsoft is working on a touch interface called "skinput" that allows users to interact by tapping their own skin	Nintendo Wii and PlayStation Move motion gaming systems work through controller-based accelerometers and gyroscopes to sense tilting, rotation and acceleration. A more intuitive type of NUI is outfitted with a camera and software in the device that recognizes specific gestures and translates them to actions. Microsoft's Kinect, for example, is a motion sensor for the Xbox 360 gaming console that allows users to interact through body motions, gestures and spoken commands. Kinect recognizes individual players' bodies and voices. Gesture recognition can also be used to interact with computers	Speech recognition applications include call routing, speech-to-text and hands-free computer and mobile phone operation. Speech recognition is also sometimes used to interact with embedded systems	Lenovo produced the first eye-controlled laptop. The Lenovo system combines an infrared light source with a camera to catch reflective glints from the user's eyes. Software calculates the area of the screen being looked at and uses that information for input	Can make it possible for someone who is paralyzed to operate a computer, motorized wheelchair or prosthetic limb through thought alone

like control over artificial control devices such as a mouse or keyboard [22]. For example, an NUI may be controlled by making a gesture or speaking a key phrase, both of which are innate human actions. In contrast, a new user must learn how to use a remote control before watching television.

Another key aspect of the NUI is invisibility [26]. The interface should not be visible to the user while they are interacting with the system. The invisibility criterion ensures that users have direct control over the system without intermediate interfaces. By leveraging intrinsic natural human action, NUIs provide users with efficient and accessible channels of direct interaction with a system or machine. Graphical user interface (GUI) allows the use of icons or other visual indicators to interact with electronic devices, rather than using only text via the command line. For example, all versions of Microsoft Windows utilize a GUI, whereas MS-DOS does not.

Challenges and Progress in Developing Virtual Patients

Despite the technology advances, researchers and developers of virtual patients often encounter some challenges and barriers when faced with developing realistic, easy-to-use interfaces. Accordingly, these challenges must be kept in mind when exploring potential advantages of developing virtual patients for VR/AR platforms. Virtual patients are complicated systems that require considerable effort to develop. Complex virtual patient architectures may consist of many different modular components for user input, speech recognition, patient response, animation, audio and lip-syncing that must work in tandem to present a realistic virtual human, potentially making the development of such a system costly and difficult [27]. Virtual patient systems may also include branching narratives which further increase the complexity of the system and the effort required to develop it, and because of this, robust branching narratives have historically been uncommon in virtual patients [28]. While complex systems offer more realistic interaction, their sophisticated architectures make authoring and adding content difficult, meaning in some instances that only developers with a deep understanding of the architecture can add new content [21].

These complexity issues have posed a barrier to entry and progression in the field, but recent development of toolkits and resources, such as the University of Southern California Institute for Creative Technology's (ICT) SimCoach [29] and the unified medical taxonomy [30], have begun to remedy this issue and make the development process less costly and time intensive. Speech recognition is continuously improving – as a result, recent virtual patient platforms such as ICT's SimSensei Kiosk boast deep natural language processing (NLP) capabilities and can parse open-ended vocal input from the user, automatically categorizing their speech and responding in real time to simulate a conversational flow [31].

In the development of SimCoach and the SimSensei Kiosk, a Virtual Human Toolkit (VHTK) has been utilized. This includes Multisense, tracks and analyses users' facial expressions, body posture, acoustic features, linguistic patterns and higher-level behaviour descriptors (e.g. attention, fidgeting); the NPCEditor, a statistical text classification algorithm that selects the character's responses based on the user's utterances; the nonverbal behaviour generator (NVBG) a rule-based system which analyses character text and functional mark-up to propose nonverbal behaviours; SmartBody, a character animation library that provides synchronized locomotion, steering, object manipulation, lip-syncing, gazing and non-verbal behaviour in real time; and vhtoolkitUnity which includes a tight integration with SmartBody, a messaging protocol, debug and authoring tools and a graphical timeline editor for creating cut scenes [32].

Natural language processing (NLP) is an important factor in the development of a natural user interface (NUI). Much has been accomplished in the field of NLP, resulting in a recent proliferation of intelligent assistants such as Amazon Echo, Siri and Google Home. Current NLP research landscape consists of hundreds of companies and continues to grow [33]. Speech recognition is continuously improving and has been integrated into many widely used applications – smartphones now allow dictation of text messages through NLP, and Windows 10 comes with the Cortana assistant which accepts natural language input [34]. In this landscape of continual research and improvement of NLP and NUI systems, it is plausible and realistic to look towards applying NLP/NUI to VR/AR virtual patient systems.

Despite these advances in extensive artificial intelligence and language processing research, natural language processing (NLP) remains one of the greatest challenges faced when developing virtual patients. Accurate natural language processing and understanding are still a challenge. Inaccurate language processing can lead to a frustrating, immersion-breaking experience that fails to simulate the flow of a clinical interview, and low-performing language systems are common, with virtual patient prototypes demonstrating 60–75% accuracy in their language processing [30]. Virtual patients may be extensively programmed to recognize words and phrases and respond accordingly, but true language understanding, conversational awareness and natural conversation flow remain largely out of reach [28]. In order to simulate a natural conversational flow, many current virtual patient systems use "pause-based" language processing which interprets and responds to the user's voice input when they stop talking for a certain length of time. This poses problems, as many phrases and statements may contain internal pauses that do not necessarily signal the end of the statement. More sophisticated language processing systems designed to deal with this problem may also struggle when a user does not pause between thoughts. Pause-based systems also suffer from latency as they measure and detect pauses before responding, slowing the flow of the conversation [35]. Some virtual patient systems circumvent the issue of natural language processing with lower-tech interfaces such as multiple-choice menus. These structured encounters are more reliable and do report positive learning outcomes but lack the robust educational/training potential of natural language input [30].

Advantages and Disadvantages of VR and AR for Virtual Patients

Both VR and AR systems have their own unique "immersion" capability, or the capability to present a convincing virtual environment to the user [36]. Where VR technologies can offer an immersive alternate reality, AR technologies can supplement a student's existing reality to provide an in situ experience such that the physical world and all accompanying real and virtual objects are perceived to exist in the same locale. Virtual objects such as 3D holograms and web pages can be positioned within the physical environment and used to interact with a virtual patient that responds to the student's actions – further providing a sense that the virtual patient is present and exists in the real world, for example, the possibility for projecting a virtual patient in a hospital room using a device such as the Microsoft HoloLens.

In head-mounted AR systems, the convergence of real and augmented environments is accomplished by allowing the wearer to see through the visor, while AR techniques involving multiple sensors, spatial mapping, computer vision and holographic positioning systems are implemented (Fig. 20.6). Retaining the ability to see the natural environment allows the physical world itself to be leveraged in development as it does not need to be recreated, only supplemented. This could allow for a greater focus on the creation of a graphically detailed virtual patient and for more attention to be given to interface, in which real or virtual elements including the virtual patient could play a role. Conversely, in VR systems one cannot see the real world through the visor, which poses potential safety hazards. VR systems provide an opportunity to create an entire alternate environment for the student, which could

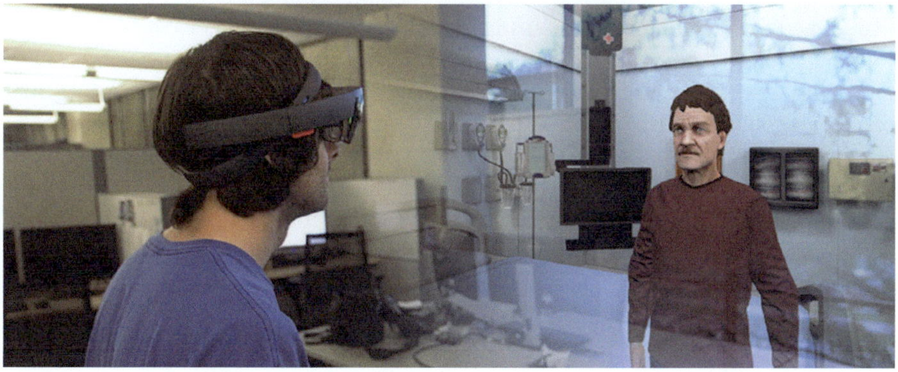

Fig. 20.6 Augmented reality technology can overlay synthetic objects onto a real-world environment. This mock-up represents the possibility for projecting a virtual patient in a hospital room using a device such as the Microsoft HoloLens. (From Zielke et al. [21], with permission)

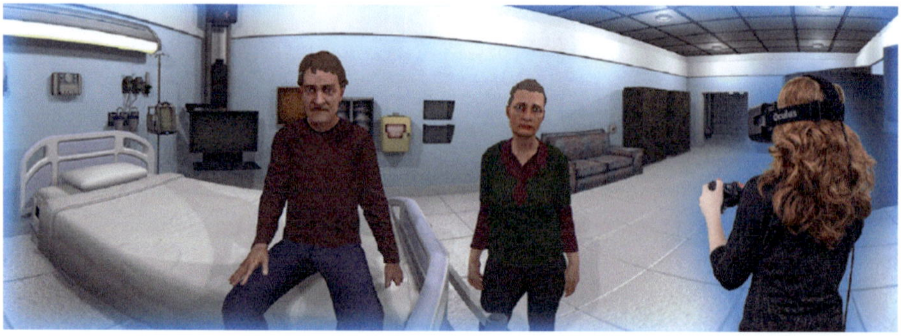

Fig. 20.7 Virtual reality technology immerses learners completely in a synthetic environment. This mock-up represents an interaction with two virtual characters, Walter and Susan, using Oculus – a VR head-mounted display device. (From Zielke et al. [21], with permission)

be used by a designer to define a smaller or larger scope for what environmental elements should be realistically present in the project, as well as to implement and control the broader visual motif (Fig. 20.7). A custom environment could offer a more consistent level of control over the student's educational experience while potentially providing a greater level of immersion.

AR can also be safer for the wearer in any existing environment as they can maintain their ability to visually navigate their natural surroundings. Additionally, though head-mounted AR device options are currently limited, some of the emerging technologies are "untethered" and do not require physical wired connections to external equipment. The elimination of external wiring further diminishes potential safety issues and could allow a student to focus more intently on the educational experience of interacting with a virtual patient. Untethered devices also reduce the time required to set up and start using a device, which could allow more flexibility regarding where and when a student may choose to learn or engage with a virtual patient depending on the device's solution for removing the wires. Some devices are untethered because they have an internal computer, while other emerging solutions for VR devices involve wirelessly connecting to an external computer providing a greater graphical capability. A gaming laptop, for example, could allow the system to remain portable while potentially still delivering a high-fidelity visual experience [21].

When presented with a completely virtualized reality, some users can experience disorientation, or a version of motion sickness known as *simulator sickness*. There are competing theories regarding the cause of the sickness, such as the sensory conflict theory and the postural instability theory [37]. Most head-mounted AR solutions do not encapsulate the user or obscure access to timely and expected visual feedback of the real world, nor do they inhibit the wearer's ability to maintain postural control, which inherently negates the likelihood of encountering simulator sickness specifically. However, strategies and best practices have been suggested for developers when creating software for VR devices to mitigate simulator sickness by properly handling issues like latency, flicker and acceleration, which have been identified as potentially contributing factors to simulator sickness [38].

While interaction with the natural environment using VR devices may be completely removed due to the encapsulating nature of the technology, AR devices allow for seamless interaction with both virtual and physical worlds. Some current AR systems are natively capable of using various predefined gestures as a natural interface to trigger interactions, as well as providing speech to text functionality that can further connect the wearer to the augmented realm through natural means. Virtual reality systems can support additions that parallel these functionalities and may have more processing power available for implementation as well, depending on the choice of external hardware. Sensors such as a microphone or a Leap Motion controller can be attached externally to some systems, and software can be extended as needed to support the desired functionality. In this way, a VR device is further able to function as a natural user interface between the student, a virtual patient and the virtualized environment.

Another feature aiding in the enhancement of some AR/VR systems as a natural user interface, as well as the creation of a sense of presence, is 3D audio. Research indicates that 3D spatialized audio is associated with higher reported "presence" or psychological sensation of physically being in a virtual space or with holographic imagery [36, 39]. Due to the head-related transfer function (HRTF) effect, everyone hears sounds differently [11]. This effect occurs because sound waves interact with other parts of human anatomy along the way into the ear canals. To account for HRTF, tiny microphones are positioned inside the ear canals of a model or a human listener, and samples are taken from many angles inside an anechoic chamber. Research indicates that HRTF audio increases users' reported presence [40]. However, most 3D audio implementations for wearable AR/VR solutions draw from existing HRTF libraries that may only be populated with measurements taken every 5° or 15° [41]. The result is that even after the required calibration of a device, the selected HRTF set may result in audible discontinuities that diminish the wearer's ability to locate virtual objects in 3D space based on sound.

In addition to the above-described potential VR/AR configurations, the HoloLens, represented in Fig. 20.6, is a potentially applicable AR solution in the implementation of a natural interface between the virtual patient, student and environment. An interesting feature of HoloLens specifically is that the calibration process for spatial audio is invisible to the user, while an algorithm uses the distance between the user's eyes as an indication of what the distance between their ear canals may be [42]. Personalized 3D audio combined with head tracking can allow a student to physically roam the mixed reality environment and gaze naturally in any direction while remaining able to locate and interact with a virtual patient using audible and visual cues. The position of the student in the space and the direction of their gaze not only changes what they hear but creates a natural interface by providing input to the virtual patient who can then respond accordingly with feedback that is meaningful to the student or changes the course of the educational experience [43–45].

Virtual Reality/Augmented Reality in Medical Education

Several studies [46–52] have documented the vital need for integrative training of medical personnel in manual, diagnostic and patient management skills. While such training is available to staffs at medical education hospitals, the access to sophisticated training by the personnel working at the remote health facility is still limited. Moreover, even in the ideal setting of a teaching hospital, training is based on "at the bedside (or in the operating-emergency room)" concept. Hence, none of the currently employed teaching methods provide satisfactory solutions for a truly well-integrated system where all aspects of medical knowledge (i.e. theoretical and practical) are employed simultaneously. Consequently, most of the currently employed teaching methods are based on flow chart (semi-static) approaches that fail to incorporate the complexity of medical reality, i.e. the environment where large amounts of information need to be instantaneously combined, analysed and transformed into a meaningful practical skills-driven activity and where time represents a critical factor [53–55].

Virtual reality (VR), as part of computer science, allows computer-based models of the real world to be generated and provides humans with a means to interact with these models through new human-computer interfaces and thus to nearly realistically experience these models [56]. This concept applies to medicine, as much as to any other field of human endeavour, where manual skills and intellectual experience need to be perfected through training in complex or potentially dangerous situations. In the medical field, creating simulations for the training of professionals offered the training students and healthcare professional a golden opportunity to enhance their skills and gain experience in different medical as well as surgical situations. Several studies documented the positive outcome of VR in surgical procedures [57]. It has also been used in recreating medical critical conditions and, in a scope with real patients, developing social and cognitive skills [52].

Emergency and trauma medicine comprise the medical specialties demanding rapid integration of discrete information elements into a coherent, outcome-oriented action subjected to a continuous modification by the variation in the nature of the incoming patient data. Virtual reality is used to replicate high-risk trauma situations from actual cases. More deeply immersive experiences let training doctors and students practice and learn in realistic workplace conditions. The training scenarios come with all the elements that healthcare providers can face in real life.

These kinds of simulations put students in situations that they may encounter in their real lives. The simulation allows, in many cases, to modify parameters, which gives rise to a new experience. They can experiment these situations without risk, in a controlled environment and with a view as realistic as you want. Such simulations improve the skills of students and their retention of knowledge [52].

Another example, aside from simulation, is exposing students to a VR session where they can directly inspect 3D models of several human organs by using virtual reality systems. Using 2D images to teach the structure of 3D objects is typically complicated, especially in courses where those 3D shapes can be hardly complex, as is the case of organs inside the human body. A recent study [58] revealed that VR to teaching anatomy is a powerful learning tool that helps to understand the anatomical structures.

Curriculum and Student Feedback

Classical teaching makes the students be passively seated in a classroom, watching a teacher explaining a power point presentation for 1 or 2 h. Instead, by using virtual reality, the students live an active experience, where immersion makes them fully engaged in the activity, without distractions. This allows them to focus all attention on what they are doing [58].

Several studies assessed how VR can be integrated into the curriculum and how it relates to the commitment of the student in learning [59]. Focusing on the learning process, an important aspect to take into account is the motivation. Motivation is defined as an internal state or condition that activates, guides and directs behaviour [60]. Training is easier if the experience is pleasant or enjoyable, which means higher level of engagement and understanding. The majority of nursing students prefer a hands-on, active approach to education [61].

Huang et al. [62] focused their work on students' attitudes towards learning environments where you use VR. To them, student's learning motivation is focused on three critical factors of VR applications: the intuitive interaction, physical sense of imagination and sense of immersion. They also say, with respect to learning, that motivation is an important cognitive factor, so that motivated students can learn more effectively.

With respect to the effectiveness of learning through the use of VR in 3D, Nicholson et al. [63] support the hypothesis that students are more receptive to understand aspects of anatomy using 3D than using 2D. In comparing the teaching of musculoskeletal anatomy through VR traditional methods, Codd and Choudhury [64] indicate that VR can serve as a complement to traditional methods of teaching anatomy. Recent studies have shown that virtual learning applications can provide the tools to learn in a quick and happy mode by playing in virtual environment [65].

On the other hand, VR use is not always capable of simulating real-life situations. Purchase of the technology can be very expensive and require ongoing updates and maintenance. Similarly, the outcomes of the exercise are only as effective as the actual training provided and the person running the simulation. Training on how to use the software and/or hardware of the simulator takes up time and costs money. The trainees need to be clinically competent and able to understand the aspects of the technical accuracy in order to provide meaningful feedback. Participants, on the other hand, may resist full engagement with the technology, thus, minimizing the potential benefits of the treatment protocol [5].

In summary, virtual reality provides technological advances regarding image and degree of immersion, which allows us to deal with restrictions that plastic models present. VR also allows us to overcome the difficulty of having access to real cadavers. Therefore, VR may provide a solution to those problems, but their use for educational purposes must begin with a solid education. In this sense, in terms of education, before choosing the technological tool, one must design, create and implement strategies that engage students in the learning process. This starts by having solid targets for each discipline and academic level.

Virtual Reality/Augmented Reality and Patient Management

Medical knowledge runs a dynamic course as it continues to progress over time leading to advances in the treatment of illness and disease. This presents a challenge to healthcare professionals who should integrate such advanced knowledge (theoretical and clinical) into their standard clinical practice to manage different cases presenting with variable manifestations. New technologies, in particular virtual/augmented reality and robotics, are expected to have a major impact on healthcare in the next decade. A recent article reviewed the use of VR in various clinical and medical settings and procedures [66, 67] which can be stratified into:

Virtual Reality Exposure Therapy (VRET)

Patients with emotional experiences, such as excessive fear and anxiety as well as posttraumatic stress disorders (PTSD) and panic disorders, may have a significant impact on the patient ability to carry out activities of daily living as well as life. In recent years, virtual reality exposure therapy (VRET) was reported as an effective novel alternative treatment tool for anxiety disorders and specific phobias. Clinicians were able to use VR technology without concerns of safety or loss of confidentiality reported in real-world exposure. In VRET, patients are immersed within a computer-generated simulation or a virtual environment where they are exposed to specific fear stimuli. Several studies revealed the positive impact of VR in such cases. Data derived from 21 studies including about 300 subjects who received VRET management revealed that VRET has a good potential as a treatment approach for several specific phobias. This was supported by better outcomes compared to traditional forms of management such as imagine exposure (where patients had to imagine feared stimulus). In another randomized trial of 97 subjects comparing VR exposure therapy to in vivo exposure for social anxiety disorder, VRET was effective for treating social fears, and improvement was maintained for 1 year [68]. VRET technique helped to introduce an environment where patients can exercise how to control their own emotional experiences which in turn increased their level of self-efficacy and confidence, hence, regain control over their own lives [69].

Virtual Reality Distraction Therapy (VRDT)

Several medical or surgical procedures may be associated with pain or discomfort. Traditionally, pain killers are usually prescribed to help with the pain. Recently, VR started to book its place in the pain management. Various psychological techniques have been suggested to help such condition. Recently, distraction using virtual environment was tried as a novel form of therapy. During VRDT the patient's attention is deviated from the harmful stimulus affecting the perception of pain. Virtual reality distraction therapy (VRDT) provides many levels of interactions to patients allowing the use of many senses, simultaneously, thus encouraging them to be immersed in the virtual world experience. Various visual and auditory senses, active emotional involvement and patient participation serve as distractors for the patient. The higher the user's immersion, the more likely the patient's attention is kept in the virtual world with less courtesy to the other painful signals. A research study using VR as a distraction intervention was conducted in two sessions over a period of 8 weeks with 28 participants (age ranging 18–23). In each weekly session, the participants were divided into two groups: baseline (control) group and VR distraction cohort. The procedure involved immersing the participant's non-dominating hand up to the wrist in a cold-pressor bath, whereas the VR cohort (using the dominating hand) had a PlayStation 2 controller as a distraction. Both groups were asked to remove their hands when they feel the pain unbearable. Time for each patient was measured with a stopwatch. Results revealed increased pain tolerance, pain threshold and decreased pain intensity, anxiety and time spent thinking about pain in the VR distraction condition compared to the baseline (control) condition that had no distraction intervention [70–76].

Cancer patients experience anxiety-filled and unpleasant moments over the course of treatment. To alleviate some of this stress, hospitals use VRDT to provide a therapeutic degree of relaxation to its chemotherapy patients [71]. Another study provided encouraging support for the use of VRDT as a technique for controlling fear and anxiety during dental procedures [74].

VR in Cognitive and Physical Rehabilitation

The use of VR has been extended into cognitive rehabilitation to treat patients with brain damage and physical rehabilitation of patients living with stroke, acquired brain damage, Parkinson's disease and other motor-related diseases. The effectiveness of VR applications can be linked to the interactive experimental medium through which VR provide a unique setting for patients to explore and act without feeling threatened. Unlike human trainers, VR provides ease of manipulation as well as consistency.

Tele-Rehabilitation

Tele-rehabilitation is another gain of VR application for patients in need to rehabilitation services. This time, the patients' management can be delivered through the Internet at the patient's home. Broeren and colleagues assessed the effect of tele-rehabilitation on 29 stroke patients, aged 45–85 years [77]. Twenty-nine stroke subjects, 17 women and 12 men, aged 44–85 years, post-stroke 1–140 months, participated in 3 different studies. Thirteen subjects underwent in- or out-patient rehabilitation at the Department of Rehabilitation Medicine, University Hospital; and 16 underwent rehabilitation in a facility for community-dwelling persons with stroke (Stroke Forum). A group of healthy individuals (self-perceived health) were recruited and served as reference subjects (range 33–85 years). A VR activity station was used, where the user stood in the real world and looked into a virtual world generated in the computer. He or she was able to reach into a virtual space and interact with three-dimensional (3D) objects through a handheld stylus (haptic device) positioned in the line of sight. It created an illusion of virtual objects for the user while the only real element was the handheld stylus and the computer equipment. Using stereoscopic shuttered glasses, the user observed a 3D image displayed above the tabletop. Every time an activity was run, data about the 3D hand movements of the patient was collected and analysed. VR motor rehabilitation application used the haptic technology (mechanical arm) that allowed the users to manipulate virtual objects using a "data glove" where both tracking and movement's sensors were embedded in the material. All participants responded favourable to the use of the VR activity station. A change of attitude took place after the subjects were exposed to playing computer games. Results from pre- and post-testing exhibited a higher median in average velocity and a decrease in median for time and hand path ratio (HPR) parameters as compared with baseline. Subjects who underwent rehabilitation in a non-hospital environment had shown excellent adherence to the rehabilitation programme thus resulting in an increased efficiency while maintaining high-quality service [77].

In concordance, pilot studies to reduce tobacco addiction showed promising results with the application of the VR affordable system: eMagin HDM. Results illustrated a statistically significant reduction in nicotine addiction, abstinence rate and dropout rate. Furthermore, knowing the benefits of VR application in medical field, diabetes technology society clinicians recently published several articles proposing studies and ideas of VR applications and their potential in obesity prevention and management [78]. Similar positive outcomes were reported on studying the impact of VR interventions in cognitive and physical impairments in brain injury patients. Therefore, VR has been suggested a new and effective tool for rehabilitation after brain injury [79]. Despite evident progress in VR-based cognitive rehabilitation systems, there is still a need for more clinical trials for its validation.

VR in Surgery, Surgical Planning and Performance

In the year 2000, the US Food and Drug Administration approved for the first time robotically assisted surgical devices for human surgery, and since that time the number of surgeries performed by this procedure has risen. Several VR simulators are now commercially available for educational and training purposes. Surgeons can perform remote tele-surgery, minimal invasive surgery, surgical pre-planning, surgical rehearsal, image-guided surgery and surgery simulation using surgery console. VR surgical simulation had been developed to perform minimal invasive surgery (MIS) partly because it requires a surgeon looking at a monitor. MIS involves performing operations through minimal incisions where the surgeon can control mechanical arms of the MIS robot, using haptic technology, while sitting comfortably in a surgical operating console [80, 81].

Currently, VR simulation is integrated in many MIS training programmes all over the world. A VR surgical planning device takes actual physical data from an individual patient and combines it with computer-generated graphical data mimicking the patient's anatomy. This allows the simulation device to plan and rehearse a surgical procedure – both for training and advanced planning of an operation. The benefits of this practice include lower infection rates, less pain, reduced morbidity, fast recovery and reduced surgical errors as compared to conventional surgical procedures [82].

VR as a Diagnostic Tool

With the ability to measure and record all behavioural responses triggered by the creation of dynamic, interactive and stimulus environments, clinicians have the privilege of having new up-to-date options for assessment and intervention options that have not available in the traditional standard practice. Technological advancement has taken diagnostic imaging to a level higher than other medical specialties. Radiological cross-sections have been used to produce a simulated three-dimensional reconstruction of organs; hence, it became a vital diagnostic tool, providing clinicians with a more naturalistic view of patient's anatomy. High-resolution data generation and collection have been made possible with the latest mixed reality technology, which can be easily navigated through, by the addition of sophisticated visualization software to the existing hardware base, offering a cost-effective valuable technology as it reduces personnel time and cost and, meanwhile, improves clinical efficacy [83]. The imaging modalities that represent computer-aided applications of VR in radiology include CT, MRI, X-ray imaging NM, ultrasound and computed radiography. VR simulation is also useful for autopsy and gross and microscopic examination and ideally suited for digital pathology. Unique applications include remote supervision and annotation, 3D image viewing and manipulation, tele-pathology in a mixed reality environment and real-time pathology-radiology correlation [84].

In conclusion, VR, AR and mixed reality are innovations that have led to a revolution in the learning environment, particularly medical learning. They have provided new opportunities for learning by doing for increased retention and proficiency, sharing valuable resources globally and offering a new style of simulated learning. The developments seen today in medical education, leveraging immersive visualizations, embodied simulations and capturing personalized analytics, could be a hallmark of what's to come as VR extends its reach through the medical as well as non-medical sciences.

References

1. Strangman N, Hall T. Virtual reality/simulations. Wakefield: National Center on Accessing the General Curriculum; 2003.
2. Mantovani F, Castelnuovo G, Gaggioli A, Riva G. Virtual reality training for health-care professionals. Cyberpsychol Behav. 2003;6(4):389–95.
3. Rasmussen K, Belisario JM, Wark PA, Molina JA, Loong SL, Cotic Z, et al. Offline eLearning for undergraduates in health professions: a systematic review of the impact on knowledge, skills, attitudes and satisfaction. J Global Health. 2014;4(1):010405.
4. Bowman DA, McMahan RP. Virtual reality: how much immersion is enough? Computer. 2007;40(7):36–43.
5. De Luca R, Lo Buono V, Leo A, Russo M, Aragona B, Leonardi S, et al. Use of virtual reality in improving post-stroke neglect: promising neuropsychological and neurophysiological findings from a case study. Appl Neuropsychol Adult. 2017;1:1–5. https://doi.org/10.1080/23279095.2017.1363040.
6. Greenleaf W. Medical Applications of Virtual Reality. http://bme2.aut.ac.ir/~towhidkhah/MI/Discussion86-1/VR%2520Med%2520overview.pdf. Accessed on 27 May 2018.
7. Pourazar M, Mirakhori F, Hemayattalab R, Bagherzadeh F. Use of virtual reality intervention to improve reaction time in children with cerebral palsy: a randomized controlled trial. Dev Neurorehabil. 2017;1:1–6. https://doi.org/10.1080/17518423.2017.
8. Van Bennekom MJ, De Koning PP, Denys D. Virtual reality objectifies the diagnosis of psychiatric disorders: a literature review. Front Psychol. 2017;8:163. https://doi.org/10.3389/fpsyt.2017.00163.
9. Augmented Reality vs. Virtual Reality – what's the difference? https://learningenglish.voanews.com/a/augmented-reality-versus-virtual-reality/3844772.html.
10. Layar App. https://www.layar.com/.
11. Milgram P, Kishino F. A taxonomy of mixed reality visual displays. In: IEICE TRANSACTIONS on information and systems. 1994. p. 1321–9.
12. Dalgarno B, Lee MJ. What are the learning affordances of 3-D virtual environments? Br J Educ Technol. 2010;41(1):10–32.
13. Psotka J. Immersive training systems: virtual reality and education and training. Instr Sci. 1995;23(5–6):405–31.
14. Schultheis MT, Rizzo AA. The application of virtual reality technology in rehabilitation. Rehabil Psychol. 2001;46(3):296.
15. Hansen MM. Versatile, immersive, creative and dynamic virtual 3-D healthcare learning environments: a review of the literature. J Med Internet Res. 2008;10(3):e26.
16. Saxena N, Kyaw BM, Vseteckova J, Dev P, Paul P, Lim KTK, Kononowicz A, Masiello I, Tudor Car L, Nikolaou CK, Zary N, Car J. Virtual reality environments for health

professional education. Cochrane Database Syst Rev. 2016;(2):CD012090. https://doi.org/10.1002/14651858.CD012090.
17. Jarmon L, Traphagan T, Mayrath M, Trivedi A. Virtual world teaching, experiential learning, and assessment: an interdisciplinary communication course in second life. Comput Educ. 2009;53(1):169–82.
18. Kurtz S, Silverman J, Draper J. Teaching and learning communication skills in medicine. Oxford: CRC Press; 1998.
19. Fertleman C, Aubugeau-Williams P, Sher C, Lim A-N, Lumley S, Delacroix S, Pan X. A discussion of virtual reality as a new tool for training healthcare professionals. Front Public Health. 2018;6:44. https://doi.org/10.3389/fpubh.2018.00044.
20. Pan X, Slater M, Beacco A, Navarro X, Bellido Rivas AI, Swapp D, et al. The responses of medical general practitioners to unreasonable patient demand for antibiotics—a study of medical ethics using immersive virtual reality. PLoS One. 2016;11(2):e0146837. https://doi.org/10.1371/journal.pone.0146837.
21. Zielke MA, Zakhidov D, Hardee G, Evans L, Lenox S, Orr N, Fino D, Mathialagan G. Developing virtual patients with VR/AR for a natural user interface in medical teaching. https://doi.org/10.1109/SeGAH.2017.7939285.
22. Falcao C, Lemos AC, Soares M. Evaluation of natural user interface: a usability study based on the leap motion device. Procedia Manuf. 2015;3:5490–5.
23. Mavromihelaki E, et al. Cyberball3D+: A 3D serious game for fMRI investigating social exclusion and empathy. In: 2014 6th International Conference on Games and Virtual Worlds for Serious Applications (VS-GAMES), Valletta. 2014. p. 1–8.
24. Kleinsmith A, Rivera-Gutierrez D, Finney G, Cendan J, Lok B. Understanding empathy training with virtual patients. Comput Hum Behav. 2015;52:151–8. [Online].
25. Raffii A, Zuccarino T. Method and system enabling natural user interface gestures with user wearable glasses. U.S. Patent 9310891. 2016.
26. "Natural User Interface". In: NUI Group. 2011. [Online]. Available: http://wiki.nuigroup.com/Natural_User_Interface. Accessed 28 May 2018.
27. Turing A. I.—Computing machinery and intelligence. Mind. 1950;(236):433–60.
28. Talbot T, Sagae K, John B, Rizzo A. Sorting out the virtual patient. Int J Gaming Comput Mediat Simul. 2012;4(3):1–19.
29. "SimCoach." 2013. [Online]. Available: http://www.simcoach.org/. Accessed 26 May 2018.
30. Donald CC, Sokolowski JA, Banks CM, editors. The digital patient: advancing healthcare, research, and education. Hoboken: Wiley; 2015.
31. De Vault D, et al. "SimSensei kiosk," International Foundation for Autonomous Agents and Multiagent Systems. 2014. p. 1061–8. [Online]. Available: http://dl.acm.org/citation.cfm?id=2617388.2617415.
32. Virtual human Toolkit. 2017. [Online]. Available: https://vhtoolkit.ict.usc.edu/. Accessed May 2018.
33. Miller D. Intelligent assistant landscape shows slow growth but huge potential. VentureBeat. 2016. [Online]. Available:http://venturebeat.com/2016/02/14/intelligent-assistance-theslow-growth-space-that-will-eventually-wow-us/. Accessed 28 May 2018.
34. What is Cortana? Microsoft support. 2016. [Online]. Available: https://support.microsoft.com/en-us/help/17214/windows-10-what-is. Accessed 28 May 2018.
35. Manuvinakurike R, Paetzel M, Qu C, Schlangen D, De Vault D. Toward incremental dialogue act segmentation in fast-paced interactive dialogue systems. In: 17th Annual Meeting of the Special Interest Group on Discourse and Dialogue. 2016.
36. Sanchez-Vives MV, Slater M. From presence to consciousness through virtual reality: abstract: nature reviews neuroscience. Nat Rev Neurosci. 2005;6(4):332–9. [Online]. Available: http://www.nature.com/nrn/journal/v6/n4/abs/nrn1651.html.
37. Johnson DM. Introduction to and review of simulator sickness research. Defense Technical Information Center; 2005.
38. Oculus VR. LLC, Simulator sickness. 2016. [Online]. Available: https://developer3.oculus.com/documentation/introvr/latest/concepts/bp_app_simulator_sickness/. Accessed 28 May 2018.

39. Hendrix C, Barfield W. The sense of presence within auditory virtual environments. Presence Teleop Virt. 1996;5(3):290–301. [Online]. Available: http://dl.acm.org/citation.cfm?id=2871028.2871031.
40. Pellegrini RS. Quality assessment of auditory virtual environments. Georgia Institute of Technology; 2001. [Online]. Available: https://smartech.gatech.edu/handle/1853/50631.
41. Oculus VR. LLC, 3D Audio spatialization. 2016. [Online]. Available: https://developer3.oculus.com/documentation/audiosdk/latest/concepts/audio-intro-spatialization/. Accessed 28 May 2018.
42. Lalwani M. 3D audio is the secret to HoloLens' convincing holograms. 2016. [Online]. Available: https://www.engadget.com/2016/11/02/microsoft-exclusive-hololensspatial-sound/. Accessed 28 May 2018.
43. Bright P. Microsoft sheds some light on its mysterious holographic processing unit. Condé Nast. 2016. [Online]. Available: http://arstechnica.com/information-technology/2016/08/microsoftsheds-some-light-on-its-mysterious-holographic-processing-unit/. Accessed 28 May 2018.
44. Xiao R, Benko H. Augmenting the field-of-view of head-mounted displays with sparse peripheral displays. In: The 2016 CHI Conference. 2016.
45. Exporting and building a unity visual studio solution. [Online]. Available: https://developer.microsoft.com/enus/windows/holographic/exporting_and_building_a_unity_visual_studio_solution. Accessed 28 May 2018.
46. Dumay A, Jense G. Endoscopic surgery simulation in a virtual environment. Comput Biol Med (United States). 1995;25(2):139–48.
47. Knuth TE, Wilson A, Oswald SG. Military training at civilian trauma centers: the first year's experience with the regional trauma network. Mil Med (United States). 1998;163(9):608–41.
48. Hoffman H, Vu D. Virtual reality: teaching tool of the twenty-first century. Acad Med (United States). 1997;72(12):1076–81.
49. Jerant AF, Epperly TD, Marionneaux RD. Medical support for operation cooperative nugget '95': joint readiness training in the post-cold war era. Mil Med (United States). 1997;162(11):702–5.
50. Pickett R. Joint readiness training center integration of live and constructive forces. I/ITSEC (CD-ROM). 1998.
51. McCarthy J, Johnston J, Paris C. Toward development of a tactical decision-making under stress integrated trainer. I/ITSEC (CD-ROM). 1998.
52. Arbor A. An immersive virtual reality platform for medical education: introduction to the medical readiness trainer. In: Proceedings of the 33rd Hawaii International Conference on System Sciences. 2000.
53. Takabayashi K, Fujikawa K, Suzuki T, Yamazakia S, Honda M, Amaral M, Satomura Y, Yoshida S, Tomioka H. Implementation and evaluation of computerized patient management problems. Medinfo (Canada). 1995;8(PT 2):1218–21.
54. Kraft S, Honebein P, Prince M, Marrero D. The SOCRATES curriculum: an innovative integration of technology and theory in medical education. J Audivo Media Med (England). 1997;20(4):166–71.
55. Kreines M, Udal'tsovlu A, Pogromov A, Ershov V, Active AS. Computer systems for medical education: approach and implementation. Vestn Ross Akad Med Nauk (Russia). 1995;10:68–71.
56. Kaltenborn KF, Rienhoff O. Virtual reality in medicine. Methods Inf Med (Germany). 1992;32(5):407–17.
57. Larsson JE, Hayes-Roth B, Gaba DM, Smith BE. Evaluation of a medical diagnosis system using simulator test scenarios. Artif Intell Med (Netherlands). 1997;11(2):119–40.
58. Fairén M, Farrés M, Moyés J, Insa E. Virtual reality to teach anatomy. Eurographics. 2017. Bourdin JJ, Shesh A, editors. 2017; https://doi.org/10.2312/eged.20171026.
59. Dickey M. Brave new (interactive) worlds: a review of the design affordances and constrains of two 3d virtual worlds as interactive learning environments. Interact Learn Environ. 2005;13(1–2):121–37.

60. Kleinginna PR, Kleinginna AM. A categorized list of emotion definitions, with suggestions for a consensual definition. Motiv Emot. 1981;5(4):345–79.
61. Boctor L. Active-learning strategies: the use of a game to reinforce learning in nursing education. A case study. Nurse Educ Pract. 2013;13(2):96–100.
62. Huang H-M, Rauch U, Liaw SS. Investigating learners' attitudes toward virtual reality learning environments: based on a constructivist approach. Comput Educ. 2010;55(3):1171–82.
63. Nicholson DT, Chalk C, Funnell WRJ, Daniel SJ. Can virtual reality improve anatomy education? A randomised controlled study of a computer-generated three-dimensional anatomical ear model. Med Educ. 2006;40(11):1081–7.
64. Codd A, Choudhury B. Virtual reality anatomy: is it comparable with traditional methods in the teaching of human forearm musculoskeletal anatomy? Anat Sci Educ. 2011;4(3):119–25.
65. Pan Z, Cheok AD, Yang H, Zhu J, Shi J. Virtual reality and mixed reality for virtual learning environments. Comput Graph. 2006;30(1):20–8.
66. Vaughan N, Dubey VN, Wainwright TW, Middleton RG. A review of virtual reality based training simulators for orthopaedic surgery. Med Eng Phys. 2016;38:59–71.
67. Aziz HA. Virtual reality programs applications in healthcare. J Health Med Informat. 2018;9:305. https://doi.org/10.4172/2157-7420.1000305.
68. Anderson PL, Price M, Edwards SM, Obasaju MA, Schmertz SK, et al. Virtual reality exposure therapy for social anxiety disorder: a randomized controlled trial. J Consult Clin Psychol. 2013;81:751–60.
69. Parsons TD, Rizzo AA. Affective outcomes of virtual reality exposure therapy for anxiety and specific phobias: a meta-analysis. J Behav Ther Exp Psychiatry. 2008;39:250–61.
70. Weiderhold MD, Weiderhold BK. Virtual reality and interactive simulation for pain distraction. Pain Med. 2007;1:182–8.
71. http://www.iactor.eu/downloads/WP%20The%20Potential%20for%20VR%20to%20Improve%20Healthcare.pdf.
72. Aim F, Lonjon G, Hannouche D, Nizard R. Effectiveness of virtual reality training in orthopaedic surgery. Arthroscopy. 2016;32:224–32.
73. Valmaggia LR, Latif L, Kempton MJ, Ruscalafell M. Virtual reality in the psychological treatment for mental health problems: an systematic review of recent evidence. Psychiatry Res. 2016;236:189–95.
74. Wiederhold MD, Gao K, Wiederhold BK. Clinical use of virtual reality distraction system to reduce anxiety and pain in dental procedures. Cyberpsychol Behav Soc Netw. 2014;17:359–65.
75. Rutter CE, Dahhlquist LM, Weiss KE. Sustained efficacy of virtual reality distraction. J Pain. 2008;10:391–7.
76. Schneider SM, Hood LE. Virtual reality: a distraction intervention for chemotherapy. Oncol Nurs Forum. 2007;34:39–46.
77. Broeren J, Bjorkdahl A. Virtual rehabilitation after stroke. Stud Health Technol Inform. 2008;136:77–82.
78. Girard B, Turcotte V. Crushing virtual cigarettes reduces tobacco addiction and treatment discontinuation. Cyberpsychol Behav. 2009;12:477–83.
79. Shin HH, Kim KM. Virtual reality for cognitive rehabilitation after brain injury: a systematic review. J Phys Ther Sci. 2015;27:2999–3002.
80. Hanna MG, Ahmed I, Nine J, Prajapati S, Pantanowitz L, et al. Virtual reality training for healthcare professionals. Cyberpsychol Behav. 2003;6:389–94.
81. Li A, Montano Z, Chen VJ, Gold JI. Virtual reality and pain management: current trends and future directions. Pain Manag. 2011;1:147–57.
82. Mejiden OA, Schijven MP. The value of haptic feedback in conventional and robotic assisted minimal invasive surgery and virtual reality training: a current review. Surg Endosc. 2009;23:1180–90.
83. Ojha U, Mohammed R, Vivekanantham S. Should there be greater exposure to interventional radiology in the undergraduate curriculum? Adv Med Educ Pract. 2017;8:791–5.
84. Pourmand A, Davis S, Lee D, Barber S, Sikka N. Emerging utility of virtual reality as a multidisciplinary tool in clinical medicine. Games Health J. 2017;6:263–70.

Part V
Mentoring: The Art and Science of Helping Adults Learn

Chapter 21
Mentoring: The Art and Science of Helping Adults Learn

Introduction

By definition, *mentor* is an experienced and trusted adviser, whereas *mentoring* is to support and encourage people to manage their own learning in order that they may maximize their potential, develop their skills, improve their performance and become the person they want to be [1]. "Mentorship" is described as a partnership between two people (mentor and mentee) normally working in a similar field or sharing similar experiences. It is a helpful relationship based upon mutual trust and respect.

The term *mentor* is derived from the Classics, as identified in Homer's Odyssey, where "Mentor", the trusted son of Alimus, was appointed by Ulysses to be tutor-adviser to his son, Telemachus, and guardian of his estates while he was away fighting the Trojan wars. Mentor became more than a guardian, teacher and adviser as he had considerable influence and personal responsibility for the development of the young Telemachus (perhaps only a few are aware that, according to Homer's epic poem, it is not Mentor who fulfilled the duty of advisor and guardian to Odysseus's son Telemachus; rather, it is Pallas Athene, the goddess of wisdom, who took Mentor's form and actually did the job of helping the young man). In concordance, the role of a mentor includes a wide range of skills. Some of these are those of facilitation, assessing and evaluation. Mentors also have to act as effective guides, supervisors and role models. In order to fulfil these roles and demonstrate the required skills, mentors must also be able to plan effectively, be organized, able to motivate as well as demonstrate competent communication skills.

The importance of mentoring in healthcare system is that we are dealing with adult learners. Malcolm Knowles [2], one of the best known theorists in relation to adult learning and adult learners, was the person who developed the concept of andragogy (practice of adult education). Andragogy is based on the assumption that adults differ in a range of ways from children in their approach to learning. As mentors deal generally with adults, it is important for them to be familiar with such concept. In his article, Milligan [3] summarized the key elements of andragogy as

Y. El Miedany, *Rheumatology Teaching*,
https://doi.org/10.1007/978-3-319-98213-7_21

"facilitation of an adult learning that can be best achieved through a student-centred approach, which enhances student's self-concept, promotes autonomy, self-direction and critical thinking, reflects on experience and involves the learner in the diagnosis, planning, enacting and evaluation of their own learning needs".

Traditionally, education in healthcare has been delivered using a predominantly pedagogical approach, i.e. in a teacher-led style with a very passive role played by the students. With the introduction of the andragogical model, and how different it is from the pedagogical teaching approach, there have been calls for changing the adult educational protocols. The andragogical concept assumes that adults become ready to learn when they experience a need to know or do something in order to perform more effectively in aspects of their lives. This will to learn motivates the adult learners to enter an educational activity with a life-centred, task-oriented or problem-focused attitude. This should reflect on the way learning experiences are organized, meaning that the curriculum should be amended to accommodate life situations rather than subject-matter items. From example, courses that might be titled "Composition I", "Composition II" and "Composition III" in a high school curriculum might be changed to be "Writing Medical Letters", "Writing Research" and "Improving Professional Communication" in the adult education programme. Another important implication is the importance of clarifying at the beginning of any learning experience what the relevance to the learner's life tasks, targets or problems is. Hence, one of the first tasks of the mentor as a facilitator is to develop the "need to know" what will be learned. The second task is to identify the "mentee's learning style".

The Science of Mentoring: Identifying the Mentee's Learning Style

The concept of learning facilitation has been increasingly used in educational contexts, advocating a change from the traditional formal teacher–student relationship to that of a more dynamic and interactive partnership between facilitator and a student. The traditional teaching approach (informative teaching) is based on a hierarchical model with the teachers having the position of power because of their knowledge and experience. On the other hand, the modern style of teaching (facilitation) promotes the ideals of sharing and partnership in the learning process where both the student and facilitator work together on a relatively equal basis to maximize the learning experience.

Learning is a lifelong process. It never makes sense to say we have learned all there is to learn or that our learning is complete. However, people vary in their preferred way of learning. Interestingly, most people are unaware of their learning style preferences. They just know vaguely that they feel more comfortable with, and learn more from, some activities than others. It would help if the learning style of the individual person could be identified, as this will reflect and consequently benefit both the mentor and the mentee. Learning styles have been identified as people repeat strategies and tactics they find to be successful and discontinue those that are not. In this way preferences for certain behaviour patterns develop and become habitual. These styles tend to be strengthened as people settle toward careers that are compatible with their preferred modus operandi (particular way or method of doing something). There are four learning styles (Table 21.1): activist, reflector, theorist and pragmatist [4].

Considering the continuous learning cycle, each learning style connects with a learning stage (Fig. 21.1). Activists adopting the approach of "I will try anything once" are well prepared for experiencing; hence come the reflectors with their fondness for contemplating data well prepared for reviewing; following who come the theorists with their need to tidy up and have answers which make them prepared for concluding; and lastly come the pragmatists with their predilection for practicality which make them well prepared for planning.

Table 21.1 The four learning styles

	Activist	Reflector	Theorist	Pragmatist
Character	Involve themselves fully and without bias in new experiences	Stand back to ponder experiences and observe them from many different perspectives	Adapt to integrate observations into complex but logically sound theories	Keen on trying out ideas, theories and techniques to see if they work in practice
Approach	Enjoy the here and now scenario and happy to be dominated by immediate experiences	Collect data, both first hand and from others, and prefer to think about it thoroughly before coming to any conclusion	Think problems through a vertical, step-by-step, logical way	Positively search out new ideas and take the first opportunity to experiment with application
Style	Open minded, not sceptical, which make them enthusiastic about anything new	Postpone reaching definitive conclusions for as long as possible (till he collects info and carry out data analysis)	Tend to be perfectionistic, does not rest easy until things are tidy and fit into a rational scheme	Tend to be impatient with ruminating and open-ended discussions. Like to get on with things and act quickly and confidently on new ideas that attract them
Tacking problems	Tackle problems by brainstorming. Their days are filled with activity. Tend to thrive on the challenge of new experiences but are bored with implementation and longer-term consolidation	They prefer to take a back seat in meetings and discussions. They are thoughtful who like to consider all possible angles and implications before making a move. They tend to adopt a low profile and have a slightly distant, tolerant, unruffled air about them	Their approach to problems is consistently logical. They like to analyse and synthesize. They are keen on keen on basic assumptions, principles, theories, models and systems thinking	They respond to problems and opportunities as a challenge

(continued)

Table 21.1 (continued)

	Activist	Reflector	Theorist	Pragmatist
Dealing with others	They are gregarious people constantly involving themselves with others, but in doing so, they seed to centre all activities on themselves	They listen to others and get the drift of the discussion before making their own points. When they act, it is part of a wide picture which includes the past, the present as well as others' observations as well as their own	They prefer to maximize certainty and feel uncomfortable with subjective judgements, lateral thinking and anything flippant	They are essentially practical, down-to-earth people who like making practical decisions and solving problems
Philosophy	I will try anything once	Be cautious	It is logical, it is good	There is always a better way, and if it works it's good

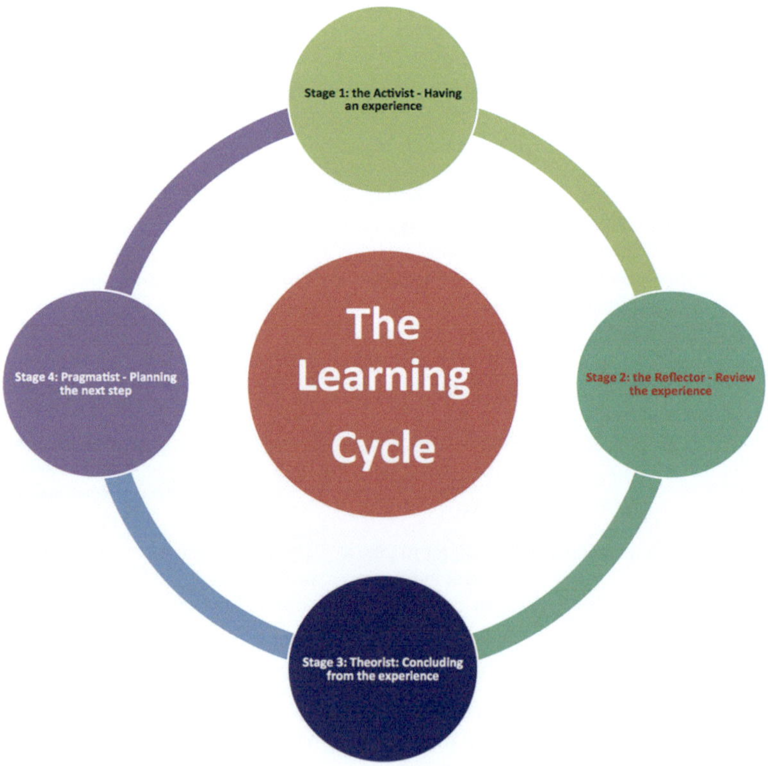

Fig. 21.1 The learning cycle: the links between learning styles and the different stages in the cycle

Mentoring, Coaching and Sponsorship

Considerable confusion exists about mentoring, coaching and sponsorship. Many people refer to coaching and mentoring interchangeably. While both processes provide personalized professional development, require special interpersonal skills and have a significant impact on an individual's career, there are some important distinctions between them. Coaching is also distinct from sponsorship, which is an advanced form of mentoring. On the other hand, the supervising process gives the supervisor authority or "positional power" over the mentee. This is a major characteristic for the supervisor, as the mentor may guide, suggest and coach but does not use power to direct actions. Figure 21.2 shows basic difference between the four items which will be discussed in the following section:

Coaching

Coaching is functional and result oriented and deals mainly with performance. Coaching helps someone become more productive and effective at a specific set of functions, tasks or practices. Therefore, coaching is more commonly seen in sports where a coach helps the individual identify and set goals in a particular area (or function) and develop a plan to achieve those goals. Then the coach gives the person the support while implementing the plan and helps to keep him/her remain disciplined and focused and consequently achieve the desired targets.

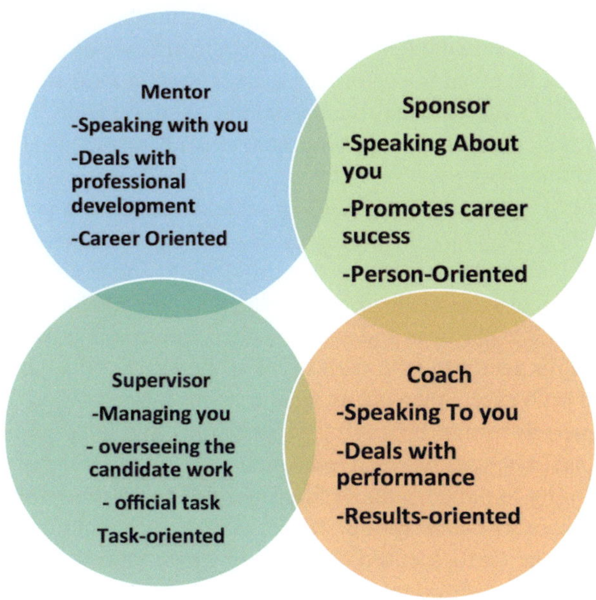

Fig. 21.2 Mentorship, coaching, supervising and sponsorship

Mentors, sponsors and supervisors might all act as coaches when they help someone improve performance or set career goals. In medical career, coaching plays an important role in the undergraduate as well as postgraduate career. Coaching is usually played by the clinical and educational supervisors and can be stratified into one of three categories: undergraduate as well as junior doctors who want to optimize their skills and clinical abilities, postgraduate doctors who want to achieve their highest level of performance and lastly the underperforming doctors who are in need to improve their performance or change certain behaviours in order to stay on track. With the expanding role of medical management in the standard practice, a large and growing number of coaches today help partners and some high-potential associates with areas like business management programmes, leadership development and leadership optimization. Hospitals also provide coaching courses in areas like communication and presentation skills, time and work management as well as team management.

Mentoring vs Supervision

Mentoring is broader, in both scope and purpose, than coaching. It differs from coaching in being more meaningful and partnership- and career-oriented. Mentoring also varies from supervision. One of the major differences between supervision/advising and mentoring is that the supervision is often task-oriented (e.g., completion of a thesis or dissertation), whereas mentoring is more about caring for an individual's long-term development. A primary aim in the mentoring relationship is for the mentee to become independent of the mentor. The supervisor/supervised relationship by its nature is interdependent. Furthermore, while the supervisor is responsible for managing the on-the-job performance of the supervised person, the mentor is not involved in performance assessment/appraisal. Mentoring covers more wide-ranging career issues than coaching or supervision, because it deals with mentees' overall professional development and advancement, not simply performance goals. Although mentor and mentee might spend time on improving performance, the relationship usually expands to larger and longer-term personal and professional career issues. Mentors often employ coaching or supervision as one of their tools, along with confidence building, role modelling, counselling and advocacy.

Within the medical career, mentors are predominantly senior consultants with greater experience and expertise than mentees. In other scenarios, peer-peer mentorship is set up to help with some of the basic skills which require closer mentoring. In both cases, they act as mentors both informally in the usual course of work and through formal mentoring programmes that have particular objectives and guidelines. They are not paid to be mentors; it is expected of them as part of their responsibility to the hospital. Mentoring is also important for career advancement. Unlike coaching or supervising, mentoring has a role in knowledge transfer and skill development, (skill-focused coaching or supervision is an exception). Mentoring, therefore, plays an important and direct role in helping training doctors become better, more highly skilled practitioners. Because they have relevant work and career experience, mentors are more likely than coaches or supervisors to use their own experiences, insights and advice to help the mentee learn and progress. Coaches can help training doctors create a plan that calls for developing certain skills and getting certain work experience, but mentors can teach and model the specified medical skills and create the work opportunities needed to achieve those goals.

Another reason mentors are so valuable is that they have good experience about the decision-making processes and managerial dynamics. Most significantly, being themselves trained as part of the medical service, mentors can transmit the medical values, culture and professionalism to younger healthcare professionals and future leaders.

Sponsorship

A sponsor is a strong advocate who has power and influence and uses that advocacy to produce positive career results. Sponsors publicly endorse the trainers' qualifications and take risks on their behalf, arguing that the person should move up to a higher compensation tier or urging their partners that he/she is ready for equity partnership or a significant leadership position. They also alert the person to opportunities and appointments to key posts. Sometimes they call in favour, put pressure on colleagues or put their reputation and credibility on the line for the person. Partners become sponsors when they perceive special value in a specific candidate and actively help him/her advance. It can occur for any number of reasons: they might see the candidate as a natural successor, as having rainmaking potential that could benefit them or as having expertise necessary to support their clients. Sponsors and champions may not guarantee success, but they make it easier and improve the person's chances of receiving a coveted leadership appointment, a fatter pay check or a new client.

Talking about modern sponsorship, it is basically mentoring at the highest level. Sponsorship is the same as the traditional concept of mentorship: a prominent and wise individual takes the candidate under his wing, supports and protects and promotes his/her career success. Current conversations about sponsorship call attention to these traditional notions of how powerful people can help others succeed in any organization. They also direct attention to a critical factor in sponsorship: the sponsor must be someone with power who purposefully champions the others' career.

Mentor Selection: The Good Versus the Bad

Just as there is no single characterisation for a mentor, there is no single personality type. However, it is clear that successful mentors characterize by having a wide range of enabling strategies, innovative ideas and skills within the mentoring relationships [5]. In considering who would be a good mentor and who might not, it is important to consider the behaviours, abilities and characteristics of those who will

Table 21.2 : Good vs bad mentors

Good mentor	Bad mentor
Motivating	*Quarterly*
Motivates individuals to set their own agenda for working or learning	Difficult to find or not accessible
	Pushing people into new role
Encourage creativity and risk taking in learning and working	Leave them to "sink or swim" strategy
Advising	*Blocker*
Advises, counsel and guides on personal, professional and career matters	Avoid meeting the others' needs by:
	The refuser: refusing requests
Assists the mentee to learn through their success and failures	The withholder: controlling through withholding information.
Develop capabilities by offering constructive feedback	The hoverer: arresting development by over supervising
Enabling	*Destroyer/criticiser*
Recognizes and supports the mentee strengths	Set out to destroy others by
Provides safe opportunities for critical reflection and professional capabilities	The underminer: subtle attacks to undermine confidence
Challenging and acts as a critical friend	The nagger: constant put downs and question abilities
Helps identify resources for learning and career socialization	The belittler: open approaches of verbal attack and argument to deliberately destroy confidence
Is an effective role model	**Is a disabling model**

be suitable for providing this role. The concept is to be a role model and be able to impose positive thinking and strategies in order to assist the educators and practitioners in making a sound selection. In contrast, in examining the nature of supportive roles, it is vital to reflect on the less positive aspects of human nature that can have a detrimental effect on others. Having identified individuals who have "disabling" behaviour or having "negative minds" (examples are the rigid mind, the ego mind and the Machiavellian mind) would help in setting up the proper mentors' team. Table 21.2 summarizes the galaxy of the good versus the bad mentors.

The Dynamic Nature of Mentoring

Mentoring is an exciting complex phenomenon that aims at benefitting individuals within a sharing partnership [6]. In the classical sense, it is much more than "the experienced guidance of the inexperienced". Mentoring is a dynamic and exciting process; not only is this attributed to its multi-coloured nature but also to its relatively complex concept. Mentoring involves the building of a dynamic relationship in which the personal characteristics, philosophies and priorities of the individual members interact to influence the nature, direction and duration of the resulting partnership (Fig. 21.3). Therefore, a mentoring

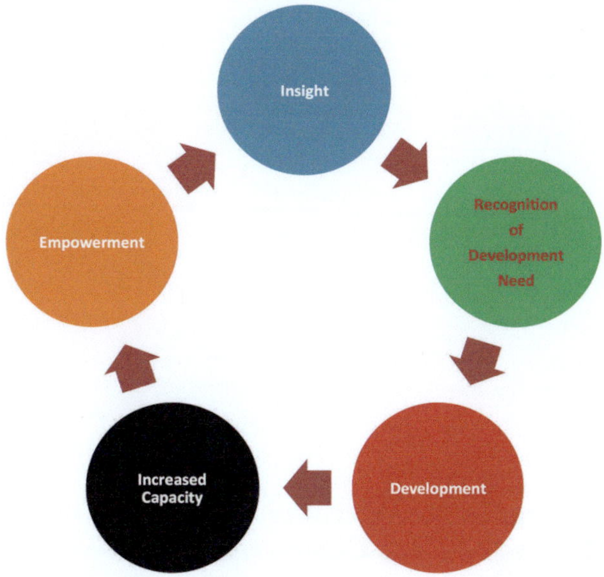

Fig. 21.3 The dynamic nature of mentoring: the mentorship cycle

relationship is one that is enabling, cultivating as well as empowering an individual within the working environment. However, it is important to clarify that a mentor is not a prerequisite for advancement or success as such events regularly occur without access to this type of significant helper. Also, it is important to acknowledge that mentors do not have that magic wand or power to fashion great individuals. However, knowing that there is someone out there willing to offer support and encouragement, endorsing the mentee's ability to come to terms with the assigned role in the organization or professional setting, in turn, enhances the mentee's self-development, self-awareness and personal fulfilment.

Individual selection of who can be a mentor is a vital process of classical mentoring as the relationship between the mentee and the mentor is dependent on the joint, dynamic, sharing characteristics of both parties for its nature and success. This relationship goes in three main phases: initiation, development and termination [7] (Fig. 21.4). The initiation phase involves the choosing process and "getting to know each other". The working phase is the main focus for individual development. The dynamics of the mentoring relationship are maintained by the interactions of both the mentor and mentee. As increasing trust as well as closeness start to build up, sharing becomes evident, and the mentee is more readily able to choose the specific helper functions that are best suited to his/her needs. The third and last stage is the "termination phase" where the mentee begins to act on his/her initiative and is in a position to begin to act independently. The termination phase can end positively as supportive friendship or negatively where there is a conflict or emotional tension or general dissatisfaction [8].

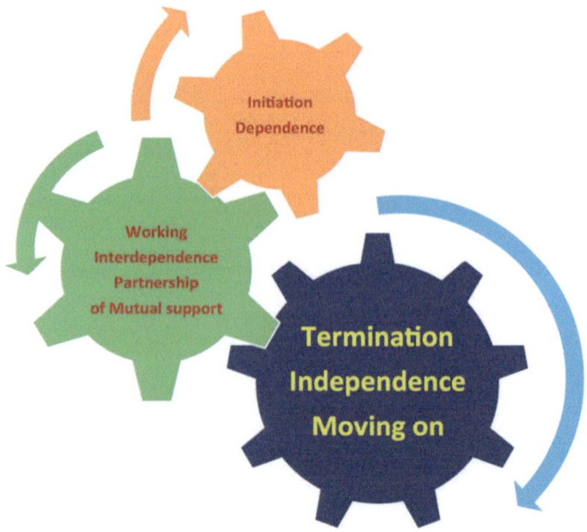

Fig. 21.4 The dynamic nature of mentoring: the three mentoring phases and the degree of dependence

Change in the Educational Tactics: Moving Toward Student-Centred Approach

In the past years, the teacher-centred approach has been the standard in the clinical education. This approach relies on direct instructional techniques and a subject orientation. The knowledge and skills to be acquired are identified by the teacher. Similarly, the evaluation is set in relation to criteria specified by a faculty [9]. On the other hand, a student-centred approach describes collaboration between students and the teacher, where educational goals and the means to achieve the goals are determined through discussion and deliberation [10]. Although the faculty define the outcome objectives to be achieved, there is much opportunity for individual earning within the broad confines of the specified objectives. Knowles [11] described the shift of the teaching-centred to the student-centred approach as a strategy in which a "content plan" is replaced by a "process plan". Meaning that instead of specifying how a body of content will be transmitted (content plan), it specifies how a body of content will be acquired by the learner (process plan). The roles of the student and teacher must shift when learning plans are introduced. The teacher becomes the facilitator of self-directed learning and content resource. The student assumes an active role in selecting objectives for learning from the pre-identified course topics and programme objectives. The outcomes for the students include expanded participation in planning learning experiences and enhanced ability for resource selection and acquisition. This comes in concordance with increased skill in self-evaluation of current performance levels. Additional benefits are increase in assertiveness and confidence that follows from the changed view of self and the modified relationships with teachers.

Rethinking Our Mentoring: Traditional Versus Modern Mentoring

Traditionally, what one would tend to think of as mentoring is a one-on-one relationship between people with differing levels of experience. However, considering the future, it is important to understand what tomorrow's leaders look like today. "Millennials" is the title given to the estimated 80–95 million future workers and leaders, born between approximately 1980 and 2000. These Millennials will dominate the workforce for the next 40 years. Millennials: the "Me Me Me" Generation are characterized by being tech-savvy, creative problem-solvers and advice seekers who are masters of the art of multi-tasking. Stephen Bell [12] discussed the Millennial generation and newer professionals seeking nontraditional relationships.

Peer-to-Peer Mentoring

Though it appears as a closely related shape to traditional mentoring, peer-to-peer model seems a good alternative. While it is based on a one-on-one relationship, often the participants are at a more similar level of experience. Similar to the model described by Kuyper-Rushing [13], the model described by Level and Mach [14] is meant to support people in the tenure process. The difference is that the people involved are at a more peer level, instead of a senior to junior level. This type of arrangement may help to ease some discomfort the mentee might feel when dealing with senior mentor, by offering a mutual coaching toward a common goal.

Cohorts

If the traditional model got mixed with the peer-to-peer model, a cohort would emerge. In this structure, there is a group of peers working together, learning from each other, and one or more people with more experience to guide the group. Mullen [15] called these "knowledgeable facilitators". A class setting is one manifestation of this programme. In an article by Mullen and Tuten [16], they used a case study of doctoral students working on a thesis. The students receive support from each other and the dissertation advisor while still working independently.

Sponsorship

The mentoring function has changed over time and has branched into two distinct types of relationship: mentoring and sponsorship. While "mentoring" relationship provides the learner with psychosocial support, "sponsorship" involves proactive instrumental help to advance a person's career [17–19]. A sponsor is someone whom the mentee seeks out, usually as a resource to a specific outcome. Golden [20] mentioned that sponsors act as a role model, cheerleader or potential door opener in a career path. While the evidence is clear that sponsorship leads to more positive career outcomes than mentoring, there are challenges in both types of support relationship. However, early experiences with most sponsorship programmes showed the need for very careful pairings and oversight [21]. Although similar to other mentoring programmes, sponsorship demands more of mentors and requires more focused effort from those being sponsored and considerable ongoing involvement by programme coordinators.

Virtual Mentorship: The Art of Modern Mentoring

"Virtual mentoring" simply refers to any mentoring activity that does not take place face to face. With today's technology there is a suite of communication tools open to this style of mentoring, including Skype, telephone, email and messaging. For candidates whose workforce is widely dispersed, or those who work in a fast-moving high-tech environment, virtual mentoring can be one of the best options available. A virtual programme has some clear advantages, for example, the ability to provide mentoring access to anyone anytime and open mentoring to people working in remote locations, who would not otherwise have access to a mentor. Participants in virtual programmes appreciate the flexibility of virtual mentoring, where there is no need to travel to an agreed meeting place or contact can be maintained even when one party is away from their usual workplace.

In a review of "e-mentoring" literature, Thompson et al. [22] noted that electronic communication forms were reported to have some advantages over traditional face-to-face mentoring. Electronic media such as email can mitigate against social cues such as status getting in the way of mentoring relationships. Being an asynchronous medium, communication by email also allows both mentor and mentee to frame and consider answers to questions rather than have to provide solutions in real time.

Some of the disadvantages of virtual mentoring are obvious. While there is a rapidly growing industry in "cyber coaching" which demonstrates that coaching relationships can be built without the richness of face-to-face interaction, some people nevertheless find it difficult to build rapport using telephone, teleconferencing, email or text. Zey [23] noted that in virtual relationships, some mentoring activities, like shadowing (where the mentee physically follows and observes the mentor in action), role modelling and attending events together, cannot be used. Thompson et al. [22], as well as Houck et al. [24], also suggested that engagement and persistence can be problematic in virtual relationships. It appears that it is easier to walk away from a "virtual" relationship than a face-to-face one.

Mentoring the Next Generation for Innovation in Today's Society

Thriving organizations recognize that every member leads and follows, directs and innovates, responds and creates in the context of relationships. It is possible that the single most important step organizational leaders can take is to ensure that their followers do not find it difficult or dangerous to innovate. Involving every member of the organization in mentoring relationships may decrease risk and increase innovation. Furthermore, it will strengthen relationships, trust and the creative environment.

To plan for the future, we need to understand what tomorrow's leaders look like today. In an innovation preparedness survey, 92% of traditionalists (which comprises employees and retirees born between 1922 and 1943), Boomers (born mostly following World War II, roughly between 1954 and 1964. The term is typically used to refer to the later years of the Baby boomer cohort) and Xers (born between 1965 and 1979) ranked the Millennials (which is a "crossover generation", born roughly between 1975 and 1985 plus or minus a few years till early years of 2000), as "high", for their ability to create and innovate [25]. Millennials are natural innovators. They just want the opportunity to do meaningful work and have a high quality of life. This is in contrast with older generations who tend to want job security, benefits, rank or prestige [26]. With several millions of Millennials currently in the workforce, there is a lot of "creative friction" requiring leaders to develop styles that focus on identifying and effectively incorporating the polarized viewpoints of employees. In a study, 50% of workers polled believe they could manage better than boss, given the opportunity [27]. Intergenerational attitudes contribute to misunderstandings in the workplace. Retention is especially difficult since Millennials have different attitudes and expectations toward work than previous generations. Reports that 66% of Millennials expect to change careers can impact negatively on the investment their superiors wish to make in them, in comparison to 84% of Boomers expect to work at their current job for the rest of their lives [28]. Mentoring relationships help intergenerational colleagues recognize and address differing perceptions about the workplace and opportunities to innovate within it.

Targeted Mentoring Model

Innovation happens in the context of relationships. They are internal and external. These relationships are with superiors, juniors and colleagues as well as in between organizations. Targeted mentoring model might be the bridge crossing over the hurdles, enhancing the relationships and consequently innovations. One longitudinal field experiment examined how a targeted mentorship programme that unfolded over 6 months boosted the development of candidates' leader efficacy and performance. Targeted mentoring was compared to leadership education delivered in a group setting. Results demonstrated that targeted mentorship intervention increased apprentice level of leader efficacy to a great degree than those participating in group training programmes [29].

The 3D Mentoring Relationship

An organization that values people recognizes each person has something to offer. Millennials are not the only members of the workforce in need of mentoring. Every employee and manager benefits from mentoring. This inclusive model recommends every member of the organization become involved in three mentoring relationships. While the model proposes to involve every organizational member in mentoring relationships, the focus here will be on benefits to the organization. Soft skills dominate the list of essential competencies for today's workplace. These include: "interpersonal and intrapersonal knowledge; skills and abilities such as ethics, personal organization and work habits; time management; teamwork and interpersonal communication; anger management; reasoning and problem solving; and managing one's learning. Mentors help younger and less experienced workers develop such skills in their personal and professional lives. These older, wiser mentors are often called "Wise Guides". Millennials show a strong need to connect their work to a higher purpose. Discussing the vision, mission, goals and direction of the organization helps new hires or members see themselves in relation to the overall direction of the organization. To cultivate Millennovators will require organization-wide involvement in a 3D mentoring relationship.

In conclusion, mentoring is the best approach to equip the healthcare professionals as well as managers with the necessary skills and knowledge enabling them to lead in complex environments. It's a low-cost and extremely effective way to prepare future leaders early on. Mentoring is as simple as a gentle push in the right direction. It's also an easy way to preserve the intangible assets of any hospital or organization – the minds and capabilities of the key young people who are the future face of any brand. Mentoring increases retention of the best and brightest, builds a reservoir of talent, speeds employee growth and shortens the learning cycle. It also engenders loyalty.

References

1. Parsloe E. Coaching & mentoring: practical conversations to improve learning. London: Kogan Page Ltd.; 2009.
2. Knowles M. Andragogy in action: applying modern principles of adult learning. San Francisco: Jossey-Bass; 1984.
3. Milligan F. In defence of andragogy. Nurse Educ Today. 1995;15:22–7.
4. Honey P, Mumford A. Setting the scene for learning styles. In: Downie C, Basford P, editors. Chapter 17 in mentoring for practice. London: The university of Greenwich; 2003. p. 241.
5. Anderson, Shannon. Towards a conceptualization of mentoring. In: Kerry A, Shelton M, editors. Issues in mentoring. London: Routledge; 1995.
6. Palmer E. The nature of the mentor. Unpublished thesis. South Bank Polytechnic, London; 1987.
7. Earnshaw G. Mentorship: the student's views. Nurse Educ Today. 1995;15:274–9.
8. Blotnick S. With friends like these. Savvy. 1984;10:45–52.
9. Bevis E, Watson. Toward a caring curriculum: a new pedagogy for nursing. New York: National League for Nursing; 1989.
10. Miller J, Seller W. Curriculum: perspectives and practice. Mississauga: Copp, Lark Pittman; 1990.
11. Knowles M. Using learning contracts, vol. 39. San Francisco: Jossey-Bass; 1986.
12. Bell S. The next generation may not want your mentoring. Leading from the library. Academic Newswire 2013. Link: http://lj.libraryjournal.com/2013/04/opinion/leading-from-the-library/the-next-generation-may-not-want-your-mentoring-leading-from-the-library/#_. Accessed 25 Jan 2018.
13. Kuyper-Rushing L. A formal mentoring program in a university library: components of a successful experiment. J Acad Librariansh. 2001;27(6):440–6. https://doi.org/10.1016/S0099-1333(01)00258-0.
14. Level AV, Mach M. Peer mentoring: one institution's approach to mentoring academic librarians. Libr Manag. 2005;26(6/7):301–10. https://doi.org/10.1108/01435120410609725
15. Mullen CA. Naturally occurring student-faculty mentoring relationships. In: Allen TD, Eby LT, editors. The Blackwell handbook of mentoring a multiple perspectives approach: Wiley-Blackwell; 2010. p. 119–38. http://tinyurl.com/p5cpw7r.
16. Mullen CA, Tuten EM. Doctoral cohort mentoring interdependence, collaborative learning, and cultural change. Scholar Pract Q. 2010;4(1):11–32. http://files.eric.ed.gov/fulltext/EJ942494.pdf
17. Kammeyer-Mueller JD, Judge TA. A quantitative review of mentoring research: test of a model. J Vocat Behav. 2008;72:269–83.
18. Allen TD, Eby LT, O'Brien KE, Lenz E. The state of mentoring research: a qualitative review of current research methods and future research implications. J Vocat Behav. 2008;73:343–57.
19. Downing RA, Crosby FJ, Blake-Beard S. The perceived importance of developmental relationships on women undergraduates' pursuit of science. Psychol Women Q. 2005;29:419–26.
20. Golden J. Mentoring as a career strategy for mid-level public library managers: a selective review of literature involving methodology and cross-disciplines. Libr Philos Pract. 2012:841–54. http://digitalcommons.unl.edu/cgi/viewcontent.cgi?article=1945&context=libphilprac.
21. Chynoweth C. Take me to your sponsor. Sunday Times, London; 2012.
22. Thompson L, Jeffries M, Topping K. E-mentoring for e-learning development. Innov Educ Teach Int. 2010;47(3):305–15.
23. Zey M. Virtual mentoring: the challenges and opportunities of electronically mediated formal mentor programs. Rev Bus Res. 2011;11(4):141–52.
24. Houck C. Multigenerational and virtual: how do we build a mentoring program for today's workforce? Perform Improv. 2011;50(2):25–30.

25. Lancaster LC, Stillman D. The M-factor: how the millennial generation is rocking the workplace. New York: Harper Collins; 2010. p. 103.
26. Schiffmann E, Tambe N, Gelles M, Azaroff R, Goldfarb E, Siemon H. Deloitte millennial model. An approach to Gen Y readiness. Deloitte Development LLC 2010: 3. Retrieved from: http://www.deloitte.com/assets/Dcom-UnitedStates/Local%20Assets/Documents/Federal/us_fed_DeloitteMillennialModelAnapproachtoGenYReadiness%20_112410.pdf.
27. Gryskiewicz SS. Positive turbulence: developing climates for creativity, innovation, renewal, vol. 346. Jossey-Bass: San Francisco; 1999.
28. Moon T. Mentoring the next generation for innovation in Today's organization. J Strateg Leadersh. 2014;5(1):23–35.
29. Lester PB, Hannah ST, Harms PD, Vogelgesang GR, Avolio BJ. Mentoring impace on leader efficacy development: a field experiment. Management Department Faculty Publications 80. 2011: 409. http://digitalcommons.unl.edu/managementfacpub/80.

Chapter 22
Mentoring in Rheumatology

Introduction

Mentoring is defined as "the process whereby an experienced, highly regarded, empathic person (the mentor), guides another individual (the mentee) in the development and re-examination of their own ideas, learning, personal as well as professional development" [1]. Effective mentoring, as reported by residents, research faculty and residency programme directors, plays an important role in the career of physicians, particularly during residency/specialty training, and is a key to career development of research faculty in clinical translational science [2–6].

Because individuals may experience mentoring at various life stages, it is not surprising that there are three distinct streams of mentoring scholarship: youth mentoring, academic mentoring and workplace mentoring. Youth mentoring involves a relationship between a caring, supportive adult and a child or adolescent [7]. Youth mentoring assumes that supportive relationships with adults are important for personal, emotional, cognitive and psychological growth [7, 8]. Academic mentoring typifies the apprentice model of education where a faculty member imparts knowledge, provides support and offers guidance to a student protégé on academic (e.g. classroom performance) as well as nonacademic (e.g. personal problems, identity issues) issues [9]. This type of mentoring may facilitate psychological adjustment and foster a sense of professional identity [10]. Finally, workplace mentoring occurs in an organizational setting, and the purpose is the personal and professional growth of the protégé [11]. The mentor may be a supervisor, someone else within the organization but outside the protégé's chain of command, or an individual in another organization [12].

Y. El Miedany, *Rheumatology Teaching*,
https://doi.org/10.1007/978-3-319-98213-7_22

Mentoring in Medicine

Mentoring has been shown to contribute to an individual's career development in academic medicine, clinical and non-clinical aspects [13–17], medical research [16, 18], career satisfaction [17] and perceived institutional support [15–19]. Academically, the mentoring process provides a means by which junior faculty can develop professional academic skills including career management, knowledge about academic medicine and collegial networking [15, 17]. Clinical mentoring is a critical approach to medical training, as it provides a bridge between didactic training and independent clinical practice. Clinical mentoring enables healthcare professionals to practice new skills in clinical settings with the support and guidance of a more specialized and experienced clinician. Intensive, practical medical training is important given the diversity of illnesses and its associated comorbidities as well as the complexity of the recently introduced medical therapies. Mentoring in research may be particularly important to new medical faculty, who often find themselves inadequately prepared for academic careers [20, 21].

The changing nature of the current healthcare environment, increased clinical and administrative responsibilities, reductions in time and collegial support for scholar activity and teaching [21] as well as lack of access to mentors can hinder faculty scholar productivity [19] and career satisfaction [22–24] and may result in attrition from academia [20]. Currently, 37–47% of physicians have reported feeling burnout [25–28]. Effective mentoring may help faculty handle these challenges and reduce their risk for burnout. Different models of mentoring are available, with each having its advantage and disadvantages (Table 22.1). Medical mentoring by itself is a good example of mentoring implementation in real-life practice. The coming section will discuss different categories of medical mentoring, its targets and the challenges it may face.

Table 22.1 Medical mentoring models

One-to-one	Team mentoring	Multiple mentors	Peer mentoring	Distance mentoring
Is individualized and personal	A mentee assembles his or her team of research investigators The mentee and mentors meet jointly as a team	The mentee has more than one mentor, and the mentors meet individually with the mentee	Involves mentoring by colleagues who are at a similar point in their career or are maybe a year or two ahead of the mentee	Mentoring via e-mail, supplemented by telephone calls and occasional visits Can be highly effective for mentees with mentors at different institutions

Table 22.1 (continued)

One-to-one	Team mentoring	Multiple mentors	Peer mentoring	Distance mentoring
Wonderful for developing a close relationship	Best approach for basic, clinical and translational research	While some of the benefits of team mentoring are lost, this method may be easier to manage, given busy schedules and the possibility that mentors are located across the country	less formal and less inhibiting than other mentoring models	Mentees to look outside their institution to find an external expert This is especially true if a particular area of expertise is needed and is not represented within the institution Other reasons for seeking an external mentor, include broadening networking possibilities and increasing contacts with others in the field
Offers only one point of view May not meet the mentee's needs if the mentor is not well versed in all of the mentee's areas of interest	This model has benefits for everyone The mentors can discover new colleagues with whom to collaborate The mentee has access to different points of view and to discussions among more senior investigators, and issues regarding conflicting advice or demands can be negotiated without the mentee feeling pulled in different directions	Having ready access to multiple mentors from different disciplines can be an ideal source of advice and guidance for a mentee on a complex research project such as: A phase 1 clinical trial with a fast-moving pace A project that requires a mentee to have several research specialists and program staff with expertise in a diverse array of fields A project in which a basic scientist is now adding a translational research component to the research portfolio and needs to learn about regulatory and statistical issues not previously encountered	Can provide important advice and guidance about negotiating in the academic world and about mentoring relationships, and this advice can be effective, but it is not sufficient as the only mentoring model Nothing can replace having one or more senior investigators work with the junior investigator and help him or her move towards a successful career as an independent investigator	Distance mentoring can be a convenient way to work with a mentor or mentee E-mails may not be the best effective communication tool and comes with a risk element If the message is not carefully written, recipients can misunderstand the message or its tone and react in a way that is not expected by the writer If a relationship has already been established between mentor and mentee, this method of mentoring may be more effective

Academic Mentoring

Academic medicine is traditionally conceived of having three main roles: teaching, service and research. These roles are changing: academic medicine still has the primary responsibility for training doctors; research remains a core role, but a major part of it is being done in institutes of biotechnology and biomedicine, whereas, most clinical service, even in academic centres, is now provided by nonacademic doctors. Traditionally academic medicine was limited to tertiary medical centres/university hospitals; however, modern evidence-based medicine has been revitalized between these three roles, and academic medicine has now extended into primary care as well as public health. The traditional "clinical service" has been reframed more broadly as "service to the health system and the patient" [29].

What Is Academic Mentoring?

Choosing your career path is a difficult one. Doing it on your own is even more difficult. Having someone to talk to and share your concerns/challenges/ideas with can be extremely beneficial, this simplify what is academic mentoring. Academic mentoring is to support the professional development of academics in their careers and to promote excellence in teaching and learning, research as well as academic leadership. In academic medicine, mentoring has an important influence on personal development, career guidance, career choice and research productivity [30]. Academic mentoring is confidential and entirely voluntary and is a partnership built upon trust and mutual respect.

Targets of Academic Mentoring

Academic mentors helped mentees flourish in the challenging environment of academic medicine by offering them emotional and moral support, working to build their personal and professional abilities and providing them with backing and protection in their academic institutions. Personal inadequacies and relational problems were identified as the main barriers to mentoring, but structural constraints such as lack of time or incentive sometimes hindered the development of functional mentoring relationships.

The Complexity of Academic Mentorship

Mentoring in academic medicine is perceived as a uniquely encompassing relationship. Considering some of the mentoring actions (such as helping the mentee to clarify feelings, motivating and fostering self-reflection) reflects the high-quality nature of the mentoring relationship. Such high level of personal involvement and commitment is required and meant to affect not only the professional but also the personal lives of the mentor as well as the mentee. The relational and reciprocal outcomes such as personal growth, interdependence and connectedness invite further exploration, especially as these types of mentoring outcomes in academic medicine have been under investigated [31].

Considering mentoring in academic medicine as a complex phenomenon mandates certain requirement to achieve its targets. Mentoring is inextricably situated in a social context and shaped by the institutional culture and climate. Successful mentoring therefore requires both commitment and interpersonal skills of mentor and mentee and also a facilitating environment of the academic medicine's institutions. Academic institutions interested in developing mentorship strategies should respect the nature of mentoring relationships, which include professional, career-related and private aspects. Future research should focus more on the separation and redefinition of mentoring relationship phases and the use a variety of qualitative methodologies and approaches to expand and deepen the body of knowledge about this important, yet elusive phenomenon [32].

Clinical Mentoring

Considered as the one of the most traditional styles of teaching in clinical medicine, clinical mentoring offers clinicians a structured and proven pathway to expand their skills, overcome obstacles and build on their strengths to make positive choices and develop their practical and business skills. Clinical mentoring seeks to strengthen district healthcare systems by providing continuing education to healthcare workers and working towards creating more efficient clinical settings. Clinical mentoring involves relationship building, identifying areas for improvement, coaching and modelling.

What Is Clinical Mentoring?

Clinical mentorship is a system of practical training and consultation that fosters ongoing professional development to yield sustainable high-quality clinical care outcomes. Clinical mentors need to be experienced, practising clinicians, with strong teaching skills.

Mentoring should be part of the continuum of the education process aiming at the creation of competent healthcare providers. It should be integrated with and immediately follow initial training, which is usually case based and participatory, based on the principles of adult learning. Mentoring is an integral part of the continuing education process taking place at the centres where healthcare professionals manage patients. It starts at the point where the initial training ends.

Viewed in this way, there should be no conflict between the local "trainer" at the district or regional levels and the clinical mentor. Often someone at the district level is assigned to coordinate or teach healthcare professionals using a standardized training curriculum. The "trainer" provides the educational foundation for the continuing education process and should work closely with the clinical mentor to coordinate activities whether in a district or region facilities [33].

Targets of Clinical Mentoring

The objectives of clinical mentoring should be clear to both the mentor and mentee to secure achieving the desired outcomes. These include supporting decentralized delivery of clinical medical care and patient management, in addition to maintaining and progressively improving the quality of clinical care. Clinical mentoring should also aim at building the capacity of first- and second-level providers to manage unfamiliar or complicated or referring them whenever appropriate. It should also support the application of classroom learning into standard clinical care and facilitate improving the healthcare workers' motivation by providing effective nonclinical support.

Clinical Supervision vs Clinical Mentoring

Clinical supervision is one of the most critical components of capacity building. Clinical supervision can be implemented in different ways depending on a number of factors such as: the type of clinical area, the culture of the organization, staffing ratios and the needs of the staff as well as the management. There is no one way to do clinical supervision, but there are a few principles which make it different from the clinical mentorship. Clinical supervision allows a person to focus on a particular aspect of their clinical practice in a way that they would not normally do. It is characterized by reflection on previous action and its implications for future action. To be able to do this, the clinical supervisor will often challenge the candidate to think outside of their current ways of working. The clinical supervisor will also offer support and advice to help the supervisee learn alternative ways of working and doing specific skills. Briefly, the clinical supervisor will be interested in the quality of the supervisee's performance and will offer constructive feedback and guidance [34].

Clinical supervision focuses on the conditions required for proper functioning of the clinic and clinical team. Are the key requirements for medical care and management prepared and ready? Is an adequate process of case management in place? Clinical supervision aims at improving the quality of medical care and treatment service delivery through joint observation, discussion and direct problem-solving, mentoring and learning from each of the topics observed and discussed as well as planning the way forward.

Although clinical mentoring and clinical supervision overlap considerably, the activities are different enough so that they will probably be implemented by different teams. Clinical mentoring focuses on the professional development of healthcare workers; clinical mentors need to be experienced, practising clinicians. Clinical supervisory is usually targeted to focused tasks and does not have the time or experience to be effective clinical mentors. Therefore, clinical mentoring and supportive supervision are complementary activities that are both necessary to build a professional system of medical care.

Medical Research Mentoring

Interest in global health has increased dramatically over the past decade among health profession trainees, including students and graduates of schools of medicine, public health, dentistry, nursing and veterinary medicine [35, 36]. Today, more and more trainees perform international research electives with the intention of dedicating their careers to underserved populations.

What Is Medical Research Mentorship?

Medical mentoring involves an engaged "mentor" who takes interest in a trainee's development. This role is critically vital for the success of that trainee's clinical research career. In clinical research, mentoring typically encompasses a number of functions and relationships, including counselling, advice, career guidance, discipline and teaching. The most commonly used definition of mentoring in medicine is from the Standing Committee on Postgraduate Medical and Dental Education (SCOPME):

> An experienced highly regarded empathic person (the mentor) guides another individual (the trainee) in the development and re-examination of his or her own ideas, learning, personal and professional development. [37]

Targets of Clinical Research Mentoring

According to SCOPME, mentors should support the trainee's career development, challenge the trainee to acquire or hone skills and foster the trainee's vision of career goals [38]. Characteristics of effective clinical research mentors include availability, insightful comments and critiques of clinical research and career activities and opportunities for trainees to develop independent clinical research careers.

The National Academy of Sciences published a practical guide to mentoring students in sciences entitled "Advisor, teacher, role model, friend: On being a mentor in science and engineering" [39]. This guide states that for trainees to pass the transition phase towards successful independent research careers, mentoring should provide an introduction to the clinical and research environments, assist with integration into the clinical research environment, provide timely guidance of research protocols and scientific papers as well as encourage the development of outstanding clinical research skills.

Finally, specific to health profession students is the goal of integrating research skills with clinical knowledge and education, the three pillars of an academic health professional [40]. The US Accreditation Council for Graduate Medical Education (ACGME) has developed a list of core competencies that provide a useful guideline for mentors hoping to impart both practical skills and a sense of social and ethical responsibility, including patient care, medical knowledge, interpersonal and communication skills, professionalism, practice-based learning and systems-based practice [41].

What Makes a Good Clinical Research Mentor?

The International Training and Education Centre for Health (I-TECH) on HIV, an organization that has delivered clinical mentoring to more than 1000 health workers at 180 facilities in a dozen countries, compiled a list of lessons learned in clinical care mentoring for both mentors and trainees [42]. These have been modified [43] to match those for clinical research mentoring and are listed in Table 22.2.

Table 22.2 Characteristics of a clinical research mentor

Establish individual tasks and duties in the mentor–mentee relationship
Outline outlooks of the research and reporting
Setting up the mentoring team
Setting up the clinical research site
Specify who needs to approve trainee project at the research site
Confirm adequate on-site supervision
Acquaint trainee with local customs
Be aware of time restraints
Help prepare ethical approval applications and confirm approvals have been obtained
Monitor progress
Aid in study design, analysis and presentation of data
Revise the abstract(s), presentation(s) and manuscript(s)
Help in setting up a research community with other trainees (and in case of international research, host-country peers)
Share research outcomes with local co-workers and research contestants
Conduct mentoring evaluations
Expand mentoring capacity
Maintain mentoring relationships

Resources on Mentorship

There are several formal useful resources for clinical research mentoring and clinical global health experiences. One such resource is the Clinical Mentoring Toolkit produced by I-TECH [42] which is a CD and DVD package that includes a step-by-step guide for starting and maintaining an effective clinical mentoring programme. The toolkit is free and includes tools for planning, assessment, training, mentoring and evaluation that can be tailored to local needs. I-TECH also conducts clinical mentoring workshops for developing mentors. The objectives of these 1–2-day didactic and interactive sessions are to provide guidelines for mentorship at international sites, to exemplify methods of good mentorship and to encourage each mentor to develop skills and resources necessary for effective mentoring.

A valuable but subjective measure of mentor training effectiveness is satisfaction with mentoring reported by trainees. Surveys containing qualitative and quantitative questions can evaluate aspects of mentoring that are functioning well and those that require corrective action. A more quantitative measure of mentoring is direct observation by a skilled mentor with use of scales to assess competence, as recommended by the I-TECH guide for clinical care mentoring [42]. Results of evaluations should be shared with programme directors to ensure each site is responsive to the trainee's needs at each international site. Evaluating mentor effectiveness typically involves qualitative scales and mentor-trainee interviews [44]. The National Institute of Health (NIH) recently initiated a programme to capture information regarding the career trajectory and academic achievement of trainees (CareerTrac) [45]; this provides a more quantitative measure that is likely an excellent surrogate for mentoring effectiveness over extended periods of time.

Finally, unlike the ethics of conducting clinical research in developing countries, the ethics of short-term clinical research projects with potentially vulnerable populations have not been well defined [46]. Similar to recommendations regarding short-term global health electives, the focus of clinical research in global health should be on improving lives through developing intentional partnerships between colleagues and institutions in resource-rich and resource-poor countries [47, 48]. Keeping this goal in mind, mentored clinical researchers should effectively train the next generation with the necessary skills to answer clinical researchers questions in global health while defining a set of ethical guidelines that will benefit future generations of trainees.

Medical Career Satisfaction Mentoring

There is growing interest in understanding the relationship between impact of mentoring and career satisfaction as well as organizational commitment in medicine. Furthermore, such increased career satisfaction reflected positively on the candidates' advancement as well as income.

What Is Medical Career Satisfaction Mentoring?

Existing evidence supports the idea that mentoring relationships can affect career development and success in academic medicine [49]. Previous research has shown that mentors influence important career outcomes, such as personal development and research productivity [50]. They can assist their protégés in various areas of career development by serving as advocates; by providing opportunities for networking; by aiding in the development of important skills such as grant writing, data analysis and manuscript preparation; and by offering personal advice and moral support [32, 51]. In addition, studies have identified a number of characteristics and behaviours that are desirable for mentors, including compatibility with their protégé, patience, generosity and trustworthiness [52]. A recent study [53] demonstrated that multiple aspects of the mentoring relationship are important correlates of career satisfaction. Because mentor behaviours – particularly the level of collegiality perceived by the mentee – do appear to be directly associated with mentees' career satisfaction, and that promotion of formal training programs that endorse positive mentor behaviours may serve as useful means to promote satisfaction and, in turn, retention in academic medical careers.

"Having the right chemistry" between the mentor and the mentee may be the cornerstone for a successful medical career. Effective mentoring necessitates a certain chemistry for an appropriate interpersonal match. Based on the Hermann four-quadrant whole brain model [54], Dr. de Boer developed a model for understanding thinking styles and the important role that they have in teaching and learning [55]. These are analytical, practical, relational and experimental. Taken that "Every classroom represents a complete spectrum of learning style preference" [54], if there was a match between the mentee learning style (Fig. 22.1) (please view the learning styles in Chap. 22) and the mentor's thinking style, successful learning will take place. This represents having the right chemistry between the mentor and mentee. Prized mentors have clout, knowledge and interest in the mentees and provide

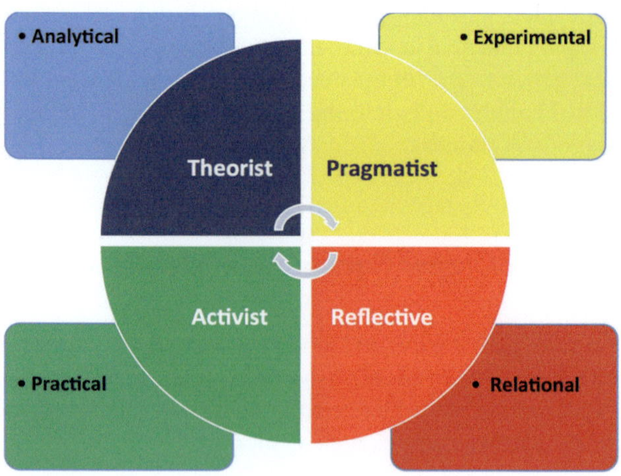

Fig. 22.1 The right chemistry between the mentor style of thinking (rectangles) and mentee style of learning (circle)

both professional and personal support. In cross-gender mentoring, maintaining clear boundaries is essential for an effective relationship. Same-gender or same-race matches between mentor and mentee were found not essential for a successful mentorship [56].

Targets and Outcomes of Career Satisfaction Mentoring

Studies carried out to assess outcomes of career mentoring tend to focus on the protégé as the main player and products such as satisfaction, increase in the number of publications and presentations, socialization of the student and improvement in student's skills as the main outcomes of the mentoring process [57–60]. Lumpkin [61] summarized the potential benefits of career mentoring as follows: (1) it facilitates the recruitment, retention and improvement of the faculty, (2) it socializes the protégé into the culture of the academic unit, (3) it increases collegial cooperation and forms a network between the protégé and the mentors, (4) it increases the productivity of the protégé and the mentor and (5) it encourages career advancement and professional improvement for both the protégé and the mentor. In another report, Cavendish [62] considered the variables of relational satisfaction, perceived time to degree, research self-efficacy and relational quality as the outcomes of mentoring relationship.

Career Mentoring Relationships

Although some studies have been conducted to evaluate the negative outcomes of a mentoring relationship, it is more likely to encounter studies explaining the positive outcomes [63]. In their meta-analysis, Allen et al. [64] revealed that protégé benefits from the mentor and that the amount of psychosocial and career mentoring the mentee received was the best predictor of objective and subjective career outcomes. Ensher et al. [65] reported that in view of the fact that mentoring relationship led to numerous positive career outcomes such as more job and career satisfaction, better organizational socialization, higher income and faster promotion rate compared to a protégé without a mentor, career mentoring has gained popularity in recent years.

The career mentoring outcomes have been endorsed by the strong relationship between mentoring and career success at workplace documented in several published studies [64–66]. Career success is defined in terms of the positive psychological and work-related outcomes produced as a result of one's work experiences [67]. In few studies examining the relationship between mentoring and student outcomes in higher education [68–70], such outcomes as the number of publications and presentations and the rate of progress have been viewed as the academic success indicators. In Dreher and Ash's study [68] on 440 graduate students at 2 US public universities, a direct positive relationship was identified between mentoring and career success. In an empirical study, Mansson and Myers [59] examined the perceptions of both 636 PhD students and 141 PhD advisors regarding the mentoring relationship, and they found that mentoring relationship was significant in terms of the academic success of the advisee.

Career Satisfaction vs Career Success

Studies assessing the strong relationship between career mentoring and career satisfaction revealed that career mentoring affected career satisfaction more than career success. The correlations between coaching, protection, exposure and visibility, challenging assignments and sponsorship subdimensions of career mentoring and career satisfaction were higher than those between the same subdimensions and career success. Mentoring relationship in standard setting is generally in the form of help that a faculty member gives to a training healthcare professional or help that colleagues give each other. The counselling given by the faculty helps the new faculty adapt to the world of academia. It also facilitates the development of good habits, improves job satisfaction and productivity, vitalizes the faculty and keeps the faculty in the organization [69, 70]. Underhill [71] reviewed 106 articles written between 1988 and 2004 on mentoring and mentoring research in the fields of nursing, education, business and psychology; she found that mentoring had a little impact on protégé's income, while it had a moderate impact on job satisfaction, the number of promotions and promotion opportunities or expectations for advancement. In the study he carried out to reveal the extent of mentoring that PhD advisors provide, Lunsford [58] found that psychosocial and career mentoring had a direct positive effect on the satisfaction with academic advisor.

Challenges in Medical Mentoring

Diversity in Medical Mentoring

There are several aspects to consider when mentors enter a mentoring relationship. Factors such as culture, background, race as well as other aspects about a person should be considered when a mentor or a mentee enters into a mentoring relationship. Mentees from underrepresented populations often face different barriers to academic success. This includes less research experience, less academic writing experience, fewer faculty role models, fewer colleagues and involvement in clinical and administrative activities as well as more obligations.

Mentors of mentees who are from underrepresented populations need to be aware of background and cultural differences and the challenges that their mentees face. As in any mentee–mentor relationship, the mentors must assess the skills and competencies and address them in a proactive and positive way. Mentors should understand that different groups face different issues and experiences, and it should not be assumed that groups or people within groups will share the same thoughts and perspectives. Furthermore, social class, geographic origin, and other demographic factors may play an important role in shaping behaviours and attitudes. The onus lies with the mentors who should remain open to ideas about race, religion and socioeconomic background and make efforts to increase their awareness and knowledge about these ideas.

Mentoring women is another special issue that needs consideration. Evidence suggests that women are less likely than men to have strong and successful mentoring relationships. Previous studies demonstrate that even promising female physician–researchers are less likely to advance in academic medical careers than their male peers [72–74]. As a result, women are less likely to be promoted to senior academic ranks, according to studies that control for the number of publications, grant support, hours worked and specialty. Women often have different issues to deal with than men do. For example, women often have to worry about managing their home life while tackling a demanding job; they may be perceiving gender bias; and they often are forced to deal with the pressures of their biological clocks [75]. Also, the mentee–mentor relationship may differ when the mentee is a woman. Women traditionally think of the mentoring relationship in terms of support and advocacy. In contrast, the traditional, male-centred version of mentoring tends to involve competition and hierarchy. In several occasions, women face several challenges with regard to establishing successful mentoring relationships. First, women and men look for different traits in a mentor. While both groups strive to find respected mentors with proven track records, women more often seek mentors who are approachable, understanding, and female. Given that fewer women are available to be mentors in academia, it's not surprising that women face difficulties finding mentors who match their needs and expectations. Second, there are inherent differences in the career paths of women and the model of academic success built around these paths. Men often begin their careers relatively unencumbered by family obligations, and they often choose to spend less time working as they get older. This traditional career pyramid is inverted for women. Women who decide to bear children do so at younger ages and face the brunt of family commitments at an earlier age. They are consequently more able and prepared to develop careers in the later stages of their life. This difference in life stage and family obligations presents another challenge, as it changes the needs of women as mentees. However, addressing the problems would help to find solutions to overcome barriers for women mentees. Knowing that women face barriers is half the battle. A mentor who has women mentees can help by being proactive and encouraging them to seek multiple mentors who can help with various aspects of their career (e.g. someone to discuss research methodology or curriculum development, someone to discuss career trajectory and someone to discuss balancing work and home life) [76].

Ethics in Medical Mentoring

Ethics involves the use of reasoned moral judgments to examine one's responsibility in any given situation. Mentors have the responsibility of teaching and role modelling the appropriate ethical behaviour of academic professionals. Mentors have the obligation to teach mentees about the responsible conduct of research as well as the ethical issues associated with being an educator. Both mentors and mentees have the responsibility of behaving ethically in their relationship.

There are certain ethical elements associated with the appropriate ethical behaviour in the mentee–mentor relationship. These include promoting mutual respect and trust; maintaining confidentiality; being diligent in providing knowledge, wisdom and developmental support; maintaining vigilance with regard to the mentee–mentor relationship (superior power increases the mentors' obligation to be aware of the mentees' feelings and the mentees' rights); acknowledging skills and experiences; as well as carefully framing advice and feedback.

These elements may expand a bit when the mentorship deals with ethical behaviour as academic professionals, to include agreeing on and abiding by rules of authorship, supporting and appreciating accomplishments, avoiding abuse of power (including exploitation and assuming credit for another's work), being alert to ethical issues and challenges, avoiding conflicts of interest (avoiding political and personal biases) and avoiding paternalism or maternalism [75].

Problem-Solving in Medical Mentoring

Whenever people work together, there are times when the relationships are challenged. Disagreements occur in even the best working relationships. In healthy situations, the issues are discussed objectively. Everyone is empowered to state his or her position and feel confident that the other is genuinely listening and wanting to understand. Possible solutions are explored with open minds, and the potential effects of the solutions are considered and weighed. It's an easy process to understand, but often it is incredibly difficult to do. People want what they want, believe what they believe, and value what they value [77]. This section will present examples of some of the problems encountered by the mentors and/or mentees and potential strategies for resolving each problem.

- *Problem: Providing inadequate support.* There are two errors a mentor can make with respect to providing support and direction. Providing too much help can stall a mentee's movement towards independence and encourage dependence. Providing too little help could leave the mentee to struggle and, again, inhibit progress towards independence.

Strategy: While it is important for the mentor to stay vigilant about his or her actions, this is probably a time when the mentee has to step up and take action.

It may be useful for the mentee to talk to peers to get a better picture of the extent of direction they are receiving. When the mentee has a good understanding of the situation and is prepared to discuss it with the mentor, the mentee should do so. Assuming that the mentee has a relationship of trust and uses good communication skills, the mentor will be responsive to the mentee's concerns [78].

- *Problem: Taking advantage of greater power.* It is important that mentors be careful about the requests they make of their mentees, since mentees are inclined to please their mentors and may perceive a request as a demand. In some cases, mentors inadvertently take advantage of their power and have a mentee take on the mentor's work. In addition to leading to fear and resentment on the part of the mentee, this could increase the mentee's workload and stall progress in his or her career development.

Strategy: It may be that the mentor is unaware of his or her use of power and that a simple conversation will solve the problem; however, it is likely that a third party will be needed to mediate the situation. If possible, the third party should be someone who is senior to both the mentee and the mentor (perhaps a division chief or department chair). A meeting of the mentor, mentee and mediator will often lead to a positive conclusion [79].

- *Problem: Dealing with conflicting demands.* Individuals at the beginning of their career have a great deal of difficulty saying "no". Junior faculty, fellows and postgraduate doctors with multiple mentors or supervisors sometimes become swamped with demands for work. Since they don't have the experience to know how to prioritize these demands, their workloads can become burdensome and a threat to their career development.

Strategy: When different mentors simultaneously want to make use of the mentee time, it is hard to decide how to prioritize the workload. The problem is often made harder because the mentee does not want to disappoint anyone. One way to resolve this dilemma is for the mentee to take the list of assignments to his/her mentors individually and ask them to help prioritize the tasks. Better yet, the mentee calls a team meeting, so the mentors can negotiate with one another about the priority of tasks [80].

- *Problem: Dealing with conflicting advice.* It is inevitable that mentees with multiple mentors and advisors receive conflicting advice with respect to research or teaching plans, writing manuscripts and other aspects of their career development. This is worth repeating: it is inevitable. Conflicting advice also inevitably leads to confusion, fear, and other negative emotions and reactions.

Strategy: Generally, most of the mentors are wise and knowledgeable, but they are not infallible. When having a conflicting advice, the mentee should think about what he/she wants to do, asking friends for their opinions and speaking to other colleagues or anyone who has been in this situation for their advice. People tend to be supportive as the mentee work out how to handle the challenge [81].

- *Problem: Lacking commitment*. On one hand, a mentor may find that his or her mentee lacks the motivation and commitment to carry out the considerable work required to develop a successful career in academia. This situation is difficult for both the mentor and mentee as the mentee has a real chance of failing and because the mentor may believe that he or she has wasted a great deal of valuable time working with the mentee. On the other hand, it is also possible that the mentee feels that the mentor lacks commitment (e.g. the mentor misses meetings or does not respond to a mentee's e-mails). The mentee's frustrations and lack of guidance can inhibit his or her movement towards independence. Because of such variances in the power between the mentor and mentee, this problem is difficult to resolve while maintaining a productive and amiable relationship.

Strategy: If a mentee is viewed as lacking commitment, it is important for the mentor to try to discern the cause. It may be that the mentee–mentor match is not working well, or it may be that the mentee has discovered that his or her career focus is no longer appealing. The junior mentees tend to be highly motivated and committed to academic careers, so while there may be an occasional case in which there is a real lack of commitment, there is usually another issue underlying the problem, and it is the mentor's job to identify it and help resolve it. Conversely, if a mentor is viewed as lacking commitment and is missing meetings and not responding to e-mails, the mentee needs to do something about it. It may be that the mentor is unaware that the mentee is feeling neglected, or it may be that the mentor is so busy with other responsibilities that there is an unfortunate lapse in mentoring. Remembering that individuals who have agreed to be mentors already have a strong commitment to the process, the mentee should raise the issue with the mentor. If it is an especially busy time for the mentor, the mentee can ask if the mentor wants to touch base or have meetings by phone for a few weeks. When discussing a problem such as this, it is helpful to have some solutions to propose [82, 83].

- *Problem: Neglecting the mentee or the mentor*. It is important to pay appropriate attention to both the mentee and the mentor. Mentees need to respond in a timely fashion to requests and recommendations from their mentors. Mentors need to be available to their mentees on a regular basis but should also be sensitive to the times when their mentees need extra support or feedback.

Strategy: It is important to maintain awareness of the other individual and what he or she is experiencing. By being vigilant, the mentor/mentee will know when something is up, and the other person may be able to offer a hand [85].

- *Problem: Crossing boundaries*. Boundaries – both professional and personal – tend to be sensitive. Crossing boundaries has the unfortunate effect of making both parties uncomfortable and has the potential for creating tension in the mentee–mentor relationship.

Strategy: To avoid this problem, the mentee and mentor should discuss boundaries at the onset of the relationship. Different people may have different ideas about what the boundaries should be. For instance, is it appropriate for a mentor to ask a mentee to babysit? This crosses the line because the power differential between mentee and mentor could result in a perception of intimidation. If the issue is work related (e.g. a mentor asks a mentee to give a talk that the mentor agreed to give), the extent to which a boundary has been crossed is less clear. Being prepared will help avoid problems down the line. It may also be useful for mentees to talk to a peer or a peer's mentors to ask for their perspectives on the issue. As in most other challenges, honest and direct communication can solve a number of problems. However, some boundaries – especially those of a sexual nature – should never be crossed [86].

- *Problem: Discovering a mismatch between mentor and mentee.* Unfortunately, a mismatch between a mentor and mentee can occur. The mismatch may result from conflicting personalities, differing career goals or areas of scientific expertise, differences in work ethic or any number of other reasons. Fortunately, the mismatch is usually discovered early in the relationship by the mentor, the mentee or both. The longer the mismatch continues, the more difficult it is to resolve.

Strategy: While finding a mismatch is regrettable, it is a problem that is relatively simple to correct. If both the mentor and the mentee believe that a switch is desirable, the mentee can work with his or her division chief, department chair and even the current mentor to help identify a more appropriate mentor.

- *Problem: Breaching confidentiality.* Confidentiality is cornerstone in the mentee–mentor relationship. A breach of confidentiality has the potential for irreversibly rupturing the mentee–mentor relationship. At a minimum, breaching confidentiality will cause considerable damage to the trust established between the mentor and mentee.

Strategy: This is a difficult problem to resolve, so it is best to avoid it altogether. At the onset of the relationship, mentees and mentors need to identify the kinds of things that should be confidential, and they need to be upfront about what is acceptable and what is not. When one party thinks there is a reason for disclosing confidential information, he or she should talk with the other to obtain permission in advance. If, however, a breach of confidentiality has occurred and it is still preferred to preserve the relationship despite the lapse in confidentiality, the person may try to rectify the situation. The mentor and mentee should make clear what they thought happened and what they can do to avoid the situation in the future. It is essential not to assume intentionality, and the mentee and mentor should try to rebuild the relationship through communication and negotiation. Rebuilding can occur only if both the mentee and the mentor want to preserve the relationship.

Why Mentoring Is Important in Medicine?

Most academics, when they graduate from medical schools, have no idea how to artfully construct a CV, apply for a position and grant or give conference presentation. It is only through networking, trial and error as well as seeking advice from senior colleagues. Such approaches help the person find relevant information and opportunities on campus and in higher education. Many academics and researchers underestimate the impact of mentoring and how far it can help them to establish and further their careers.

Though it would be impossible to create a blueprint for good mentoring because, ultimately, it's about human relationships and every relationship is unique, it is still possible to explore the attitudes, expectations and activities that are worth adopting, as well as give some guidance on how to build relationships that will be mutually beneficial. It is also worth considering the different ways of giving and receiving support [84].

Mentoring in Rheumatology

As the population ages, the demand for rheumatologists worldwide is increasing; however, the gap between the number of rheumatologists in training and the number needed continues to widen [85]. Simultaneously, rheumatologists struggle to maintain a clinical as well as academic research career due to time demands, insufficient funding, clinical workload and relative lack of mentorship [86, 87]. Sustaining a research workforce pipeline is essential to advancing our understanding of the pathophysiology, prevention and treatment of rheumatic diseases.

In a trial to help combat such negative workforce trend, the American College of Rheumatology, through interviews with past preceptorship student recipients, discovered that most of the students who participated in a preceptorship program knew very little about rheumatology before they began. Unless they were personally affected by a rheumatic disease, it was a mentor who introduced them to the field and opened their eyes to a specialty that they previously would not have considered. The American College of Rheumatology also found that early exposure, clinical mentors, and clinical rotations are the most important factors that influence fellows when choosing a specialty like rheumatology. Similarly, in Europe, a survey on mentoring in rheumatology was distributed to young clinicians and researchers in rheumatology among 30 European countries [88]. The aim was to explore perceptions of, participation in and satisfaction with mentoring programmes among young clinicians and researchers in rheumatology. Results revealed that career mentoring, especially in the clinical setting, was recognized as a major unmet need of existing mentoring programmes in rheumatology in Europe. Gender-specific differences were identified in the expectations from mentoring. Given this and the importance of mentoring for career prosperity of young physicians and scientists, the survey highlighted the importance of developing and refining mentoring programmes in rheumatology in Europe.

The Value of Mentoring in Rheumatology

Mentoring is a reciprocal, long-term relationship with an emotional commitment that exists between a novice (protégé) and experienced (mentor) healthcare professional; mentoring implies a knowledge or competence gradient, in which the teaching–learning process contributes to a sharing of advice or expertise, role development and formal as well as informal support to influence the career of the protégé. Mentoring provides protégés and mentors with opportunities for professional growth and career satisfaction. Lack of such satisfaction with a career in medicine may contribute to healthcare professional leaving the profession.

With the predicted shortage and anticipated need for rheumatologists in healthcare and academia in the future, it is more important than ever to explore career satisfaction, not just job satisfaction, for rheumatologists. Career satisfaction is defined as the contentment that a healthcare professional feels as a rheumatologist in terms of intrinsic and extrinsic rewards [82]. Career satisfaction concerns the rheumatologist's feeling about the choice of rheumatology as a career. Job satisfaction is related to the satisfaction a rheumatologist has with a current position as a healthcare professional; career satisfaction encompasses more than just the rheumatologist's job. It refers more broadly to satisfaction with a career in musculoskeletal medical care and may be a critical element in retaining the rheumatologist in the profession. Rheumatologists who have a sense of career satisfaction and feel more fulfilled may contribute to the growth of the profession. Mentoring may be a strategy that can contribute to career satisfaction for both the mentor and protégé.

The Rheumatology Mentoring Path

Similar to the mentoring path in medicine, the rheumatology mentoring path can be grouped into three categories: faculty–undergraduate student mentoring relationship, faculty–graduate student mentoring relationship and the mentoring relationships among faculty members [85]. Mentoring in higher education institutions is traditionally formed as either an informal or a planned program. In formal mentoring programs, novice faculty works with experienced faculty in a one-to-one program [86]. Faculty mentoring relationship spreads over several years, during which the relationships go through initiation, cultivation, separation and redefinition phases [84]. Initiation phase lasts for about a year, and depending on the efficiency of the mentor, the support given to the protégé and counselling competence, the protégé starts to respect and admire the more experienced organizational member. In this phase, both the mentor and the protégé begin to establish some expectations regarding a future mentoring relationship. During the cultivation phase, which occurs in the following 2–5 years, the mentor and the protégé test the expectations formed in the first phase. The mentor generally deals with the protégé's career mentoring and psychosocial mentoring. The career-related function of mentoring relationship enables the protégé to develop his or her career by learning everything related to work and to improve within the organization. The psychosocial function, on the other hand, refers to the aspect of mentoring which is affected by human values. These values are related to the psychosocial development of the protégé and aim at empowering the person in terms of competency, identity and professional role. During the separation phase, which lasts between 6 months and 2 years, the mentor and the protégé re-evaluate the need for maintaining the mentoring relationship as the protégé becomes less dependent on the mentor [59]. During this phase, the mentor starts to provide less career and psychosocial mentoring. Finally, in the redefinition phase, the relationship changes from mentoring relationship into a peer or friendship relationship.

Alleviating the Gap in Rheumatology

Mentoring has been identified as the key factor to inspire rheumatology's next generation. A broad range of mentoring programs have been developed and sponsored within institutions and by professional organizations in the United States and Europe [89–92]. AMIGO is an inter-institutional mentoring program for early-career paediatric rheumatologists developed by the American College of Rheumatology Special Committee on Pediatrics together with the paediatric rheumatology research organization ("Childhood Arthritis and Rheumatology Research Alliance", CARRA). The success of the AMIGO program demonstrated that such a mentoring program embedded within a professional organization can influence the overall "culture of mentoring" [93].

Using the lessons learned from this study and borrowing the framework established by the AMIGO program, it is expected that a similar inter-institutional mentoring program for adult rheumatologists can be successfully created. Both the American College of Rheumatology and British Society for Rheumatology have launched a new mentoring scheme which is a flexible and open platform that matches developing professionals to trusted mentors with relevant skills and knowledge. This service is offered completely free in Britain. The scheme offers the newly qualified consultants a unique opportunity for career development.

Similar peer-to-peer mentoring for individuals with early inflammatory arthritis was assessed. A study [94] was carried out to examine the feasibility and potential benefits of early peer support to improve the health and quality of life of individuals with early inflammatory arthritis. Results revealed that mentees experienced improvements in the overall arthritis impact on life, coping efficacy and social support (effect size >0.3). Mentees also perceived emotional, informational, appraisal and instrumental support. Mentors also reported benefits learnt from mentees' fortitude and self-management skills. The training was well received by mentors. Their self-efficacy increased significantly after training completion. Participants' experience of peer support was informed by the unique relationship with their peer. All participants were unequivocal about the need for peer support for individuals with early inflammatory arthritis.

An adult inter-institutional mentorship program would need to provide training for both mentors and mentees, templates for mentor–mentee interactions (e.g. how to establish expectations) and an example agenda (already available through AMIGO) [95]. Benefits for mentor participation in such a program also need to be considered [96–98]. Foundational material for the relationship would be an example "road map" for understanding career development in rheumatology research. A face-to-face meeting in addition to regular meetings via phone may have a role also be important for the success of the program. Additional challenges may need to be considered such as potential conflicts (and how to resolve conflict) between institutional-based and remote mentors.

Why to Be a Mentor: What Is in It for Me?

Despite the abundance of evidence on the advantages of having a mentor, there is a paucity of literature on the benefits the mentor might gain. Sambunjak et al. [30] performed a systematic review of mentorship programs and pointed out that the mentoring relationship is subject to the time pressures and commitment of both protégés and mentors. In a formal needs assessment, Ramani et al. [99] outlined strategies to become an effective mentor and proposed that the mentors take pride in developing the next generation and meeting new colleagues. Others have reported mentors are generally "satisfied" with their roles by being able to keep up with advances in research techniques [100] or feeling like they belong to a network to share ideas [101]. Omary [102] pointed out that documentation of formal mentorship is important in securing federal funding for research. On another front, mentors enjoy increased salary by performing the added responsibilities and can count on a loyal base of support from their junior colleague protégés. Annual appraisals and job performance evaluations typically reflect the extra-educational role carried out by the mentor. Brown et al. [103] and Penner et al. [104] reported in the psychosocial literature that mentors enjoy improved mental health as a result of helping people and a healthier immune system.

In conclusion, mentoring is an important contributor to success in medicine in general and rheumatology in particular. Increasingly, institutions have begun to address this need by building formal mentoring programs for their trainees and junior faculty. Proper mentoring programs might be the magic wand to inspire rheumatology's next generations. However, formal evaluation of these mentoring programs remains challenging and requires more research activities. Mentorship in the medical arena can produce positive outcomes. Mentors in academic medicine can expect to derive personal satisfaction, improved scholarly productivity and widespread networks of loyal supporters who share similar interests and values.

References

1. Standing Committee on Postgraduate Medical and Dental Education (SCOPME): 22 SCOPME Report. 1998. http://www.mcgl.dircon.co.uk/scopme/mentor5.pdf.
2. Feldman MD, Huang L, Guglielmo BJ, et al. Training the next generation of research mentors: the University of California, San Francisco, Clinical & Translational Science Institute Mentor Development Program. Clin Transl Sci. 2009;2:216–21.
3. Stamm M, Buddeberg-Fischer B. The impact of mentoring during postgraduate training on doctors' career success. Med Educ. 2011;45:488–96.
4. Feldmann MD, Arean PA, Marshall SJ, Lovett M, O'Sullivan P. Does mentoring matter: results from a survey of faculty mentees at a large health sciences university. Med Educ Online. 2010;15:5063.
5. McKenna AM, Straus SE. Charting a professional course: a review of mentorship in medicine. J Am Coll Radiol. 2011;8:109–12.
6. Donovan A. Views of radiology program directors on the role of mentorship in the training of radiology residents. AJR Am J Roentgenol. 2010;194:704–8.
7. Rhodes JE. Stand by me: the risks and rewards of mentoring today's youth. Cambridge, MA: Harvard University Press; 2002.
8. Ainsworth MDS. Attachments beyond infancy. Am Psychol. 1989;44:709–16.
9. Jacobi M. Mentoring and undergraduate academic success. A review of the literature. Rev Educ Res. 1991;61:505–32.
10. Austin AE. Preparing the next generation of faculty. J High Educ. 2002;73:94–122.
11. Kram KE. Mentoring at work. Glenview: Scott Foresman; 1985.
12. Eby LT. Alternative forms of mentoring in changing organizational environments: a conceptual extension of the mentoring literature. J Vocat Behav. 1997;51:125–44.
13. Palepu A, Friedman RH, Barnett RC, et al. Junior faculty members' mentoring relationships and their professional development in US medical schools. Acad Med. 1998;73:318–23.
14. Stange KC, Heckelman FP. Mentoring needs and family medicine faculty. Fam Med. 1990;22:183–5.
15. Morzinski JA, Diehr S, Bower DJ, Simpson DE. A descriptive, crosssectional study of formal mentoring for faculty. Fam Med. 1996;28:434–8.
16. Rogers JC, Holloway RL, Miller SM. Academic mentoring and family medicine's research productivity. Fam Med. 1990;22:186–90.
17. Pololi LH, Knight SM, Dennis K, Frankel RM. Helping medical school faculty realize their dreams: an innovative collaborative mentoring program. Acad Med. 2002;77:377–83.
18. Jackson VA, Palepu A, Szalacha L, Caswell C, Carr PL, Inui T. "Having the right chemistry": a qualitative study of mentoring in academic medicine. Acad Med. 2003;78:328–34.
19. Woods SE, Reid A, Arndt JE, Curtis P, Stritter FT. Collegial networking and faculty vitality. Fam Med. 1997;29:45–9.
20. Cadman EC. The academic physician–investigator: a crisis not to be ignored. Ann Intern Med. 1994;120:401–10.
21. Illes J, Glover GH, Wexler L, Leung AN, Glazer GM. A model for faculty mentoring in academic radiology. Acad Radiol. 2000;7:959.
22. Edwards K. "Short stops": peer support of scholarly activity. Acad Med. 2002;77:9.
23. Bligh J. Mentoring: an invisible support network. Med Educ. 1999;33:2–3.

24. SCOPME An Enquiry into Mentoring. Supporting doctors and dentists at work. London: Standing Committee on Postgraduate Medical and Dental Education; 1998.
25. Kohrs FP, Mainous AG. Retention of family medicine faculty development fellows in academic medicine. Fam Med. 1999;30:23–7.
26. Shanafelt TD, Sloan JA, Habermann TM. The well-being of physicians. Am J Med. 2003;114:513–9.
27. Deckard GJ, Hicks L, Hamory BH. The occurrence and distribution of burnout among infectious disease physicians. J Infect Dis. 1992;165:224–8.
28. Whippen DA, Canellos GP. Burnout syndrome in the practice of oncology: results of a random survey of 1000 oncologists. J Clin Oncol. 1991;9:1916–20.
29. Wilkinson D. International working party to promote and revitalise academic medicine. ICRAM (the International Campaign to Revitalise Academic Medicine): agenda setting. BMJ. 2004;329(7469):787–9.
30. Sambunjak D, Straus SE, Marušić A. Mentoring in academic medicine: a systematic review. JAMA. 2006;296:1103–15.
31. Townsend KC, McWhirter BT. Connectedness: a review of the literature with implications for counseling, assessment and research. J Couns Dev. 2005;83:191–201.
32. Sambunjak D, Straus SE, Marusic A. A systematic review of qualitative research on the meaning and characteristics of mentoring in academic medicine. J Gen Intern Med. 2010;25(1):72–8.
33. WHO recommendations for clinical mentoring to support scale-up of HIV care, antiretroviral therapy and prevention in resource-constrained settings (2005). file:///F:/Teaching%20 Rheumatology/Mentoring/WHO%20recommendations%20for%20mentorship.pdf.
34. Fowler J. Supporting self and others: from staff nurse to nurse consultant. Part 5: clinical supervision. Br J Nurs. 2011;20(13):830.
35. Drain PK, Primack A, Hunt DD, Fawzi WW, Holmes KK, Gardner P. Global health in medical education: a call for more training and opportunities. Acad Med. 2007;82(3):226–30.
36. Ravdin JI, Peterson PK, Wing E, Ibrahim T, Sande MA. Globalization: a new dimension for academic internal medicine. Am J Med. 2006;119(9):805–10.
37. SCOPME. Standing committee on postgraduate medical and dental education. An enquiry into mentoring. A SCOPME report. London: London Department of Health; 1998.
38. Bower DJ, Diehr S, Morzinski JA, Simpson DE. Support-challenge-vision: a model for faculty mentoring. Med Teach. 1998;20(6):595–7.
39. Sciences NAO. Advisor, teacher, role model, friend: on being a mentor to students in sciences and engineering. Washington, DC: National Academy of Sciences; 1997.
40. Manabe YC, Jacob ST, Thomas D, Quinn TC, Ronald A, Coutinho A, Mayanja-Kizza H, Merry C. Resurrecting the triple threat: academic social responsibility in the context of global health research. Clin Infect Dis. 2009;48(10):1420–2.
41. Stewart MG. Accreditation council on graduate medical education core competencies. 2001. Accessed on 4 Feb 2018. Available at http://www.acgme.org/acWebsite/RRC_280/280_coreComp.asp
42. I-TECH. Clinical mentoring toolkit. 2008. Accessed on 4 Feb 2018. Available at www.go2itech.org/resources/toolkits.
43. Shah S, Nodell B, Montano S, Behrens C, Zun J. Clinical research and global health: mentoring the next generation of health care students. Glob Public Health. 2011;6(3):234–46.
44. Berk RA, Berg J, Mortimer R, Walton-Moss B, Yeo TP. Measuring the effectiveness of faculty mentoring relationships. Acad Med. 2005;80(1):66–71.
45. NIH. Careertrac. 2009. Available at https://careertrac.fic.nih.gov/Welcome.do?recordSet=trainee.
46. Singer PA, Benatar SR. Beyond Helsinki: a vision for global health ethics. BMJ. 2001;322(7289):747–8.
47. Abbasi NR, Godkin M. Limits on student participation in patient care in foreign medical brigades. Virtual Mentor. 2006;8(12):808–13.

48. Drain PK, Holmes KK, Skeff KM, Hall TL, Gardner P. Global health training and international clinical rotations during residency: current status, needs, and opportunities. Acad Med. 2009;84(3):320–5.
49. Palepu A, Friedman RH, Barnett RC, et al. Junior faculty members' mentoring relationships and their professional development in U.S. medical schools. Acad Med. 1998;73:318–23.
50. Sambunjak D, Straus SE, Marušić A. Mentoring in academic medicine: a systematic review. JAMA. 2006;296:1103–15.
51. Straus SE, Chatur F, Taylor M. Issues in the mentor–mentee relationship in academic medicine: a qualitative study. Acad Med. 2009;84:135–9.
52. Cho CS, Ramanan RA, Feldman MD. Defining the ideal qualities of mentorship: a qualitative analysis of the characteristics of outstanding mentors. Am J Med. 2011;124:453–8.
53. De Castro R, Griffith K, Ubel P, Stewart A, Jagsi R. Mentoring and the career satisfaction of male and female academic medical faculty. Acad Med. 2014;89(2):301–11.
54. Herrmann N. The whole brain business book. New York: McGraw-Hill; 1996.
55. De Boer A, Steyn T, Du Toit PH. Whole brain teaching for whole brain learners. S Afr J High Educ. 2001;15(3):188–93.
56. Lechuga VM. Faculty-graduate student mentoring relationships: mentors' perceived roles and responsibilities. High Educ. 2011;62:757–71. https://doi.org/10.1007/s10734-011-9416-0.
57. Lunsford L. Doctoral advising or mentoring? Effects on student outcomes. Mentoring Tutoring: Partnership Learn. 2012;20:251–70. https://doi.org/10.1080/13611267.2012.678974.
58. Mansson DH, Myers SA. Using mentoring enactment theory to explore the doctoral student–advisor mentoring relationship. Commun Educ. 2012;61:309–34. https://doi.org/10.1080/03634523.2012.708424.
59. Ogunyemi D, Solnik JM, Alexander J, Fong A, Azziz R. Promoting residents' professional development and academic productivity using a structured faculty mentoring. Program, Teach Learn Med: Int J. 2010;22:93–6. https://doi.org/10.1080/10401331003656413.
60. Lumpkin A. A model for mentoring university faculty. Educ Forum. 2011;75:357–68. https://doi.org/10.1080/00131725.2011.602466.
61. Cavendish SE. Mentoring matters: the influence of social support and relational maintenance strategies on critical outcomes in doctoral education (Unpublished PhD thesis). Kentucky: University of Kentucky; 2007. Retrieved from http://uknowledge.uky.edu/gradschool_diss/498.
62. Gibson SK. Being mentored: the experience of women faculty. J Career Dev. 2004;30:173–88. https://doi.org/10.1023/B:JOCD.0000015538.41144.2b.
63. Allen TD, Eby L, Poteet ML, Lentz E. Career benefits associated with mentoring for protégés: a meta analysis. J Appl Psychol. 2004;89:127–36. https://doi.org/10.1037/0021-9010.89.1.127.
64. Ensher EA, Thomas C, Murphy SE. Comparison of traditional, stepahead, and peer mentoring on protégés support, satisfaction, and perceptions of career success: a social exchange perspective. J Bus Psychol. 2001;15:419–38. https://doi.org/10.1023/A:1007870600459.
65. Judge TA, Cable DM, Boudreau JW, Bretz RD. An empirical investigation of the predictors of executive career success. Pers Psychol. 1995;48:485–519. https://doi.org/10.1111/j.1744-6570.1995.tb01767.x.
66. Seibert SE, Kraimer ML. The five-factor model of personality and career success. J Vocat Behav. 2001;58:1–21. https://doi.org/10.1006/jvbe.2000.1757.
67. Dreher GF, Ash RA. A comparative study of mentoring among men and women in managerial, professional, and technical positions. J Appl Psychol. 1990;75:539–46. https://doi.org/10.1037/0021-9010.75.5.539.
68. Mathews P. Academic mentoring: enhancing the use of scarce resources. Educ Manag Adm Leadersh. 2003;31:313–34. https://doi.org/10.1177/0263211X03031003007.
69. Schrodt P, Cawyer CS, Sanders R. An examination of academic mentoring behaviors and new faculty members' satisfaction with socialization and tenure and promotion processes. Commun Educ. 2003;52:17–29. https://doi.org/10.1080/03634520302461.

70. Underhill CM. The effectiveness of mentoring programs in corporate settings: a meta-analytical review of the literature. J Vocat Behav. 2006;68:292–307. https://doi.org/10.1016/j.jvb.2005.05.003.
71. Ley TJ, Hamilton BH. The gender gap in NIH grant applications. Science. 2008;322:1472–4.
72. Jagsi R, Motomura AR, Griffith KA, Rangarajan S, Ubel PA. Sex differences in attainment of independent funding by career development awardees. Ann Intern Med. 2009;151:804–11.
73. Jagsi R, DeCastro R, Griffith KA, et al. Similarities and differences in the career trajectories of male and female career development award recipients. Acad Med. 2011;86:1415–21.
74. Pohlhaus JR, Jiang H, Wagner RM, Schaffer WT, Pinn VW. Sex differences in application, success, and funding rates for NIH extramural programs. Acad Med. 2011;86:759–67.
75. Martinez ED, Botos J, Dohoney KM, et al. Falling off the academic bandwagon. Women are more likely to quit at the postdoc to principal investigator transition. EMBO Rep. 2007;8:977–81.
76. Institute for clinical research education. University of Pittsburgh. https://www.icre.pitt.edu/index.aspx. (Accessed on 4 Feb 2018).
77. Benner P. From novice to expert: excellence and power in clinical nursing practice. Menlo Park: Addison-Wesley; 1984.
78. Benner P. From novice to expert: excellence and power in clinical nursing practice. Upper Saddle River: Prentice-Hall; 2001.
79. Peplau H. Interpersonal relations in nursing: a conceptual frame of reference for psychodynamic nursing. New York: Putnam; 1952.
80. Peplau HE. Interpersonal relations: a theoretical framework for application in nursing practice. Nurs Sci Q. 1992;5(1):13–8.
81. Peplau HE. Peplau's theory of interpersonal relations. Nurs Sci Q. 1997;10(4):162–7.
82. Vance C. A group profile of influentials in American nursing, M.S. dissertation, Columbia University Teacher's College. 1977.
83. Darwin A, Palmer E. Mentoring circles in higher education. High Educ Res Dev. 2009;28:125–36. https://doi.org/10.1080/07294360902725017.
84. Kram KE. Phases of the mentor relationship. Acad Manag J. 1983;26:608–25. https://doi.org/10.2307/255910.
85. Rheumatology ACo. 2015. Workforce Study [cited 2016 Dec 8]. Available from: http://www.rheumatology.org/Learning-Center/Statistics/Workforce-Study.
86. Ogdie A, Shah AA, Makris UE, Jiang Y, Nelson AE, Kim AH, et al. Barriers to and facilitators of a career as a physician-scientist among rheumatologists in the US. Arthritis Care Res. 2015;67(9):1191–201.
87. Wilkes M, Feldman MD. Mentoring clinical trainees: a need for high touch. Lancet (London, England). 2017;389(10065):135–7.
88. Frank-Bertoncelj M, Hatemi G, Ospelt C, Ramiro S, Machado P, Mandl P, Gossec L, Buch MH. Mentoring of young professionals in the field of rheumatology in Europe: results from an EMerging EUlar NETwork (EMEUNET) survey. Clin Exp Rheumatol. 2014;32(6):935–41.
89. Kashiwagi DT, Varkey P, Cook DA. Mentoring programs for physicians in academic medicine: a systematic review. Acad Med: J Assoc Am Med Coll. 2013;88(7):1029–37.
90. Silet KA, Asquith P, Fleming MF. Survey of mentoring programs for KL2 scholars. Clin Transl Sci. 2010;3(6):299–304.
91. Meagher E, Taylor L, Probsfield J, Fleming M. Evaluating research mentors working in the area of clinical translational science: a review of the literature. Clin Transl Sci. 2011;4(5):353–8.
92. Chen CM, Lou MF. The effectiveness and application of mentorship programmes for recently registered nurses: a systematic review. J Nurs Manag. 2014;22(4):433–42.
93. Moorthy LN, Muscal E, Riebschleger M, Klein-Gitelman M, Nigrovic LE, Horon JR, et al. Efficacy of an interinstitutional mentoring program within pediatric rheumatology. Arthritis Care Res. 2016;68(5):645–51.
94. Sandhu S, Veinot P, Embuldeniya G, Brooks S, et al. Peer-to-peer mentoring for individuals with early inflammatory arthritis: feasibility pilot. BMJ Open. 2013;3:e002267.

95. Rheumatology ACo. AMIGO 2016 [cited 2016 Dec 14]. Available from: http://www.rheumatology.org/Get-Involved/Mentoring/AMIGO.
96. Maisel NC, Halvorson MA, Finney JW, Bi X, Hayashi KP, Blonigen DM, et al. Institutional incentives for mentoring at the US Department of veterans affairs and universities: associations with Mentors' perceptions and time spent mentoring. Acad Med: J Assoc Am Med Coll. 2017;92:521–7. Epub.
97. Feldman MD, Steinauer JE, Khalili M, Huang L, Kahn JS, Lee KA, et al. A mentor development program for clinical translational science faculty leads to sustained, improved confidence in mentoring skills. Clin Transl Sci. 2012;5(4):362–7.
98. Ogdie A, Sparks JA, Angeles-Han ST, Bush K, Castelino FV, Golding A, Jiang Y, Kahlenberg JM, AHJ K, Lee YC, Machireddy K, Ombrello MJ, Shah AA, Wallace ZS, Nigrovic PA, Makris UE. Barriers and facilitators of mentoring for trainees and early career investigators in rheumatology research: current state, identification of needs, and roadmap to an inter-institutional adult rheumatology mentoring program. Arthritis Care Res (Hoboken). 2017; https://doi.org/10.1002/acr.23286.
99. Ramani S, Gruppen L, Kachur EK. Twelve tips for developing effective mentors. Med Teach. 2006;28:404–8.
100. Taherian K, Shekarchian M. Mentoring for doctors. Do its benefits outweigh its disadvantages? Med Teach. 2008;30:e95–9.
101. Connor MP, Bynoe AG, Redfern N, Pokora J, Clarke J. Developing senior doctors as mentors: a form of continuing professional development. Report of an initiative to develop a network of senior doctors as mentors: 1994–99. Med Educ. 2000;34:747–53.
102. Omary MB. Mentoring the mentors: another tool to enhance mentorship. Gastroenterology. 2008;135:13–6.
103. Brown SL, Nesse RM, Vinokur AD, Smith DM. Providing social support may be more beneficial than receiving it. Psychol Sci. 2003;14:320–7.
104. Penner LA, Dovidio JF, Piliavinn JA, Schroeder DA. Prosocial behavior: multilevel perspectives. Annu Rev Psychol. 2005;56:365–92.

Part VI
Education: The Art and Science of Facilitating

Chapter 23
How to Be a Good Educator

Introduction

The educational process is composed of three main foundations: the curriculum, the student and the teacher. Much attention has been paid to the curriculum including the different approaches to teaching, learning and assessment, as well as the students' selection and how they can learn more effectively. On the other hand, less attention has been paid to the teacher. The teacher or educator is a key element in the creation of the condition in which learning occurs. Lawrence Stenhouse, an education guru, suggested that there could be no such thing as curriculum development without teacher development [1]. Good teachers have a range of technical skills, an understanding of basic educational principles, an enthusiasm and passion for teaching as well as a commitment to evaluating and improving their own teaching. The acquisition of these abilities by a teacher is important.

Teachers nowadays have a challenging and multifaceted role. Teaching is about much more than the transmission of information to the learner. Teaching encompasses the complex tasks of planning, preparing and delivering a learning program as well as assessing whether students have achieved the expected learning outcomes. To support the students' learning, the good teacher must have in addition to the necessary subject knowledge, technical skills required for lecturing, facilitating small group discussions, providing feedback and assessing the students' competence. They should also demonstrate the necessary attitudes and professionalism for the job. It is now recognized that the effective successful teacher requires a combination of technical competence and an appropriate teaching and professional approach. Lastly, what is required of a good teacher will vary also to some extent depending on the subject being taught and in which part of the world, teaching is taking place. Though the teaching principles mostly remain the same, the approaches, views and contexts may vary. This chapter will present the science and art of teaching, principles of outcome-based education and what makes a good educator. It will also discuss ways to bridge the gap between education theory and practice.

Y. El Miedany, *Rheumatology Teaching*,
https://doi.org/10.1007/978-3-319-98213-7_23

The Science of Teaching

A professional teacher does not operate using a cookbook approach, blindly following a set of rules or procedures. Good teaching, just like any other field of professional endeavour, is best delivered when there is an understanding of the underlying process. Educational researchers have described a variety of theories and factors that influence learning. There are, however, some general principles about learning that can inform what can be done by medical teachers. The study of the educational theory and science of teaching [2, 3] reveals that there are four key principles reflective of effective education to which teachers can relate in their day-to-day practice:

- Feedback: Give feedback to students as they progress.
- Activity: Engage the student in active rather than passive learning.
- Individualization: Relate the learning to individual needs.
- Relevance: Make the learning relevant to the student in terms of their career objectives.

Over time, there has been a shift in the teaching science. Teaching has moved from "opinion-based" to "evidence-based" style. Evidence-based teaching is a philosophy that has two elements: First, it involves teachers not taking for granted that their current practice is optimal. Second, evidence should be sought that will inform decisions as to the most effective teaching approach. There is a widely held view among clinicians, medical researchers and medical teachers that evidence to inform decisions relating to teaching is not available. This is not the case. Often those who are concerned about the lack of evidence have either not looked for it or have looked in the wrong places! Systemic reviews and collaborations have identified approaches to help teachers make decisions about their teaching practice based on the best evidence available. Educational strategies such as feedback, simulators as well as assessment methods, e.g. OSCE, can help teachers base their practice on available evidence.

The aim is that the teaching and professional judgement should be combined with the understanding of the best evidence available so that the teacher can make the correct decision, adopt the proper teaching strategy and take the appropriate action.

Outcome-Based Education

Traditionally, medical education has focused on teaching methods such as the lecture and small group work, on the design of the curriculum as well as the assessment of the learner (using different approaches). Over the past years, there has been a move in the education system towards an outcome-based approach where the emphasis is on the product of the learning rather than on the process.

Outcome-based education is a performance-based approach at the cutting edge of the curriculum development and offers a powerful way of changing and managing medical education. The learning outcomes define the process of what is taught, how it is taught and how it is assessed. Based on that, the outcome-based education has three main pillars: learning outcomes identified, the curriculum and educational strategy as well as commitment (Fig. 23.1).

Implementing outcome-based learning in the medical education process had led to a major move in the educational concepts. Medical educators adopting this approach are motivated to specify the instructional objectives for their learning programs. This enhances the modification of the "ownership of outcomes" concept into partnership of students and teachers or what can be described as "ownership of the process". Consequently, adopting outcome-based education has shown several advantages with growing calls for adoption on a wider scale in medical education. Knowledge in the medical field is nearly doubling every 18 months. Therefore, it is no longer feasible given this information explosion, to cover all aspects of a subject. Adopting such approach will help in tailoring the medical education to meet the targeted aims and help the students achieve their goals and reach the expected level of competency. However, while the approach offers many advantages, it has also been criticized by some teachers and educators. Some of the concerns expressed about the approach are presented also in Table 23.1. However, it is important to recognize that these criticisms relate more to how outcome-based education is implemented in practice rather than to the principle itself. Furthermore, most of the provided challenges can be avoided, and the increasingly documented benefits of the approach outweigh the disadvantages [4].

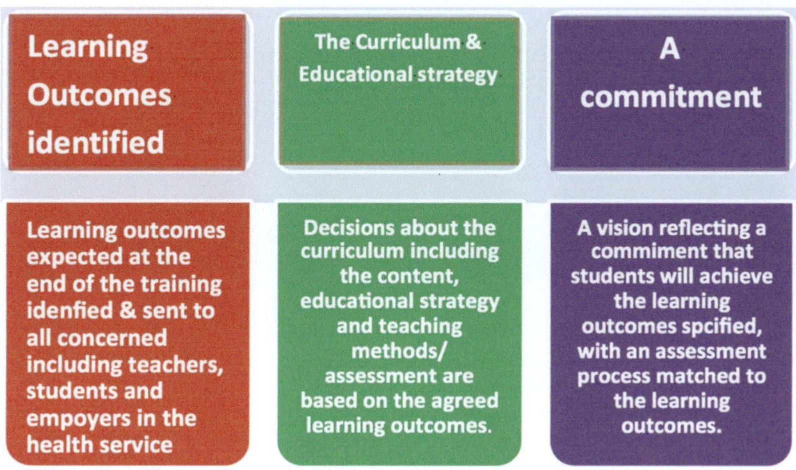

Fig. 23.1 Requirements of outcome-based education: outcome-based education is based on three main pillars. The learning outcomes should be identified and specified. Decision about the curriculum and educational strategy should be based on the specified outcomes, as well as a commitment with vision towards achieving the educational targets

Table 23.1 Advantages and disadvantages of outcome-based learning

Advantages of outcome-based learning	Disadvantages of outcome-based learning
Highlights competencies to be achieved (e.g. the doctor's knowledge, skills and attitude rather than they were trained)	*Lack of research base* that demonstrates the effectiveness of implementing outcome-based learning
Able to meet the rapid developments in medicine	*Demands are imposed on the teachers implementing outcome-based learning* (teachers should specify learning outcomes, link these outcomes to teaching, learning and assessment)
Potential consideration of important but neglected topics (e.g. communication skills, breaking bad news, patient safety)	*Change the concept of the teacher to "education technician"* implementing a non-malleable model
Points the students in the right direction (a move towards student-centred approach, the outcome-based education works as a glue that holds the curriculum together)	*The outcome-driven curriculum limits the learner ability to create or innovate*
Emphasizes accountability and transparency in medical education	
Provides the basis for allocating the resources to individual courses (by considering the overall learning outcomes of the course, the providers can ensure the time and resources to individual teaching sessions)	
Ensures all assessments are valid (the approach is a move towards more performance-based assessment and facilitates an assessment-to-a-standard approach)	
Ensures the continuity across the continuum of medical education (ensure continuity between undergraduate, postgraduate and continuing medical education)	
Flags up problems in the curriculum (ensures evaluation of the curriculum. Failure to meet the outcomes and identifies problem(s) with the curriculum)	
Helps teachers to select the topics to be taught in a teaching session (considering the expected learning outcomes and guides the teacher to the topics to be covered)	
Enable the comparison of all curricula worldwide. (In Europe, the tuning project aims at establishing a learning outcome framework for primary medical degree qualification)	

What Makes a Good Educator?

Teaching is a profession that requires mastery of both the subject matter that is being taught and approaches to teaching, with a major outcome which is students' effective and efficient learning. Teaching is a complex and multifaceted activity that involves a wide range of competencies and attributes. To meet their responsibilities, teachers require a range of technical skills, conduct small group sessions and facilitate student's learning, together with regular assessment of the students in a range of contexts. To be a good educator, teachers should also take responsibility for their personal continuing professional development and regularly assess and review their own competence.

Assess Own Competency

As a professional, a key task for educators is to take responsibility for the quality of their teaching and for the assessment of their own competence. The educator may believe that he/she has given an outstanding lecture, while in practice students find the lecture incomprehensible, boring or irrelevant. There are several ways to help educators assess their teaching process:

- Reflection on own performance as a teacher
- Attain feedback from colleagues
- Videotape or record their own teaching
- Analysis of the students' feedback
- Evaluate whether students have achieved the projected learning outcomes
- Study measurements of the educational environment (in the local institution)
- Judge the impact on the student's or trainee's career
- Attend/actively contribute in conferences on medical education events

Keeping Up to Date

Like all branches of medicine, medical education is constantly changing and developing. Over the past decade, significant developments have taken place with curriculum planning including move to "outcome-based education" and "inter-professional education". The portfolio has also expanded to include assessment, developments to the standard setting as well as implementation of new learning technologies, such as simulated teaching, virtual patients, e-learning and the use of the Internet [5].

There are different ways of keeping up-to-date, and the educator should choose whichever approach works well for him/her:

- Textbooks
- Journals
- Newsletters
- Guides and reports
- Online information
- Conferences and meetings
- Courses on medical education
- Membership of professional education associations or communities

Teamwork Player

The moves towards more vertical and horizontal integration in the curriculum, to outcome-based education and problem-based learning, necessitate basic scientist and clinician teachers working more closely in a team. The greater emphasis on inter-professional education and work-based learning requires collaboration between educators and practitioners in the different professions. An atmosphere of collegiality among teachers is important and has been shown to contribute to student achievement. Teachers need to be supportive and respectful to each other and demonstrate that they work together as a member of a team. An evaluation some years ago of a UK government teaching and learning technology initiative found that only projects that had content, education and technology experts collaborating together were successful [6].

Bridging the Gap Between Education Theory and Practice

Implementing Outcome-Based Education Approach in Practice

In contrast with the students, who rely heavily on the curriculum and targeted outcomes as their best approach to their learning and passing the assessment tests, teachers' response differs when it comes to implementing outcome-based education as their standard teaching approach. Figure 23.2 shows the different teachers' styles and how they react to preparing learning outcomes or incorporating them into their teaching [7].

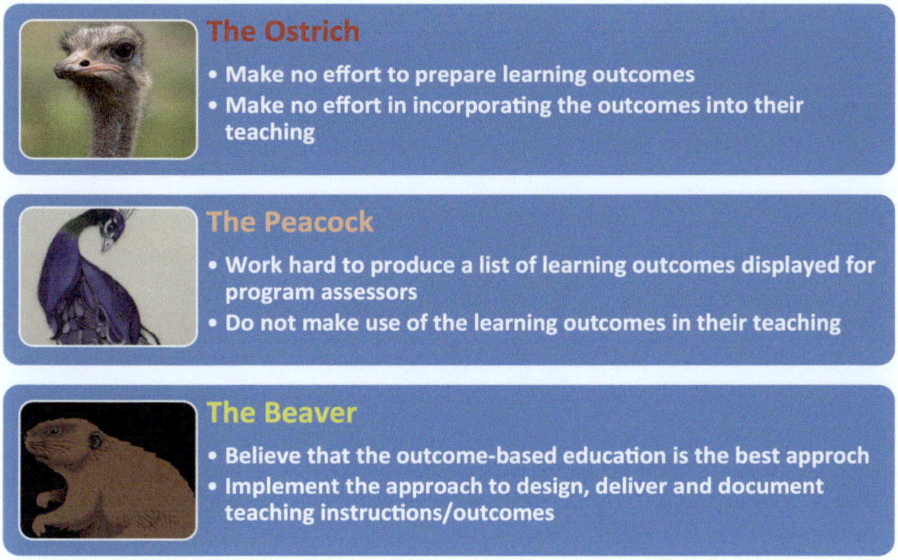

Fig. 23.2 Implementing outcome-based education in practice: different styles of teachers

Planning an Outcome-Based Education Program for Medical Education

Any outcome-based education curriculum should start with the question "what are the expected learning outcomes to be achieved by the end of the programs and what capabilities should the graduate have as a practicing doctor?" Figure 23.3 summarizes the steps to plan an outcome-based education program. This starts with identifying an outcome framework to describe the broad targets and performance capabilities aimed for. For example, in the broad domain of musculoskeletal examination, more detailed learning outcomes include taking history, morning stiffness (interpreting the value of asking about duration of morning stiffness and its reflection on the underlying pathology), assessment of health-related quality of life, social domains, medication history, the nature of the underlying pathology (e.g. identifying whether the pathology is a soft tissue or joint problem, inflammatory or mechanical joint pain), response to previous medical or physiotherapy management as well as patient-reported outcomes. After defining the exit learning outcomes and working backwards, outcomes are specified for each of the courses in the curriculum. These will highlight how the course will contribute to the overall medical school's

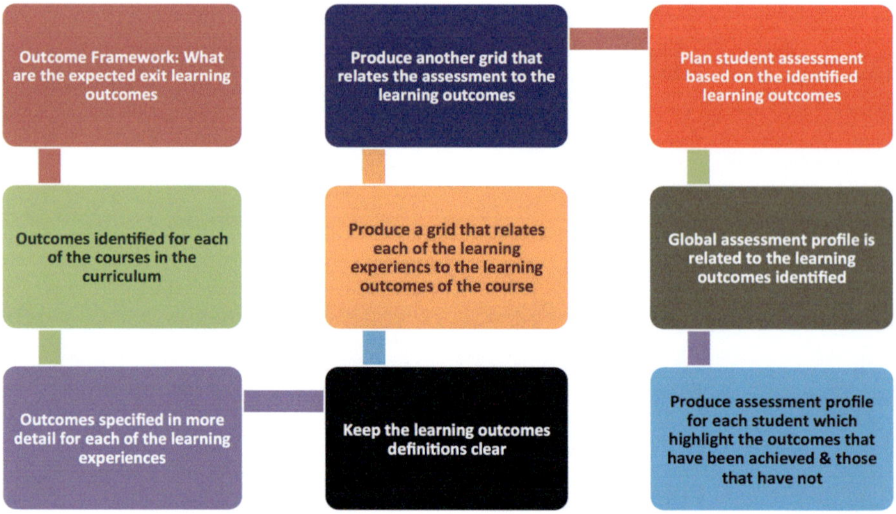

Fig. 23.3 Implementing an outcome-based education approach in practice: planning an outcome-based education program

exit learning framework [8]. The outcomes are detailed and specified further for each of the learning experiences in a course, e.g. a lecture or a clinical session. A grid that related each of the learning experiences to the course learning outcomes is put. Another grid should be produced relating the learning outcomes to the students' assessment. Keeping the definitions clear as much as possible would help planning an effective student assessment. Based on the outcomes to be evaluated, the appropriate assessment tools are identified. A global assessment profile is identified in relation to the learning outcomes, followed by an individual assessment profile for each student which outlines the achieved outcomes and those which have not.

The Curriculum Content Sequencing

While the attention has been focused on the overall organization and elements comprising the medical curriculum (including the learning outcomes, the curriculum contents, methods of teaching, educational strategy and assessment), less consideration has been given to the learning sequence within the curriculum. It is a basic concept that if the learners could not see the value of the courses being taught and its relevance to the expected eventual goals, they may lack the motivation, and the learning process becomes ineffective. Perhaps, this is one of the main reasons for the move to include clinical courses and experiences earlier in the medical curriculum.

While some logistics may influence the sequencing in some centres, the general rule of sequencing includes (1) the prerequisites (the required knowledge or skill needed to be attained before the student go for the course), (2) the contents of the course (what should the student study to achieve the targeted learning outcomes) and (3) application of the learning gained and value of continuing to learn after finishing the course). Throughout this path of learning, the educational tactics should follow a simple logic approach: (1) from simple to complex, (2) from general to specific or detailed information as well as (3) from basic theory principles to clinical application.

The Spiral Curriculum

Relevant to the sequencing concept, is the approach where an iterative revisiting of topics, subjects or themes is adopted, which fits with the spiral curriculum model (Fig. 23.4). However, a spiral curriculum is not simple reiteration of the subject taught. With each teaching cycle, there is deepening of the students' understanding, building up on the previous phase of learning. Figure 23.5 shows the main features of the spiral curriculum, namely, (1) revisiting the taught topics, (2) gradual increase of difficulty, (3) new learning linked to previous learning and (4) increase of the students' competence [9].

The Transition Between Phases

As the students proceed along the curriculum, it is vital that the transition between the different phases appears as seamless and relevant as possible. To smooth this transition process, bridging courses may be required. These transition programs should consider the individual students' achievements as well as competencies and make sure that the required prerequisites have been achieved before they move to the next phase of the learning process. Complementary learning courses can be offered to fill the gaps, in case deficiencies have been identified. Transition

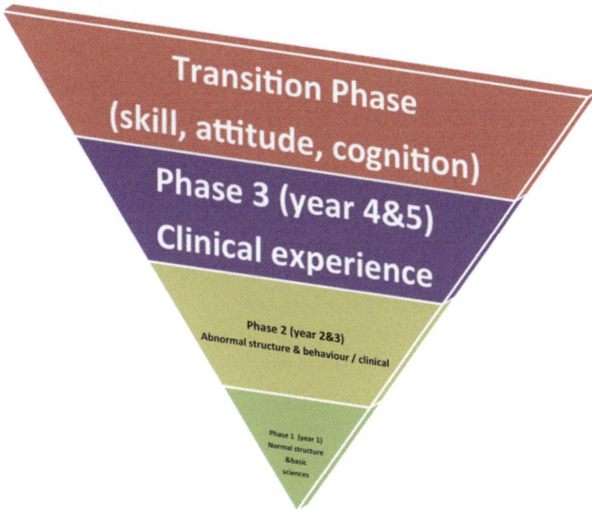

Fig. 23.4 The different phases of spiral curriculum. (Modified from Harden and Stamper [9] with permission)

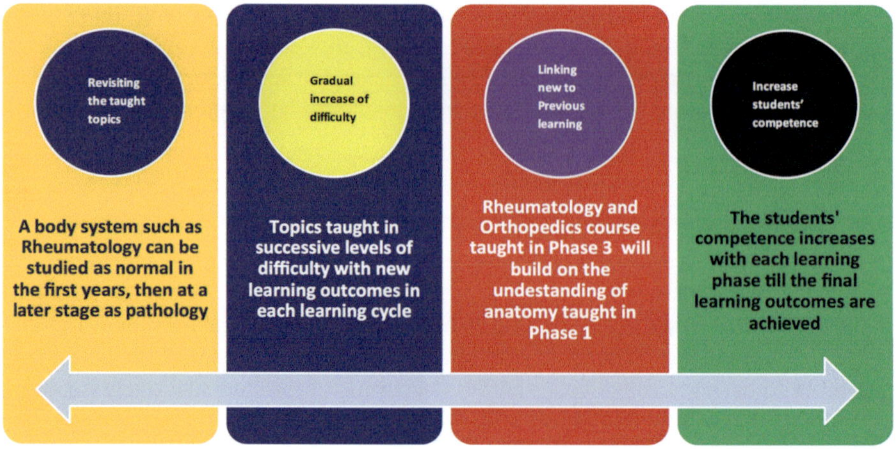

Fig. 23.5 Main features of the spiral curriculum

programs are essential, particularly at the interface between under- and postgraduate phases before the students start their first medical appointment as trainee doctors [10]. Such transition program should include induction workshops including handover and team working, shift working, sleep and health as well as stress and resilience. The program should also include a period during which the training undergraduate students shadow a senior doctor to get acquainted to the practical skills, administrative and procedural arrangements expected from him/her as a junior doctor with remediation wherever required.

Moving from Teacher-Centred to Student-Centred Learning

Over the past few years, there has been a significant shift in the attention from the teacher to the student. This move from teacher-centred to student-centred learning entailed a change from the informative teaching style "sage on the stage" to a facilitator style of learning "guide on the side" (Fig. 23.6). Perhaps one of the main reasons for such move is todays' consumer-driven society. Currently, there is more interest in the student as a consumer of the learning. Medical schools ranking has changed, and todays' medical schools are ranked based on their students' feedback and employability. An example of this ranking system to measure the best medical school is the medical school rankings in the United Kingdom which has been set to be judged using the following criteria: (1) Complete University Guide overall score; (2) Guardian score, largely based on student perspective; (3) graduate prospects, a measure of graduate employability; and (4) student satisfaction, borrowed from the National Student Survey [11].

Earlier work revealed that student-centred approach is more motivating for students [12]. In fact, the concept of outcome-based education involves a commitment

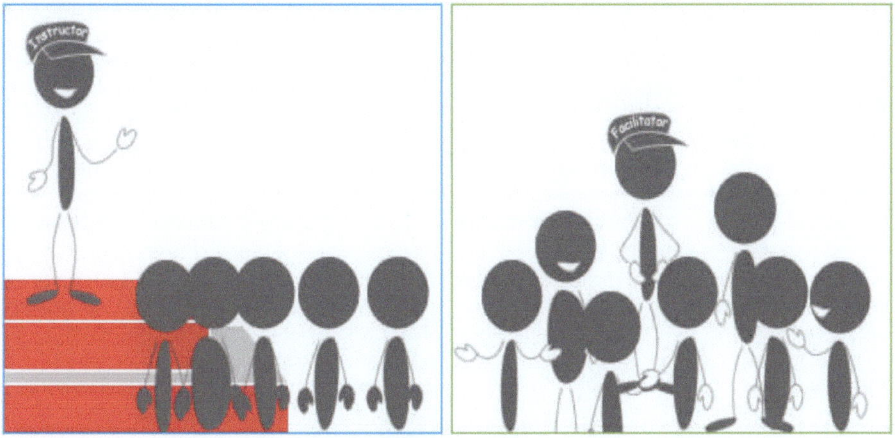

Fig. 23.6 Moving from teacher-centred approach to student-centred approach

to ensure that all students achieve the expected learning outcomes as well as prepare the students to continue their medical education after finishing the undergraduate phase. Furthermore, the new teaching approaches such as simulated teaching and flipped learning are based on the student. Such approaches motivate the students to show a positive reaction when allowed to share in the decision-making process regarding their learning. Table 23.2 shows a comparison of the pros and cons of teacher-centred versus student-centred learning approaches.

Which Educational Strategy Should Be Adopted?

Pressure has been mounting to move the medical education programs towards better integration of basic and clinical science throughout the medical curriculum. Much of the impetus has come as a result of the need to manage the ever-increasing medical knowledge domains, increased recognition of the importance of imparting students with independent learning skills and demonstrating the application of knowledge, skills and attitudes inherent in the practice of medicine. Traditionally, medical schools used curricula that were based on discipline/department approaches to medical education relying heavily on assimilative learning (the acquisition of additional knowledge in isolation) [13]. It became apparent that this approach often placed too much emphasis on the basic sciences and not enough on the clinical sciences, as these courses were taught in isolation. Human organ-based curriculum models were developed in part to address this isolation, creating an organizational structure that de-emphasized individual department or course material. A number of schools have since adopted a human organ-based or systems-based learning structure that encourages the "elaboration of knowledge in richer and wider contexts" [14, 15]. Recently, many schools have moved towards a more integrated approach

Table 23.2 A comparison of pros and cons of teacher-centred and student-centred learning approaches

Teacher-centred		Student-centred	
Pros	Cons	Pros	Cons
Teacher takes the responsibility and assumes all students will understand	Table of the host menu (no options for the students, it is what the teacher offer)	A la carte menu. (the students choose what they want to learn)	Some students prefer to work alone, so group work can become problematic
As the teacher direct all classroom activities, there are no concerns that students will miss an important topic	The teaching is not linked to the learning outcomes	Students have responsibility to direct their own learning, reflect on the content, ask questions and complete tasks independently	Because the teacher doesn't always deliver instruction to all students at once, some students may miss important facts
Classroom remains orderly, students are quiet and the teacher retain full control of the classroom and its activities	Doesn't allow students to express themselves, ask questions and direct their own learning	Students learn important communicative and collaborative skills through group work	Because students are talking, classrooms may often be noisy or chaotic
Decisions regarding the course, learning approaches and deadlines are made by the teacher	Students are not engaged in the decisions about the learning process	Students are engaged in the content and decisions about the curriculum	Teachers may have to attempt to manage all students' activities at once, which can be difficult
Decisions regarding the learning and its outcomes are taken by the teacher	No integration of the assessment with the learning	Assessments are integrated with the learning process	

to teaching scientific and medical knowledge along a continuum from normal body to abnormal body [16]. This continuum allows for less fragmented learning opportunities for students where they can benefit from a more transformative learning approach (the building of new knowledge onto already existing knowledge) [17]. Other medical schools still retain a "two-by-two" curriculum where students focus on classroom-based learning in the first 2 years and hospital or clerkship learning in the second 2 years.

The content arrangement, its sequence and which educational strategy have been recognized as the main pillars of a curriculum. However, when teachers are offered "a new innovative curriculum" or "a traditional curriculum", they tend to reject the innovative approach. The reason given is that one or more components of it seem inappropriate in their own situation. An example of curriculum planning has been detailed in the SPICES model [18]. The model identifies six educational approaches and presents each on a continuum. Table 23.3 summarizes the different SPICES educational strategies. Based on their current educational approaches and the targeted outcomes, medical schools or individual teachers can decide where they stand and which particular educational strategy they want to implement.

Table 23.3 The SPICES model of curriculum strategies

	Student-centred	Problem-based / task-based	Integrated or inter-professional	Community-based	Elective-driven	Systematic
Style	Teacher-centred	Information-oriented	Discipline-based	Hospital-based	Uniform	Opportunistic/ apprenticeship
Focus	What students learn	A clinical problem	Body systems, e.g. CVS/ MSK Integration of basic and clinical sciences	Only hospital-based setting	Include both core elements common to all students and electives or student-selected components	Learning outcomes, teaching and assessment
Students	Students given more responsibility	It is what the students need to know to understand the problem that drives their activities	Make sense to the students. Students also develop team work skills	Not favoured. Students find it more attractive to experience both hospital- and community- based learning	Students have the choice of topics for their study	The students are attached to their master(s) and acquire skills by following the master. The students can be attached to one teacher or clinical unit or hospital ward for a period
Teaching	Teachers are challenged to ensure they meet the individual student needs in terms of content, learning approach and time taken to complete	1. To use problem based learning to develop a usable body of integrated knowledge 2. To develop problem-solving skills	Moving from the building block principle where each subject has its own block of time and restricted to one part of the course, into the teacher taking responsibility for this integration so the subjects are presented to the student as a meaningful whole	Better contact with the community where they are trained to serve Primary care has been seen as the weak link in the health-care system	The student is given the opportunity to study a subject, in depth, of their own choosing which has not been covered in the program	Teaching and learning experiences should be planned and recorded. This should be included in the students' learning program

Student Progression in an Outcome-Based Education Curriculum

It is accepted and acknowledged that students' perception and progression vary towards the targeted exit learning outcomes. In the era of student-centred education, the students' attainments of the learning outcomes can be implemented to monitor and design a strategy for their progression through the curriculum. Assessing how a learner can apply their learning towards a specific outcome, which is called "Mastery", can be a prerequisite before the learner is permitted to progress from one section of the medical course to the following one (e.g. a student should show competency/mastery not only in basic sciences but also in communication skills to be allowed to proceed to clinical courses in the later years of medical school). Progression can also be projected across the education continuum from undergraduate to postgraduate state then to the continuing medical education stage.

Four dimensions can be considered with regard to the learners' achievements of learning outcomes and their progression through the course [8]. These are increased breadth, increased difficulty, increased utility and application in practice and lastly increased proficiency (Fig. 23.7). The sequence of courses in the curriculum should enable the learners to progress positively towards the exit learning outcomes with the learning outcomes at each stage being challenging and achievable.

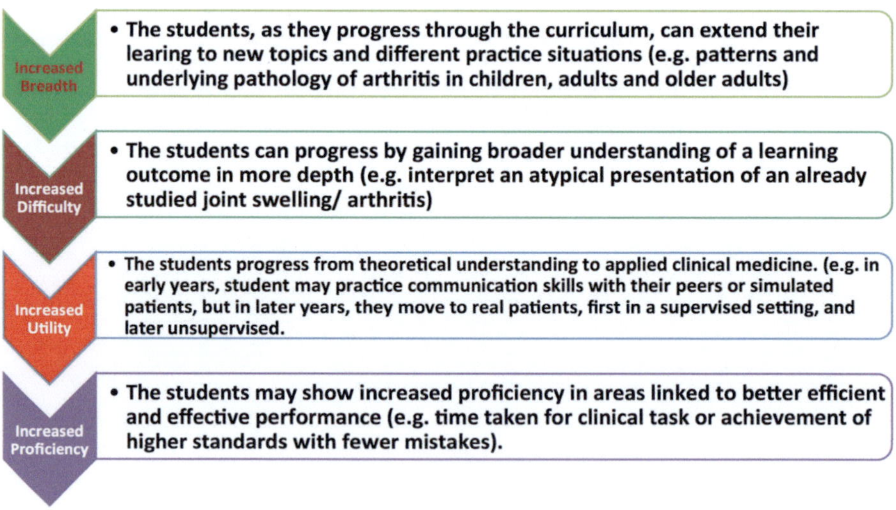

Fig. 23.7 Students' progression: The sequence of courses in the curriculum should enable the learners to progress positively towards the exit learning outcomes with the learning outcomes at each stage being challenging and achievable. Four dimensions have been identified in relation to the student's progression through the curriculum

Assessment in Medical Education

Competence in medicine has been defined as "the habitual and judicious use of communication, knowledge, technical skills, clinical reasoning, emotions, values, and reflection in daily practice for the benefit of the individuals and communities being served" [19]. In the United States, the assessment of medical residents, and increasingly of medical students, is largely based on a model that was developed by the Accreditation Council for Graduate Medical Education (ACGME). This model uses six interrelated domains of competence: medical knowledge, patient care, professionalism, communication and interpersonal skills, practice-based learning and improvement and systems-based practice [20]. While competence is not an achievement but rather a habit of lifelong learning [21], assessment plays an integral role in helping physicians identify and respond to their own learning needs. Ideally, the assessment of competence (what the student or physician is able to do) should provide insight into actual performance (what he or she does habitually when not observed), as well as the capacity to adapt to change, find and generate new knowledge and improve overall performance [22].

Goals of Assessment

Over the past decade, medical schools, postgraduate training programs and licensing bodies have made new efforts to provide accurate, reliable and timely assessments of the competence of trainees and practicing physicians [23]. Such assessments have three main goals: to optimize the capabilities of all learners and practitioners by providing motivation and direction for future learning, to protect the public by identifying incompetent physicians and to provide a basis for choosing applicants for advanced training.

Types of Assessment

Assessment can be formative (guiding future learning, providing reassurance, promoting reflection, and shaping values) or summative (making an overall judgment about competence, fitness to practice or qualification for advancement to higher levels of responsibility). Formative assessments provide benchmarks to orient the learner who is approaching a relatively unstructured body of knowledge. They can reinforce students' intrinsic motivation to learn and inspire them to set higher standards for themselves [24]. Although summative assessments are intended to provide professional self-regulation and accountability, they may also act as a barrier to further practice or training [25].

Assessment Tools

Assessment is vital for the process of medical education. Several assessment methods have been developed and implemented by different medical school [26]. These include:

1. *Written exercises*
   - Multiple-choice questions (either single best answer or extended matching format): assess knowledge and ability to solve problems.
   - Key feature and script concordance questions: assess clinical reasoning, problem-solving ability and ability to apply knowledge.
   - Short-answer questions: assess the ability to interpret diagnostic tests, problem- solving ability and clinical reasoning skills.
   - Structured essays: assess synthesis of information and interpretation of medical literature.
2. *Assessment by supervising clinicians:*
   - Global rating with comments at the end of rotation: assess clinical skills, communication, teamwork, presentation skills and work habits.
   - Structured direct observation with checklists for rating (OSCE): assess communication skills and clinical skills.
   - Oral examination: assess knowledge and clinical reasoning.
3. *Clinical simulations:*
   - Standardized patients and objective structured clinical examination (OSCE): some clinical skills, interpersonal behaviour and communication skills.
   - Incognito standardized patients: assess actual practice habits.
   - High-technology simulation: assess procedural skills, teamwork and simulated clinical dilemmas.
4. *Multisource (360°) assessment:*
   - Peer assessment: professional manner, work habits, interpersonal behaviour and teamwork.
   - Patient assessment: assess the ability to gain patients' trust, patient satisfaction and communication skills.
   - Self-assessment: assess knowledge, skills, attitude, belief and behaviour
   - Portfolios: assess all aspects of competence, particularly appropriate for practice- based learning and improvement as well as systems-based practice.

The use of multiple observations and several different assessment methods over time can partially compensate for flaws in any one method [27]. Van der Vleuten [28] described five criteria for determining the usefulness of a particular method of assessment: reliability (the degree to which the measurement is accurate and reproducible), validity (whether the assessment measures what it claims to measure), impact on future learning and practice, acceptability to learners and faculty and costs (to the individual trainee, the institution and society at large).

Challenges in Assessment

New Domains of Assessment

There are several domains in which assessment remains problematic and requires further evaluation. Quality of care and patient safety depend on effective teamwork, and teamwork training is emphasized as an essential element of several areas of competence, yet there is no validated method of assessing teamwork [29]. Also professionalism remains another challenge. So far there is no definition for professionalism agreed by the experts. Traditionally, it is left to the examiner to evaluate and score it [30]. Though, dozens of scales that rate communication are used in medical education and research [31], there is little evidence that any one scale is better than another. Furthermore, the experiences that patients report often differ considerably from ratings given by experts [32].

Multidimensional and Longitudinal Assessment

In contrast to longitudinal assessment which involves collection of student work created in response to specific, known instructional objectives and evaluated in relation to the same criteria, the use of multiple methods of assessment can overcome many of the limitations of individual assessment formats [33]. Variation of the clinical context allows for broader insights into competence. Consequently, the use of multiple formats provides greater variety in the content areas to be evaluated. Furthermore, input from multiple observers provides information on distinct aspects of a trainee's performance. Longitudinal assessment avoids excessive testing at any one point in time and serves as the foundation for monitoring ongoing professional development.

The Art of Diagnosis

The combination of the multimethod assessment outcomes (e.g. including direct observation of the student interacting with several patients, MCQ examination, an encounter with a standardized patient followed by an oral examination, written essays as well as peer assessment) into a portfolio resembles the art of diagnosis; it demands that the student synthesize various bits and types of information in order to come up with an overall picture. A good number of medical schools have implemented longitudinal assessments that use multiple methods in their students' evaluation [34].

Standardization of Assessment

Although accrediting organizations specify broad areas that the curriculum should cover and assess, most of the medical schools make their own decisions about methods and standards of assessment. This model may have the advantage of ensuring consistency between the curriculum and assessment, but it also represent a challenge when comparisons are made between students across medical schools for the purpose of subsequent training [35].

Assessment and Learning

It is generally acknowledged that assessment drives learning; however, assessment can have both intended and unintended consequences. Students study more thoughtfully when they anticipate certain examination formats [36], and changes in the format can shift their focus to clinical rather than theoretical issues [37]. Assessment by peers seems to promote professionalism, teamwork and communication [38]. The unintended effects of assessment include the tendency for students to cram for examinations and to substitute superficial knowledge for reflective learning.

Assessment of Expertise

The assessment of trainees and physicians who have higher levels of expertise presents a challenge. Expertise is characterized by unique, elaborated and well-organized bodies of knowledge that are often revealed when they are triggered by characteristic clinical patterns [33, 39, 40]. Thus, experts who are unable to access their knowledge in artificial testing situations but who make sound judgments in practice may do poorly on some tests that are designed to assess communication skills, knowledge or reasoning. Furthermore, clinical expertise implies the practical wisdom to manage ambiguous and unstructured problems, balance competing explanations, avoid premature closure and note exceptions to rules and principles, even when under stress. Testing either inductive thinking (the organization of data to generate possible interpretations) or deductive thinking (the analysis of data to distinguish among possibilities) in situations in which there is no consensus on a single correct answer presents formidable psychometric challenge.

Assessment and Future Performance

The evidence that assessment protects the public from poor-quality care is both indirect and scarce. Few studies have shown correlations between assessment programs that use multiple methods and relatively crude estimates of quality such as diagnostic testing, prescribing and referral patterns [41]. Correlating assessment with future performance is difficult not only because of inadequacies in the assessment process itself but also because relevant, robust measures of outcome that can be directly attributed to the effects of training have not been defined. Current efforts to measure the overall quality of care include patient surveys and analyses of institutional and practice databases. When these tools are refined, they may provide a more solid foundation for research on educational outcomes.

In conclusion, in contrast to the past when teaching was a skill that the doctor was expected to possess or acquire, effective teaching techniques are now a requirement for doctors and can be learnt and perfected like any other medical skill. Every doctor is expected to deliver teaching, whether to medical students, allied health professionals or postgraduate doctors. Furthermore, there is an expectation to show formal training in teaching methods. A passionate teacher will be an asset to any medical department. This, coupled with the personal satisfaction of being an effective teacher, is the motivation to become a better medical educator.

References

1. Harden R, Laidlaw J. Essential skills for a medical teacher. The roles and competencies of a good teacher (chapter 1). Edinburgh: Churchill Livingstone Elsevier; 2012. p. 3–8.
2. Kauffman DM. Applying educational theory in practice. In: Cantillon P, Wood D, editors. ABC of learning and teaching in medicine. 2nd ed. Oxford (chapter 1): Wiley-Blackwell; 2010.
3. Haig A, Dozier M. Systemic searching for evidence in medical education. BEME guide no 3. Dundee: AMEE; 2003.
4. Hodges BD. Cracks and cervices: globalization discourse and medical education. Med Teach. 2009;31:910–7.
5. Carr D. Professionalism and ethics in teaching (professional ethics). London: Routledge; 2005.
6. Mc Gaghie WC. Scholarship, publication and career advancement in health professions education. AMEE education guide no 43. Dundee: AMEE; 2010.
7. Harden RM. Outcome based education – the ostrich, the peacock and the beaver. Med Teach. 2007;29:666–71.
8. Harden RM. Learning outcomes as a tool to assess progression. Med Teach. 2007;29:678–82.
9. Harden RM, Stamper N. What is a spiral curriculum? Med Teach. 1999;21:141–3.
10. Dornan T, Littlewood S, Margolis SA. How can experience in clinical and community setting contribute to early medical education? A BEME systematic review. BEME guide no. 6. Med Teah. 2006;28:13–8.
11. Medical school ranking in 2018. https://www.themedicportal.com/application-guide/choosing-a-medical-school/medical-school-rankings/.

12. Cheang KI. Effects of learner-centered teaching on motivation and learning strategies in a third-year pharmacotherapy course. Am J Pharm Educ. 2009;73(3):42.
13. Seel N. Assimilation theory of learning. In: Seel N, editor. Encyclopedia of the sciences of learning. New York: Springer; 2012. p. 324–6.
14. Davis MH, Harden RM. Planning and implementing an undergraduate medical curriculum: the lessons learned. Med Teach. 2003;25(6):596–608. https://doi.org/10.1080/0142159032000144383.
15. Dent J, Harden RA. A practical guide for medical educators. 4th ed. London: Churchill Livingstone/Elsevier; 2013.
16. Harden RM, Davis MH, Crosby JR. The new Dundee medical curriculum: a whole that is greater than the sum of the parts. Med Educ. 1997;31(4):264–71.
17. Gullo C, Dzwonek B, Miller BA. Disease-based approach to the vertical and horizontal integration of a medical curriculum. Med Sci Educ. 2015;25(4):1–11.
18. Harden RM, Sowden S, Dunn WR. Some educational strategies in curriculum development: the SPICES model. ASME med education booklet no 18. Med Educ. 1984;18:284–97.
19. Epstein RM, Hundert EM. Defining and assessing professional competence. JAMA. 2002;287:226–35.
20. Batalden P, Leach D, Swing S, Dreyfus H, Dreyfus S. General competencies and accreditation in graduate medical education. Health Aff (Millwood). 2002;21:103–11.
21. Leach DC. Competence is a habit. JAMA. 2002;287:243–4.
22. Fraser SW, Greenhalgh T. Coping with complexity: educating for capability. BMJ. 2001;323:799–803.
23. Leung WC. Competency based medical training: review. BMJ. 2002;325:693–6.
24. Friedman Ben-David M. The role of assessment in expanding professional horizons. Med Teach. 2000;22:472–7.
25. Sullivan W. Work and integrity: the crisis and promise of professionalism in America. 2nd ed. San Francisco: Jossey-Bass; 2005.
26. Epstein RM. Assessment in medical education. N Engl J Med. 2007;356:387–96.
27. Wass V, Van der Vleuten C, Shatzer J, Jones R. Assessment of clinical competence. Lancet. 2004;357:945–9.
28. Van Der Vleuten CPM. The assessment of professional competence: developments, research and practical implications. Adv Health Sci Educ. 1996;1:41–67.
29. Committee on Quality of Health Care in America. Crossing the quality chasm: a new health system for the 21st century. Washington, DC: National Academy Press; 2001.
30. Ginsburg S, Regehr G, Lingard L. Basing the evaluation of professionalism on observable behaviors: a cautionary tale. Acad Med. 2004;79(Suppl):S1–4.
31. Schirmer JM, Mauksch L, Lang F, et al. Assessing communication competence: a review of current tools. Fam Med. 2005;37:184–92.
32. Epstein RM, Franks P, Fiscella K, et al. Measuring patient-centered communication in patient-physician consultations: theoretical and practical issues. Soc Sci Med. 2005;61:1516–28.
33. Norman GR, Van der Vleuten CP, De Graaff E. Pitfalls in the pursuit of objectivity: issues of validity, efficiency and acceptability. Med Educ. 1991;25:119–26.
34. Epstein RM, Dannefer EF, Nofziger AC, et al. Comprehensive assessment of professional competence: the Rochester experiment. Teach Learn Med. 2004;16:186–96.
35. Colliver JA, Vu NV, Barrows HS. Screening test length for sequential testing with a standardized-patient examination: a receiver operating characteristic (ROC) analysis. Acad Med. 1992;67:592–5.
36. Hakstian RA. The effects of type of examination anticipated on test preparation and performance. J Educ Res. 1971;64:319–24.
37. Newble DI, Jaeger K. The effect of assessments and examinations on the learning of medical students. Med Educ. 1983;17:165–71.

38. Nofziger AC, Davis B, Naumburg EH, Epstein RM. The impact of peer assessment on professional development. Presented at the Ottawa Conference on Medical Education and Assessment. Ottawa, 2002.
39. Schmidt HG, Norman GR, Boshuizen HP. A cognitive perspective on medical expertise: theory and implication. Acad Med. 1990;65:611–21. [Erratum, Acad Med 1992;67:287]
40. Bowen JL. Educational strategies to promote clinical diagnostic reasoning. N Engl J Med. 2006;355:2217–25.
41. Tamblyn R, Abrahamowicz M, Dauphinee WD, et al. Association between licensure examination scores and practice in primary care. JAMA. 2002;288:3019–26.

Part VII
The Essence of Teaching

Chapter 24
Reclaiming the Art and Science of Teaching

Good teaching has a balance of powers and skills. The arts and science are often thought of as polar opposites. While the science component of teaching is about exciting research that examines what tends to work best in the classroom and the rigorous methodology of constant improvement, the "act" of teaching a student is an "art", and for every educator, teaching is a performance and the lessons are the script. However, is teaching an art or a science? There are several publications written trying to answer the question of whether teaching is a science or an art. Interestingly, it seems many conclude that teaching is both a science and an art.

The Enduring Relationship of Science and Art

Viewing teaching as part art and part science is not a new concept. Indeed, effective teaching is a dynamic mixture of expertise in a vast array of instructional strategies combined with a profound understanding of the individual students and their needs at different points in time. The individual teacher must sift through a myriad of research and opinions to build a local knowledge base for interacting with the students in his/her class. This is similar to medical practitioners who go through a myriad of research studies and views to build a local knowledge base for interacting with their patients. Educational research is not a blunt tool that smashes all doubt about best practice. However, it provides general direction that must be interpreted by individual teachers in terms of their unique circumstances.

Although research will never be able to identify instructional strategies that work best with every student in every class, what the best research can do is tell us which strategies have a good chance (i.e. high probability) of working well with students. Individual teachers should consider which strategy to adopt with the right students at the right time. In a nutshell, a good part of effective teaching is an art – based on science, hence the title, The Art and Science of Teaching.

Y. El Miedany, *Rheumatology Teaching*,
https://doi.org/10.1007/978-3-319-98213-7_24

Science, Art and Quality Teaching Standards

Quality framework of andragogy as well as pedagogy is so important to ensure that the integrity and quality of the teaching profession is uniform across classrooms. The way in which a teacher teaches has a dramatic impact on achieving their education targets and learning outcomes. Tutors who merge science and art in teaching can be considered as role models for demonstrating what a high level of quality in learning looks like; therefore the quality teaching standards set the bar for teachers and consequently students. There are three dimensions of andragogy/pedagogy, closely linked to style of teaching. The three dimensions are:

- Intellectual quality: which refers to producing high levels of intellectual thinking. Teachers must ensure that they treat knowledge as a basis for setting challenging work that requires a deeper understanding and ability to problem-solve and engage in higher-order thinking through connections between ideas.
- Quality learning environment: refers to a positive environment which offers high support for learning. Teachers have high expectations that their students will achieve good results in their on-task ability, student engagement and quality of work.
- Significance: Teachers make meaningful and engaging learning experiences. Teachers recognize that learning becomes clear when teachers link work to out-of-class contexts so that learning becomes important to students.

This quality framework of teaching is important to ensure that the integrity and quality of the teaching profession are uniform across different classes. In the meantime, it gives the teacher the chance to implement the science and art in the teaching process. The way in which a teacher teaches has a dramatic impact on their quality of achieving learning outcomes.

Science, Art and Technology

Over the past few years, a new "power" has shown its face and booked its place in the teaching algorithm. Today's generation of students are growing up in a digital world. Using digital devices is a huge part of their everyday experience out of school/university. Through Google they have access to a wide wealth of digital information, content and resources. With all of this so intrinsic to their "outside school/university" experience, modern technology gave the "3D" style to the teaching process. The challenge for the teaching profession is how to optimize the use of science and art to harness all this for learning within the classroom and at home. This generation of "digital natives" has much lower need for libraries, the traditional resource used by students half a generation ago. Learning styles are changing, and teachers need to adapt their teaching styles accordingly.

With the change in learning styles, the role of the teacher is changing too. In addition to being a presenter of lesson material, the teacher should act as a facilitator/coach in an increasingly collaborative learning environment. These two key styles of learning – presenting and collaborating – link directly to the science and art in teaching. Implementing different types of technology in the classroom mandated different styles of teaching. Interactive whiteboards have been the bastion of the presenting style of learning, where the teacher is at front of class and all students are involved in interactive learning. For the more personalized learning, laptops, netbooks and tablets are increasingly pervasive in the classroom.

This new expansion in technology represents a challenge to modern teaching with its both pillars: the science and art. The crucial point is that the teacher will still want and need to deliver his teaching task while he remains in charge of the classroom. Teachers may swap part of the science or art skill to let students use technology for some parts of a lesson while they continue to be the centre point of attention. This may be at the front of the classroom or, as is becoming more relevant, to be able to move around the classroom and, still, remain in control. In these styles of classroom environment, clearly the ability of devices to talk to each other, i.e. the seamless connectivity between student tablets and front-of-class display, becomes increasingly a key. The concept of the "flipped classroom", discussed earlier in this book, is a method of teaching which is turning the traditional classroom on its head. Students do not need a teacher there when they are just viewing a lecture which can be done at home, perhaps by watching a video created by the teacher, or when they are completing an assignment. In fact, the modern gadgets and mobile PCs (laptops, netbooks, tablets) truly unleash the full potential of 1:1 learning, allowing a fully personalized learning experience for each student.

Integrating the Art and Science in Medical Practice

Practicing medicine is an art, based on science. The concept of an art is placed in the core of practicing medicine and comes up in a variety of situations. In fact, medicine can be considered as "applied science". The first and the most compelling aspect of the art of medicine involves communication. This is usually encountered in the standard clinical practice where medicine is always painted in a positive light. During the consultation, the doctor is implementing the best of his/her knowledge and the use of critical thinking in the approach to patient care. However, the art of medicine is not only focussed on the positive aspects. It also includes showing compassion and concern when dealing with the patients, having a good bedside manner, respecting patient autonomy and giving the patient enough time to raise their concerns or queries then answer them professionally using the evidence-based medicine algorithms as a guideline, educating the patients, sharing with them the decision-making process regarding their management and lastly coming up with a mutual agreement on a plan of action.

In conclusion, to be an effective teacher, one must not only stay up-to-date of the latest research in the field of education but must also continually practice the art of applying this information, assessing what works and refining the teaching approach, enhancing it with modern technology, in order to create an effective learning environment.

Index

Y. El Miedany, *Rheumatology Teaching*,
https://doi.org/10.1007/978-3-319-98213-7

MIX
Papier aus verantwortungsvollen Quellen
Paper from responsible sources
FSC® C105338

If you have any concerns about our products,
you can contact us on
ProductSafety@springernature.com

In case Publisher is established outside the EU,
the EU authorized representative is:
Springer Nature Customer Service Center GmbH
Europaplatz 3, 69115 Heidelberg, Germany

Printed by Libri Plureos GmbH
in Hamburg, Germany